P9-DIB-135

Contributors

FRED L. ALLMAN, JR., M.D.

Director, Sports Medicine Clinic, Atlanta, and
Orthopaedic Consultant, Georgia Tech and the
Atlanta Public Schools, Atlanta, Georgia.

Rehabilitation Following Athletic Injuries

GAEL R. FRANK, M.D.

Orthopaedic Staff, Research Hospital,
Kansas City, Missouri. Consultant Staff,
Orthopaedic Division, Kansas City
General Hospital, Kansas City, Missouri

Injuries of the Hand

BOB J. RUTLEDGE, M.D.

Clinical Professor of Neurosurgery and
Chairman of the Department, University of
Oklahoma, Oklahoma City, Oklahoma.

Craniocerebral Injuries During Athletics

C. P. WILKINSON, M.D.

Clinical Associate Professor of
Ophthalmology, University of Oklahoma,
Oklahoma City, Oklahoma.

Injury in the Vicinity of the Eye

TREATMENT OF INJURIES TO ATHLETES

DON H. O'DONOGHUE, M. D.

Professor Emeritus of Orthopaedic Surgery
University of Oklahoma Medical School
Oklahoma City

Third Edition   illustrated

W. B. SAUNDERS
Philadelphia • London • Toronto

W. B. Saunders Company: West Washington Square
Philadelphia, PA 19105

1 St. Anne's Road
Eastbourne, East Sussex BN21 3UN, England

1 Goldthorne Avenue
Toronto, Ontario M8Z 5T9, Canada

Library of Congress Cataloging in Publication Data

O'Donoghue, Don H

Treatment of injuries to athletes.

Includes index.

1. Sports — Accidents and injuries.   I. Title. [DNLM:
   1. Sport medicine.   2. Athletic injuries — Therapy.
   QT260 026t]

RD131.03 1976   617'.1027   74–17760

ISBN 0–7216–6927–1

Treatment of Injuries to Athletes   ISBN 0-7216-6927-1

© 1976 by W. B. Saunders Company. Copyright 1962 and 1970 by W. B. Saunders Company.
Copyright under the International Copyright Union. All rights reserved. This book is protected
by copyright. No part of it may be reproduced, stored in a retrieval system, or transmitted in any
form or by any means, electronic, mechanical, photocopying, recording, or otherwise, without written
permission from the publisher. Made in the United States of America. Press of W. B. Saunders
Company. Library of Congress Catalog card number 74-17760.

Last digit is the print number: 9   8

This book is dedicated to the delightful and devoted members of my personal staff whose unstinting efforts made the preparation of this third edition not only possible but pleasurable.

PREFACE TO THE THIRD EDITION

In considering the purpose of a preface for this third edition many thoughts come to mind. The first one is to acknowledge my profound admiration for my confreres involved in the development of the specialty of sports medicine. Within the last relatively few years sports medicine, which had been considered a hobby for the frustrated athlete who had not quite gotten over his pregraduation days, has blossomed to include some of the most sophisticated procedures and certainly has supported some of the most important precepts of the physician.

With each new edition I ponder the problem of a bibliography. A bibliography is extremely important in noting the sources of information, more detailed information than is permissible in a single volume. On the other hand the specialty has developed so rapidly with so much talent that I find myself at a complete loss to know what to recommend and what to omit. Perhaps I do not solve anything by omitting all of it, but as I look through some of the modern articles and notice references to 200 or more sources I wonder how much this really contributes to the practical knowledge of the physician who is going to treat the injured or ill athlete. Hence, for this reason and also, I suppose, for an inherent compulsion not to credit the wrong person with the right thing, I have omitted the bibliography. I refer the reader to the Bibliography of Sports Medicine prepared under the auspices of the Committee on Sports Medicine of the American Academy of Orthopaedic Surgeons, which does list a great many authoritative articles on the subject. This volume is available from the American Academy of Orthopaedic Surgeons, 430 North Michigan Avenue, Chicago, Illinois, 60611, and is well worth the minimum charge.

Originality I do not claim. As I have said before, everything I know I learned at my mother's knee or some other joint. Seriously, however, I do bow long and deep to the many capable, earnest, enthusiastic, altruistic, dedicated, young and old, orthopaedists, and others, who have involved themselves in the care of the athlete. As I have not personally credited my many friends for their contributions, so I do not myself expect any credit for the material published in this book. Originality of a certain procedure is not my interest; rather, it is its application and sustained effectiveness in the care of the athlete that is important.

I still greatly appreciate the American athlete. The exigencies of my personal situation have made it possible, and desirable, for me to travel with the University of Oklahoma football team on their weekends away from home. No more delightful group of people could be assembled. If there ever was a day of the football bum, this day has long since passed. We see the cream of American manhood involved in a highly competitive situation with innumerable examples of total unselfishness and dedication to the greatest good for the greatest number. Their ready acceptance of the fact that the doctor is on their side and is dedicated to doing what is best for them as a person is, indeed, reassuring. My association with the University of Oklahoma Department of Intercollegiate Athletics continues to be a highly salutary one, a unit to which I owe a debt of gratitude for their complete cooperation in our study of and advancement of the care of the American athlete.

Again, a word of appreciation to all of my long-suffering staff who have personally helped me in the revision of this book. My secretaries, my radiology technician, my surgical nurse, and my long-time secretary-manager, without whom I could not function, have especially been involved in the work we have been carrying on. Their organizational ability, their memory, their careful preservation of specific cases, and their patience have rendered this research much easier.

Then, finally, to the many orthopaedic surgeons who have unstintedly shared their feelings, beliefs, problems and cases with me, particularly to the Sports Medicine Committee of the American Academy of Orthopaedic Surgeons and to the newly formed but very viable American Orthopaedic Society for Sports Medicine, I express my gratitude. Without these people this work would not have been possible.

DON H. O'DONOGHUE, M.D.

PREFACE TO THE FIRST EDITION

I have given a great deal of thought to the advisability of including a bibliography in this volume. The material in this book is in large part basic. No claim is made for originality of concept or of procedures. Indeed, it is so fundamental that proper acknowledgment is well nigh impossible. I give full credit to my confreres, both present and past, for all I know about the subject. I had at first considered that I might credit those procedures which are generally understood to have been advanced by a specific man. Further consideration made it seem unjustifiable to credit some things but to leave the greater number unacknowledged. So a very grateful bow is offered to those members of the medical profession who take the pains to reduce their thinking to print and so make it available for all who want to, and can, read. By the same token, the thoughts in this book are freely available to anyone and no credit need to given me. My reward will be in your perusal of this book.

I also owe a debt of gratitude to the American athlete. That which in the beginning was an interesting sideline in a life devoted largely to pediatric orthopaedics, has burgeoned to become perhaps my major interest. The young athlete with his tremendous enthusiasm and his desire to recover is a stimulation to anyone who has the privilege of caring for him. He makes a splendid antidote to the rapidly increasing group of "free loaders" who would rather be supported by their brothers than return to work.

Finally, I must express my sincere appreciation to the Athletic Department of the University of Oklahoma, which has to my personal knowledge never permitted selfish considerations to interfere in any way with the proper medical management of its athletes. It has presented a shining example which has spread throughout our state and has been particularly valuable in our successful efforts to improve the overall care of the young athlete in our public schools. The combined efforts of school administrators, teachers, coaches, trainers and physicians are resulting in a steady improvement in this vital area which will be rewarded manyfold by notable improvement in the physical condition of our people.

DON H. O'DONOGHUE, M.D.

Oklahoma City, Oklahoma

ix

The BILL OF RIGHTS for the SCHOOL and COLLEGE ATHLETE

Participation in athletics is a privilege involving both responsibilities and rights. The athlete has the responsibility to play fair, to give his best, to keep in training, to conduct himself with credit to his sport and his school. In turn he has the right to optimal protection against injury as this may be assured through good technical instruction, proper regulation and conditions of play, and adequate health supervision. Included are:

Good Coaching:

The importance of good coaching in protecting the health and safety of athletes cannot be minimized. Careful conditioning and technical instruction leading to skillful performance are significant factors in lowering the incidence and decreasing the severity of injuries. Also, good coaching includes the discouragement of tactics, outside either the rules or the spirit of the rules, which may increase the hazard and thus the incidence of injuries.

Good Officiating:

The rules and regulations governing athletic competition are made to protect players as well as to promote enjoyment of the game. To serve these ends effectively the rules of the game must be thoroughly understood by players as well as coaches and be properly interpreted and enforced by impartial and technically qualified officials.

Good Equipment and Facilities:

There can be no question about the protection afforded by proper equipment and right facilities. Good equipment is now available and is being improved continually; the problem lies in the false economy of using cheap, worn out, outmoded, or ill-fitting gear. Provision of proper areas for play and their careful maintenance are equally important.

Good Health Supervision ... Including:

FIRST . . . a thorough preseason history and medical examination. Many of the sports tragedies which occur each year are due to unrecognized health problems. Medical contraindications to participation in contact sports must be respected.

SECOND . . . a physician present at all contests and readily available during practice sessions. It is unfair to leave to a trainer or coach decisions as to whether an athlete should return to play or be removed from the game following injury. In serious injuries the availability of a physician may make the difference in preventing disability or even death.

THIRD . . . medical control of the health aspects of athletics. In medical matters, the physician's authority should be absolute and unquestioned. Today's coaches and athletic trainers are happy to leave medical decisions to the medical profession. They also assist in interpreting this principle to students and the public.

American Medical Association
Committee on the Medical Aspects of Sports

9801—141F: 369-2M-D243 OP-37

CONTENTS

CHAPTER 1

INTRODUCTION

INTRODUCTION TO THE THIRD EDITION

Time marches on and with it marches the care of the athlete. Further advances in organized efforts have occurred in the past five years. The American Orthopaedic Society for Sports Medicine has been organized to encourage dissemination of knowledge among the orthopaedists. The AOSSM is particularly designed to provide a forum for orthopaedists who are interested in improvement of health care to the American athlete. The drive of this important new society has been to alert the orthopaedist, primarily but not exclusively, to the proper means by which improved care can be provided the athlete. Several foundations that are dedicated to the health of the athlete are operating for the common good. The activities of the Sports Medicine Committee of the American Academy of Orthopaedic Surgeons, which was formed in 1962, have greatly expanded from the original one postgraduate course per year, until in 1975, eight courses were presented in diverse parts of the country.

Sports Medicine is coming of age but I see no signs of senescence. On the contrary, a great number of eager young orthopaedists are pushing the older group and are receiving proper recognition for their efforts for the good of the athlete. Much in this Third Edition evolves from past volumes, since basic principles do not change. An effort has been made to provide more clarity, to establish principles, and to make room for new concepts as they develop. We are trying hard to eliminate old eponyms and to prevent the establishment of new ones, since semantics is a very important factor in education.

Since the previous editions of this book have been published, there has been marked change in the athletic picture, particularly related to female contestants. Importance has always been attached to the female contestants through the many years in which records were kept. There has always been, however, a slight reserve about whether or not the distaff side of the show should be granted equal time with the spear side. There must be many areas in which the competition can be equal. Certainly up to the age of puberty, the girls may be further developed than the boys, but from then on, the males begin to get more physical characteristics, and the females more romantic ones. In this work we have made no effort to discriminate between male or female. Since the book is basically on athletic injuries, there is little here that applies to the male that doesn't apply equally as well to the female. Since there is, to my knowledge, no short word to imply "he" or "she," my "he" and "his" will refer to both sexes to the disparagement of neither. I love them all.

Since rehabilitation has become of maximum importance in the treatment of the athlete, whether he be young or old, we have included a chapter devoted to rehabilitation. Fred Allman, the author of this chapter, has devoted a major part of his professional life to the advancement of this aspect of treatment of musculo-skeletal conditions and I extend a most grateful thanks to him for his help in adding this aspect. Dr. Allman has also been kind enough to add shorter sections on rehabilitation in regard to specific injuries, particularly some of the more common ones. Once again, Dr. Gael Frank has cooperated very much in the preparation of the material on the hand and I appreciate his efforts in this direction. The section on craniocerebral injuries has been carefully reviewed with the idea of some more definitive recommendations. This has been done by Dr. Bob Rutledge, an eminent neurosurgeon at the University of Oklahoma School of Medicine, with my sincere appreciation. For the first time we have included some authoritative material on treatment of injuries to the eye. Although this is an infrequent injury, it is one that causes great dismay on the part of the team physician who is hard put to decide just what level of care this requires. Ophthalmologist Dr. Pat Wilkinson, who has a long background in athletics, has contributed to this effort and has our heartfelt thanks for giving authenticity to an area in which my personal opinions are far less than authoritative.

INTRODUCTION TO THE SECOND EDITION

I had intended to completely rewrite the introduction to this second edition. However, I find the comments made in the introduction to the first edition as valid today as they were when written a number of years ago. The principles remain the same.

In the intervening years there has been a vast expansion of athletic participation and, I am happy to say, an even more comprehensive program to improve the young athlete. Most of the points referred to in my introduction to the First Edition have developed amazingly well. The educational programs have vastly expanded as will be noted. Many excellent books and articles have been published. There has been a notable expansion of the breadth of participation. Most responsible athletic programs today make a real effort to provide participation for every young person who desires it. Responsible medical organizations have awakened to realize not only the tremendous increase in the importance of trauma in relation to economic loss, morbidity and mortality, but that sports medicine has attained great stature. The same precepts which serve to make sports medicine unique have contributed to the development of methods of prevention, diagnosis, and treatment which can be and have been applied to nonathletic situations.

There has also been a sweeping evolution in the medical care of the young athlete. Led by the American Medical Association Committee on the Medical Aspects of Sports, many organizations throughout the United States have organized very active committees dedicated to the health of American youth. This A.M.A. committee has invited the participation of other organizations with interest in sports medicine. Under this committee's aegis a coordination committee has been formed with representation from similar committees of other associations, medical and non-medical, concerned with the problem. Annual meetings of this group committee have been held since 1964. The total number of associations represented in this group is rapidly approaching 50. A subcommittee on standard sports nomenclature from the A.M.A. committee has published a thesaurus of definitions in an attempt to clarify the language and so improve communications. I shall follow this terminology in so far as it is possible in this book.

Led by the Sports Medicine Committee of the American Academy of Orthopaedic Surgeons, which was activated in 1962, the orthopaedic aspects of this development have greatly expanded. The Committee promotes instructional courses, presents exhibits and encourages scientific study of musculo-skeletal conditions relative to sports. The American Academy of Orthopaedic Surgeons Committee has encouraged and promoted programs for coaches, trainers, team physicians and orthopaedists all about the country. More recently the Committee has presented an increasing number of postgraduate seminars developed for orthopaedic surgeons. This interest is not confined to orthopaedic surgeons, however. It has been taken up by internists, pediatricians, physiatrists, physiologists, neurologists, and indeed the whole gamut of the medically oriented professions. Sophisticated courses are given for specialists, more practical ones for generalists, and still others directed to trainers and physical therapists. In fact, at this time the coverage of the field seems complete. In spite of all this, each new program develops new ideas which may bring about some breakthrough in treatment, conditioning or prevention.

My present effort is to try to bring this volume up to date and in line with the progress made in this and other fields. Methods change, but general principles are remarkably constant.

Finally, a few words of appreciation for the many colleagues who have contributed to this volume. They shall remain largely anonymous, but without this constant contact I should have little to offer. Most of the actual cases are my own, since I find that I write better and with more confidence about cases with which I am wholly familiar. I shall never fail to appreciate the many contacts that I have had with members of my profession, both in the United States and abroad, by personal association, by direct correspondence and by study of their excellent reports. I cannot close this introduction without acknowledging a great debt of gratitude to my dedicated and long-suffering personal staff who serve as my memory for cases and who patiently put up with my constant desire for improvement by substituting new material at the last minute. Without their efforts this book would have been impossible.

INTRODUCTION TO THE FIRST EDITION

A book devoted entirely to injuries to a special group must have justification. Why injuries to athletes alone? Why not just injuries in general? Certainly the athlete is a human being, subject to the same frailties as the rest of the race, and one might reasonably expect him to be treated in the same manner. Could not the physician refer for guidance to one or more of the multitude of books that have been written on the subject of injury?

The very fact that you are reading this book to some extent justifies it. Obviously you recognize the athletic injury as a special situation—an area in which we as physicians can render a unique service. I believe that a few paragraphs explaining our approach to this stimulating subject will give added meaning to the later sections on specific injuries.

There is, indeed, real significance in the fact that a separate volume on the subject of injuries to athletes is considered to be warranted. Ten years ago this would not have been likely. Lately, however, there has been a tremendous upsurge of interest in this subject, not only among orthopaedists, but among physicians in general, and indeed among the laity. An increasing number of postgraduate seminars and medical sessions have been concerned with it. At a postgraduate course on athletic injuries sponsored by the University of Colorado at Denver less than four years ago, at which from 30 to 40 registrants were expected, an amazing total of almost 300 very interested and enthusiastic physicians, orthopaedists, coaches and trainers appeared. In the following years the attendance was markedly increased. The injuries discussed at this and other meetings have been largely those of college athletes, but there is presently a ground swell in various parts of the country to develop these educational sessions to include secondary school and even grade school athletics.

Organized athletics has been extended to involve a major segment of our youth. In many areas not only the junior high schools but the grade schools participate in competitive sports. Whether or not this is good, it must be recognized as a fait accompli which cannot be ignored. There is no present trend toward less athletics. On the contrary, the trend is toward a more inclusive program. Indeed, one of the major criticisms leveled at athletic programs has been their tendency to include the few to the neglect of the many. It should be recalled that in this country the various types of organized athletics, many of them competitive, must serve almost the whole function of physical conditioning, whereas in other countries there are various health clubs, hiking clubs, ski societies, etc. Organizations of the latter type have not been popular in the United States. Our citizens are a keenly competitive group and exercise for exercise's sake; the calisthenic drill, the regimentation into marching clubs, has not appealed to them, one reason being the fact that in other countries these various groups have been used as springboards for political activity. Our youth have an almost paranoid dislike of anything smacking of regimentation. The effort, therefore, must be not to decry athletics and demand less participation but, on the contrary, to demand greater participation and then see to it that the whole background of organized athletics is improved.

There can be no denying that competitive athletics has a great appeal to the mass of our people. However, the public is more inclined to look at the score, to observe the outstanding player, and to foster the competitive contest than to direct its attention toward those facets of the program which are best calculated to return the major good to the greatest number. Comparatively little attention outside the confines of sport itself has been paid to conditioning or to prevention of injury. An occasional blare of publicity follows a major injury to a stellar athlete or the untimely death of a budding prep school player. Occasionally this triggers a lay magazine article on the importance of equipment or the value of physical conditioning as important factors in the prevention of injury. The greater emphasis, however, is placed on the injury itself. The sports pages eagerly play up injury to the star. Wryly enough, the reporter moans that the star has been disabled by his operation rather than by his injury.

In the final analysis, however, the lay public and, I fear, the majority of our medical profession have little knowledge of the actual processes of training and the actual mechanics of injury.

COMPETITIVE ATHLETICS: BENEFITS AND RISKS

Why is it important for young men to participate in athletics? Certainly it does carry an element of risk. Perhaps the solution to the problem of athletic injuries lies in the prayer of the timorous mother that her boy not compete. Abandonment of sports would certainly be the quickest way to prevent injury to the contestant.

In common with many others, I believe there are tangible benefits to be derived from athletic competition that greatly outweigh the element of risk. Certainly some of them are obvious. No one seriously doubts that the athlete does develop a stronger, healthier body. Most of the myths of catastrophic sequelae from strenuous athletic activity have been dispelled. The "athlete's heart" is a bogeyman which has finally been exorcized. The ex-athlete who "turns to fat" has at least postponed his impending adiposity throughout his years of training. The trained athlete is superior to his more sedentary fellow in drive and stamina, and better fitted for both work and play.

I think most of us would agree that competitive athletics does have a salutary effect upon the character of the participant. This is particularly true if the program is managed so that the major emphasis is placed on the development of the ability in the athlete to value his own, and respect his opponent's, capabilities rather than to win at any cost. The player learns the importance of team participation, that he must sacrifice immediate gain to the final end, that

desire is one of the key factors in success. The fact that the word "sportsmanship" seems trite has in no way changed its reality as a trait of character. Team effort as opposed to individual glory, ability to take a job and to follow it through, the necessity for taking it as well as dishing it out, are all basic lessons learned by the successful athlete.

There are certainly material benefits for the athlete in our present educational system that have much importance. Many a young man goes to school because of his athletic ability. Much has been said about scholarships, especially by those who know the least about them. Suffice it to say that the athletic scholarship does permit many a lad to finish his education who otherwise would have dropped out of school long before. Who are we to say that the athletic scholarship is not as worthwhile as the scholarship for merit in other fields? In most of the better schools of the country the scholarship athlete has to maintain a scholastic average higher than the average of his school. A good estimate of the quality of the scholarship program in a given institution can be made from the proportion of the scholarship boys who go ahead to graduation.

So much for the benefit of athletics to the student in school. But after graduation, what? It has been said that the athlete out of school is as a fish out of water. Not so! Many athletes develop their careers in some form of physical education or a related field. The conditioning of our youth depends upon the organized type of athletic training which he gets in the elementary and secondary schools and in such organizations as the Y.M.C.A. and the Boy Scouts. Without the trained athlete to provide capable leadership these programs would be in sorry straits, indeed. We need these people. Indeed, we will find that much of the physical education of our youth is in the hands of the former athlete. On a more personal plane, many an athlete makes contacts during his school years with men who are seeking his very type of qualifications to man the leading jobs in industry. In many years of knowing athletes I have seen most of them display the same fine enthusiasm and attain the same success in life that they did in school. Certainly there are real advantages to an athletic program from many standpoints.

Why then is there such bitter opposition to organized competitive athletics as such? Not because of any interference with scholastic pursuits, not because of any moral implications, not because the aftereffects of training impair the physique in later life, but because of one principal thing, namely, physical injuries. Do athletes get physical injuries? The answer is "Yes, they do." Here is a very real objection to the athletic program—in fact, almost the only real objection. Our youngsters do get injured—on occasion even seriously or fatally injured. It must be the duty of the medical profession to accept this challenge and do everything in its power to minimize those things which interfere with the goals of the athletic program.

THE ROLE OF THE PHYSICIAN

What can we as physicians do to prevent injury, to minimize temporary disability and to prevent permanent disability? Much indeed has been accomplished in the past few years toward these ends. A few years ago the trainer in the average scholastic institution was a fugitive from the supply room, having graduated into the "wrapping and taping" club largely by osmosis. He had no real knowledge of injuries and his main concern actually was to "keep 'em rollin'." We all remember the famous men who attained a great deal of notoriety by reason of their ability to keep the athlete in the game. Too many times this goal of immediate playing was a more vital one than the final goal of complete recovery of the patient. During this era the doctor was a necessary evil. The player felt that once he reached the doctor his days as an athlete were over. In too many instances this feeling was justified for two very pertinent reasons. First, since the doctor was the last resort, he did not see the player until long after treatment should ideally have been instituted. Second, and I think of almost equal importance, was the sad reality that it was not of any immediate concern to the doctor whether or not the patient was an athlete or was able to remain one after treatment was completed. All too often the first recommendation the doctor made was "Well, give up football," or "You must not play any more baseball." This simply tended to confirm the conviction of the player, the coach and the public that athletes and physicians were incompatible. Also, in the past there has been a tendency on the part of the coaching staff to demand that the player continue in spite of injury or be labeled "yellow." The trainer was urged to "tape her up" and "run him back in"—often to the detriment of the player, the team and the game. In our major institutions this is no longer true.

A more enlightened approach has demonstrated that everyone is better served by having the injured player promptly and ably treated, thereby obtaining recovery before he does himself irreparable damage. The successful coach seeks to protect the player and seeks to prevent damage to either body or mind. In the well-run athletic program of today, the coach, trainer, team physician and specialist *all* combine in one effective unit designed to keep the player well equipped and in ideal condition. In fact, more emphasis is placed, and actually more time is spent, on preparing a player to participate and on preventing his injury than is spent on treatment. The player, coach, trainer and physician are no longer working at cross purposes in most institutions. Athletic injuries are much less frequent and they are less severe than in the past. The period of disability is shorter. The degree of recovery is more complete. Many factors have combined to cause this vast improvement in the one area where it must be conceded that athletics may have a bad effect.

Se we find that once again the physician must become not only the doer but the teacher. The physician with an especial interest in athletes must prepare himself to handle their injuries, and he must in turn pass this information on to other physicians. It must be recognized that there is one overriding difference in the management of injuries to athletes. That is, the patient must get complete recovery from his injury or he is no longer an athlete. True enough, this axiom *should* apply to any injury the doctor sees, but nowhere else is it dramatized quite so constantly as in the care of the athlete.

DIAGNOSTIC JUDGMENT

The outstanding consideration in the treatment of athletic injury is early detection not only of the nature of the injury but of its degree. The optimum time to examine an athlete for injury is as soon as possible after he is hurt. There must be no compromise with this statement. It may be impossible to examine the patient or to make a complete diagnosis at once, but if it can be done precious time has been saved. Frequently the initial examination is by the coach, the trainer or the physician on the field. Whoever this is, he must make as careful an evaluation of the injured player's condition as he is capable of doing and must pass this information on to each succeeding link in the chain of therapy. The doctor must conscientiously and objectively examine the player. Does the injury seem serious enough that the boy should not return to the game, or should he be strapped up and allowed to play? To err is human, but the margin of error can be drastically reduced by comprehensive consideration of the patient's injury. There is no place here for wishful thinking. The player is eager to continue and should not be deprived unnecessarily of this privilege. On the other hand, if continued competition adds to the hazard of injury, he should not be permitted to compete. It is, of course, always better to err on the side of conservatism.

After the injury sidelines the player, what then? The prevalent habit of packing the injured part in ice and delaying examination until a convenient time the next day, or even later, is to be deplored. Your examination as a physician should be done at the earliest possible moment even at considerable inconvenience to yourself, the coach or the player. It should be obvious that the part should be undressed, all taping or strapping removed, and a meticulous examination carried out. Frequently the diagnosis, which will be easy in the early stage, becomes exceedingly difficult as pain increases apprehension, and swelling, edema and hemorrhage interfere with an accurate evaluation of the injury. If consultation with a specialist is needed, seek it promptly so that the specialist, too, may be able to take advantage of the optimum time for treatment. The specialist should have enough integrity to be able to cooperate with the referring physician and to "take the monkey off his back," as it were, in regard to the severity of the injury. This is particularly true of the decision on whether or not the player should be allowed to compete, either at once or later.

CONCEPTS OF TREATMENT

Once treatment is decided upon, the physician should proceed to carry it out with confidence. If the treatment is within the capabilities of the team physician, he should be permitted to conduct it. If the specialist's attention is required, the specialist himself should not hesitate to say so. The physician should be encouraged to seek the specialist's advice early, and this will be done only when there is good rapport between the player, the referring physician and the specialist.

The following concepts ("Five A's") of treatment have proved to be of great value: (1) accept athletics; (2) avoid expediency; (3) adopt the best method; (4) act promptly; (5) achieve perfection.

1. *Accept athletics.* The physician—not the player, not the coach, not the parents, but the physician—must recognize the value of competitive athletics. He must believe that it is vital to this particular patient to be restored to competitive athletics. If the physician fails in this, the patient-doctor relationship suffers and rapport is lost. The doctor who deprecates the player's ambition should not be treating him.

2. *Avoid expediency.* Outside influence must not be permitted to outweigh sound medical judgment. Many pressing factors will tend to influence the doctor's decision. All concerned are extremely unwilling to believe that the player is really hurt. The boy's desire to compete, his fear of failing his teammates, the parents' desire to see their son excel, the coach's hope that the player is not really hurt—all must be ignored if the proper conclusion is to be reached. Procrastination, vacillation and so-called "conservative" attitudes must not prevail. Temporary convenience must be sacrificed for the ultimate goal.

3. *Adopt the best method of treatment.* Medical evaluation of the nature and extent of injury must be the controlling factor in the choice of treatment. A temporizing attitude will not accomplish the best results. If you really believe that one method is distinctly better than another, you should recommend it and then carry it out. This must be an entirely objective decision. How often do we hear the statement "Well, perhaps it would be better to operate on this knee, but I'll put it in a cast" or "We really should have put the boy on crutches, but. . . ."

4. *Act promptly.* A definitive decision as to the proper method of treatment must be made at the earliest possible moment and then that method must be carried out. We have been able to show conclusively that delay very often spells the difference between success and failure of treatment.

5. *Achieve perfection.* Make complete recovery your goal. While this may not be possible in any given case, it must always be the goal. The athlete is basically in good condition and can well tolerate any reasonable measure if it serves to increase his chances for a complete recovery.

Will such a program be accepted? Yes, but not without some educational effort on the part of the doctor. He must be able to show conclusively that the program is better not only for the doctor, but for the school, the coach and especially for the player. This will require time. He must be interested and capable. As his program develops, those most concerned will recognize the benefits. They will observe that the sprained ankle responds to treatment, that a short, complete layoff is followed by normal ability as opposed to an ineffectual season. The coach will note that prompt treatment restores the player more rapidly and permits more actual playing in the long run and so is better for the team. The player will not fear the doctor who has a sympathetic and understanding attitude. He notes that his buddy gets well. He also expects to get well and will accept the physician's recommendation for treatment. He may fear some specific part of the treatment, such as the insertion of a needle into a joint, but never to the extent of failing to return or refusing the treatment provided he believes that the doctor is sincerely trying to restore him to his normal ability.

These are not idle dreams of Utopia. The type of program described is practical and has been established in a number of institutions. It must be our aim to make it the rule, not the exception. Nor is a full scale, university-type training program necessary. The program does require an able, conscientious coach and a physician who will interest himself in the peculiar problems of the athlete.

PART I

PREVENTION OF INJURIES

CHAPTER 2

PREVENTION OF INJURIES

The prevention of injuries should be the major goal of anyone responsible for the physical and mental conditioning of athletes. If we grant that the athletic program is important from the standpoint of the improvement of the physical and mental condition of our young people, we must adopt every possible means to see that there is no detrimental effect from the athletic program. There may be differences of opinion concerning the benefits of athletics, but one cannot deny that almost the only deleterious effect is physical injury. We spend much time devising ways and means to relieve the effects of injury. If we spent even a small percentage of this time in striving to prevent the injury from occurring, a major portion of our problem would be solved.

Prevention of injuries has many facets. In a university-type training program, more attention will be given to prevention of injuries by one means or another than to their treatment. In the secondary school programs, someone must be made responsible for the physical welfare of the players. There has been a steady improvement in this facet of the problem for many years. The

trainer has become a skilled professional person. Unfortunately, most secondary schools cannot afford full-time trainers. The role of the physician here must be that of advisor to whatever amateur trainer is available. It is neither fair nor advisable to put the whole responsibility of physical conditioning upon the busy coach, however capable he may be. The coach must of necessity concentrate his attention on the practice session or on the game. His training duties must be incidental to this. The team physician should be the one who is especially interested in this problem. He must be willing to accept the responsibility for it even at some inconvenience to himself. It may seem very tedious to supervise the details of strapping, wrapping, equipment, weight control and all of the other areas of training, but the team physician is not worthy of the name if he is not willing to do it. This is particularly important in the preseason training period. Prevention of injury is as much the sphere of the doctor as is prevention of disease. The overall aim of the athletic program is to improve the participant. If the program leaves the participant in poorer condition than

13

when he started, it has failed regardless of how many games have been won.

THE INDIVIDUAL PLAYER

PHYSICAL CONDITION (GENERAL HEALTH)

Before the prospective player is permitted to enter an athletic program, he should have an intelligent and complete physical examination. It is not necessary to take a multitude of laboratory tests. The general physical examination should, however, provide leads to needed supplemental measures. For example, if there seems to be a defect in vision, a detailed examination of the eye should be recommended. If a cardiac murmur is discovered, it should be investigated. It is not enough simply to examine a player and record the findings. The physician should be willing to give an opinion as to the boy's physical ability to participate in the sport concerned. If he does not feel himself capable of doing this, he should recommend special examinations. It is not proper to request a boy to drop the program simply because the physican does not know whether or not he has a physical defect which would contraindicate his participation. It is almost as bad to err by overconservatism as it is to overlook serious hazards. Does this functional heart murmur really constitute a hazard? Can this boy's adiposity be controlled? Are this young man's bones to be judged overbrittle because he has had several fractures? To each individual the answers are extremely vital. They must be vital to the examining physician as well.

Once it has been decided that the candidate may compete in athletics, every effort must be made to *improve* his physical condition. He should be given advice as to his diet and told to avoid faddish eating, to avoid overeating and to eat regularly. He should be advised not to snack between meals at the expense of his regular meal. Many young people are subject to constipation. This can usually be completely controlled by regulation of the diet, which is far better than the habitual use of laxatives. An effort should be made to determine the proper weight for the individual player, and his diet then is regulated to reach this weight by high caloric regimens for the undernourished and low caloric, high protein diets for the adipose. On every squad there will be several players who are in dire need of regulation in dietary matters.

The player should be instructed in good living habits. He should get plenty of rest and sleep. The two are not necessarily synonymous. If he has irregular study and sleeping hours, an effort should be made to find a schedule more in keeping with his general surroundings. There is no point in forcing him to go to bed early and to get up early if the habit of his family is to go to bed late and to get up late. There is nothing magical in certain specific hours of sleep. The benefit is in the number of hours and the degree of relaxation. The well-regulated program should permit the player to have 30 to 40 minutes of relative relaxation between practice or competition and eating. It goes without saying that he should be instructed not to eat just before strenuous practice periods. Great emphasis is put on regulating eating before an actual game, but too often the practice session is not so well regulated. The player's blood may be concentrated in his muscles by extreme physical exercise when it should be busy aiding in the digestion of his food.

The player should be instructed to avoid all drugs except on the specific prescription of a physician. This includes intoxicants and nicotine. Stimulants are not only useless but may cause irreparable overexertion. Various fads should be discouraged.

CONDITIONING

The physical conditioning of a player should be a continuous thing. If the player can be kept in good condition throughout the year, one of the major goals of the athletic program will have been accomplished; namely, the improvement of the general condition of the youth of America. Nonetheless, there are certain sports that require concentration of conditioning far beyond the others. Ideally, the conditioning should be fitted to the sport. In our University of Oklahoma program, for example the football player is urged to keep in condition the year round. It is fully understood that he probably will not keep in game condition for the full 12 months, but it is fatuous to believe that he can be put in game condition in two or three weeks. Hence, each individual player is instructed when he leaves school on exactly what he should do that summer. The following summer conditioning program for high school athletes is recommended by Mr. Ken Rawlinson, Head Trainer, University of Oklahoma, and is quoted directly from his book:*

A Recommended Summer High School Conditioning Program

It is my belief that a high school athlete needs even more incentive to carry on a summer conditioning program than a college athlete. There follows a summer or off-season conditioning plan that can be inaugurated in any high school.

  I. Squad meeting—end of school—tell boys why of everything.
    1. Start in June—peak in August.
    2. Calisthenic program.

----

*Rawlinson, Ken: Modern Athletic Training. Englewood Cliffs, New Jersey, Prentice-Hall, Inc., page 25.

    3. Weight training program.
    4. Isometric program.
    5. 6:30 mile.
    6. Wind sprints.
    7. Run circles, figure 8's.
    8. Stadium steps.
    9. Rope skipping.
   10. Rehabilitative exercises.
   11. Temperate living.
       A. Sleep—"the great restorer"—a minimum of nine hours. Two hours before midnight is better than four after.
       B. No intoxicants. The A.M.A. has stated that "alcohol is a detriment to the human organism. Its use in therapeutics, as a tonic, food, or stimulant has no scientific value. It attacks the central nervous system. It is not a food; it is a poison."
       C. No smoking. Nowhere is there any medical evidence that states that it improves an athlete's ability. It actually slows him up. Nicotine is a poison. If one smokes a pack of cigarettes a day for a week, he inhales 400 mg. of nicotine, which in a single injection would kill him instantly.
       D. No drugs. The United States Olympic Committee has recently ruled that any competitor who uses drugs, stimulants, or other substances known as "dope" for any purpose will be disqualified.
       E. Good diet.
   12. Possibly assign weight for first practice.
   13. Date and place of physical exam.
   14. Pre-season physical test.
       6:30 mile
       Push-ups—30
       Sit-ups—50
       Pull-ups—10
 II. Personal letters in summer—incentive, challenge.
    1. Season's objectives (offense, defense, etc.)
    2. Conditioning hints.
    3. Rehabilitative exercises.
    4. Physical exam—reminder.
    5. Pre-season physical condition test.

"What Makes a Champion" by Bud Wilkinson

1. Condition.
2. Will to win.

3. Physically tougher than opponent.
4. Execution of fundamentals.
5. Fewer errors.

A Recommended Summer College or University Conditioning Program

Short sprints develop speed. Distance running develops endurance. Running in circles, figure 8's (around goal posts), strengthens ankles, knees, hips and back.

JUNE:

Daily exercises (see below).
Run 2 to 3 days a week—distance running, 440's—jog 1, walk 1, etc. Minimum 2 miles.

JULY:

Daily exercises (see below).
Run 3 to 4 days a week—distance running plus a few sprints, 880's—jog 1, walk 1, etc. Minimum 2 miles. Sprints: 10–20–30 yards. Three of each at ½ speed.

AUGUST:

Take your salt tablets daily. If possible work out at 4:00 p.m. daily—climatic conditions are thus about equal to our practice sessions. Work 5 to 7 days a week with emphasis on:

A. Daily exercise program.
B. Sprints (10–20–30 yards—start with 5 of each at ¾ speed and work up to 10 at full speed).
C. Be able to run a mile. Objective: backs, 6:00; lineman, 6:30.
D. Football drills (wave, quarter eagles, pass cuts, etc.).
E. You should be within 3 pounds of your assigned playing weight by August 1.

Daily Exercises

Follow the daily exercise program during June, July and August (increase tempo in August). For a variation on many of the daily exercises you may use the INTENSITY SYSTEM—maximum effort over a limited time (example: number of push-ups you can do in 20 seconds—decrease time interval as you progress).

EVERYDAY:

1. Rope jumping (objective: 15 minutes).
2. Step bench. Using an 18 to 21 in. bench or chair, do at least 45 steps each leg once a day.

3. Wrestlers bridge. Position: Weight supported on feet and head—rotate in circles to right and left.
4. Weight training—at least three times a week.

DAILY EXERCISE GUIDE

Do five exercises per day for six days a week during the months of June and July. Increase the tempo in August. These exercises are set up specifically to reach every area of the body and can be done daily in the athlete's room or back yard. He should start exercises by jumping rope.

MONDAY:

Side Bender. Position: Stand with feet apart, hands clasped overhead, arms straight. Bend sideward to the right, bending right knee and slowly going as far as possible. Repeat to left. Repeat ten times each side.

Knee Stretcher. Position: Stand with feet apart, knees slightly flexed and hands on outside of knees. Press knees together with hands, knees offering resistance. Repeat outward 20 times.

Shoulder Hang. Position: Grasp an overhead crossbar, ladder, treelimb, etc., and hang, elbows straight. Hang one minute, relax, and repeat ten times. Especially good for boys with acromioclavicular, muscular or nerve shoulder trouble. (If shoulder will permit, walk hand-over-hand across overhead ladder.)

Hurdle Spread. Position: Sit in hurdle position with right leg forward. Bend trunk forward and touch right foot with both hands. Repeat 40 times, then extend left leg and repeat 40 times.

TUESDAY:

Groin Stretch. Position: Stand with feet apart, hands on groin. Bend body obliquely to right and left (forward and backward). Stretch it out.

Bicycle Ride. Position: Support body on shoulders with elbows on ground and hands on hips supporting the body. Move feet and legs in motion necessary for riding a bicycle as rapidly as possible for count of 40. Repeat four to five times.

Stomach Drill. Position: Flat on back with hands under hips, with legs straight together and toes pointed. Raise feet slowly with a slow count of ten until the legs are perpendicular to the ground, lower them slowly halfway and stop; here spread the legs and bring them together eight times, then lower legs to within six inches from the ground and repeat the spread eight times. Raise legs slowly to the perpendicular position and lower them to the ground very slowly. Repeat eight times.

Leg Flexing. Position: Sitting position. With both hands grasp left leg and pull knee up to ear. Relax and repeat with right leg. Repeat rapidly for count of 100.

WEDNESDAY:

Wood Chopper. Position: Stand with feet apart, trunk turned right, hands together and over right shoulder. In a chopping movement bring arms down vigorously between the legs. Uncoil over left shoulder and repeat. Repeat 20 times each side.

Push Up or Push Up and Clap. Position: Flat on stomach push up with toes dug in and hands flat on ground, clap hands and catch on hands without allowing body to contact ground. Repeat 10 to 15 times.

Quarter Eagles. Position: Feet width of shoulders, parallel, and heels on ground. Bend at knees so thighs are parallel to ground. Maintaining the above base, jump 1/4 turns to right and left.

Belly Rock. Position: Face down, hands back of neck. Raise head, chest and legs and rock back and forth 75 times.

THURSDAY:

Trunk Twister. Position: Stand with feet apart, hands clasped behind head and elbows back. Bend and bounce downward and simultaneously rotate trunk far to left. Recover and repeat to right. Repeat 15 times to each side.

All Fours. Position: Face down. Weight on hands and feet, and walk forward, backward, sideward, etc.

Burpee. Position: Assume squat position with hands on ground, elbows inside knees. Thrust feet and legs backward, weight supported on hands and toes. Return to squat position, then to starting position. Repeat 20 times.

Sit Up and Paw Dirt. Position: Flat on back with arms extended overhead. Sit up, thrust arms forward and touch toes, knees straight. Return to starting position. Swing legs overhead until feet touch ground behind neck. Dig the dirt with running motion of legs, for 15 counts. Return to original position and repeat.

FRIDAY:

Mountain Climber. Position: Squatting with hands on ground, right leg drawn up to chest and left leg extended to rear with knee straight. With a fast cadence extend right foot backward and bring left leg to chest. Repeat 25 times.

Leg-Back Stretch. Position: Flat on back with arms bracing shoulders against the turn. With knee stiff, raise one leg to perpendicular position and swing it across body until foot touches hand on opposite side, shoulders flat throughout. Repeat 20 times with right, left and both legs (good for low back injuries).

Toe and Heel Dance. Position: One-half squat position with trunk erect. Remaining in this position, jump with the right heel extended in front and the left toe extended behind. Jump again, reversing the order of the feet. Repeat rapidly 40 times. From same position jump with the right heel to the side and left foot in place. Repeat to left.

SATURDAY:

Sacroiliac Stretch. Position: Sitting with knees drawn to chest. Lock arms around knees and roll back onto shoulders. Continue to roll and tighten the grip of the arms.

Leg Stretch. Position: Stand erect with hands at sides. Bend forward without bending knees, and touch toes. Repeat 20 to 30 times. Repeat same with legs crossed.

High Step-Dive. Position: Stationary high step run-dive forward, weight on hands and let chest strike ground lightly, then abdomen, thighs and feet. Jump to feet and repeat 15 times.

SUNDAY: Optional.

The major portion of this conditioning must be carried out by the athlete himself. He cannot be expected to do it without proper direction and instruction. Each boy is given a set of exercises which he is to use three or four times a week until the first part of August and then daily until the beginning of the fall practice. He is encouraged to supplement these exercises by jogging, running for endurance, wind sprints and other types of exercise. He is encouraged to maintain, at least to some degree, his training program by getting rest, sleep, proper food and by avoiding dissipation throughout the summer. Furthermore, each boy is assigned the weight at which he is expected to be when he reports for the first day of practice in the fall. The player is told that he should report in such condition that he could play a game on the first day of practice.

Obviously, such a program cannot be fitted entirely to the secondary school. However, the essence of the program is there. If the boy is to participate in football, he should start conditioning himself early in the summer. It will not suffice simply to tell him to keep himself in shape. He must be given a specific program to follow. Most of the eager young athletes will be glad to carry out such a program if they know what is really expected of them. There is probably less trouble with physical conditioning for football than for any other sport since this is recognized as a rugged sport. It is equally important for the player to be conditioned for such games as basketball, baseball and particularly for track. Many a track career has been nipped in the bud because the participant has not been "brought along" by gradually increasing effort. A single major effort by the broad jumper or the sprinter may be responsible for losing the whole season of competition since he may develop tenosynovitis of the tendo Achilles or a strain of the hamstring muscle or a *stress* fracture of the foot or fibula (Fig. 49, page 86). A runner should not be permitted to run the mile under competitive conditions until he has many times paced himself through this same distance at a gradually accelerating rate. The baseball player who needs to get his arm as well as his legs in top shape may require a wholly different set of exercises, although the goal remains the same. He must not be permitted to exert the maximum strength of any muscle until it has been suitably conditioned for this effort. This is well known as it applies to the pitcher, but it may be equally disastrous for the outfielder or third baseman to start his practice with maximum throws to the plate or across to first. These fac-

tors are particularly pertinent in secondary school players, who have a maximum of desire and a minimum of regulatory common sense. They require supervision and this is one of the major advantages of organized athletics. In a regulated program the player can have supervision and so be developed gradually until his full potential is reached.

It should be noted that the doctor has a real responsibility to eliminate any exercise that he feels to be bad, no matter how traditional or popular it may be. Any orthopaedist handling injuries knows all too well the danger of the popular "deep knee bends" and "duck waddle." In these exercises as the heel is forcibly jammed against the buttock, there is a real danger of a posterior tear of the medial or lateral meniscus. They have no advantage over three-quarter knee bends. Obviously, all doctors will not agree on which exercises are particularly bad and which are good. The doctor must first inform himself and then have the strength of his conviction in offering his advice to the athletic administration.

The following examples of exercises for conditioning for certain sports were also developed by Mr. Ken Rawlinson and published in his book.*

Conditioning Athletes' Bodies

For top performance, body conditioning is absolutely necessary. A conditioned boy is less susceptible to injuries. Conditioning affects:

1. Ability to play.
2. Mental attitude.
3. Determination.
4. Teamwork.
5. Spirit.

Many fail to make the team because they do not have the desire. They will not pay the price to get themselves into shape both physically and mentally. Mental conditioning is a phase often overlooked, but it is

---

*Rawlinson, Ken: Modern Athletic Training. Englewood Cliffs, New Jersey, Prentice-Hall, Inc., Chapter III.

very vital. Many athletes do not think it is important, but it goes hand-in-hand with physical conditioning. If an athlete is going to be great, he must have both.

Conditioning at Oklahoma

The conditioning program for the fall season at the University of Oklahoma begins at the close of spring football practice (approximately the middle of May). This portion of the conditioning program must be carried on by the athlete himself. He cannot be expected to do this without proper direction and instruction. It is our firm conviction that if athletes have the desire to be great, they must be, and are, willing to pay the price to help accomplish their goal.

Basic Principles of Running

An important phase of conditioning is running. Every athlete should learn how to run correctly. Anyone can be taught to run a little faster, if he has the desire. Following are a few suggestions:

1. Relax. The body must be supple to attain best performance.

2. Run on the balls of the feet.

3. Point the toes straight ahead. You lose at least one-half inch on each step if toes are not straight ahead.

4. Run in a straight line. It is the shortest distance between two points.

5. Develop your proper stride. The average stride is the height of your body. Lengthen your stride as much as possible but do not overstride. It is worse than an understride.

6. Running angle is important; body leaning, head up, ankles, hips, shoulders and head in a straight line. Do not bend too far backward. You should be in the proper running angle and with the proper stride 12 to 15 yards from the starting point.

7. Arm action is very important; opposite arm and leg move in unison. Keep arm relaxed and shoot uppercuts to height of shoulder and not beyond center of body. Bring arm back so hand does not go beyond crest of hip, a relaxed piston-like movement.

* * *

Short sprints develop speed.

Distance-running develops endurance.

Running in circles and figure 8's strengthens ankles, knees, hips and back.

* * *

The yearly conditioning program at the University of Oklahoma follows. (Take into consideration that we work on rehabilitation the year round.)

JUNE:

Run two or three times a week, distance plus exercises.

JULY-AUGUST:

Five weeks before the start of fall football practice we send each boy a weekly post card of activities that we request be performed daily. The cards are to be properly marked and returned to our office at the close of each week. A sample of the daily activities are:

Mile jog.

15 minutes of calisthenics and stretching exercises.

10 to 30 yard quick starts.

Mile at a good pace.

By the first day of fall football practice each athlete should be in condition to play a regulation game if it were necessary. If he watches his weight and works hard and faithfully, he will have no trouble reporting back in tip-top condition. The athlete should post the daily exercises in his bedroom.

If Post-Season Game:

December — practice.

January — nothing.

February — March — an organized off-season conditioning program (HPER 103) which meets three times a week for a period of 50 minutes of all-out activity. The class consists of strength, quickness, mat, running, and agility drills. Weights are assigned for spring practice.

If No Post Season Game:

December — nothing.

January — run, exercises, handball, weights, etc.

February-March — same as above.

April-May — spring practice: Tuesday, Wednesday, Thursday and Saturday for five weeks. Assign weights for fall practice.

Weight Lifting as Part of the Program

Weight lifting, like any other activity, is an ideal form of exercising if not carried to an extreme. Weight lifting alone is not recommended. It should be a part of an over-all program.

In regard to agility, muscle mass and endurance, Dr. Robert Brashear, orthopaedic surgeon of Knoxville, Tennessee, made the following comments in his booklet on "Athletic Injuries": "Whether one is trying to rebuild a weakened muscle postoperatively or whether one is trying to develop a boy's muscles, he must strain his muscles to the ultimate if he is to build muscle mass. We develop grace and agility by handball and boxing, by fancy diving, by the trampoline and even by doing the jitterbug. We develop endurance by running up and down the stadium steps, but we never develop muscle mass except by strain."

A suggested weight-lifting program for football players is as follows:

BUILDING STRENGTH, POWER, BODY BULK

Breathe in deeply when lifting, exhale when lowering. In the first six exercises below, start with 40 to 50 pounds and increase the weight five to ten pounds per session. Athletes should build up to maximum weight, with 15 repetitions of each exercise done in three series of five each. These exercises should be done three times a week, with adequate warm-up before each exercise (running, stretching exercises, and rope-skipping).

1. To develop spring, initial charge, ankles, body balance and strength:
   Calf Raises. Place a weight on back of neck, feet eight inches apart, body straight. Raise up on toes as high as possible.
2. To develop leg power and strength, back strength, explosive power, increase size of thoracic cage (good weight-gaining exercise):
   Knee Bends. Place a weight on back of neck, feet 12 to 14 inches apart, heels flat on ground, toes pointed slightly outside, head up, shoulders back, buttocks low. Squat down *three-fourths* knee flexion, return to starting position. If weight is too heavy, do only a half squat. (Do not do a deep knee bend.)
3. To strengthen upper back muscles, pulling power, shoulder snap, fingers and wrist:
   Rowing Motion. Feet 24 to 30 inches apart, head up and foward, knees straight but not stiff. Lift weight from ground to chest and return.

4. To strengthen lower back, shoulders, wrist and fingers:
   Stiff-Legged Dead Lifts. Bar on floor in front of feet, feet 12 to 15 inches apart, legs and arms straight. Bend at waist and grasp bar in middle of hand grip. Straighten back and lift weights up to low abdomen. Lower weights to ground in same manner as they were picked up.
5. To develop upper body, shoulders, chest, forearm, and elbows:
   Bench Press. Lie flat on back (on bench), with feet on ground. Grasp bar on outside edge of grip of bar. Elbows are placed wide and along line of bar. Lift weights straight up, extend elbows.
6. Best all-around strength exercises. Neck, arms, back and legs:
   Place feet under bar and about 12 inches apart, toes slightly outward, head high, back and arms straight, heels down. Bend at knees and grasp bar, arms and back straight. Lift bar to low abdomen, keeping arms and back straight. Lower to ground with same body movements.
7. To build up knee and thigh:
   Quadriceps Lift. Use iron boot or table. Sit on table, knee bent. Lift foot, knee straight. Use maximum weight and lift three series of ten (30 lifts total).
   Hamstring Lift. On stomach or standing, use iron boot and raise knee to right angle. Same technique as quadriceps lift.
8. To build up or prevent shoulder injury:
   Bar Hang. Five chins and two minutes of hanging at arms' length.

Heavy resistance with low repetitions builds strength and high repetitions with less resistance builds endurance.

THE INGREDIENTS OF GREATNESS

As part of athletes' mental conditioning, the following qualities and applications can be posted in the training room.

C-oncentration
H-eart
A-ttitude
M-odesty
P-ractice
S-acrifice

COACHING

The coach himself has a responsibility in the program of prevention of injury that can be exercised by no one else. A great deal of the time and effort of the coach must be spent on fundamentals. The player must be taught to improve his agility. He must have extensive work on coordination. He must be instructed as to the proper stance. The player who is constantly alert, whose muscles are in balance, who is prepared for motion in any direction will usually not be hurt. The injury most often comes at a moment when the player is off guard and unprepared for the blow. The coach should instruct him in the way to protect his head and neck in tackling; will show him how to block most effectively and to avoid injury to himself; how best to avoid the bruising block or the damaging tackle. The rules of sport are so designed as to minimize injuries and the coach will advise the players to obey the rules, not only because it is proper but because if everyone obeys the regulations, there is less chance that anyone will be hurt. An illegal maneuver by one player invites retaliation by another. Proper coaching will keep this to a minimum.

ATTITUDE

The attitude of the player is all-important from the standpoint of prevention of injuries. Here the combined efforts of the whole organization are important. The coach, the trainer, the physician, the specialist—each has his part to play. Attitude is, however, the primary responsibility of the coach and the trainer. The player's desire to play, to excel, to do a good job will stimulate him to carry out those things needed to reach this goal. In order to play well he will recognize that he must be in good condition, and recognition is the first step toward accomplishment. The player must have confidence in his own ability. This confidence arises from his knowledge that he is in excellent condition and that he can put out maximum effort without exhaustion or injury. The player must be tough. This does not imply that he must be mean or dirty. It simply means that he must be physically tough so that he can take whatever physical punishment is required to accomplish the desired end. He must be physically stronger per pound than his opponent. This can come only from excellent conditioning. Given the desire to play, self-confidence, mental alertness and a tough physical condition, he must then learn to play with "carefree abandon." This does not mean he should be reckless, but that he should not be apprehensive and fearful. If the coach can inculcate this spirit in the minds of his players, he will find a sharp decrease in the number of disabling injuries among them. This is an extremely important product of physical conditioning.

ENVIRONMENT

It is also important that proper environment for athletics be available since this can be a major deterrent to injury.

ARTIFICIAL TURF VS. NATURAL GRASS

In the last several years, there has been a great drive to install artificial turf, and so have the advantage of a uniform and constant playing surface. This was initiated in the football field, but soon expanded to include track and some other sports. A major selling point has been that the frequency of injuries can be decidedly reduced by artificial turf. This is particularly applied to knee injuries. Controversy still continues as to the relative merits of artificial vs. natural turf. One problem in collecting statistics on the injury rate is the fact that there are so many variables involved, and one cannot make a constant out of so many variables. One can't compare the stadium playing field that is restricted to football—and then only to six games—that has tender loving care the year around, to a field that is used for multiple purposes and is ill kept, and come up with any reliable figures as to injury rates. If we cannot define the typical natural field, how can we compare the natural field with the artificial turf?

So, too, there are several varieties of artificial turf that have different characteristics. It would appear now (1976) that we have a somewhat different set of injuries on the artificial turf than we do on the natural grass. Shoulder girdle injuries seem to be more frequent owing to the hardness of the surface compared to good grass well kept. Various foot conditions, such as large toe injuries from snubbing—including the toenail, the interphalangeal joint, etc.—seem to be more frequent (Fig. 1). We do not as yet have any reliable statistics that indicate that the incidence of knee injuries has been decreased either in number or in severity by the artificial turf.

The final decision in each individual case must be based on a comparison of the artificial turf with whatever other surface may be made available. To clarify this point, it might well be that a field that is poorly kept, or possibly, a field that is hard pan and is played on constantly, would be a better candidate for artificial turf than a better kept area. This problem will soon reach the public schools, and one can imagine the competition that may arise once the high schools join the fray. Hopefully, we may have some more compelling figures to clarify the validity of the present

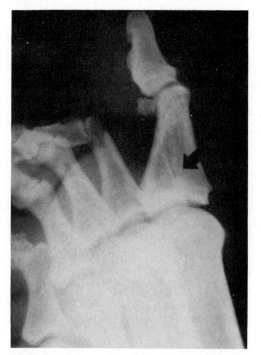

Figure 1. Linear fracture extending obliquely into the MP joint as a result of jamming the big toe against the shoe. The shoe stopped and the toe jammed forward into the shoe. This type of injury seems more prevalent on the artificial turf.

assumptions, pro and con, in regard to artificial turf.

THE PLAYING FIELD

The university programs lay great stress on the condition of the field—not only the game field, which is often reserved for weekends, but particularly the practice field. The secondary schools do not have the advantage of adequate funds for constant supervision of their play areas. However, a little rudimentary care and common sense will accomplish the greater part of the same objectives. Each sport has its individual field requirement.

In *football* the practice field should be level and preferably firmly sodded. At the beginning of the season the field should be carefully screened for all foreign material before it is used. If necessary, the squad can fan out and cover the field to remove rocks, boards, tin cans, paper, all the objects which may have accumulated on the field during the summer when it was out of use. Whoever mows the area should be instructed to remove all such foreign material, not just avoid it. Of perhaps even greater importance is the necessity for leveling of the field. This does not simply mean that it should not be put on a hillside. It means that small imperfections should be filled. A person is more likely to receive an injury stepping into a gopher hole than he is running into a trench. He can avoid the larger imperfections but may fail to see the smaller ones. A few hours spent in so conditioning the field will be well worthwhile. It may be impossible to do much about the firmness of the terrain once the season starts. However, a little effort in the spring may pay dividends in the softening of the soil and obtaining cover with grass. Watering the field, if possible, helps immensely. A good playing surface is far more important than fancy stadiums, decorated goal posts, and the like, and comparatively little money spent on the field will produce gratifying results.

I do not believe anyone uses lime to mark the fields any more. Certainly its use should be condemned. Ample room should be provided at the sidelines so that the player does not crash into obstructions such as stakes, brick piles, or fence rails as he runs out of bounds. Similarly, ample room should be provided at the ends of the field, extending well beyond the end zone so that the pass receiver does not charge into a stone wall or fall over the curb of the running track. Safety equipment around the field is important. The markers should be nontraumatic. There should be no stakes driven into the ground as permanent markers unless they are flush

with the surface. The "chain gang" should be instructed to throw their rods flat on the ground if the play approaches the side line. Wooden benches should be kept well away from the sidelines. All these things seem quite rudimentary but a season never passes that someone does not receive a serious injury from hazards that could have easily been removed.

Other sports, too, have their problems. The *basketball floor* should be smooth and free from splinters and not too slick. There should be ample room along the sidelines even at the penalty of making the court narrower. Charging into a wall can account for breaking an arm, leg or skull since the basketball player does not wear much protective equipment. The practice of hanging the goal at one end of the court just at the front of the stage is a dangerous one. There should be ample room to run under the basket at the ends. No foreign material should be allowed on the floor.

The *baseball field* presents equally important problems. Much attention is usually paid to the infield, and rightly so since irregularity of the infield causes many "bad bounces" and this is of interest to everyone. Too many times the outfield is a weed patch. Grass is allowed to grow tall enough to conceal bricks, cans and stones, which are definite hazards. The sprinting fielder stepping into a hole in the ground receives the same type of injury as the football player but is less able to cope with it because he has less protective armor. The interest of the school in the baseball team can be stimulated by having the younger boys police the outfield.

In *track,* attention should be paid to the running surface. The curb should either be high enough that the runner will avoid it or else low enough that he will not flip his ankles if he hits it.

You may say that these things are not the responsibility of the physician.

They are the responsibility of the physician if he feels himself responsible for the prevention of injuries. There is little accomplished by conditioning a player well and then having him break an ankle as he steps into a hole where a dog has dug up a bone.

If it is necessary for play to take place on inadequate areas, certain precautions must be taken. There is no excuse for leaving debris around. This can always be removed. It may be necessary, however, to play basketball on concrete or blacktop. It may be that some of the football fields are "hardpan" and cannot be remedied. In these circumstances more contact padding should be provided. Knee and elbow pads are mandatory. The wearing of full-length stockings may prevent painful abrasions on the legs. Long-sleeved shirts serve a similar purpose.

BALANCED COMPETITION

There is considerable controversy over the desirability of competitive athletics in the younger age groups. It is my personal belief after many years of an active orthopaedic practice that the youngster is in much less danger under controlled competitive conditions than he is in ordinary backyard play. Certainly this is true from a physical standpoint. We see relatively few grade school youngsters with injuries from football. We see many with injuries from incidental things. The energy of the youngster is such that he is going to expend it doing something. He is safer under supervised athletics than he is walking along the top of a fence, climbing trees or playing in the streets. Neither do I go along with that group of my pediatric colleagues who believe that competition is dangerous for the youngster. From a practical standpoint the youngster is competitive soon after he is born. If the competition can be directed into proper channels, it can be a healthy thing and much more educational than being beaten up by the neighborhood bully. To a youngster the frustration of losing a game is no more severe than that of the baby who breaks a rattle, and it is equally short-lived. This is particularly true if his competition has direction and understanding. He is taught to recognize that someone must lose each time someone else wins.

Competitive athletics does have a real responsibility with regard to equalization of the competitors. Most of the organized programs do this very well. The youngster is regulated not only according to age but according to size, so that the 200 pound 14 year old does not compete with the 85 pound 12 year old. This is a distinct improvement over the casual sandlot games which are catch as catch can and usually are dominated by some prematurely developed youngster.

Balanced competition is particularly necessary in the grade schools but also is important in the high schools. A small high school that is dependent upon a relatively small squad must of necessity have boys on the team who have something less than Olympic capacity. Hence, care should be taken in scheduling games that a team of immature boys does not compete with a juggernaut of excellent, well-trained athletes. This is not nearly as pertinent now as it has been in the past. Comparatively few teams now schedule a so-called "warm-up" or "breather." They usually start right out in competition with their equals. Much credit is due to the secondary school conferences, which make a real effort to match teams of equal capacity against each other. The danger of injury is thus minimized.

Many sports medicine committees which have studied the problem carefully, including the Sports Medicine Committee of the American Academy of Orthopaedic Surgeons, have stated that properly controlled competitive athletic programs are not only permissible but are desirable for the youngster. The well-organized programs will control the factors stated previously. Such programs should be particularly concerned with overemphasis on winning, poor participation of players, overenthusiasm by parents, and overambition on the part of the coach.

EQUIPMENT

Athletic equipment has a great deal to do with prevention of injury. This is especially true of football, and most of our attention will be given to this sport. Good equipment is a must for a football program. We immediately run into the obstacle of an inadequate budget in many schools and for these a happy medium must be sought.

The physician must take a decisive part in directing the equipment phase of the preventive program. To do so he must inform himself, since ill-founded advice based on personal bias is a poor substitute for well-informed judgment. The first step is to determine what things are necessary and are within the budgetary capacities of the particular program. There are two somewhat competitive facets of this problem. Certain items of equipment will add to the ability of the player and so are very desirable from the standpoints of both coach and player. However, one should not allow too much emphasis to be placed upon this facet to the disadvantage of protective measures.

For convenience the items of equipment for the football player will be discussed beginning with the headgear and working down. I believe that this plan will serve our purpose better than to attempt to grade them according to necessity. Indication will be given as to the relative importance of the various pieces of equipment.

There have been vast improvements in *headgear* in recent years and these continue. The old felt headgear that fit like a skull cap did little more than dull the blow and is a far cry from the modern plastic suspension helmet of today. The most important single element of the helmet is the system of webbed suspension straps. These straps must fit the head and keep it from contact with the plastic shell, else the whole function of the suspension is lost. The player himself should be instructed about this, since only he can really tell whether the fit is proper. The helmet should protect the back of the neck, and should fit so that when the neck is extended the helmet does not drive into the back of the neck but rather slides down it. The front of the helmet should protect the forehead. The ear pieces should fit well over the ears. The orifice for hearing should coincide with the external auditory canal. It is obligatory that some sort of a bar be worn to protect the face. There has been much experimentation with these bars. One of the most effective is a single bar so placed as to make it difficult for the knee or elbow to reach the eye or nose, yet it protects the mouth. Double bars are more expensive and probably are not necessary for routine use, although they may be needed in specific circumstances. Attempts to use a wide plastic bar have failed because the player tries to see through the plastic with resultant distortion of vision. The headgear is the most important single piece of equipment.

The player with a fractured nose or malar bone will require a double bar or "bird cage" to more fully protect the area around the front of his face. The player with an injury to the jaw will need a bar placed lower to protect the mandible. Incidentally, the players must be sternly instructed that they must not grab the bar of their opponent. All of this is designed to protect the wearer of the helmet. Currently there is considerable agitation over the hardness of the helmet as related to the opposing player. The plastic shell is extremely hard. Its blow is cushioned somewhat by the fact that it is not at the end of a rigid pole so that there is a certain recoil element when the head of the player hits the opponent. At present, work is being done to design a helmet with an outer covering that is less traumatic and yet is not too heavy (Fig. 2). The use of a mouthpiece is universally accepted as being mandatory for the football player. Most of the high schools, and many of the football conferences in college, require it. Some of the players don't particularly like to wear a mouthpiece. I think this depends to a considerable amount on

how well it is fitted. The dentists now have a very quick and accurate method of making these mouthpieces, and the mouthpiece should be made and fitted for each individual player. It used to be the mark of an athlete to have his two front teeth knocked out, but this is no longer true—nor is it necessary, since the mouthpiece will effectively prevent it.

Injuries to the *neck* are relatively common in football. Most of them are minor but may be quite distressing. Obviously the player should not play with a serious injury to his neck. After a sprain or during the recovery period it may be desirable to protect his neck against excessive motion. This cannot be done well with adhesive, which is widely used elsewhere in the body, but quite effective use can be made of the so-called "cotton collar." This is actu-

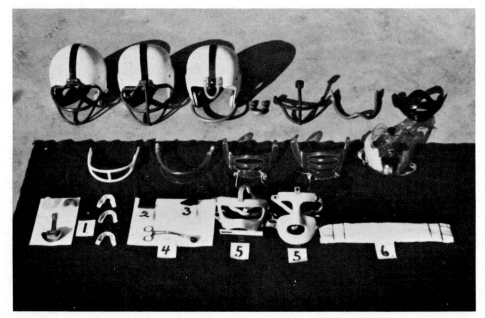

Figure 2. Protective equipment—neck, face and head. Upper two rows illustrate different types of football face protection. (Courtesy of Rawlinson, "Modern Athletic Training," © 1961 by Prentice-Hall, Inc.)

1. Mouthpiece	4. Tongue forceps
2. Headgear snubber—protects bridge of nose	5. Face guards for sports other than football
3. Oral screw	6. Rolled towel

ally a quilted pad narrower at one end than the other, wrapped around the neck and fastened with suitable straps to support the chin, mandible and occiput. A very simple substitute is an ordinary turkish towel (Fig. 2) folded lengthwise to about the width of the distance from the angle of the jaw to the shoulders and then wrapped firmly around the neck. This is quite effective for the player who occasionally gets a "pinched nerve" in the neck, since it serves to prevent the motion that causes the pinching. A resilient "horse collar" is commercially available and is also effective.

Most modern *shoulder* pads are effective in preventing injury to the shoulder girdle. Ideally they should be designed to protect the sternum and clavicles and particularly the acromioclavicular areas. The cap that extends over the deltoid serves to prevent painful contusions in this area. The most important attribute of any shoulder pad is that it fit the wearer. Too frequently the player picks his own pads out of a pile and he is unable to judge a proper fit. Someone should see that the pad actually fits to protect the parts it is designed to cover. A common injury to the front of the arm is the so-called "blocker's spur," which may often be caused by the edge of the shoulder pad itself rather than by the opponent. If the shoulder has been injured, more adequate support can be obtained from the so-called "Big Boy," or a double cantilever pad. A properly fitted foam rubber or plastic pad may be placed judiciously to protect bruised areas. Straps and strings should all be intact (Fig. 3).

Elbow pads are usually not worn unless there is a specific indication. The person with an olecranon bursitis, abrasion over the elbow or anything else of this nature should wear a suitably fitted pad. This applies to basketball as well as football.

Simple coaptation foam rubber or plastic splints may be used on the *arm* or *forearm* to protect an injured area (Fig. 4). No unyielding fiberboard or plastic splint may be used below the elbow.

A suitable protective pad should be applied to the *hand* over injured areas. Again, great care must be exercised. No rigid pad is permissible. The protective wrapping of the normal hand utilized by the professionals is not popular in high school or university programs. A recently developed plastic foam pad serves to protect the back of the hand and leave the front of the hand free.

Properly fitted shoulder pads protect the upper part of the *chest* quite adequately and we would not ordinarily recommend supplemental chest pads. Fractured ribs are best protected by circumferential strapping or rib binder (Fig. 4). Two points should be stressed. In the first place, circumferential strapping is not compatible with the deep breathing necessary for active participation. In fact, it is designed to prevent deep breathing. In the second place, the fractured rib is not well protected by a contact pad at the tender site since pain in the ribs comes as much from compression or expansion of the chest in any diameter as it does from a direct blow. Indeed, compression injury is more likely to hurt than a blow over the tender area. Contusions, however, are troublesome since any direct contact with them causes pain. The contusion may involve the skin or underlying bone and both can be well protected by a fiber pad, one of the most effective being the pad with a sponge rubber or plastic doughnut around its margin, which holds the pad away from the injured part. A supply of this type of contact pad is inexpensive and will add to the ease and comfort of the competitor.

Since the *abdomen* is essentially soft there is no requirement for contact

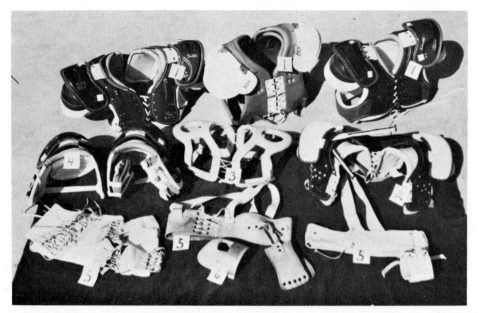

Figure 3. Protective equipment — shoulder, arm, elbow and hand. (Courtesy of Rawlinson, "Modern Athletic Training," © 1961 by Prentice-Hall, Inc.)
1. Heavy duty linebacker, big boy shoulder pads
2. Double cantilever shoulder pad (two rolls of paper denote the double cantilever)
3. Protection for under a shoulder pad
4. Home-made bruise pad — takes pressure off the shoulder
5. Shoulder harnesses (dislocations, strains and sprains)
6. All-purpose injury pad with hole cut in top

padding here. The player with deep abdominal tenderness, as from liver or spleen injury, should not compete. The back of the abdomen or flanks is best protected by pads built into the pants or a belt type pad that incorporates two contact pads running along either side of the spine to protect the so-called "kidney area" (Fig. 5). The football pants themselves contain padding for the iliac crest and trochanters. Here again, well arranged contact pads may protect tender areas, provided always that the underlying pathologic condition is not such that competition should be prohibited. The athletic supporter is a must and no player should be allowed to practice or compete without one. The popular jockey shorts are not an adequate substitute for a well fitted athletic supporter. If there has been injury to the genitalia with a painful testicle, some of the more protective type supporters may be utilized, although they are not particularly comfortable and seem awkward to wear.

Most of the football pants incorporate a quadriceps pad that covers the front and lateral aspects of the *thigh*. Many of these pads are quite inadequate. If they are built into the pants leg, the latter should fit very snugly or the pants should be strapped down with adhesive. A loose thigh pad does far more harm than good since its edge may cause the very injury it is designed to prevent. In case of painful injury the pad may be strapped to the thigh with adhesive, preferably elastic in type. Anything constrictive around the thigh has the potential of reducing its blood supply and causing muscle cramps. This

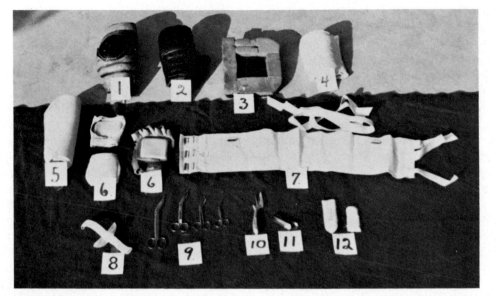

Figure 4. Protective equipment—shoulder, arm, elbow and hand *(continued)*. (Courtesy of Rawlinson, "Modern Athletic Training," © 1961 by Prentice-Hall, Inc.)

1. Elbow bruise pad
2. Fracture glove
3. Sternum or chest injury pad—lace to shoulder pads
4. Upper arm bruise pad—fiber and sponge rubber
5. Forearm pad
6. Hand pads
7. Rib belt
8. Resusitube Airway
9. Bandage scissors
10. Tape cutter
11. Handle of a spoon made into a finger splint
12. Felt thumb pads

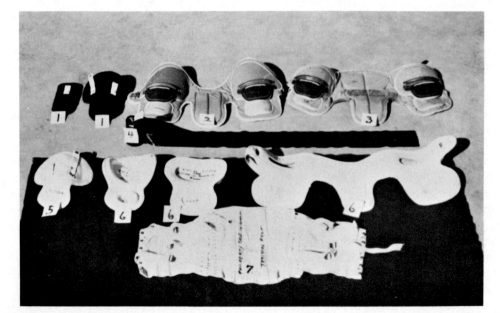

Figure 5. Protective equipment—groin, pelvis, buttocks and back. (Courtesy of Rawlinson, "Modern Athletic Training," © 1961 by Prentice-Hall, Inc.)

1. Tail piece and hip pad
2. Hip injury pad
3. Low back injury pad
4. Rubber slingshot bandage
5. Hip pad
6. Pads for protection of a bruised hip
7. Back brace

is not nearly so frequent in the thigh as in the calf, but it may occur. The strapping should be snug but not tight. The protective pad prevents contact injury only. If the muscle itself is damaged, active movement of the muscle is the danger and this is not prevented by any pad. Similarly, contact pads are useless in protecting the hamstrings against strain either at their attachment to the pelvis or at the musculotendinous junction in back of the thigh.

The normal *knee* is usually not strapped to prevent injury. Occasionally the boy who has grown rapidly to 6 feet or so but still has immature joints may feel that his knees are insecure and want to wear some type of protection. It is extremely difficult to protect the knee against the most common type of injury, namely, injury to the medial collateral ligament mechanism due to external rotation of the leg with the knee slightly flexed, with or without forcible contact against the lateral aspect of the knee. The ordinary pull-on elastic bandage is worthless protection here. It may add to the player's feeling of security, but if tight enough to do much good it may also constrict his circulation.

If the knee has been injured the protective wrapping becomes important. It then has some design, namely, to prevent recurrence of a particular type of stress injury. Here again, the pull-on or wrap-on elastic bandage is of little value since it does not in any way protect against lateral or rotary stress. One must also question the value of an elastic pull-on bandage that incorporates a short metal bar or hinge either on one or both sides. The bar is not long enough to prevent leverage action of the leg and thigh. It is cumbersome and at best is inconvenient to wear. There are almost as many modifications of knee braces as there are people treating injured knees, a sure indication that none of them is particularly good. Recent developments

aim to produce a corset-like brace that is longer and so more effective than those currently available. My own preference is for the octopus type which to some extent simulates the support given by adhesive strapping.

Many players with greater or lesser knee disabilities are attached to one or another type of support. If this support gives them confidence and they feel it helps, I think it is permissible to use it. It will not prevent re-injury. If there is swelling in the knee, particularly effusion, and this is mild enough to permit the player to participate, it is proper for him to wear a pull-on or wrap-on elastic bandage in order to prevent further stretching of the suprapatellar pouch. All of these bandages have the doubtful virtue that they restrict flexion of the knee and so may to some extent prevent overstrain by the deep knee bend or duck waddle position.

If the knee actually needs protection for a weak ligament, for example the medial collateral, this can be best obtained by adhesive strapping. Cross strapping of the knee either on one or both sides as illustrated (Fig. 6) gives considerable protection against the knee "springing open" on the injured side. Owing to the bipod nature of the femoral condyles, it is usually necessary that the condyle of the femur and the tibial plateau actually separate to put stress on the medial collateral ligament, and this can be minimized by adequate strapping. The cross-hatch strapping also to some extent restricts rotation of the leg on the thigh and so the familiar position of external rotation-abduction is prevented. We now believe that the medial collateral ligament capsular fibers can be damaged without an actual separation between femur and tibia. The taping described helps to prevent the rotation that may cause the tearing.

If the injury to the knee was caused by hyperextension, strapping to prevent

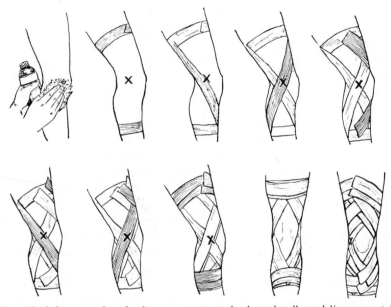

Figure 6. A method for strapping the knee to support the lateral collateral ligaments (x). The criss-cross straps should cross in the midline. Maximum support for this dressing is medially and laterally, but it is also effective against rotatory stress between tibia and femur, especially if both sides are taped as illustrated here.

hyperextension (Fig. 7) will be much more effective than any permissible brace. Each trainer has his own methods of strapping and one who intends to do this sort of preventive strapping should familiarize himself with the various methods and practice them. Some prefer regular adhesive, others, elastic adhesive. Actually, I believe a combination of the two is probably best. The newer type of elastic tape that stretches laterally rather than length-

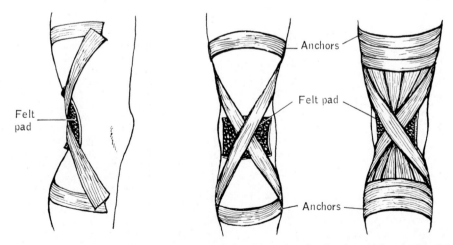

Figure 7. Strapping of knee to prevent hyperextension. Note that the leg is positioned with the knee slightly flexed. A convenient way is to have player stand on the table with a 3 or 4 inch block under the heel.

wise gives much firmer support than the regular elastic type and conforms well to the rounded surfaces. By the very virtue of its firm support, it allows somewhat less mobility.

The knee also needs to be protected against direct contact. Most football pants have a knee pad, although in most cases it is woefully inadequate. However, it is far better than nothing and I think every school should have a rigid requirement that these pads be worn. This is even more important in a secondary school. I insist on this requirement in the secondary schools because in these young people the cartilage of the patella and of the femoral condyle is more susceptible to injury, and irreparable damage may be done to these areas by direct impact. This is particularly pertinent because many of the fields of play are very hard, and the youth is likely to pay for his indiscretion not only by a ruined football season but by permanent damage to the knee. It is the responsibility of the physician, trainer or coach to insist on the wearing of proper protection of the knee against direct contact.

In most sports *leg* protection is not necessary. The exceptions are such games as soccer and hockey. Certain special categories as the baseball catcher are self-evident. Painful areas in the legs may be protected by contact pads.

There has been constant debate as to the virtue of support of the *ankle* during competition. It is my considered opinion that in football every player should have his normal ankles wrapped for every practice or game session. Many players will resist this since they feel it may diminish their agility. When the situation is explained to them, they will almost always accept the wraps gratefully. It is very easy to learn to put on an ankle wrap. The Louisiana wrap (Fig. 8), or some modification, is perfectly adequate. The wraps are inexpensive. They can be laundered easily and there is no excuse for not insisting on them if the athletic administration concerned agrees they are valuable. The ankle wrap does not restrict ankle motion per se at all since ankle motion is simply dorsal and plantar flexion. It does restrict lateral motion somewhat,

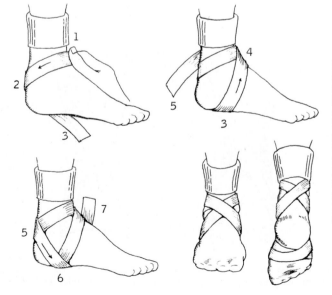

Figure 8. Louisiana ankle wrap. This requires a 100-inch web ankle bandage. The start of the wrap is shown in the upper left drawing and is continued at the upper right, then lower left. At 7 the starting point is reached. The wrap is continued in this same fashion, with overlapping of turns, until the bandage is exhausted. Directly to the right, one complete turn of the bandage is shown. This is not the whole wrap. The bandage may be applied over a heavy sock, as shown, but wrinkles must be avoided.

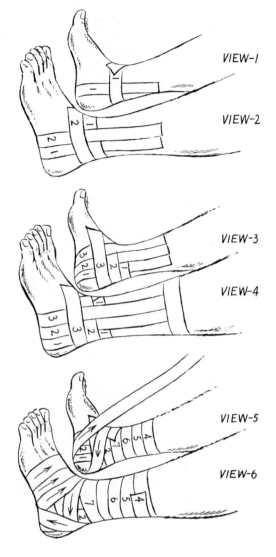

Figure 9. Taping procedure. If this taping is for a previously injured ankle, the long strips should extend higher on the leg. Views 3 and 4 are direct Gibney strapping. Views 5 and 6 add the "heel lock," View 5 to help prevent eversion and View 6 to help prevent inversion. The two combined give much better stability but also less mobility. (Courtesy of Rawlinson, "Modern Athletic Training," © 1961 by Prentice-Hall, Inc.)

but even tarsal motion is not greatly restricted. It is protective against excessive tarsal motion, however, and so will effectively reduce the danger of sprain. It is difficult to sprain an ankle that is protected by a well-placed ankle wrap unless the force is a major one sufficient to tear the wrapping.

If the ankle has been previously injured, the ankle wrap probably will be inadequate, and one should resort to adhesive tape. One should familiarize himself with a good standard method for taping and learn to do it well (Figs. 9 to 14). The tape has the advantage that it may be extended up as high on the leg as is desirable. The greater the protection needed, the higher the strapping should go. Since the tape is placed on the skin, there is a certain amount of "give" in the bandage, but the further the strip extends up to the leg the less the resultant play and the firmer the fixation. If the strapping is applied because of an old injury, it should vary according to the part to be protected, since

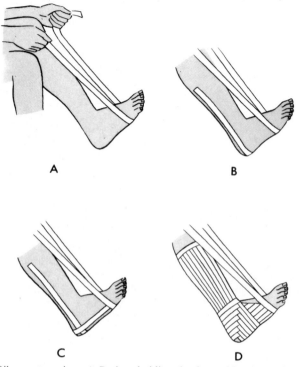

A   B

C   D

Figure 10. Typical Gibney strapping. *A*, Patient holding the foot with a loop of muslin to keep it at the right angle and inverted or everted as the case may be, depending on the location of the sprain. *B*, First strip of one-inch adhesive tape that begins well back on the calf, at the bulge of the calf, extending down under the heel and up the opposite side. If the sprain is a lateral sprain, the strip should start on the medial side and come to the lateral side. *C*, Other portion of the weave, a strip running from the base of the first toe around the ankle and back to the base of the fifth toe. *D*, Application of successive strips, as many as necessary to reach the front of the foot. The horizontal strips should not overlap in front. If the strapping is for a chronic case where swelling is not a factor, it would be more secure to overlap the strips in front. The whole thing is secured by a circumferential strip around the top of the dressing and then further secured by gauze bandage. It should be emphasized again that in an acute case there should be no circumferential wrapping overlapping on the front of the foot or on the front of the ankle. Note that the foot is held at a right angle to the leg and inverted or everted, depending upon the location of the sprain.

different types of strapping will be required for the lateral and the medial ligaments (Fig. 10), the arch (Fig. 11), the metatarsal area (Fig. 12), the tendo Achilles (Fig. 13) and the dorsiflexors (Fig. 14).

The type of *shoes* is a debatable question. There is no doubt that the high shoe protects the ankle and foot better than the lower one, but many players feel that they are much more active in a low cut shoe. Presumably a low cut shoe plus the ankle wrap should be adequate. However, the high shoes do

not replace the ankle wrap. The player cannot be relied upon to lace his shoes tight enough to give support and yet not so tight as to be uncomfortable. I believe the ankle or foot that has been injured should be fitted with a high shoe.

So, too, there is considerable argument about the type of cleat. The value of certain types of cleat will depend a good deal upon the terrain. Many factors argue against long, pointed cleats. They have a real disadvantage upon frozen surfaces or hard ground, as well as upon matted bermuda, which may

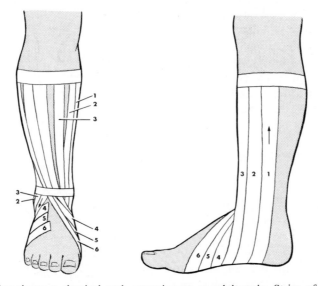

Figure 11. Drawing shows a classical arch strapping on an adult male. Strips of one-inch adhesive tape are necessary. Strip 1 starts just above the lateral malleolus and passes under the heel up the inner side of the foot to above the bulge of the calf. Strips 2, 3, and 4 pass up the leg in a similar course; the number of strips used depends somewhat on the size of the leg. As strips 5, 6, and 7 reach the front of the ankle, they are then twisted across the front of the leg to the lateral side. Five or six strips are utilized with the arch strapping extending clear up and clear forward to the base of the head of the metatarsals. Strips are anchored at the calf and above the ankle with one or more circumferential strips. If the injured arch is high, a felt pad should be inserted under the arch and held in place by short strips of tape, particularly if a flat support shoe is worn. This felt pad is probably not necessary in a shoe having a heel and a good support.

catch the cleat. Some players feel that the hold secured by the pointed cleat on the sod will prevent injury, whereas the proponents of the opposite view believe that its fixation to the ground may encourage injury. In any event the cleat, whatever type is used, should be properly placed on the shoe and should be

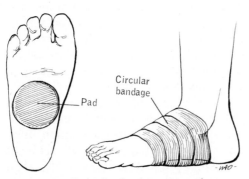

Figure 12. Strapping for the metatarsal area.

intact. A broken cleat is a danger not only to the opponent but also to the player himself, since it gives him insecurity when he expects security. The football shoe leaves an unprotected peg sticking out of the shoe when the cleat breaks off. This is indeed a lethal weapon. Also, running on this peg concentrates the force on a very small area and is likely to result in a disabling bruise of the plantar surface of the foot.

There has been much indecision as to the proper shoe for artificial turf. Certainly the long pointed cleat is not the best. The present trend (1976) is toward the soccer type shoe with multiple, short cleats. It also makes some difference whether the field is wet, or cold, or both. Sometimes in these instances a basketball type shoe will grip better.

It is extremely important that the shoe be well fitted, since a shoe that is too tight or too loose will inevitably give trouble. This is true whether it be football, basketball, baseball or track.

The feet are extremely vulnerable to minor ailments, such as blisters, athlete's foot, stone bruise, and so forth, and the player should be instructed early in his career as to their proper care.

Although the education of the player in aspects of injury prevention may seem to be a forbiddingly comprehensive problem, it acutally will require relatively little time. Much of the instruction can be given en masse to the whole squad, and a few minutes explaining to the players that prevention is to the individual interest of each one and should be his responsibility will be of great value. This must be followed by inspection. At first this should be carried out at relatively frequent intervals.

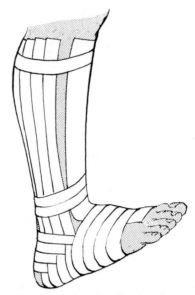

Figure 14. Strapping for the dorsiflexors. The dorsiflexion is overdone in this drawing and will interfere with running. Neutral position (right angle) is desired.

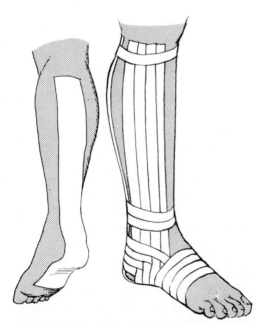

Figure 13. Strapping for the Achilles tendon. This is strapping of the ankle in plantar flexion: a strip extends from the toes, under the arch of the foot and up the back of the leg. The posterior strip of two inch tape is the most important here. The other strips give added security and help fix the initial strip.

Once the season is under way, however, the routine will be so established that only an occasional inspection will suffice, and this can be done in the course of other instruction with the expenditure of little extra time. For example, a method to determine whether or not the athletes actually have their ankles wrapped properly during the practice session is to have them remove their shoes on the field while the coach is talking to them at the end of practice. The players who have their ankles properly wrapped are permitted to go on in and shower at the conclusion of the talk. Those who have not must remain for another work-out. Such measures are not unduly punitive but serve to call attention to the fact that observance of the regulations is important to the staff.

There is nothing more rewarding than to conclude a football season with the players in better condition than when they started. As in all fields of medicine, prevention is far better than cure.

PART II

GENERAL PRINCIPLES
OF TREATMENT

CHAPTER 3

PRECEPTS AND EXAMINATION

Some of the principles of treatment mentioned in the Introduction merit repetition here. The basic treatment of the athlete is that of any young, healthy human. The most important consideration is that recovery be prompt and, above all, complete. Later in the book the specific treatment for certain conditions will be detailed, but the same basic principles apply to each, modified according to the location and the degree of the injury.

PRECEPTS FOR THE CARE OF THE ATHLETE

The Five A's
1. Accept athletics.
2. Avoid expediency.
3. Adopt the best method.
4. Act promptly.
5. Achieve perfection.

PROMPT EXAMINATION IS MANDATORY

Prevention is better than cure; but if injury occurs, the first step must be early recognition of the nature and the severity of the damage. There is usually no better time to determine the extent of an injury than when it happens. The practice of waiting to see is not compatible with the first principle of treatment of athletes, namely, prompt and specific care. As time passes, edema and inflammation supervene to cloud the picture. A careful, complete examination, done early, will often permit definitive treatment days, or even weeks, earlier than the "wait and see" method. Saturday's injuries should not be examined on Monday morning just to suit the convenience of the doctor or others. Once a decision concerning treatment is reached, it should be carried out confidently and completely. If a specialist is needed, he should be consulted early. It is disheartening to examine a patient weeks after his injury and find that the time for proper treatment is long past.

BELIEVE IN THE VALUE OF COMPETITIVE ATHLETICS

The physician must recognize that to this patient it is vital that he be restored to athletic competition. If the pa-

39

tient believes that the doctor disparages the importance of athletics, a sympathetic link between patient and doctor is lost. A master violinist would not trust the treatment of his hands to one who believed fiddle playing to be unimportant.

Avoid Expediency

Too often outside influences may overbalance sound judgment. The player's desire to compete, overoptimism, failure to admit the extent of the damage, or hesitation to interfere with school attendance may lead one to adopt a "middle of the road" course. Strict medical evaluation, not temporary convenience, must be the deciding factor.

Adopt the Best Method of Treatment

Here too a temporizing attitude is fatal to good results. If you really believe the patient needs a cast, use it! If you think he should be on crutches, insist on it! If his ligament needs surgical repair, see to it! The best treatment is early treatment. Time is of the essence in obtaining a complete recovery in most injuries. It is particularly important in ligament and muscle-tendon injuries.

Above All, Treatment Must Be Prompt

Unnecessary delay is not compatible with good results in ligament, muscle-tendon and vascular injuries. "Don't hurry but don't fiddle" is as applicable here as it is in the operating room.

The Goal Must Be 100 Per Cent Recovery

It may not be possible to attain a perfect result in a given case, but if we do not try for it, we will never reach it. The young, well-conditioned athlete will tolerate whatever reasonable measures are necessary to give him complete recovery, and the doctor must resist compromise or unjustified complacency that tends to negate this goal.

The foregoing precepts will simplify the care of the athlete so that the physician, instead of dreading this responsibility, will learn to look forward to the patient who gives such prompt and gratifying results. It is an interesting fact that most of the principles set forth here are readily applicable to other aspects of medical practice.

EXAMINATION

Time

The optimum time for the first examination of the injured athlete is as soon as possible after the injury. The prevalent custom of making a superficial and hasty examination (often on the field) and then sending the player to the ice bag for several hours is certainly to be deplored. It may not be possible to examine the player at once, but the goal should be to examine him as soon as it can be done properly.

Place

Obviously, the first superficial examination of a player will be done on the field or on the sidelines. This can be little more than a cursory evaluation of the severity of the injury. If the injury is of any consequence, proper facilities must be available to make a detailed examination away from the crowd, preferably in a suitable examining room. At this time it will be possible to remove all of the clothing from the part and all of the protective strapping. The knee cannot be examined, for example, through a pair of football pants or over adhesive or elastic strapping. It follows that arrangements must be made to transport the player to suitable surroundings. It is highly desirable that this examination be carried out without the usual cluster of players, parents and fans gathering around and offering gratuitous advice.

Manner

In order to treat injuries to athletes successfully one must cultivate the practice of detailed, meticulous examination. In the case of an extremity injury, an examination should first be carried out on the uninjured extremity for the purpose of comparison. This procedure also can allay to some extent the apprehensions of the injured player and prepare him for the type of examination that is to be carried out on the injured part. Then the examination itself must be performed in a tender manner, taking care to show the injured person that you have great concern for him and his injury. More detailed suggestions will be made under the appropriate headings.

History

The first step in the examination is the history. Try to obtain as accurate a story as possible from the player or other people concerned as to the mechanism of injury. Did the injury appear to be severe or did it seem mild? Was disability immediate or delayed? Was deformity originally present and later reduced either spontaneously or with help? Did the player feel something slip or tear? Obtaining a careful history may give a vital clue as to the nature of the pathologic condition.

Physical Examination

By *observation* note the general appearance at the site of the injury. Observe the location of the swelling, any possible deformity, any damage to the skin or evidence of a direct blow.

By *palpation* determine the degree of underlying tension in the tissues, possible fluctuation caused by hematoma formation, and the presence of local heat, tenderness or crepitation.

By *manipulation* determine the range of pain-free motion, the location of pain on motion, significant instability or abnormal motion. For any given area it is well to develop a routine for examination designed to check all the stabilizing elements of that particular joint. For example, a knee should be checked not only for lateral stability in extension but also for lateral stability in partial flexion and for anteroposterior or rotatory stability. By overlooking any one of these, vital information may be missed in the course of the examination.

X-ray examination should be carried out where fracture is manifest or only suspected. In this day and age there is little excuse for failure to obtain x-ray visualization since this is so readily available. X-ray examination is an art in itself, but it should be noted here that it is of little value to take excellent radiographs if they are not carefully studied and properly evaluated (Fig. 15). (See X-Ray Examination, below.)

With a complete examination of this character it is the unusual case that will not present a definite clue as to the proper diagnosis. If, for one reason or another, diagnosis cannot be made at the time of the first examination, repeated examinations must be made until the diagnosis is clear. Every effort should be made to make a definitive

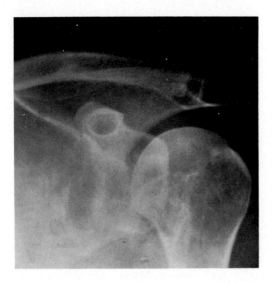

Figure 15. A radiograph of the shoulder showing posterior dislocation. On casual glance, no lesion is apparent. Careful inspection will reveal the head of the humerus medial to the glenoid convexity. In this case special views not routinely made will confirm the diagnosis.

diagnosis at the first examination since this will permit the institution of specific treatment at once. In any event, re-examination should be made from time to time in order to obtain an exact picture of the progress of the condition. Details of examination of individual parts will be given under appropriate sections. It cannot be overemphasized that successful treatment depends upon accurate diagnosis, which in turn depends upon a careful, all-inclusive, atraumatic examination of the injured part.

X-ray Examination

X-ray visualization is taken so much for granted now that one cannot justify the omission of this examination if there is any possibility of positive findings. It follows, therefore, that there will be many negative and, to some extent, useless x-ray examinations carried out. However, even if the examiner ignores the medico-legal complications (which he would indeed be bold to do), there is a good argument for generous use of x-ray visualization. The current agitation against overuse of x-ray need not apply to films made for diagnostic

purposes, provided they are made under proper control with suitable equipment. The extremely rapid x-ray film in common use today causes minimal radiation exposure. A few confident words of explanation to the timorous will allay fears of over-radiation. One is justified in refusing management of a case in which x-ray visualization is not permitted.

However, it is not sufficient simply to order that the part be x-rayed. Routine x-rays, while they may be of some beauty and value, may not serve at all to rule out the presence of a lesion. The "as is" film may be extremely enlightening. Simply place the injured part over the x-ray film and take a picture of it without any positioning, holding or restraint. After this picture is made then make the standard views. Very often the "as is" picture will be more enlightening than any other (Fig. 16).

The prevalent habit of sending a patient to x-ray and having the film made by the technician or even the radiologist, who has no actual knowledge of the injury suspected, results in many faulty interpretations. The physician should know what he is looking for on the film and so advise the radiologist. He should himself be prepared to position the part to demonstrate the lesion he suspects. If anteroposterior and lateral views are not sufficient, other views should be made (Fig. 18). If abnormal motion is suspected, stress x-rays may be desirable. If the original films are negative, repeat films after seven to ten days may be diagnostic (Fig. 17). Once the x-ray is made it should be carefully studied, not only immediately but after the film is thoroughly dried and prepared for viewing. If doubt remains, views of the opposite extremity may be valuable or further views of the injured part may be desirable. If the original film is inadequate technically because of overexposure, underexposure, poor

positioning, or blurring due to motion, one should not hesitate to request repeat films. With such careful planning and adequate follow-up by the doctor, the x-ray may indeed be a valuable adjunct to the management of a given case. Definite suggestions as to positioning and the use of multiple views will be made when considering specific injuries. (See Fig. 18.)

Laboratory Examination

The laboratory examination has taken a larger place in athletic medicine in recent years. It is particularly important in the preliminary examination to determine whether or not the player

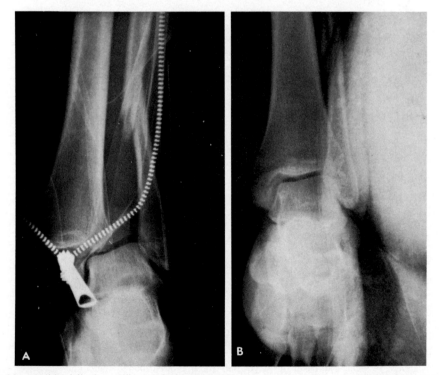

Figure 16. *A*, "As is" view. Film made in an air splint reveals complete dislocation of the talus, rupture of the tibiofibular ligament, fracture of the medial and posterior malleoli of the tibia and a fracture of the fibula. Note the clarity with which all of this pathology is demonstrated. *B*, Anteroposterior view after careful positioning shows there to be a fracture of the medial malleolus and a fracture of the fibula. While this would suggest the injury revealed in *A*, further testing is not necessary by manipulation to determine the pathology since the "as is" view demonstrates it exactly.

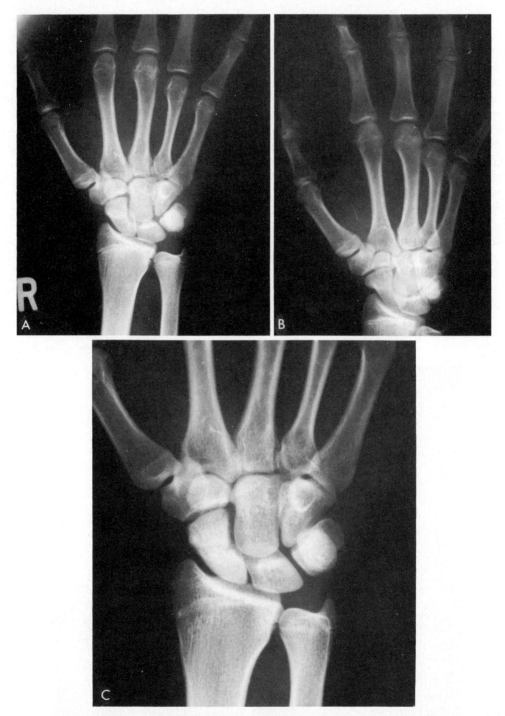

Figure 17. This 16 year old baseball player fell on the outstretched hand and received a painful "sprain" of the wrist. X-rays *A* and *B* were interpreted as being negative. *C*, X-ray 10 days later shows definite fracture through the navicular. This boy wore a protective splint during this interval. If there is any doubt about the possibility of fractured navicular, a splint should be worn until recheck x-rays are made.

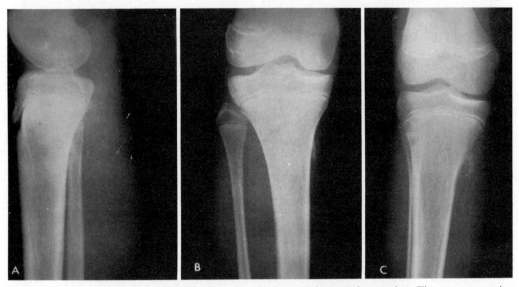

Figure 18. Case 1. Exostosis of tibia. Note that the lateral view (*A*) is negative. The anteroposterior view (*B*) is inconclusive as to the nature of the mass, whereas the oblique (*C*) reveals the tumor very distinctly.

Legend continued on following page

should compete. Routine tests are not mandatory, yet it is quite simple to obtain a blood and urine evaluation. The electrocardiogram is valuable in suspected heart lesions and so forth.

The laboratory may be quite valuable in the treatment of special conditions as will be indicated in the text.

The electroencephalogram in a head injury, cultures of infected wounds, and tests for gout in severe joint inflammation are examples. Each of these tests involves some expense and should be used only if indicated. They should be used unsparingly when a necessary part of the treatment.

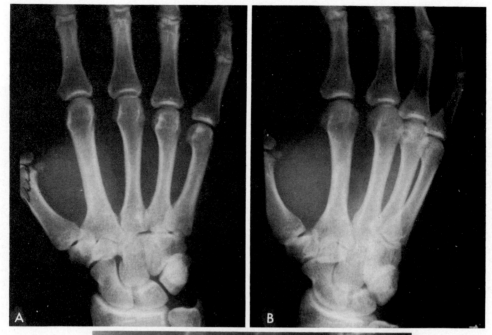

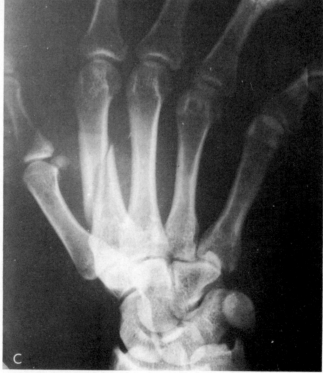

Figure 18 *(Continued).* Case 2. During blocking drill, this 22 year old football player felt something snap in his right hand. It swelled up and an x-ray was made, which was interpreted as being normal. *A,* Straight AP view shows a little change of density of the index metacarpal, as does the oblique *B. C,* Special oblique view clearly reveals the nature of the pathology, the spiral, oblique fracture with displacement.

CHAPTER 4

PRINCIPLES IN THE MANAGEMENT OF SPECIFIC INJURIES

CONTUSION

A contusion may be defined as a direct blow against the integument, causing bruising of the skin or underlying tissues. This results in capillary rupture and an infiltrative type of bleeding followed by edema and inflammatory reaction. The result is local swelling which may be superficial or deep depending upon the nature of the object striking the blow and the location involved. Thus the blow of the patella against the hard ground catches the skin between two hard objects and the resulting damage is to the skin and subcutaneous areas and possibly to the patella. On the other hand, the blow of a hard headgear against the unprotected thigh will catch the muscle between the headgear and the femur. The resulting damage is to the muscle, since the underlying soft tissue effectively protects the skin. The basic pathologic change is the same regardless of the area involved or the type of blow.

Proper *treatment* consists of limitation of bleeding by application of cold and a pressure bandage in the early stages for 12 to 24 hours, together with immobilization and protection to prevent further injury. This is followed by measures to encourage healing. Local heat, rest and protection are vital at this stage. The area involved and severity of the involvement will determine the specific method utilized in a given case. Basically, the part must be protected from further damage by another direct blow or from overfunction, and/or from injudicious methods of treatment. Faradic stimulation, for example, should not be used early in a severely bruised muscle. Unless the bleeding is considerable and of major proportions, the local infiltration of hyaluronidase or local anesthetic is not justified. In extensive contusion, particularly of the thigh or back, systemic medication with the various enzyme preparations may be of value. *Rehabilitation* should begin slowly within the limitations of pain and should progress in parallel with the healing. Obviously a simple contusion may require little treatment or rehabilitation, whereas an extensive contusion in a vital area may tax one's ingenuity to restore function while continuing protection.

HEMATOMA

The athlete is particularly prone to hematoma formation, since he regularly exposes himself to the type of trauma likely to cause hematomata. For this discussion a hematoma will be defined as a collection of pooled blood within a relatively restricted area (Fig. 19, *A*). Pooled blood is not blood which has infiltrated through soft tissues but rather blood which has collected in a localized area and maintained its identity as blood. It can readily be appreciated that this pooling will occur in many situations, in many locations and from varying types of trauma, since the basic condition from the pathological standpoint is bleeding within the tissues. We do not ordinarily refer to bleeding within an anatomically closed space as a hematoma, as for example in a joint or bursa or within a hollow viscus. In hematoma formation bleeding takes place into the tissues and by virtue of pressure from the hemorrhage the blood makes a space for itself which it wholly fills by

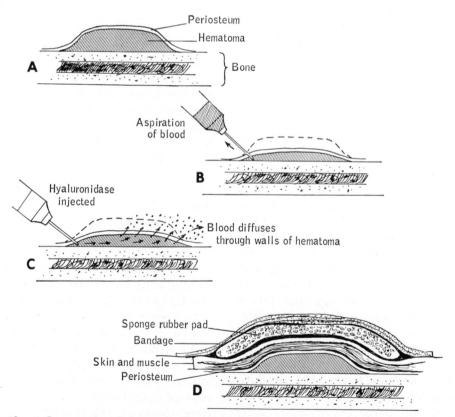

Figure 19. *A*, Cross section of a hematoma. In this instance the skin and subcutaneous tissue overlie bone and there is a collection of blood underneath the periosteum, well walled off.

B, Needle extending into the hematoma with the blood aspirated and the walls partially collapsed.

C, Showing hyaluronidase inserted into the hematoma with little arrows indicating the blood that then diffuses through the walls.

D, Same hematoma with overlying pressure dressing, indicated by sponge rubber pad and bandage in cross section.

pushing other tissue away. This may be extremely extensive as in hematoma formation up and down the fascial planes of the back following a serious vessel rupture in the vicinity of the spine, or it may be extremely localized as in the collection that forms between the skin and the periosteum over the shin.

DIAGNOSIS. A superficial hematoma is easily recognized, but the diagnosis of a deep-seated hematoma may be difficult. Fluctuation is pathognomonic, but its presence may indeed be difficult to determine deep in a muscle mass. In doubtful cases diagnostic aspiration is justified.

TREATMENT. The treatment of hematoma must of necessity vary widely according to its location and extent. Treatment may be directed toward elimination of the hematoma itself or toward relieving pressure caused by it on an adjacent structure. The general principles of treatment consist of (1) prevention of further bleeding; (2) evacuation of the blood; (3) encouragement of absorption of the blood and (4) protection of the part until healing takes place.

During the diagnostic phase, even before definitive treatment is begun, pressure dressings should be applied to prevent further bleeding. An ice pack is used for the same purpose. Once it is determined that there is an aspirable quantity of blood present, one may appreciably shorten the convalescent time by removing the blood (Fig. 19, B). Aspiration demands surgical aseptic technique. A large 15 or 16 gauge needle should be employed since one could hardly expect to evacuate old blood through a 22 gauge needle. Following aspiration the area should be infiltrated with hyaluronidase (Fig. 19, C), which tends to break down the confining wall and hasten the absorption of blood. Any attempt to aspirate a hematoma under any but the most aseptic conditions

must be condemned. The dressing room or indeed the average training room is not the place for aspiration because the possibility of infection is particularly great in extravasated blood.

The center of a hematoma is to some extent like the center of an abscess. It may be quite avascular so that the circulating blood does not reach it, and many months may be required for absorption of the blood even in the absence of infection or other complication. The speed of absorption of the hematoma may be increased by diffusion of the hematoma, which is aided by the administration of hyaluronidase and the application of a pressure bandage (Fig. 19, D). These measures lead to more rapid absorption by bringing about greater exposure of the hematoma to the circulating fluids of the body. It has been said that it is unwise to aspirate a hematoma until one is sure the bleeding has stopped because increasing pressure of the hematoma itself will tend to discourage further bleeding. This is fallacious reasoning since the same amount of pressure can readily be applied by external means. The hematoma should be evacuated as completely as possible even at a very early stage, and then a pressure bandage will actually keep more pressure on the area than intrinsic pressure from the blood alone could be expected to do.

Under certain circumstances surgical evacuation of a hematoma may be justifiable. Certainly if the blood has coagulated, and consequently is not aspirable, removal will shorten the recovery period. Various factors must affect the decision to operate. The extent of the surgical approach necessary, possible further damage to tissue already involved, damage to new areas by the approach, and above all the condition of the skin should be weighed carefully against the possible benefits of evacuation. The utmost care must be taken to prevent infection. Any compromise in this area may lead to disaster.

When the area involved is an actively moving part of the body it should be protected not only against a direct blow but also against motion, since motion tends to break down the clot within the vessels and to perpetuate the bleeding. Motion also tends to cause irritation throughout the lesion and to encourage overreactive scar formation, calcification, or ossification. Many a potential case of myositis ossificans has been aborted by careful protection of the part after proper local treatment. It is particularly important in muscle bleeding not to employ the "work it out" technique by massage, since this simply encourages further bleeding and promotes ossification. Absorption is also accelerated by the application of heat, which tends to improve the circulation of the area.

Protection against contusion should be continued as long as the area is symptomatic. However, protection against motion may be terminated much sooner. If the hematoma involves muscle or joint or a moveable part, mobility can be resumed *within the limits of pain* almost at once. Voluntary pain-free contraction will tend to aid absorption, but forcible exercise of a muscle containing a hematoma will only aggravate the pain. The dividing line between what is a good level of activity and what is deleterious may be very fine indeed. In many instances the athlete will be prone to minimize his symptoms in order to step up his activity, so that real acumen is required in judging how soon full activity may be permitted. Hematomata of more static areas, as under the skin, require protection during periods of bodily contact. The compression bandage should be removed whenever it is obvious that the liquid hematoma is no longer present, unless further support is needed because of circulatory embarrassment. It should be noted that following a relatively superficial hematoma there will be gross discoloration of the skin and that this may migrate a considerable distance if a pressure bandage is used. It is not at all unusual in the case of a hematoma over the shin or calf for ecchymoses of the skin to appear about the ankle or even in the foot. This occurrence is oftentimes alarming to the patient, and he should be reassured that it only represents a late stage in the absorption of his hematoma and does not indicate that his condition has grown worse or has extended. It is wise to warn the patient early that he may develop severe discoloration in the skin and that this may take weeks to disappear.

To recapitulate:

1. Diagnosis should be prompt, with aspiration if necessary to make a final determination.

2. The volume of contained blood should be reduced by aspiration, hyaluronidase, pressure, cold first, then heat, and closely controlled activity.

3. Re-injury should be prevented by protection against trauma or against excessive activity.

4. Resorption should be encouraged by exposing the hematoma to a larger surface area of circulation, by improving the local circulation, and by maintaining the general circulation.

Excessive scar formation, ossification, or calcification can oftentimes be prevented by these measures.

MYOSITIS OSSIFICANS

Myositis ossificans is a frequent complication of the combination of contusion and hematoma involving the muscle near its origin on bone. The term is often used to include several conditions which may differ considerably. The name would imply inflammation of a muscle followed by ossification. I do not think this often happens. Much more commonly there is ossification of infiltrated blood along the muscle origin on the bone. The condition may appear as a simple exostosis having a broad base with a sharp extension into the muscle and may seem to be an involvement of the periosteum rather than the muscle (Fig. 20). The muscle is merely displaced by the ossifying mass. In this type of case the etiology is probably partial avulsion of the muscle fibers from the periosteum or a simple contusion of bone causing a subperiosteal hematoma. The mass is true bone and is firmly attached to the parent bone. In another type of so-called myositis ossificans there is actually a plaque of bone lying within the muscle and separated from the bone by a layer of muscle. It is difficult to determine here just what causes the ossification. The most likely assumption is that some periosteal cells invade the hematoma at the time of injury with formation of true bone and

that the condition is not a metaplasia of muscle into bone. A third condition which is also called myositis ossificans is the ossification about a traumatized joint or a fracture site. A hematoma in these locations will ossify as a result of the repeated insult to healing tissue (Fig. 21). In these instances there is no involvement of muscle whatever.

ETIOLOGY. Trauma is almost always the initiating cause of myositis ossificans. In the case of the long muscles the cause may be repeated trauma such as occurs to the upper arm as a result of the constant blows of the blocker in football (Fig. 20). It may be a single forceful blow, as on the quadriceps lateralis or intermedius (Figs. 22 and 24) in the anterior thigh, followed by active use. It may be caused by unwise or excessive manipulation of a fractured bone (Fig. 21). In all these conditions one underlying factor is present, namely, repeated chronic irritation of an area al-

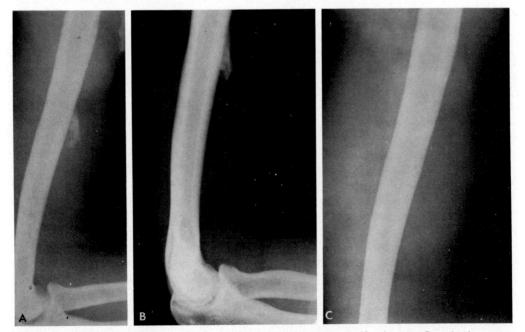

Figure 20. Myositis ossificans. *A,* Well developed, but immature ossification. *B,* Completely mature ossified mass with wide base attached to the bone and spurlike projection into the muscle. *C,* One year after removal. No evidence of recurrence.

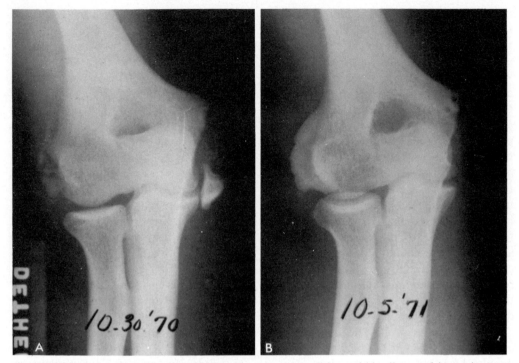

Figure 21. A year prior to the first examination, this patient dislocated his elbow and it was in a cast for 9 days. One year later he dislocated his elbow again, and it was again in a cast for 9 days. He returned to practice in one month and dislocated it once more. With each episode he had marked swelling. With his last injury eight days ago he had numbness of the ring and little fingers that gradually cleared up. *A*, X-ray from initial examination shows the ossification on the lateral side of the elbow. This is characteristic of repeated injuries with inadequate immobilization. It also shows an avulsion of the epiphysis of the medial epicondyle on the inner side. The fragment was removed and the muscle mass was secured to the epicondyle through drill holes. *B*, One year later. Note maturity of the ossification laterally, but with a large mass of bone. At this time he is asymptomatic except for restriction of motion due to the lateral mass.

ready damaged. If blood infiltrates into the muscle and the muscle is put at rest, the chances are that this blood will be absorbed without further complication. If the muscle continues to be irritated by active use, by repeated blows, by unwise manipulation or by massage, these repeated insults superimpose a new injury over the early repair and the result is ossification.

PATHOLOGY. The process begins as an infiltrating hemorrhage either subjacent to bone or directly involving it. As healing progresses, instead of the orderly formation of scar to be replaced to a greater or lesser extent by normal tissue, osteogenesis occurs in the tissue and it is transformed into bone. This may be an extensive process or a very mild one, depending more upon the extent of the repeated insults than upon the original injury. This process tends to continue as long as the irritation continues. When the part is put at rest and the blood supply is improved by local heat, the ossifying process may be arrested. In many instances the bone will be absorbed and the mass will shrink in size and disappear. In other instances as the bone formation matures it becomes smaller (Fig. 24) and terminates as normal bone in the form of an exostosis.

DIAGNOSIS. Diagnosis is not difficult once the ossification has matured. It is much more important to recognize the impending pathologic condition. If following a bruise on the thigh or arm a diagnosis is made of contusion with hematoma formation, and this condition does not promptly resolve, one should be on guard against formation of bone within the area. This explains why, in the discussion of contusion and hematoma, we insisted that rehabilitation should be carried out within the limits of pain and that reactivation of the area should depend not upon any predetermined time but upon the subsidence of symptoms. X-rays made early will be negative and should be repeated after two or three weeks if the symptoms persist. I have seen many cases in which the clinical examination demonstrated to my satisfaction a calcified mass within the muscle, but the x-ray showed only a little cloudiness (Fig. 22). The

symptoms disappear under proper management and the result is a small flake of ossification either on the bone or in the underlying muscle. More often it is complete resolution (Fig. 23).

TREATMENT. The early treatment of myositis ossificans is preventive and not surgical. *There is no place for operative treatment in the early stage of myositis ossificans.* As the impending condition is recognized the muscle should be put at rest. Physical therapy in the form of heat is permissible but no passive manipulation should be done. Some active motion may be permitted within the restriction of the splint, but only if it is painless. So treated, the condition may well subside and become asymptomatic. Granted, there may be considerable temporary stiffness of the

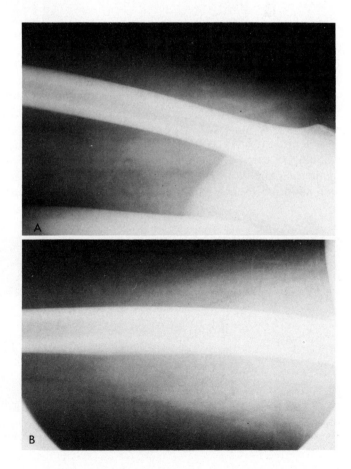

Figure 22. *A*, X-ray four months post injury, showing the definite osseous shadow along the proximal third of the femur. *B*, Six months later, this has almost completely regressed and disappeared.

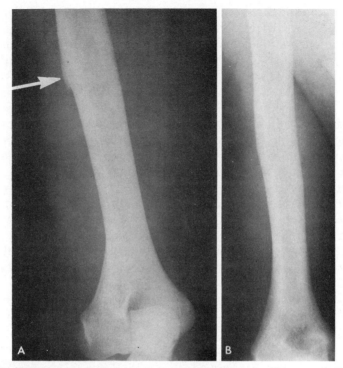

Figure 23. *A*, Ossification in midarm that matured and disappeared within a year (*B*). This probably represented bleeding into the periosteum.

part and much time will have elapsed, but a crippling condition will have been averted.

REHABILITATION. Rehabilitation should be carried out well within the limits of pain, at least for the first several months. (See Chapter 22.) Should the patient be seen after the ossification has occurred, the same treatment is instituted, namely, rest and inductive heat.

In the early stage, particularly in myositis ossificans about a long bone, the appearance is frequently that of a new growth, with characteristic lamina-

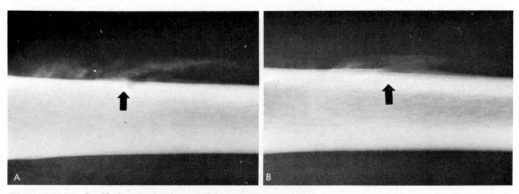

Figure 24. *A*, Ossified mass in the quadriceps intermedius muscle overlying the anterior femur at six weeks (arrow). *B*, Six months later, following immobilization and controlled rehabilitation. Note regression of mass (arrow).

tions of ossification or sometimes the stellate sunray effect which may simulate osteogenic sarcoma. One should not ignore the history of trauma in a case of suspected bone tumor. There have been many cases of myositis ossificans mistakenly treated by operation for bone tumor and major tragedies have resulted. This is particularly prone to occur because the biopsy of an early myositis ossificans will reveal actively growing young bone, very similar to callus. This may be indistinguishable by the pathologist from a neoplasm. Careful attention to the symptoms and above all to the course of the lesion is of value. Since myositis ossificans runs a relatively short course, at least in the expanding stage, a period of watchful waiting is justified in case of any doubt. In the meantime the part is put at rest and films are made at two-week intervals. Myositis will show diminution of ossification or maturity of the margins, quite different from the development of an osteogenic type tumor. Operation even for the purpose of biopsy may be disastrous (Fig. 25). A few weeks delay probably will be of little importance in the development of an osteogenic tumor.

As the healing progresses and the bone becomes more mature, more activity can be permitted, again restricted by pain. There is no place for passive stretching, certainly within six months, and the physiotherapist or trainer must be carefully instructed so that his urge to hasten rehabilitation will be controlled. One must rigorously resist the use of the knife. Under the exigencies of sport, everyone is anxious to have the player rehabilitated and may feel that the sooner the operation is done the quicker will be the recovery. This is one instance in which the reverse is true. Recovery will be quite prompt following removal of a mature exostosis, whereas it will be indefinitely postponed by an attempt at removal of forming bone.

OPEN WOUNDS

This category of injury includes a wide range of conditions of varying severity from a simple scratch on the skin to a compound fracture. A simple classification of breaks in the skin begins with an *abrasion*, which may be defined as a scraping and sliding injury to the

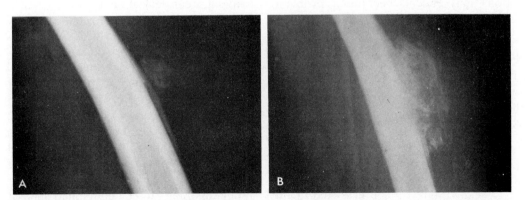

Figure 25. *A*, Early myositis ossificans. Rather typical case but operated on elsewhere when misdiagnosed as a malignancy. *B*, X-ray a few weeks postoperative showing marked increase in the size of the mass due to the meddlesome surgery. This should be left alone for at least six more months or longer if the mass does not appear to be mature. (Note two types of involvement in the first view: ossification along the periosteum and the oval mass completely separated from the periosteum.) Resection of mass after maturity resulted in good function.

skin usually accompanied by a contusion as the integument is caught between an external object and underlying structures. In the ordinary abrasion the full continuity of the skin has not actually been broken through. A *laceration* is a wound of the skin caused by a relatively sharp object so that the skin is actually cut through its full thickness. A *puncture wound* is one made by a penetrating object which pierces all layers of the skin. *Vesiculation* is blistering caused by mechanical, thermal or chemical burning in which the layers of the skin are separated by an exudation of fluid.

ABRASION

An abrasion, which is defined as a scraping injury to the skin, may be of any grade of severity from a simple excoriation of the skin by the opponent's headgear to very extensive damage. The major abrasions will occur over areas of the body where there is firm underlying tissue, particularly bone. Areas commonly injured are the shin, the knee, the iliac crest, the elbow and the back of the hand. Abrasions in themselves are not particularly serious but their complications may indeed become a problem. The most immediate consideration, once injury to the deeper structures has been ruled out, is the prevention of infection. It cannot be overemphasized that the player should be carefully instructed to report any break on the skin that occurs on the playing field. The combination of an open wound and mother earth has very serious connotations from the standpoint of local and generalized infection.

TREATMENT. The first step in the management of abrasion is prevention by providing adequate playing fields. Contact sports should not be played on concrete, cinder tracks, or rough irregular ground with rocks and glass in the soil. The requirements for player protection will vary directly with the nature of the terrain. Thus a player on a well groomed, heavily sodded playing field may need but little protection, whereas one playing on hard, poorly sodded ground or on abrasive surfaces should have protection such as elbow pads, long sleeved jerseys and long socks.

Once an abrasion occurs it should be reported promptly and as promptly treated. When this is done an abrasion usually is of little importance. The first step in treatment is to clean the skin and there is no better cleansing agent than soap and water. There seems to be no real virtue in a surgical soap (such as the hexachlorophene soaps) for a single wash since the unique value of these preparations is in the build-up of the antiseptic in the skin by repeated washings. Ordinary bland white soap and water is entirely adequate, thorough cleansing being the important factor. The soap acts as a solvent for grease and embedded dirt. If necessary one can brush out ground-in dirt with a soft brush so that when the washing is complete the wound is fresh looking with no embedded foreign material. Some attention to detail at this first washing will save a great deal of later effort.

If a wound has been properly cleaned the application of a topical antiseptic is of doubtful value. In the ordinary abrasion we do not recommend painting with iodine, merthiolate or other chemical. If the surface is not too moist a protective spray such as tincture of benzoin may be applied, in order to reduce pain. Such a spray tends to seal the wound and yet permits exudation of fluids. The application of collodion over such an area is to be condemned since it may simply seal in the infected fluids. The use of a bland ointment with a water-soluble base is recommended if the surface is "weepy." Greasy ointments should be avoided. An antibiotic ointment such as sulfathiazole in Aquaphor, or Furacin may be used. It should be borne in mind that such preparations may cause sensitivity and local reaction and even delay healing.

A suitable dressing and pad are applied to prevent re-injury since disability from an extensive abrasion that has been repeatedly crusted over and peeled off may last for several weeks and materially impair the activity of the athlete, particularly if the abrasion is on an area such as the knee, ankle or hand. The amount of protection necessary will vary a great deal with the severity of the abrasion, its location and its extent. Protection must be (1) against direct trauma and (2) against active overuse of the skin. The latter is particularly pertinent in an abrasion over the extensor surface of a joint such as the knee. Should infection ensue, warm moist packs, rest, elevation and suitable antibiotics are indicated. Great care should be taken in the dressing room in handling the infected wound since one infection may spread to many other players.

LACERATION

As defined, a laceration is a separation of the skin with relatively sharp edges. Ordinarily in athletics this is not a cleanly incised wound as with a knife or razor blade; instead, it is a combination of a contusion and a lacerated wound in which the lacerated edge is jagged and irregular. These wounds, too, may be of any degree, from an extensive tearing of the skin with considerable separation of the skin edges to a fissure-like injury with but little external evidence of damage.

TREATMENT. After it has been determined that there is no underlying injury, the first goal in management is to obtain a clean wound. A laceration caused by a blow of a blunt object against a sharp underlying bone as in the eyebrow represents simply a splitting of the skin without penetration and is probably amply cleaned by the bleeding which accompanies it. On the other hand, a laceration caused by a broken cleat or the sharp equipment of the opposing player is potentially dirty and should not be closed without ample cleansing. A wound that has had direct contact with the ground must be promptly and thoroughly cleansed. The player should be taken to the dressing or treatment room and the wound very carefully explored for foreign material. If necessary, procaine may be injected along the wound edges to facilitate this examination. If the wound appears clean with no penetrating foreign matter, it is unwise to scrape out the interior of the wound with an abrasive — and a gauze compress qualifies as such. Simple flushing of the wound with saline or 0.5 per cent procaine solution will usually be adequate.

Next, the wound edges are carefully inspected. Often the wound is not cut cleanly through the skin at a right angle but is a slicing type with a very thin edge on one side and a thick sloping edge on the other. In this instance careful minimal trimming of the skin margins in order to get sharp edge-to-edge contact will speed up healing and prevent excess scar formation. If it is felt essential that the player return promptly to the game, he may have a preliminary suture and then a definitive suture immediately after competition is over. From the medical standpoint this course is much inferior to proper closure of the wound in the first place, but it is to be preferred to leaving a jagged wound imperfectly sutured. If there are undermined edges with considerable soft tissue damage beneath the skin, the wound may require drainage. It is better to put in a small wick that permits exudation than to allow fluid to accumulate. Frequently such accumulation can be prevented by direct, suitably placed pressure on the wound. Direct pressure also serves to prevent edema of the wound edges, which may cause considerable tension on the sutures and finally disrupt them.

In suturing the wound, swelling and edema should be anticipated. Only enough sutures are used to obtain accurate wound approximation. This principle accounts for the emergency room aphorism that "the slicker the wound looks immediately after suture, the sloppier it looks the following day." This is not to imply that the repair should be careless but simply that one should not place multiple small, shallow sutures in an effort to obtain fine approximation since these will inevitably pull out as swelling ensues.

The wound should be carefully inspected daily over a period of several days, since it is potentially infected and should be treated as such. If there is any suggestion of a collection of fluid in the wound, one or more stitches should be removed and the wound allowed to drain freely. The question of further participation in athletics before it has healed must depend entirely upon its location and extent. In many body areas the laceration can be adequately protected against both trauma and undue stretching of the skin and there is no reason why further participation cannot be permitted. Once there is evidence of any complication, more protection should be utilized and the inflamed wound must be treated by the usual measures of immobilization, warm wet dressings, antibiotics and general support.

Careful primary attention to the lacerated wound will give very gratifying results. A tetanus toxoid booster should be given. Antitetanic serum of human origin is now almost always available and should be used if toxoid immunity has not been developed previously. The danger of anaphylactic reaction to horse serum outweighs the importance of giving antitetanic horse serum, except in the most unusual circumstances.

PUNCTURE WOUND

This condition has been defined as a wound by a penetrating object. The object may be small, as a splinter or nail, but even a rather broad object may penetrate the skin, making a relatively small opening and continuing deeper into the soft tissues. This has the potentiality of a puncture wound and should be treated as such. Such wounds are not common in athletics but should be promptly and adequately treated when they do occur. The author recalls one instance during a track session when one of the participants was kneeling on one knee with the other thigh thrust forward when he received an errant javelin in his anterior thigh. This not only caused a puncture wound through the skin and ruptured the muscle mechanism but split the shaft of the femur.

Of first importance are the severity of the wound, the depth of the penetration and the possibility of underlying damage to the joints or bone, but particularly to the blood vessels or nerves. A penetrating wound over a joint should be assumed to have entered the joint without proof to the contrary because the potentialities of joint penetration are of major importance. A history is carefully taken as to the nature of the penetrating object, the depth of the penetration, whether or not it went through clothing, and whether the entering body was contaminated, as in the case of the peg of a broken cleat or piece of wire or nail which happened to be on the playing field. It will not suffice to wash off the skin, apply protective dressing and "wait and see." It may be necessary to wait and see, but this decision should be made only after careful history, thorough examination and some effort to explore the wound. If there is underlying damage which will require surgical repair, this repair should be done at once since the wound is potentially infected. Even a few hours delay will change it from a potentially to an actually infected wound. After that, definitive surgery is extremely hazardous.

TREATMENT. After one has satisfied himself that there is no underlying damage, the wound itself is treated. The skin will often be puckered and discolored around the margin, which indicates that the hole at one time was considerably larger than it is at the time of examination. The skin tends to stretch and tent inward under pressure of the blow, so that when the point does penetrate the stretched skin, it may make a fairly large hole. When the skin returns to its normal tension this hole will shrink and appear minute. The importance of determining the nature of the object and the depth of penetration is obvious.

If the object was contaminated and penetrated deeply, it will be wise to split the skin, examine the underlying tissue, clean out the sinus tract and then decide whether or not to carry out primary closure. Primary closure may be carried out if the wound has been treated promptly and satisfactorily lavaged. The use of a drain will depend upon the degree of damage and whether or not one expects continued oozing and collection of fluid. It is much better to let the fluids seep outside through a tissue drain than to accumulate in the wound to make an ideal medium for infection. Only if the wound seems minor, the penetrating object small and the depth not great is one justified in simply cleansing the skin and observing. If the decision is made to observe the wound, exactly that should be done—and frequently. It is not proper to wait until secondary symptoms demand attention, for by this time a definite infection will be developing. A tetanus toxoid booster should be given. (For tetanus serum see page 62.)

BLISTERS

MECHANICAL CAUSES. Blisters on the skin may occur under varying circumstances, the most common being friction from an ill-fitting shoe or a wrinkle in the sock. Another frequent source is irritation by adhesive tape or by friction between the tape and skin due to the fact that the tape was poorly applied, or it has been under undue tension, or the individual has perspired and so separated the tape from the skin in certain areas while it remains adherent to the skin in others. In any event the resulting traction on the skin tends to separate its superficial layers from the underlying dermis, the area fills with exudate and the blister forms. While the blister itself may be a relatively simple and apparently minor ailment, its location may be such as to make it a problem of some magnitude. A blister on the back of the heel, for example, may handicap the player throughout the season. Extensive vesiculation under the adhesive tape may render it impossible to use adhesive in that particular area of the body, and so vital protection may have to be discontinued with resultant injury to the unprotected joint or ligament beneath.

Another disabling area of vesiculation is the sole of the foot where it is not uncommon to have a blister directly under the first toe or first metatarsal head. This is particularly common in the track man who runs in light shoes with very pointed spikes, so that he may get direct pressure in a single area of the sole. This constant sliding of the skin on itself results in blistering. The skin of the sole is thick and a very deep blister under the skin (Fig. 26) may go unrecognized and be treated as a simple contusion. I have seen such a blister enlarge until it separated a large portion of the calloused skin under the forefoot. This condition manifestly is not compatible with competition.

The best treatment of blisters is *prevention.* Carefully fitted shoes and clean, wrinkle-free socks are extremely important. If strapping or wrapping is used, it should be carefully placed and its location changed if it begins to irritate the skin. Careful preparation of the skin before application of adhesive will often prevent irritation either by reaction to the tape or by partial slipping of the tape on the skin. A simple wrinkle in the tape in a weight-bearing area of the body may cause prompt blistering beneath it. If an irritated area develops which appears to be the prelude to a blister, careful protection should be used either by very thin, smooth tape applied directly to the skin or by soft padding to prevent friction between the skin and equipment. An ounce of prevention is certainly worth a pound of cure here.

Once a blister develops, proper *treatment* is of considerable importance. Here again the location of the lesion makes some difference in the type of treatment instituted. If the blister is located in an area where there ordinarily is no friction, as the thigh or calf, the top of the blister may be removed, the area carefully cleansed and the resultant abraded area treated appropriately (with benzoin spray, for instance). This management, however, is not practicable for a blister caused by pressure from a shoe or another piece of equipment. In this instance it is quite important to protect the skin over the blister. The blister should be treated by passing a hypodermic needle through the adjacent skin and into the blister to drain the fluid and relieve the pressure. This is particularly applicable on the plantar surface of the foot so that some of the callus can be preserved until such time as the floor of the blister develops some resistance of its own. Once the roof of the blister is broken, it is well to trim it all away and treat the floor by benzoin solution, proper protection, etc. The ragged edges of the top of the blister not only irritate the lesion further but serve to form pe-

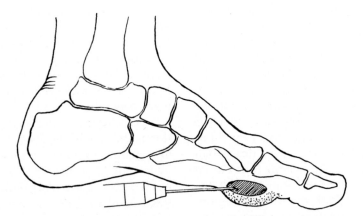

Figure 26. Cross section drawing of the vicinity of the first metatarsal head, showing the heavy epidermis of callus with a blister lying between this and the underlying dermis. A needle has been inserted to draw out the fluid. (Needle inserted away from the blister margin, through intact skin.)

ripheral pockets containing infected fluid.

CHEMICAL CAUSES. Chemical blistering is not frequent since the marking of fields by lime is no longer common practice. It does have the added complication of irritation of the surrounding skin and should be treated by protection by bland emollients much as in a thermal burn. The *thermal burn* has no particular application to athletic injuries but occasionally occurs as a result of carelessly applied physical therapeutic measures and as such may be extremely distressing. The burn from the ultraviolet machine is of course similar to sunburn and should be treated as such. Injuries from the infrared or electric heating pad and various types of hot packs are true thermal burns and may cause vesiculation, but usually remain a local reaction. These direct heat applications usually cause sufficient pain that the treatment is stopped before the burn is severe. The result is usually first degree or at the worst a mild second degree burn with only moderate vesiculation. The deep electrical burns caused by diathermy or other inductive agents may be extremely severe. A diathermy burn should be very carefully investigated to determine whether or not the damage is limited to the skin. It may well be so, since oftentimes the burn is secondary to the condensation of fluid between the applicator and the skin; thus it actually is from hot water. If it is a true electrical burn the deep tissues may indeed be burned more severely than the skin. An electrical therapeutic appliance is no plaything, and its indiscriminate use by untrained personnel should be frowned upon. The patient should be instructed not to put too much faith in the dials of the machine, and he should be told to report the slightest discomfort, since it is neither safe nor desirable to have the heat reach

the level of discomfort to the part being treated.

SKIN INFECTIONS

Skin infections secondary to direct trauma are oftentimes the bane of the training room, because they may start in one player and spread like wildfire through the whole squad. Any skin infection, however superficial, should be very carefully washed, the surrounding skin cleansed, protective dressing applied and great care taken not to reinfect the skin by use of dirty clothing. It is obvious that once suppuration occurs, the pimple or boil should be opened under aseptic technique and the area of surrounding skin protected by careful cleansing with antiseptic solution and protective dressing. The dressing should be destroyed and not indiscriminately tossed to the floor. Many of the so-called eczemas are indeed skin infections, and therefore the affected player's clothes should be isolated from the remainder of the squad.

Fungus infections are particularly distressing and are prone to develop under adhesive tape applied to the feet. Occasionally on removal of the tape the whole plantar integument will peel off as a result of extensive fungus undermining. Application of proper fungicidal measures will clear up the local lesion quite adequately. The big danger is that casual handling of the socks, contamination of the floor and common shower stalls will spread the fungus from the player who is relatively immune to his own fungus to his neighbor who has no resistance to this particular organism. While it may be an entirely latent infection in one player, his locker mate may develop a virulent infection. Ordinary rules of cleanliness, soap and water, clean socks and some type of bath shoes will help to minimize this problem. If it becomes epidemic in a given situation, special measures will be necessary to sterilize the shower stalls and locker room floors. Enteric drugs are promising, and one of the oral fungicides should be used if the infected area is extensive or resistant to local measures.

TETANUS PREVENTION

The problem of tetanus is very important in the athletic program in spite of its great rarity. It is one condition in which prevention is almost completely effective and treatment is relatively ineffective, therefore little justification exists for not employing preventive techniques.

TOXOID. Every athlete should have tetanus toxoid injections prior to his participation in sports. These injections have been well proved, were adopted by the armed forces and have been extremely effective in eliminating the danger of tetanus from questionable wounds. There is ordinarily no reaction to toxoid injections and it is entirely feasible at the beginning of the school year to insist on the series for each athlete. If the patient has had toxoid within the year, one can relax about the ordinary skin involvement. If he sustains a particularly virulent type of puncture wound, as by a rusty nail, injection of a booster dose of toxoid can be given at that time with no danger of reaction and with complete effectiveness, since tetanus develops rather slowly and the toxoid booster can develop the antibodies much more rapidly than the organism develops its toxin.

ANTITETANUS SERUM. If the injured player has not had toxoid, the toxoid series should be started at once. It probably will not be effective for the current lesion. Antitetanic human serum is usually available and should be used in a prophylactic dose in all penetrating wounds. Horse serum should be used only under the most urgent necessity. The dangers of anaphylaxis either at the time of initial administration or at a later exposure are so great, and the reaction so dangerous, that routine use of antitetanic serum in horse serum is not recommended. If it is necessary to use antitetanic serum, a careful sensitivity test should be run and given at least one hour to react before the serum is injected. The patient should be carefully watched for at least 24 hours, and he should be warned that he is subject to anaphylactic reaction as long as two or three weeks following the injection. He should also be warned that another injection of horse serum may be particularly dangerous. If the wound really seems to be a dangerous one, it should be opened freely and thoroughly lavaged. Massive antibiotic dosage should also be given.

STRAIN

Injuries to the Muscle-Tendon Unit

For the purpose of this discussion it is important that we make a clear distinction between strain and sprain. The subcommittee on Athletic Nomenclature of the A.M.A. Committee on Sports Medicine has confirmed that strain should apply to the muscle-tendon unit and sprain to the ligament injury. These structures are quite distinct, the muscle-tendon units including a motor element whereas the ligament is primarily a stabilizer.

Strain may be defined as damage of some part of the unit (muscle, tendon or the attachment) occasioned by overuse (chronic strain) or overstress (acute strain). So we properly have mild (first degree), moderate (second degree) and severe (third degree) strain of the unit. The strain will occur at the weakest link of the muscle-tendon unit at a given time. Under a given stress the tendon may rupture, the muscle-tendon junction may give way or the damage may be to the muscle itself or to its bony attachment.

There has been a tendency to consider muscle and tendon in different categories; frequently injuries to the tendon and injuries to the muscle are described in separate chapters. More recently, proper emphasis has been placed on the fact that the muscle-tendon mechanism is indeed a unit which consists of a muscle arising usually from bone which terminates in a tendon, or tendons, which itself attaches to bone. Such a unit crossing a joint or joints serves a double purpose: (1) it acts to stabilize the joint in this case combining with its antagonist to prevent motion; and (2) it serves as a motor to accomplish a certain motion. Under this conception it can be seen that functionally it is a unit. Impairment of any part of the unit affects the whole. Each part must be restored to its normal condition if normal function is to be maintained. It is bootless to speak of injury to the muscle and of injury to the tendon as separate elements. Injury to the unit is of two types: (1) strain and its consequences; and (2) contusion and its complications. (See page 47.)

CHRONIC STRAIN. Chronic strain from overfunction causes fatigue of the muscle and its sequelae — muscle spasm, myositis, and ischemia. It may also result in irritation at the musculotendinous junction or tenosynovitis along the course of the tendon or inflammatory reaction at the tendinous attachment. Although these seem to be different conditions, they are basically the same and require basically the same treatment: specifically, rest, local heat, local injection, and protection against strain. General measures such as antispasmodics may be of some value if the area involved is a major one such as the hip, thigh or back. In this condition prevention is of more importance than cure. In the athlete, the whole purpose of his long training is to build up the musculotendinous unit gradually so that it is able to withstand a progressively heavier work load, thus increasing its strength, endurance and ability to avoid strain. Once the strain occurs the problem is magnified by the fact that relief will require a sharp reversal of the activity cycle. A period of complete rest must be followed by the same gradual progressive build up. This is very onerous to the athlete and his impatience to resume activity often results in recurrence of this injury with an even more frustrating period of disability. Prevention of recurrence is a major problem in any strain of the muscle tendon unit. Often the anatomical or physical condition of the athlete will make him more vulnerable to overstress of the muscle. If his hamstrings are tight and short, if his calf is so short he cannot dorsiflex his foot, if his back is so tight he cannot touch his fingers to the floor, a course of stretching exercises may be very fruitful in preventing recurrence of the strain or, indeed, in preventing strain in the player who has not yet developed the condition. (See Chapter 22.)

The extent of disability and the difficulty of maintaining adequate protection will vary considerably with the unit involved and also with the type of activity to be restored. For the track man, a strain of the musculotendinous unit of the calf may be completely disabling. To the baseball player, it may be the triceps that throws him out of action. The rower may be disabled because of strain to his back. In every instance the strain has resulted from the very activity which is important to this individual. As such it poses a major problem in rehabilitation.

The complications of such a condition may be major. The baseball pitcher, for example, may develop painful myositis which progresses to ossification and spur formation at the origin of the triceps from the glenoid (Fig. 27); it may continue until pitching is impossible. A tenosynovitis may develop in a tendon, particularly one which is surrounded by a sheath. The recurrent irritative strain of the biceps tendon passing through the bicipital groove is a classic example. Chronic strain may be caused by prolonged overuse or by a single episode of overactivity. It is not

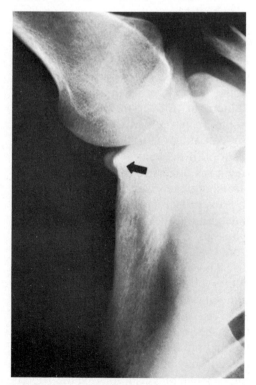

Figure 27. Baseball pitcher who developed ossification at glenoid attachment of triceps brachii. Nonsurgical treatment consisted of patient's retirement from pitching for one season.

caused but may be initiated by an acute injury. The result is an inflammatory reaction between the tendon and the sheath, congestion with inflammation, oversecretion of fluid and increase in fibrin content which causes sticky adhesions between the tendon and the surrounding synovium. If the strain is not eliminated in the early stages, the tenosynovitis progresses to a chronic inflammatory reaction with swelling, edema, pain and possibly painful crepitation. If the tendon continues to slide up and down its sheath, irritation is increased until a constrictive or adhesive tenosynovitis results which may completely arrest the motion in this particular tendon and sharply interfere with function of this muscle-tendon unit. Although this may seem to be a specific condition, the same thing may happen in the muscle and will require the same treatment, this time directed to the tendon rather than to the muscle itself. Indeed, the treatment may finally have to be surgical resection of the tendon sheath or possibly transference of a tendon to a less constricted area. Again, the classic example is the bicipital tendon at the shoulder, which on the one hand, is likely to advance to adhesive or constrictive tenosynovitis. On the other hand, the tendo Achilles, lacking the specific sheath, may have the inflammatory symptoms but not the complication of constriction. Chronic strain is not likely to result in hemorrhage into the muscle. The calcification resulting from chronic strain will be in the origin of the muscle or at the insertion of the tendon.

ACUTE STRAIN. Acute strain, in distinction to chronic strain, is the result of a single violent force applied to the muscle; for example, the violence of the sprinter coming out of the blocks when his muscles contract violently against the resistance of the block. It may be the result of resistance to a force. For example, with the muscles contracted, a

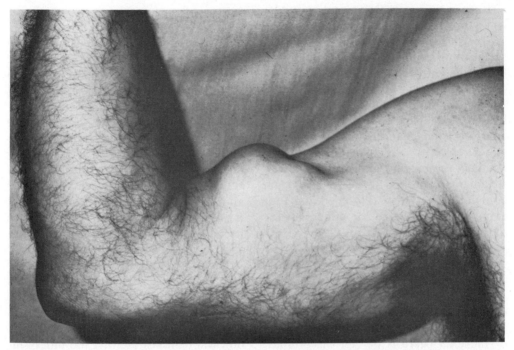

Figure 28. Rupture of long head of biceps brachii caused by patient's awkward catch of partner in gymnastics. Note bunching up of muscle attended by complete loss of function of long head. Condition was resolved by reattaching long head, which would no longer reach to bicipital groove, midway down shaft of humerus. Symptoms were relieved and some function was restored.

violent force is applied which is greater than the unit's ability to withstand. This is exemplified by the strain to the biceps brachii resulting from trying to support a weight with the flexed forearms that is greater than the biceps unit will tolerate (Fig. 28). The injury is likely to be localized and may occur in any part of the unit. One can see that inflammation in the origin of the muscle and strain at the attachment of the tendon to bone appear to be, and indeed are, identical injuries. So also are injuries to the musculotendinous junction or injuries in the muscle belly itself. The injury occurs at a certain location simply because at this given moment it is the weakest link in the chain. It must be obvious that the amount of damage (mild [first degree], moderate [second degree] or severe [third degree]) that occurs is contingent on the violence of the force

and the strength of the resistance. The pathological feature consists of disruption of some of the fibers of the unit. There may be rupture of a few muscle fibers or of the entire muscle. The tendon may be partially avulsed from the bone or completely torn away.

Whereas the treatment of chronic strain is rest and avoidance of the activity that caused the strain, the treatment of acute strain must be restoration of the integrity of the unit. This may require, in one case, simple protection against additional stress until healing occurs or, in another, surgical restoration. In the great majority of instances the injury is minimal and recovery is prompt. As the individual steps on the curb of the running track, his ankle is forced sharply into dorsiflexion and he has pain localized at the junction of the calf muscle and the tendo Achillis. He has sharp pain, sits down and rubs his leg, exercises his foot up and down and is able to resume walking. If he tries to sprint or to dorsiflex his foot violently, he will have discomfort. The following day the area will be sore. The muscle will be contracted and dorsiflexion will be resisted. This is caused by some degree of damage to the muscle and tendon fibers with attendant bleeding, inflammatory reaction and protective resistance to motion. The subsequent course of the injury will depend on the extent of damage and the effectiveness of treatment.

MILD (FIRST DEGREE) STRAIN. In this degree of strain there is no appreciable disruption. Pathological changes are confined to a low grade inflammatory process with swelling, edema and some discomfort on function of tendon or muscle. There is neither discernible loss of strength nor any restriction of motion. Early examination will elicit pain on active motion or passive stretching which is sharply confined to the area of damage. Later as muscle spasm occurs exact localization may be difficult. Localization of the point of stress may be important in treatment. Mild strain is very distressing to the athlete. Hamstring strain may sideline the sprinter even though the injury is mild. The baseball pitcher is a classic example of chronic strain of the arm, wherein the strain is not severe enough to restrict motion or strength but may sharply reduce endurance.

Treatment of the acute strain must be rest of the unit and protection against active use. Local injection may be hyaluronidase in the muscle, lidocaine in the tendon sheath. There is no place for steroid injection in the acute injury. The most important treatment is protection which must vary with the amount of damage. In one case it may consist of immobilization and in another, of simple avoidance of violent activity. Enteric acute inflammatory agents, such as aspirin or phenylbutazone, may be useful. Muscle relaxants will help control spasm.

MODERATE (SECOND DEGREE) STRAIN. The distinction between first and second degree strain lies in the extent to which pathological development has occurred. Whereas in a mild strain there is no loss of strength but only irritation, in moderate strain there has been actual damage to the muscle, tendon or attachment which definitely compromises the strength of the unit. There is not complete disruption as in severe strain but there is definite loss of strength; whether 90 per cent or 10 per cent is the problem. Diagnosis depends upon a careful evaluation of the unit—all symptoms are more severe than in mild strain, yet careful examination will demonstrate that the unit is intact.

Treatment of this injury must be more definitive. Whereas in mild strain the treatment is largely symptomatic, in moderate strain we predicate specific weakness but no loss of continuity. Local treatment is by ice pack and injection (lidocaine). This, together with protection, will give symptomatic relief. Since there has been definite damage to some part of the unit, *protection* becomes all important. Since protection means cessation of violent muscle activity it follows that splinting, taping and so on are important. Tendons and muscles heal slowly so protection must be prolonged for several weeks. If activity is resumed too soon, at best the muscle spasm recurs, at worst the unit may rupture (Fig. 29). Consequently activity must be carefully resumed and kept within the limits of pain. The part must be protected against further injury. The situation is frustrating to the athlete, the doctor and the coach. In the final analysis adequate treatment is largely protective

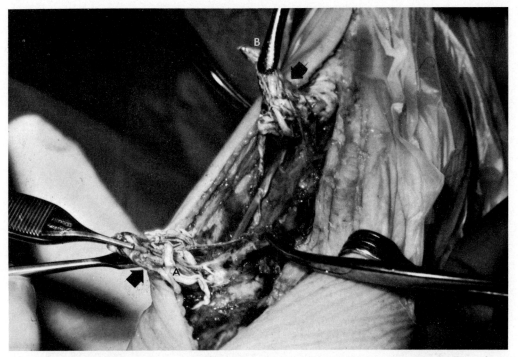

Figure 29. Professional football player injured calf six weeks prior to surgical procedure shown here. Symptoms, which subsequently subsided, included swelling, pain, and tenderness at muscle-tendon junction of calf. Six weeks following initial trauma, patient, running down a ramp, slipped, heard something snap, and felt acute pain in the back of the lower leg. Loss of function of the calf was essentially complete with a defect at the muscle-tendon junction. At time of surgical repair, roughly half the tendon was found to have been torn six weeks previously whereas the remaining half showed a fresh tear. Repair and reconstruction using the peroneus brevis was carried out with apparent success. Photograph shows earlier "A" and later "B" pathologic changes at torn ends of tendon and extensive disruption of tendon with early degenerative changes (arrows).

and will result in complete recovery. Inadequate care will result in a chronic, more or less crippling impairment of the unit which is devastating to the athlete.

SEVERE (THIRD DEGREE) STRAIN. Rupture of any component of the unit is usually the result of violent contraction against firm resistance: for example, the irresistible force and the immovable object. It may be preceded by damage to a lesser degree which has improperly healed. The tendon may give way or separate at the muscle-tendon junction, or the muscle itself may rupture. When the forces applied are greater than the strength of the unit, something must give. In a first or second degree strain

the primary treatment is protection. In a complete (third degree) tear it must be restoration of the unit.

Diagnosis depends upon recognition of the loss of function of the unit. This may be quite deceptive. On the one hand, muscle spasm may render the unit inoperative although it is actually intact. On the other, the unit may be disrupted, a condition that may be very difficult to detect. Sometimes the actual defect may be palpated in the muscle-tendon unit (Fig. 30). At other times the muscle may bunch up as in rupture of the long head of the biceps brachii, the rectus femoris or the hamstrings (Figs. 31, 32).

TREATMENT. If detected early, re-

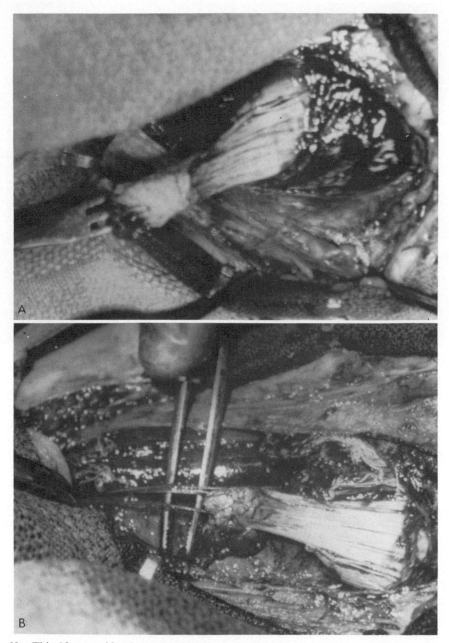

Figure 30. This 20 year old pole vaulter had severe pain in his groin as he thrust off the ground. He was no longer able to run or vault without immediate swelling in the area. An ice pack was applied and he was examined the following day. There was swelling in the groin, with palpable muscle separated from the pubis. When the thigh was adducted against resistance, the adductor muscle bunched up, and this mass traveled distally. *A,* At surgery, the incision parallels the adductor longus distal to the pubis. The tenaculum holds the avulsed tendinous end of the adductor longus muscle. *B,* Mattress sutures were placed in this mass allowing it to be pulled up to its origin on the pubic bone and fastened through drill holes. A plaster spica cast was applied, to be worn for eight weeks, but after six weeks the patient and his local doctor removed the cast. The muscle attachment seemed firm and the cast was left off. Six months postoperatively, the adductor was intact and there was no bulging of the muscle; the patient was asymptomatic and was released for sports activity. Note: Knee to right of picture, pelvis to left.

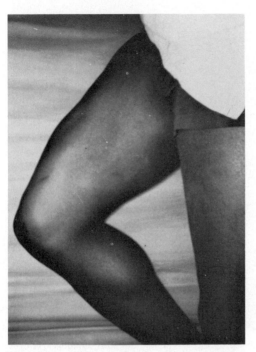

Figure 31. While straining against opponent, professional football player felt painful snap in "groin"; swelling was massive. Patient treated for "hematoma." "Bunching up" of rectus femoris in front of thigh with extensor stress one year later is obvious. Condition was only mildly disabling and no treatment was recommended.

pair of the unit is quite feasible whether it is tendon or muscle, and it is even more important to repair these injuries early than those of ligament or bone. Every effort must be made to determine separation of the muscle or tendon. If it can be diagnosed early, surgical repair will give the best results (Fig. 33). If it cannot be diagnosed, treatment as for moderate strain should be carried out until the accurate pathological condition is demonstrable. Often it is then too late for repair because of muscle spasm and shortening. Athletic activities must be eliminated until healing has occurred (eight to ten weeks). Too often resumption of the activity that caused the trouble will cause recurrence. Late reconstructive procedures may be necessary and will be described in relation to specific areas. In far too many instances

this will be a procedure of salvage and cannot be expected to restore normal function.

DISCUSSION OF MUSCLE-TENDON INJURIES

Successful treatment depends upon an accurate diagnosis of the location and extent of the injury. It has been emphasized that in ligament injuries the doctor must be able to make a definitive decision concerning the best treatment based on a true recognition of the pathological process present. In muscle early treatment is even more important than it is in the ligament or tendon. An early muscle rupture can be readily repaired. It may be impossible to suture a ruptured muscle after a lapse of as little as two weeks (Fig. 34). Consideration of the problem will show why this is true. The muscle-tendon unit is normally in constant tension. The tone of the muscle is such that it keeps the tendon taut and ready for function. In a normal unit at no time is the tendon relaxed in the sense of a slack rope. Consequently when the muscle is ruptured the fibers immediately separate. At this time, however, no actual contracture has developed. The fibers have simply shortened and can readily be pulled back to their normal length if it is done early. By the same token, the muscle itself is in good condition. Edema and necrosis have not occurred and ordinarily successful suture can be made even in the belly of the muscle. Within a very short time the contraction of the muscle becomes a contracture and it is impossible to get the ruptured ends together, particularly since the local condition is such that the suture will not hold. This also applies to avulsion of the muscle from bone. However, when the muscle is avulsed from its origin, a fragment of bone, or at least periosteum, frequently

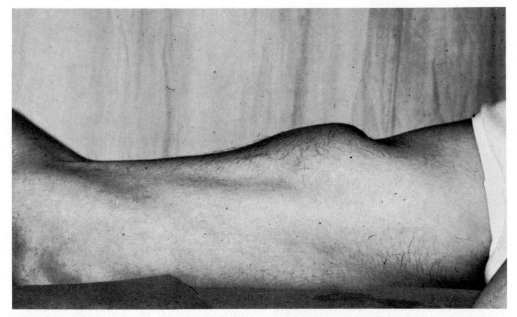

Figure 32. Sprinter felt something "give way" in back of thigh and had to stop running. He was treated for hematoma in muscle. Figure shows "bunching up" of muscle under stress (six months following injury). Any stress of the hamstrings caused pain between the bunched up muscle and the fibrous band running from muscle toward ischium. Reattachment of torn muscle to adjacent hamstring muscle was required.

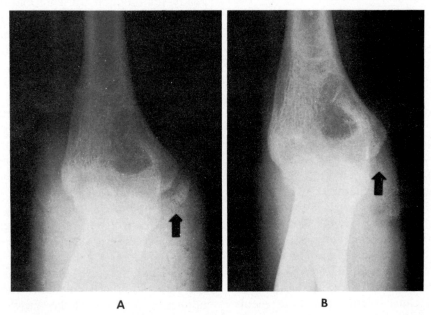

A   **B**

Figure 33. Patient fell on outstretched arm while performing gymnastic maneuvers. *A*, Avulsion of flexor pronator attachment at internal condyle occurred. *B*, Fragment of bone was removed and attachment to condyle repaired. Patient regained normal function of arm.

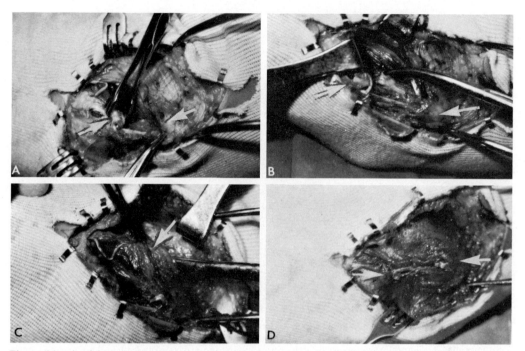

Figure 34. Avulsion of a portion of the flexor pronator muscle attachment to the medial epicondyle. This was an old injury resulting in disability. On exposure of the epicondyle, the detached bundle of muscle including the flexor carpi ulnaris and portion of the flexor profundus is shown. *A,* The tenaculum grasps the avulsed muscle end. The hemostat indicates the medial epicondyle about 2 inches away. *B,* The avulsed muscle is in the retractor. The larger (upper) hemostat indicates the pronator radii teres. The smaller (lower) hemostat is on the epicondyle. *C,* The pronator radii teres is mobilized but not detached from the condyle ready to shift into the space left by the avulsed muscle. *D,* The repair. The avulsed end is sutured into the angle formed by the pronator above and the flexor bundle below. The arrow indicates the end of the avulsed muscle with the pronator above it and the undamaged muscle below it. The condyle is at the right arrow. Patient has resumed his activity as a professional quarterback.

is peeled away with it. This gives an additional base for retention of sutures so that it may be possible to reattach a muscle to its origin somewhat later than it is to suture the muscle itself (Fig. 35). It still becomes increasingly difficult with the passage of time and before many weeks repair will become impossible (Fig. 36). In an avulsion of the tendon from bone there is considerably more leeway since the tendon gives fixation for the suture and the muscle itself is normal and has less tendency to fibrose than if it is torn (Figs. 37 and 38). Ironically, however, it is relatively easy to diagnose rupture of the tendon or avulsion of tendon from bone whereas it may be very difficult to diagnose muscle

rupture. A little consideration will verify this observation. Frequently the tendon is in a position wherein it can readily be palpated since the muscle is intact and its tendency to *bunch up* on contraction may be obvious. Also, this is not screened by the inflammatory reaction within the muscle itself which occurs when the muscle is damaged.

The ultimate fate of injury to the muscle-tendon unit depends upon the ratio of the severity of the injury and the acuity of the diagnosis (Fig. 39). If the injury is not severe, the diagnosis may never need to be made and recovery, although incomplete, may eventually occur (Fig. 40). Unfortunately, the severe injuries may be more difficult to

Text continued on page 76

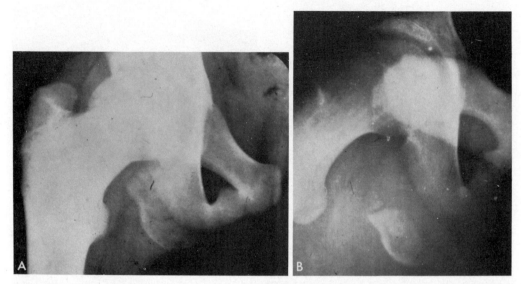

Figure 35.   Three weeks before, this 16 year old boy had severe pain when hurdling. He did not fall but immediately had to stop. X-ray shows an avulsion of the ischium including the biceps and semitendinosus origin. *A,* Neutral position. *B,* In abduction showing the gross displacement. This required open reduction and internal fixation to assure good healing. Overcoming the contracture was easy because of bone fragment that permitted firm traction by the suture.

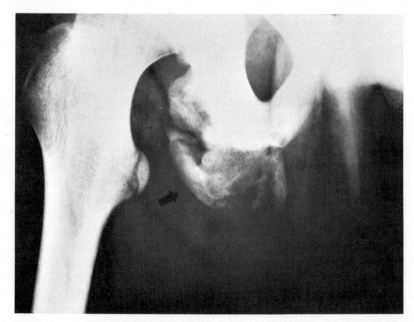

Figure 36.   Excessive ossification from untreated avulsion of hamstring muscles from the ischium. This extremely painful mass required resection and repair and caused more than one year's disability.

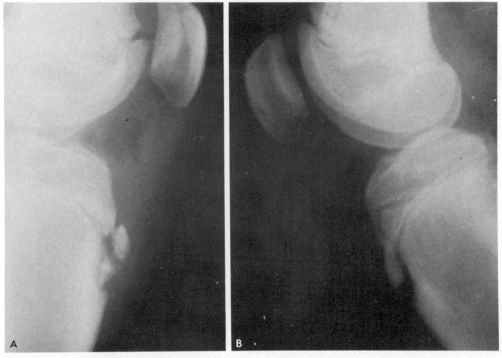

Figure 37. Avulsion of central portion of the patellar tubercle by acute trauma. X-ray shows central fragment is avulsed. The operation revealed this to be a block of bone with almost the entire patellar tendon attachment. The block was resected and the tendon attached to the underlying bone. No growth disturbance occurred. *A*, Displaced central portion of the patellar tubercle apophysis. *B*, The opposite side for comparison.

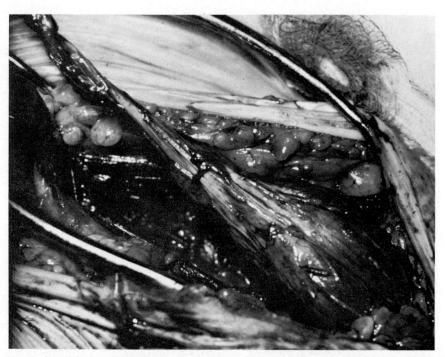

Figure 38. Patient fell between two trucks, catching himself with right arm overhead and taking his whole weight with the arm stretched up. Despite severe pain in shoulder, patient continued working. Roughly one month following initial trauma, he noticed knotting of muscle in arm upon contraction. Condition gradually worsened until he was unable to lift anything overhead and experienced weakness and pain in arm when stress was placed on arm in flexion. Examination revealed bunching up of biceps brachii in lower arm upon contraction to flex elbow. Photograph shows mass of biceps just proximal to elbow with rupture of long tendon at, roughly, level of bicipital groove. Since tendon could not be extended upward to bicipital groove, it was fastened through a hole drilled in humerus at junction of upper and middle thirds. Function improved and pain lessened but muscle continued to bunch up. Rupture of the tendon near its attachment permitted a better result than if tendon had pulled off muscle junction or if muscle had ruptured through its own substance.

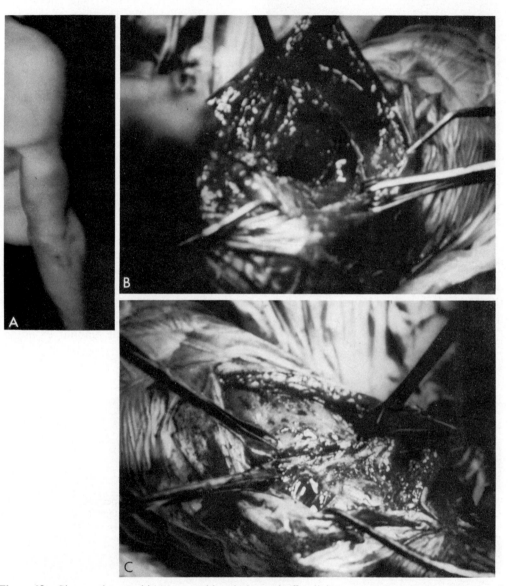

Figure 39. Six months ago this 14 year old male jumped off a diving tower, a wet rope caught around his upper arm, and he hung by his arm. There was immediate bulging of the muscle with gross indentation. His doctor advised him to wear a sling for 12 days. *A,* At examination six months later, he had a notable indentation with bunching up in the mid arm. He still favored the arm and experienced tiring on prolonged use. At surgery, there was a gross defect transversely across the medial and long heads of the triceps with retraction of both ends, the interspace being a very thick walled bursa. *B,* The gaping hole between the muscle heads, held in the tenacula. *C,* The two ends apposed, held in the tenacula. These were repaired by direct suture. Good function of the long head was restored with less definite contraction of the medial. Some of this deep furrowing in the arm persisted owing to loss of subcutaneous fat.

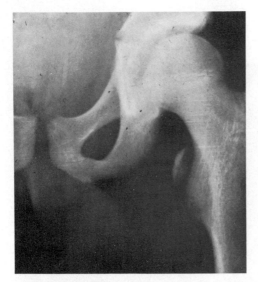

Figure 40. Avulsion of the lesser trochanter by the psoas tendon. It was treated by immobilization with fibrous union, asymptomatic.

diagnose than the less severe ones since the area involved will be greater and the local reaction more severe (Fig. 41). One can only urge that when the physi-

cian suspects injury to the muscle-tendon unit he at least make those rudimentary tests which may determine whether or not the function of this unit has been changed. This may seem elementary but the observance is often honored only in the breach. The injury occurs, there is obvious disability, diffuse tenderness and considerable pain. The involved area may be wrapped, strapped, or splinted or the patient put to bed without any actual effort to determine the exact diagnosis (Fig. 42). During the examination every effort must be made to localize the pathological condition to a specific area.

A rather common injury occurs to the thigh adductor muscle group (Figs. 43 and 44). This area may be quite difficult to examine since in such an injury the player tends to keep his thighs together and resist abduction since this causes pain. A little careful persuasion will ordinarily permit manual examina-

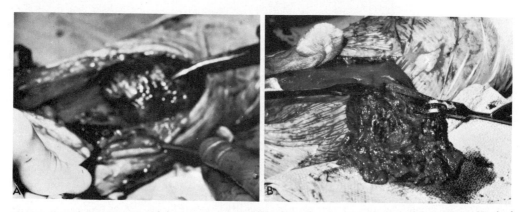

Figure 41. Eighteen year old boy was water skiing four days prior to surgical treatment. He had looped the handle of the tow line around his flexed left elbow, was thrown head over heels, the rope locked around his arm, and he was dragged through the water. The following morning extensive swelling was present in the entire arm. The nerve and blood supplies in the hand were intact. A balled mass that could have been either muscle or hematoma was present just above the front of the elbow. However, unlike an ordinary muscle, the mass did not contract when the elbow was flexed. Because patient was unable to define the exact site of pain, surgical exploration was temporarily deferred. Three days following initial trauma, a defect in the upper arm in the region of the biceps brachii was detected. Surgical treatment was performed on the fourth day following injury. *A,* The exposed mass is the belly of the muscle with the fibers and muscle bundles running transverse to the arm at right angles to the biceps. Releasing it from below, we flipped the end up and found that the proximal end was tucked under the distal portion. Nerve and blood supplies were completely severed, accounting for inability of muscle to contract. *B,* Necrotic mass was removed. NOTE: Elbow to the right of picture, shoulder to the left.

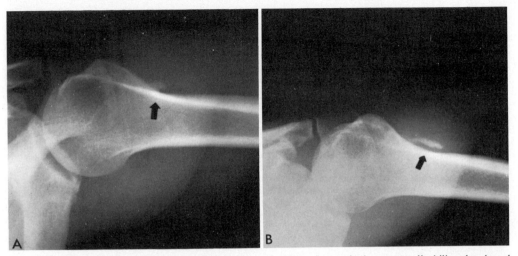

Figure 42. Shoulder x-ray of 20 year old wrestler in whom increasingly severe disability developed over many months. *A*, X-rays reveal calcification along margin of bicipital groove which was found at surgery to be calcification within the partially avulsed attachment of the teres minor at the lateral side of the groove. Resection of mass resulted in relief of patient's symptoms. *B*, Some postoperative recurrence with return of symptoms.

tion at which time a defect in the tendon can be noted, the location of tenderness may be defined and by careful testing interference of function of a specific muscle may often be determined. Active contraction or passive stretching of the unit will elicit pain at the site of injury. If active adduction of the thigh causes pain along the descending ramus of the pubis or in the vicinity of the ischium, one should suspect muscle damage in this area, particularly if the injury consists of overabduction. Careful palpation may actually localize the muscle involved. After careful physical examination, x-ray examination is valuable. It should be borne in mind, however, that routine views may be very unenlightening. Anteroposterior view of the pelvis for avulsion of the semimembranosus tendon may be completely negative whereas the flake of bone avulsed will show quite readily in the oblique or tangential views.

Treatment of these conditions is very rewarding. It may be enough simply to put the muscle at rest in the position in which the muscle is the shortest.

In rupture of the adductors, for instance, the patient could be placed with the knees together. This will not suffice if complete rupture has occurred since the very tone of the muscle will shorten it beyond its normally relaxed position.

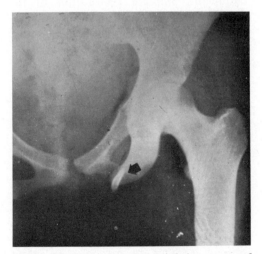

Figure 43. Avulsion of the inferior ramus of the pubic bone by the adductor muscle attachments following a fall by patient "attempting to do splits." Cartilaginous end of pubic epiphysis was palpable under the skin. Injury was treated by open reduction and internal fixation.

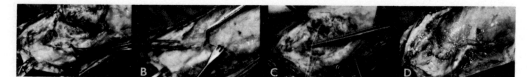

Figure 44. Surgical slides show exposure of thigh of 26 year old male who, while running relay, felt something snap on back of his thigh with attendant balling of muscle. Subsequently, he experienced posterior thigh pain. Although he was able to run moderately, he experienced a catching pain in this region whenever he attempted to sprint. Although desirous of playing professional football, he was unable to engage in even ordinary athletics. The injured muscle is exposed by a longitudinal incision along the back of thigh parallel to it. (For orientation, the right side is toward the trunk, the left is toward the knee.) *A,* The end of the ruptured long head of biceps femoris muscle is held by two tenacula. Towel clamp in center is on conjoined raphe of the long and short heads, the short head being intact. *B,* The two heads opposed. Tenacula now hold ruptured long head against its tendinous insertion. *C,* Mattress suture placed through muscle in three layers and passed up and through aponeurosis. *D,* After sutures are tied, biceps is restored to its normal attachments. Suture was possible after six weeks, since tendinous fibers were present with muscle mass.

For example, in the avulsion of the distal attachment of the biceps brachii, the arm may be placed in complete flexion so that the hand is on the shoulder and yet the avulsed tendon end will not lie in its normal position since the shortening of the muscle will draw it away from its bed. In the great majority of instances, complete rupture of the tendon unit requires surgical repair for normal function. Results of early repair are extremely gratifying. The difficulties of delayed repair are enormous and seldom result in complete restoration of the muscle unit. In many instances complete removal of the muscle units will be required because of functional interference by other adjacent groups.

SPRAIN

Injuries to the Ligament

DEFINITION

A sprain may be defined as an injury to a ligament resulting from overstress which causes some degree of damage to the ligament fibers or their attachment. A ligament is designed to prevent abnormal motion of a joint while permitting normal functional motion. Certain ligaments may bind two bones firmly together with relatively little motion, such as the tibiofibular syndesmosis which permits slight rotatory motion while preventing separation of the two bones. Other ligaments serve to reinforce a joint and permit a rather wide excursion of normal motion but prevent motion in an abnormal direction. Fundamentally, abnormal motion to a degree beyond the power of a ligament to withstand it will cause a sprain. This is to be contrasted with a direct blow over a ligament which may cause a contusion. As abnormal force is applied the ligament becomes tense and then gives way at one or the other of its attachments or at some point in the substance of the ligament (Fig. 45). If the attachment pulls loose with a fragment of bone, it is called a "sprain-fracture," but the mechanism is the same. The location of the damage will depend upon the weakest link in the chain of the ligament, which may be within the ligament itself or at one of its attachments, possibly at the site of an area of previous damage. The extent of the damage depends upon the amount and duration of the force. If the abnormal force is arrested or terminated promptly, there may be little actual functional loss to the ligament and only a few of its fibers may be involved. In this instance there is localized hematoma formation with prompt deposit of fibrin in the hematoma. The fibrin is invaded by fibroblasts, and as the reparative process proceeds the final termination is restoration of a normal ligament. If the damage is more severe, so that there is actually more disruption of ligament fibers, there may be considerable functional loss. Where the ligament is completely torn, all function is lost. In this case the findings will depend upon the location of the tear. Ordinarily there will be relatively extensive hematoma formation with swelling and edema. The process of

repair will be much slower and much less complete and, if untreated, will result in scar formation rather than restoration of normal ligament. The ligament may heal overlong and hence be slack and be subject to repeated stress. This will ultimately terminate in instability causing degenerative changes in the joint.

DEGREE

For the purpose of this discussion sprain will be divided into three dif-

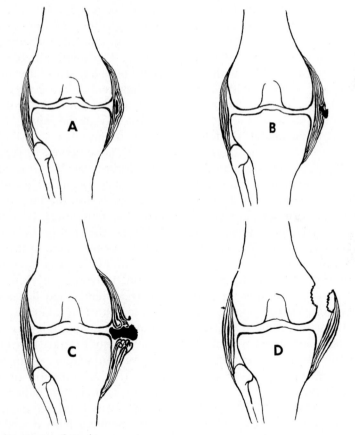

Figure 45. Various types of sprain.

A, Mild (first degree) sprain, in which there is a little hematoma in a very localized area in the ligament with only a few fibers separated.

B, Moderate (second degree) sprain, a more severe tear of the ligament but with at least half of the fibers remaining intact.

C, Severe (third degree) sprain. Complete tear through the ligament with separation of the ends.

D, Sprain-fracture. The ligament is torn off bone with a fragment of bone.

ferent categories according to the severity of the injury.

MILD (FIRST DEGREE) (FIG. 45, *A*). This is a sprain in which some fibers of a ligament have been torn with a little resultant hemorrhage into the ligament but with no actual functional loss. There is no demonstrable diminution in strength in the ligament. This is of considerable importance from the standpoint of treatment since the factor of protection is not important. The ligament is not weakened. Treatment is symptomatic only.

MODERATE (SECOND DEGREE) (FIG. 45, *B*). A moderate sprain is one in which some portion of the ligament is torn and some degree of functional loss is present. The amount of damage may vary from tearing of a relatively small portion of the ligament to almost complete avulsion — from "mild" with no functional loss to "severe" with complete functional loss of the ligament. The emphasis here must be on protection since one may be unable to determine the actual extent of the damage. One would not expect wide retraction of the torn ligament ends in a moderate sprain. Union can therefore proceed in an orderly manner with replacement of fibrous scar by ligament during the process of repair. If the damage is relatively severe, however, there may be considerable permanent scar formation with resultant weakness in this segment of the ligament. Obviously, protection here is mandatory to promote efficient repair and prevent permanent weakness. "Once a sprain always a sprain" is an aphorism not acceptable in the modern concept of therapy.

Yes, a sprain may heal. The greatest challenge to the physician in the treatment of sprain is in the moderate type. Most orthopaedists now accept surgical treatment as being necessary for the complete recovery of a complete ligament tear. The fact that it takes 6, 8, or 10 weeks for the ligament to heal after surgical treatment is readily accepted by both doctor and patient. The ligament is protected for this period.

Not so the moderate sprain. For the ligament to heal properly, the ligament ends must be apposed and held there until they have healed. In the moderate (second degree) sprain the ligament ends have not been widely separated since the remaining portion of the ligament has prevented dislocation of the joint. Hence, the ligament ends are presumably close together. It will, however, require the same length of time to heal, (namely, 6, 8, or 10 weeks) and probably will require 4 months to become secure. In the case thus treated nonsurgically, the symptoms of pain, swelling, and edema subside in 2 or 3 weeks. The joint is stable. Normal motion and even stress are pain free. Yet, the ligament is in the very early stage of healing, and not really any stronger than on the day of the injury. The player returns to play. The so-called "healed ligament" is subjected to repetition of the very forces that hurt it in the first place. The injury recurs. This often happens repetitively and the joint that was stable after the first injury becomes unstable. Witness the influx of unstable joints sent in for treatment at the season's end.

The player may have had excellent treatment for the early, brief period; yet the treatment failed because protection was too short. It takes as long for a ligament to heal as it does for a bone.

SEVERE (THIRD DEGREE) (FIG. 45, *C*, *D*). In severe sprain there is complete loss of function of the ligament due to a force that either tears it completely away from one or the other of its attachments or pulls it apart somewhere within its substance. One must presume that there has been at some time wide separation of the ligament ends, else the tear would not have been complete. Since efficient repair is dependent upon apposition of the torn ends of the ligament, it becomes vitally important to replace the ligament ends in approximation. We have been able to show experimentally in the dog that if the torn ends of the ligament are placed together the tissues heal by ligament fiber. On the other hand, ligaments which heal across a gap by scar formation never take on the characteristics of normal ligament.

It can be seen, therefore, that in first degree sprain *treatment* is relatively unimportant and is designed mostly toward prevention of pain; and that in second degree sprain the critical factor in *treatment* is protection in order to permit repair. On the other hand, in third degree or severe sprain the emphasis must be placed on reapposition of the ligament ends in order to assure a ligament that not only heals in its normal length but with its normal strength. It follows that diagnostic acumen is of great importance in the management of ligament injuries, since treatment depends upon the nature of the lesion rather than upon the patient's progress following injury.

DISLOCATION

Dislocation, or luxation, may be defined as an actual displacement of the opposing contiguous surfaces making up a joint. This, of necessity, presumes loss of function of some of the ligament structures of the joint since the ligaments are designed to prevent displacement or abnormal motion. *Subluxation* is a partial dislocation. In acute sprain when the ligament finally tears, the joint subluxates either by a slipping of the bone ends on themselves or by a separation of the bone ends. If the force continues until the joint actually is disrupted there is a dislocation. This may be spontaneously reduced or the bones may lock in the dislocated position (Fig. 46); in either instance there is loss of function of the ligament.

It is possible to have a chronic dislocation without fresh damage to the ligament. In this case one presupposes that the ligament has been previously torn or stretched to the point that dislocation of the joint occurs within the capacity of the surviving ligament. However, in acute dislocation or acute

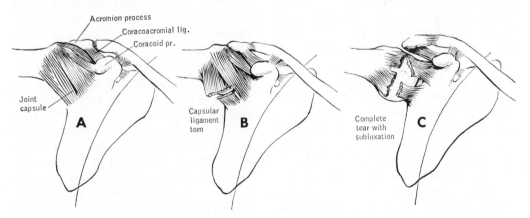

Figure 46. Complete dislocation showing attendant ligament damage.
A, First stage of dislocation of the shoulder. The arm is externally rotated and abducted, tightening up the anterior and inferior capsular ligaments. The tuberosity hinges on the acromion.
B, Continuation of the force with the tuberosity locked firmly against the acromion. The ligament fibers tear antero-inferiorly and the head begins to subluxate.
C, Head subluxating downward and further away from the acromion. Complete rupture of the capsular ligaments.

subluxation the ligament must tear. This is of considerable importance from the standpoint of treatment, because if, in an acute dislocation, one visualizes a complete tear of one or more ligaments, the advisability of surgical repair must certainly be considered seriously.

Treatment. Since dislocation is simply the end result of a severe sprain, it can be treated as such. Thus, protection is essential until the ligament has healed, regardless of the method used to secure its repair. For example, if a shoulder dislocates it may promptly be reduced either by a teammate, the coach or the physician. The fact that it remains out of joint 30 seconds or 30 days is no indication of the extent of ligament damage, although it may have vast effect on the end result. Even if the joint dislocates and immediately reduces itself, nonetheless there is ligament damage and treatment must be designed to further the repair of this tear. In some instances surgical repair will be advisable, while in others it will not be necessary. In either event the importance of carrying out protection until the ligament completely heals cannot be overemphasized.

Dislocations as a group are vastly undertreated and as a result are notorious for poor results. The dislocated finger may be promptly reduced, but if the player continues to play or goes without medical care or without splinting of the finger, permanent disability of the involved joint almost inevitably results. Either a painful, swollen joint with restricted motion or a weak, relaxed joint with recurrent dislocation is often the consequence of a nonprotected dislocation. A minimum of six weeks is needed for a ligament to repair even under optimum circumstances. Even at six weeks the actual strength of the repaired ligament does not approach normal, so suitable protection should be continued. After the six weeks of complete immobilization of the involved joint the finger may be fastened to the adjacent one by tape loops or other bands so that the finger flexes, and extends but lateral stress is eliminated. (See Knee Dislocation, p. 600.)

TENOSYNOVITIS

Tenosynovitis may be defined as inflammation of the synovium surrounding a tendon. This inflammation is usually due to strain from unaccustomed overuse but may be due to a direct blow or to infection. The result is reaction of the normally avascular synovium with increased blood supply, invasion by inflammatory cells, oversecretion of synovial fluid and increase in fibrin content causing "sticky" adhesions between the tendon and its surroundings. The exact manifestations vary greatly, depending upon the tendon involved, and will be considered in some detail under various headings. Actually the symptoms are those which would be expected to result from irritation of inflamed tissue by motion of the tendon. The first manifestation is pain on function, which may progress to the point of constant pain even at rest. Crepitation is frequently present. As the tendon slides up and down it adheres to the synovium causing so-called "snowball crepitation," which can be felt by placing the fingers over the involved tendon while it slides up and down. As the condition progresses, the adherence between the tendon and synovium becomes more firm and may finally result in complete loss of the gliding capacity of the tendon within its sheath. This is particularly true in areas where there is a true tendon sheath (such as the long head of the biceps at the shoulder) and is not common where mesotendon is concerned as in the tendo Achilles. *Treatment* is directed toward the pathological disorder and the principles of treatment are rest, local heat and local injection. The specific treatment will vary according to the site of the condition. Steroids should not be used topically for acute conditions.

SEQUELAE OF TENOSYNOVITIS

Under ordinary circumstances and with proper care, the tenosynovitis will subside completely and normal function results. In certain cases, however, either because of the severity of the condition or as the result of inadequate treatment or the anatomical characteristics of the area involved, complications may arise which may cause severe and permanent disability.

The first of two common sequelae of chronic tenosynovitis is *adhesive tenosynovitis*. As the name implies, the tendon and its surrounding sheath become bound in an inflammatory mass leading to actual adherence between the two,

which interferes with the normal gliding motion of the tendon (Fig. 47). This restriction of motion may be complete or only partial. The degree of disability will depend upon the location of the involved tendon. If it is in an area where there is a true sheath, such adherence will prevent motion completely and the muscle-tendon unit loses its function in regard to this particular area. On the other hand, if it is in an area not constricted by a true sheath, the adherence may simply result in traction strain and possibly some restriction of function rather than complete loss. Treatment for true adhesive tenosynovitis is difficult, since if the adhesions are trimmed away they may promptly reform. However, resection of the sheath or transferring the tendon to a less constricted area may be effective remedies.

The second common sequela is *constrictive tenosynovitis* caused by thickening of the walls of the sheath with resultant narrowness of its lumen. This frequently occurs in an area where

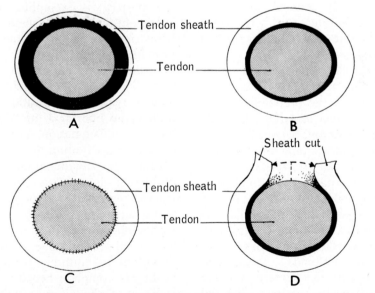

Figure 47. Tenosynovitis. *A,* Drawing showing the tendon lying in the sheath with some irritation of the inner wall of the sheath. *B,* Same area, showing the tendon sheath and underlying tendon both swollen and the sheath very tight. *C,* Same area, showing the sheath and tendon adherent to each other. *D,* The area after sectioning of the sheath and releasing of the pressure.

more than one tendon passes through the same tunnel or sheath. In such an instance the tendon itself is not adherent to the sheath, but the sheath is so tight that the tendon will not slide through it. This may start as an initial snapping, such as a trigger finger, and may terminate in complete loss of gliding of the tendon through this tunnel. Whereas adhesive tenosynovitis is difficult to treat adequately, this constricting type is readily relieved by simply enlarging the tunnel surgically by resection of a part of the sheath. These conditions will be discussed in some detail in relationship to specific areas in the body.

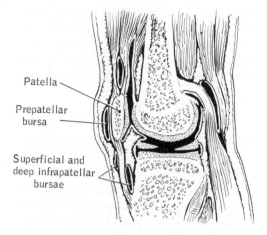

Figure 48.   The patellar bursae.

BURSITIS

Bursitis is an inflammatory reaction within a bursa. It may vary in degree from very mild irritative synovitis with discomfort to suppurative bursitis with actual abscess formation. A bursa is specifically designed to facilitate motion between contiguous layers of the body, and the athlete with his violence of motion is particularly prone to bursal involvement resulting from repetitive local trauma due to tissue friction or from direct blows.

The examples of bursitis are legion. The bursae most frequently damaged by direct trauma are the prepatellar, lying between the patella and the skin (Fig. 48) and the olecranon, between the olecranon process of the ulna and the skin. The trauma is usually repetitious, resulting in synovial irritation with thickening of synovium and formation of excess fluid. A large sac of synovial fluid is contained within the bursa. By virtue of the increased tension in the bursa, additional direct trauma tends to further distend its walls until the bursa may reach an amazing size. *Treatment* is directed toward prevention of repeated injury and reduction of the irritation within the

bursa. Aspiration of fluid, local injection of corticoids, protection against direct trauma and application of a pressure bandage to appose the walls of the sac are in order. If the condition becomes chronic and the synovitis is persistent, surgical removal of the bursa may become necessary.

Bursitis caused by friction between moving parts is exemplified by that occurring in the bursa beneath the internal hamstring tendons at the knee. Here the principal manifestation of bursitis will be pain on motion of the knee, tenderness over the bursa and local inflammatory reaction. Aspiration will be of little value but local injection may reduce the inflammation. *Treatment* must consist in preventing the motion that is causing the inflammation rather than protecting it against direct trauma. Local injection of a long-acting anesthetic agent plus a corticoid together with application of local heat and a protective splint is of value. Here again it is important to continue protection until healing is complete because recurrence is likely if the activity that originally caused the inflammation is resumed earlier.

SYNOVIAL HERNIA
(GANGLION)

Another condition involving the tendon sheath and sometimes the joint is the synovial hernia or so-called *ganglion*. This condition as a rule results from a defect in the fibrous sheath of the joint or tendon that permits a segment of underlying synovium to herniate through it. In the athlete it usually follows a mild sprain, although it may also be degenerative in nature. The irritation accompanying this herniation results in continued secretion of fluid so that the sac gradually fills up and enlarges. In some instances it may reach an alarming size.

As a rule the synovial hernia will appear as a small, discrete, sometimes extremely hard nodule lying directly over the tendon or the joint capsule. It is often impossible to tell whether the primary involvement is tendon or joint. The consistency of the tumor may vary from that of bone to that of a soft, fluctuant, obviously liquid mass. This difference in consistency is more apparent than real and is due to the degree of tension within the sac, since the sac uniformly will be found to contain a clear, gelatinous, viscous fluid which is blood-tinged only following aspiration or recent trauma. Certain areas of the body have a particular predilection for synovial hernia, notably the wrist.

The *differential diagnosis* is that of a tumor mass and is not unduly difficult. Synovial hernia may be confused with a dislocated bone such as the semilunar at the wrist. It must be distinguished from a neoplasm. Its general location, the lack of local symptoms, the consistency—all are definite diagnostic leads. The mass will ordinarily be translucent to transillumination, but this may on occasion be extremely difficult to demonstrate by this procedure owing to unfavorable location. Pain is not a notable factor. The complaint usually is that of a sprain of an adjacent joint. There may be pain and aching on overuse. Frequently extremes of motion may cause considerable discomfort, particularly if the protrusion is recent and rather tight.

Treatment of synovial hernia is essentially surgical. Although these masses do tend to come and go and so may respond to periods of splinting and protection or snug wrapping, these measures do not usually solve the problem. They merely postpone it. I have, however, known of many cases in which the ganglion has spontaneously regressed and to my knowledge never recurred. When it is symptomatic enough to interfere with athletic activity, it should be removed. In surgical excision great care must be taken to remove the whole mass. The defect in the capsule or sheath must be repaired since recurrence is very likely after incomplete removal. The prevalent habit of making a ½ inch incision and popping the mass out like a cyst is really no more effective than the time-honored method of beating it with the edge of a book and is doomed to failure. I well recall a romance that was blighted when I temporarily cured a ganglion over the dorsum of the lady's foot by a sharp blow with the edge of a frying pan.

Aspiration followed by injection of corticoids has been recommended. In my experience this has been unsatisfactory. However, it may serve to postpone definitive treatment until a more suitable time. To the athlete such a time is at the termination of his season of activity. Under these circumstances the joint should be carefully protected against overstrain. There is no objection to adequate strapping and continued participation provided this can be made pain-free. Following successful surgical removal, rehabilitation should be as careful as following any joint surgery and protective strapping should be used throughout the remainder of the season since there is some weakness of the joint inherent in this condition.

STRESS FRACTURE*

With the increasing involvement in sports activities by non-athletes that seems to characterize this era, the non-conditioned participant is exposed to the same hazards of injury as is the trained athlete. Alas, he is ill-equipped physically to withstand the forces to which his weekend activities will expose him. A particularly puzzling condition is the stress, or fatigue, fracture.

During World War I, many young men were put into uniform with ill-fitting shoes and a pack on their back and were required to take long hikes over rough terrain. Metatarsal bones were not prepared for this excessive stress. The term "march fracture" was coined to describe the fracture of the metatarsal shaft that was caused, not by acute injury, but by repeated stress (Fig. 49). The condition is peculiarly deceptive, since there is no history of injury, early x-rays are negative, and yet the symptoms persist. "Goldbrick" is a common label that is dispelled only by the appearance of periosteal new bone formation that develops at the site of the insult.

Nor is the appearance of this new callus a wholly unmixed blessing, deceptive once again because of the absence of injury, early negative x-ray, and persistent local tenderness and pain in the bone. The delayed appearance of periosteal new bone formation mimics that of dread bone sarcoma (Fig. 50). Biopsy is particularly misleading since early callus is often indistinguishable from early tumor.

---

*Printed in part in O'Donoghue, D. H.: The Deceptive Stress Fracture. Consultant Magazine, Vol. 13, #11, pp. 106–111, Nov., 1973.

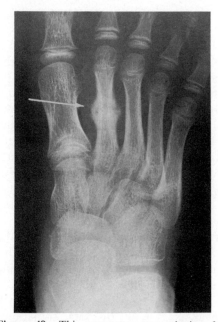

Figure 49. This youngster was playing football and complained of soreness in his right foot. He had no history of any specific injury. There had been three weeks of continued crippling when this x-ray was taken. Note complete absence of any fracture line as such. This is a typical "stress" fracture in that there was no definite injury, no specific moment of disability. Although his lesion was fairly mature when first seen, he was treated with a boot cast because he was still symptomatic. Uneventful recovery.

As this condition has become better understood, it is recognized that a little patience will reveal the progression of early callus to mature bone with healing of the stress defect (Fig. 51). Ofttimes this may occur without an actual fracture line ever appearing across the shaft.

While this condition is very common in the foot, this stress or fatigue fracture can appear almost anywhere and under the most confusing of circumstances (Figs. 52 and 53). A high index of suspicion plus a careful examination that reveals painful stress and tenderness over the bone occurring without specific trauma, but under rather unusual stresses, adds to the diagnostic picture.

Once suspected, x-ray examination, repeated at weekly or bi-weekly intervals, will secure the diagnosis. I must repeat that one must resist the temptation to biopsy. An early biopsy may lead to tragedy. If the mass is really

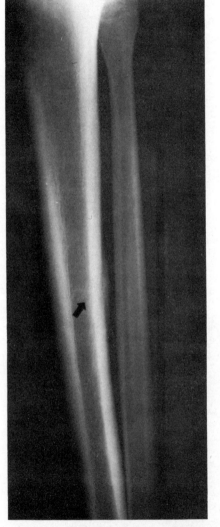

Figure 50. This long distance runner began to have cramping in his calf and pain in his leg that was increased by exertion. X-ray made after several weeks shows periosteal proliferation back of the tibia and a transverse line of sclerosis across the bone indicating the original stress fracture. Because of his persistent complaint and the appearance of the x-ray, he was biopsied elsewhere one week later. The biopsy report was "proliferation of new bone, probably callus." This is a rather classical instance of stress fracture that is quite common in track athletes and is frequently confused with tumor.

malignant, the 2 to 4 weeks delay necessary to permit callus to mature will not adversely affect the progress of the tumor. It may well prevent a diagnostic and therapeutic error. If biopsy is carried out, the pathologist will be faced with a real dilemma. It may not be possible for him to differentiate between early callus and new growth of a tumor. Recommendations for amputation have bèen made and, indeed, carried out when it seems, in retrospect, that the pathology was probably a stress fracture rather than a malignancy.

No age is spared. While the condition is common in young athletes, it may also occur at any age (Fig. 54). Only very occasionally will stress fracture progress to actual separation of the fragments. Stress fracture is not the same condition as the incomplete fracture occurring after an acute injury. In the acute injury, the fracture line may not be immediately recognizable and the patient may be treated for sprain. The history of the acute injury, however, renders the problem less confusing and subsequent x-rays will confirm the diagnosis. The uncertainty about the diagnosis of a true stress fracture is in the absence of a history of acute injury.

The treatment is protection against stress until the lesion has solidly healed, followed by gradual resumption of activities in order to build up strength and resistance in the involved area. Since weight-bearing bones are subject to the most stress, i.e., foot, tibia, fibula (Fig. 55), femur, pelvis, and back (Fig. 56), prevention of weight-bearing may be necessary. A walking cast may not suffice in leg bones. Pain is the indicator. If it hurts to walk, walking must be interdicted until it becomes pain free as the healing progresses. Since the diagnosis may not be confirmed for 2 or 3 weeks, it follows that treatment of the painful extremity—with possible history of some unusual activity, followed by ach-

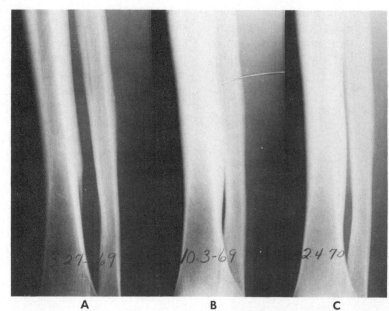

A   **B**   **C**

Figure 51. Six months ago this 17 year old male, while running in track, started having pain in the right shin. This continued to get worse and interfered with his running. *A,* The original x-ray three weeks post onset shows early callus with bone production around the distal third of the tibia. He was advised that he had a stress fracture but there was no treatment. He continued to have trouble off and on all summer; lately, so severe, he could not run at all. Examination revealed tenderness in the distal third of the tibia, particularly posteriorly. *B,* Six months after the onset, x-ray shows increased maturity of the bone. Since he was still quite symptomatic, a plaster cast was applied at this time with symptomatic improvement. *C,* One year later, x-ray shows complete maturity. Patient asymptomatic.

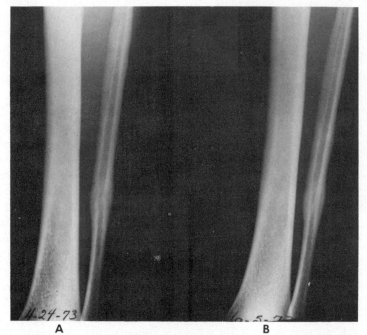

A   **B**

Figure 52. This 18 year old male injured his left fibula in the middle third six months before. X-ray negative. No treatment. The leg improved and apparently healed. Three months later he started running and began to have increasing pain so that finally he could not run. Examination revealed tenderness over the distal third of the shaft of the fibula with some thickening of tissue and some enlargement around the bone. *A,* X-ray six months subsequent to the injury revealed a typical stress fracture at the junction of the middle and lower thirds. *B,* Two months later, x-ray shows the resolution and maturity of the callus.

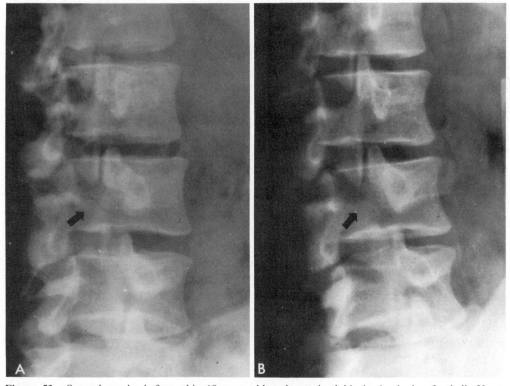

Figure 53. Several weeks before, this 19 year old male strained his back playing football. X-rays were reported negative. He continued to have a painful low back that was relieved some by a brace. One week later he tried to play, collapsed, and had to be helped from the field because of severe right lumbar muscle spasm. Routine AP and lateral x-rays were negative. *A,* Right oblique view shows stress fracture of the pars interarticularis of L-3 Right. *B,* Uneventful recovery following conservative treatment. If routine x-rays do not reveal the pathology, special views should be made. (Standard AP or PA oblique views will illustrate this while usual AP and lateral films will not.)

Figure 54. This 56 year old lady took an unaccustomed long hike. Toward the end of the day she noted increasing pain on the top of the foot, more severe during the night. Examination revealed tenderness over the second metatarsal with swelling. Clinical diagnosis was stress fracture. *A,* X-ray negative. She was placed in a walking cast for six weeks. *B,* X-ray six months later shows minimal mature callus. Uneventful recovery. I believe the early immobilization accounts for the minimal callus formation.

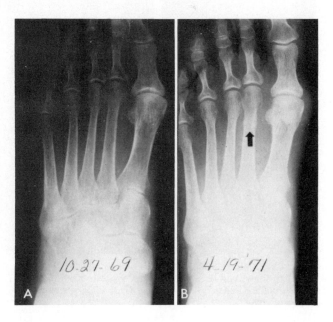

ing pain, becoming more severe, remaining quite localized, and accompanied by tenderness on the bone—should require non-weight-bearing and whatever degree of immobilization is necessary to relieve the pain. There is no reason to postpone the initiation of treatment until the x-ray is positive, since this only prolongs the period of disability. Surgery has no place in the diagnosis or treatment of this condition. Spare the scalpel!

FRACTURE

There is nothing particularly unique in the *treatment* of fractures of the athlete. The general principles previously mentioned must be constantly borne in mind, for while one should always attempt to get the best result in the quick-

est time with a minimum of interference of activity, this becomes particularly pertinent in the athlete. By and large, a definite fracture is usually adequately treated, since the injury is severe enough to make the diagnosis obvious. The use of x-ray examination is so universal now that the ordinary fracture is recognized early.

Certain exceptions to the previous statement will be discussed in detail under proper headings. I should like to mention specifically fracture of the navicular at the wrist, "march" fracture of the metatarsals (Fig. 49) and fatigue fracture of the fibula (Fig. 55). These conditions are all too frequently overlooked because the immediate symptoms may be chronic in nature. Invaluable time is lost during which the crippled athlete believes he has a strain or a sprain. The ideal time for treatment

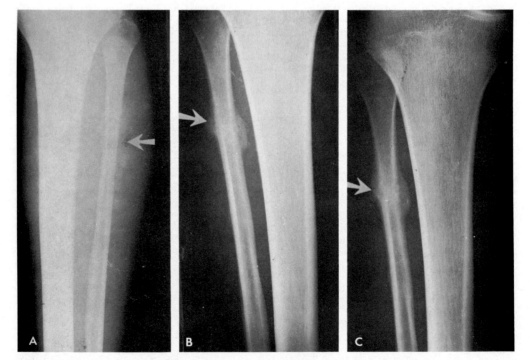

Figure 55. Fatigue fracture. This fracture may be mistaken for myositis ossificans or a tumor. *A,* Early film shows periosteal proliferation suggestive of tumor. *B,* There is increased periosteal proliferation but the fracture line is now appearing. *C,* Healing stage. The fracture line is disappearing. Notice consolidation of callus.

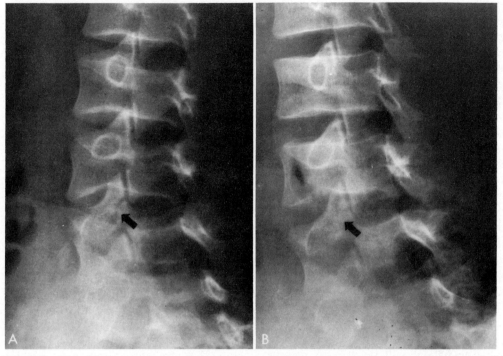

Figure 56. This 16 year old male pulled a muscle in his back while wrestling six weeks before. It did not seem too severe and he was treated by the usual heat modalities. He had some improvement. Two days ago he was running and had recurrence of severe intractable pain in the back with muscle spasm in the back extending into either hip. Examination revealed pain in the right lumbar muscle mass with spasm. *A,* X-ray reveals a fracture across the pars interarticularis over L-5 on the right. *B,* Two months later his cast was removed and he had solid union. Asymptomatic.

has frequently passed when the condition is finally recognized.

Another type of fracture that may easily be overlooked is the avulsion fracture. The athlete is subject to sudden spurts of violent activity that may forcibly avulse a fragment of bone either at a tendon or a muscle attachment (Fig. 57). The condition is primarily one of muscle-tendon injury, the bone fragment being incidental. Its treatment should be that of the primary condition. Neglect or oversight may cause long periods of chronic disability. This is particularly true since this fracture is very prone to calcification or ossification of the accompanying hematoma.

The optimal treatment of fractures depends upon prompt and definitive

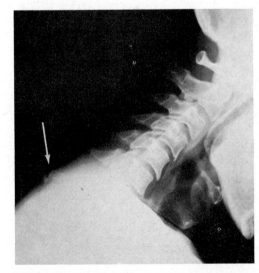

Figure 57. Fresh injury of the neck showing avulsion fracture of the tip of the seventh cervical spinous process.

diagnosis. Since these patients are in good health and in splendid physical condition, one may almost always use the best method of treatment without that compromise necessitated by the patient's poor condition, which is so often necessary in regular practice. Hence, we are more prone to carry out open reduction of the various fractures where indicated, not only because the general condition of the patient will permit it but because by firm internal fixation we are oftentimes able to start rehabilitation at once. We may even be able to entirely avoid external fixation involving the adjacent joints.

REHABILITATION. The great importance of maintaining the athlete in good physical condition, if he intends to resume his athletic activity in the near future, must be borne in mind. If we presume in the case of a certain fracture that the patient will be able to resume athletic activity in four weeks, he will be wholly unable to do this if he has not in the meantime continued his rigorous training. For example, a minimal fracture of a malleolus without displacement may require fixation in a cast for four weeks. Throughout this interval the patient should be actively exercising his opposite extremity and his upper extremities. He should keep up exercises vigorous enough to maintain his endurance to some extent and keep on his training diet in order to avoid gaining weight. It is important also that the muscles of the involved extremity should be actively exercised. In this instance the boot cast itself can serve as a weight to permit exercise of the quadriceps, hamstrings, hip, abdomen and back. It is not so commonly recognized that by isometric contractions of the muscles within the cast he may also keep the muscles of the lower leg and foot in tone.

Again depending upon the location of the fracture, it may be possible to apply protective splints or a protective

dressing in such a way that he can resume competition. With judicious application of proper equipment, participation, even in football, may be permitted.

It can be seen that the whole success of such a program depends upon prompt, definitive diagnosis so that healing may progress rapidly and efficiently. Adequate protection must be maintained to minimize irritation at the fracture line which may result in overcalcification or delayed union. A prompt return to athletic competition will be hastened by early diagnosis, accurate repositioning, firm fixation, either internal or external, continuing rehabilitation and protective dressing. The doctor who is capable of treating fractures should have sufficient ingenuity to devise a specific program for each definite condition.

This book will make no attempt to cover the whole field of fractures but some that are more common to athletes will be discussed in considerable detail. An effort will be made to point out methods of treatment which have stood the test of time in regard to acceleration of physical activity following particular fractures.

CHONDRAL AND OSTEOCHONDRAL FRACTURES*

Although chondral and osteochondral fractures have been to a large extent overlooked in the management of these injuries involving the joint, more attention has been paid to them in the last few years. This is particularly pertinent in regard to the knee and ankle, since by far the greatest number of injuries occur in these two joints. Since the initial symptoms of the injury are often

*Printed in part in O'Donoghue, D. H.: Chondral and Osteochondral Fractures, Journal of Trauma, 6:469–480 © 1966, The Williams & Wilkins Co., Baltimore.

obscure and the immediate disability slight, an early definitive diagnosis may be difficult. By the time a proper diagnosis is made, the condition may have advanced from an acute injury to a chronic condition. Indeed, the initial injury may have been or may be completely overlooked or its significance minimized.

This whole question of separation of cartilage from bone with or without a bony fragment has been buried in a morass of contradiction. Osteochondritis dissecans, chondromalacia (particularly of the patella), joint mouse, idiopathic synovitis with effusion, chronic sprain and, in fact, many other lesions of the knee not initially diagnosed may well have originated as a chondral fracture. The diagnosis is frequently so delayed that the original injury may have been forgotten, particularly by the young athlete who is subject to multiple injuries and whose memory for them, at best, is none too good (Fig. 58). Many cases of so-called osteochondritis dissecans lesions originate as chondral or osteochondral fractures. This may be an avulsion fracture caused by traction of the posterior cruciate ligament at its femoral attachment (Fig. 59, Case 1). It

may be by the direct contusion of a blow driving the patella against the femur (Fig. 60). It may be a shearing fracture (Fig. 61) which occurs in the patella or in the lateral femoral condyle as the patella is dislocated over the lateral condyle. These injuries often cause relatively few early symptoms. The x-ray may well be entirely negative. There is too great a tendency for the x-ray to be considered the ultimate diagnostic instrument (Fig. 62). As a result, the patient goes along for weeks or months, his injury classified under various diagnoses indicated previously. Yet, there has been no real recognition of the true nature of his lesion nor any effort to determine the exact etiology.

This subject naturally divides itself into two categories, one the *acute fracture*, the other the *late manifestations*. The former must be differentiated from acute injuries to the ligaments, to the menisci, to the synovium or to the periarticular structures of the knee. The latter must be distinguished from other chronic intrinsic conditions of the knee.

No such simple division can properly be made, however, since it is apparent that the two groups are one and the same, the latter being the logical sequela

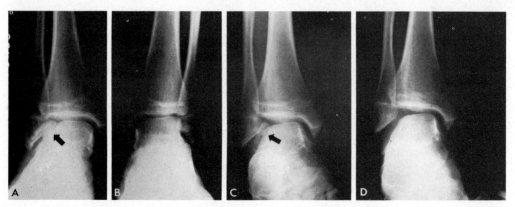

Figure 58. Fourteen year old girl seen with swelling of the ankle and persistent pain and disability, especially after prolonged standing. A fall, two years before, had been treated as a slight sprain. *A,* Shows osteochondral fracture at the dome of the talus, laterally. *B,* Normal ankle. *C,* Inversion view demonstrating fragment. *D,* Two months after surgical removal of fragment. No resultant instability but some persistent discomfort.

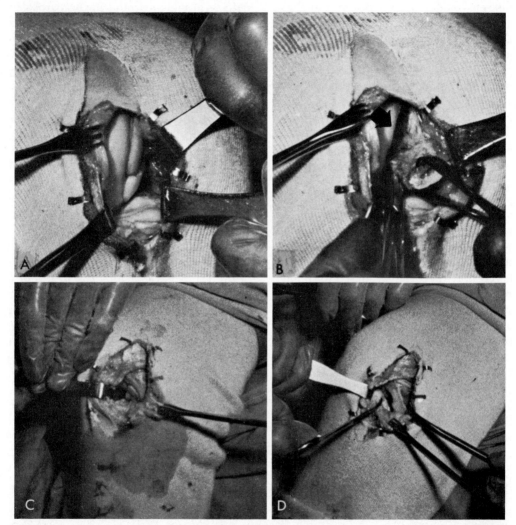

Figure 59. Comparison of acute and chronic chondral fractures of the femoral condyle. Case 1 (top). Injury to the knee at four weeks with continued disability and hemarthrosis. Surgery reveals a large osteochondral fragment containing two thirds of the femoral attachment of the posterior cruciate ligament. There is relatively fresh granulation tissue on both the fragment and the bed. *A*, Typical appearance of osteochondritis dissecans. *B*, The fragment with its vascular bed. Treatment was removal of the fragments and repair of the ligament into the bed by drill holes. Uneventful recovery. This is a chondral fracture, sub-acute.

Case 2 (bottom). Similar case at 18 months with intermittent effusion and moderate disability, and showing increasing synovitis. *C*, Surgery reveals fragments at the same location as in *A*, Case 1. Fragments and bed are quite sclerotic. The posterior cruciate ligament attaches to the fragments. *D*, Removal of the fragment and repair of the ligament through drill holes. This is a typical osteochondritis dissecans and would seem to have the same etiology as the Case 1 fracture. (From O'Donoghue, The Journal of Trauma, Vol. 6, 1966.)

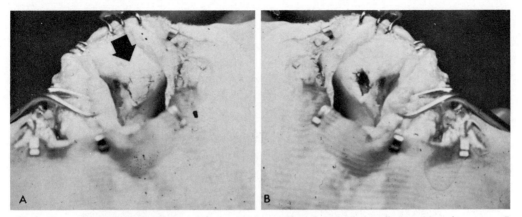

Figure 60.   *A*, Acute injury by direct fall on the flexed knee with bloody effusion. Negative x-ray. *B*, The defect after removal of the fragment showing the fresh vascular bed with blood that has infiltrated the cartilage. (From O'Donoghue, The Journal of Trauma, Vol. 6, 1966.)

of the former. Whether or not the acute fracture results in the chronic condition often depends directly upon the treatment or lack of treatment given the original condition. Chronic chondral fractures do not occur as such. They must evolve from an acute injury.

Once the chronic condition develops, it may be classified under a wholly different category. The acute fracture of the patellar cartilage be- comes patellar malacia (Fig. 63). Avulsion of the femoral articular cartilage by the posterior cruciate ligament attachment becomes osteochondritis dissecans (Fig. 59, Case 2). The displaced chondral fragment becomes the joint mouse (Fig. 64). Indeed, I believe that many, if not the majority, of cases of joint mouse, patellar malacia and osteochondritis dissecans occurring in young people are really chondral fractures.

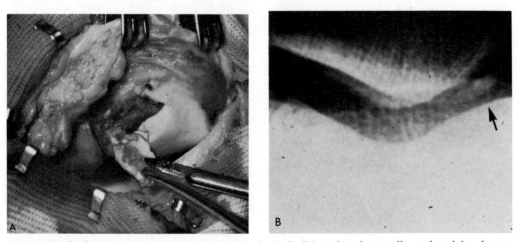

Figure 61.   Patient was blocked from behind in football dislocating the patella; reduced by doctor, no support. Examination four weeks later revaled gross swelling, hemarthrosis, and pain. Patella not loose or malaligned. *A*, The obviously fresh injury with fresh granulating bed caused by shearing force of the patella against the femoral condyle. *B*, Silhouette showing the osteochondral fragment (arrow). (From O'Donoghue, The Journal of Trauma, Vol. 6, 1966.)

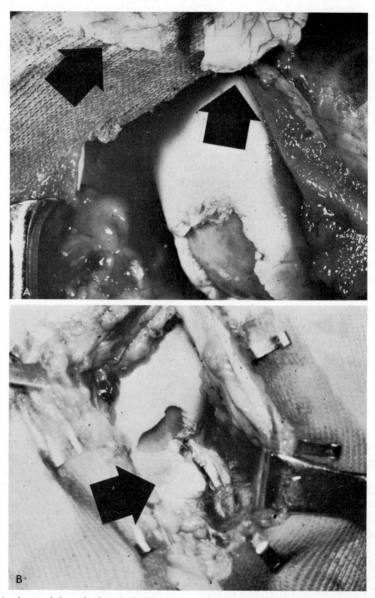

Figure 62. *A.* Acute injury in baseball from sliding into second base with direct contusion of the knee. Note fresh vascular bed and mosaic of blood through the avulsed fragment. *Negative x-ray. B,* A similar older injury in which the fracture bed is sclerotic and the fragments of cartilage are necrosed. This would be called *osteochondritis dissecans.* If fragments were completely loose, it would be called a *joint mouse.* Negative x-ray. (From O'Donoghue, The Journal of Trauma, Vol. 6, 1966.)

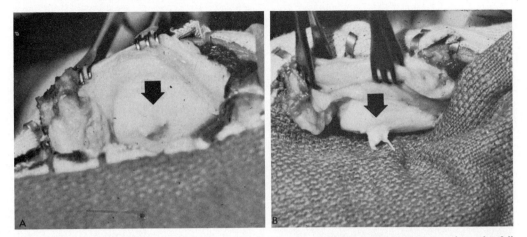

Figure 63. *A,* One year after direct fall on the knee, with chronic patellar symptoms since the fall. Note central area with degenerative cartilage similar to Figure 60*A*. *B,* "Shaving brush" protrusion of the cartilage. Note similarity of the lesion shown here with that in Figure 60: Both are chondral fractures, the one acute, the other chronic. (From O'Donoghue. The Journal of Trauma, Vol. 6, 1966.)

Acute Chondral Fracture

Mechanism of Chondral Fractures
1. Compaction
   A. Patella—direct trauma
   B. Tibial plateau—by femoral condyle
   C. Patellar groove of femur—by patella
2. Shearing force
   A. Patella—over femoral condyle
   B. Femoral condyle—by patella

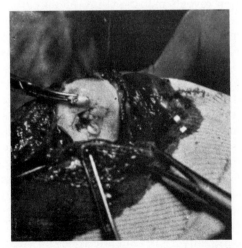

Figure 64. Acute traumatic dislocated patella. Note the acute chondral fracture in the middle third of the patella resulting from the forceful blow of the patella against the femur. (From O'Donoghue, The Journal of Trauma, Vol. 6, 1966.)

C. Condylar margin—by direct trauma
3. Avulsion
   A. Upper tibia—by anterior cruciate ligament
   B. Medial femoral condyle—by posterior cruciate ligament
   C. Patella—by quadriceps tendon, by medial retinaculum, and by patellar tendon

These fractures result from three main types of trauma: compaction, shearing and avulsion. *Compaction* fractures result from direct force applied vertically to the joint surface. The mechanism of compaction fracture is exemplified by the direct blow over the patella, crushing the patellar cartilage against the femoral cartilage. The femoral cartilage being convex is better able to withstand the injury, and the cartilage under the patella is compressed or compacted (Fig. 65). Similarly, the same type of injury which may cause a plateau fracture of the tibia may be limited in its force and cause compaction of the tibial cartilage as the convex femoral condyle crushes into it. The femoral condyle itself may be damaged by either the patella or the tibia by the same mechanism.

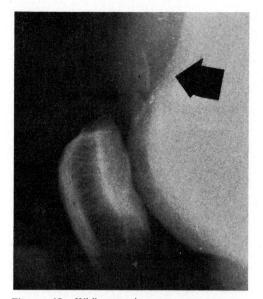

Figure 65. While running cross-country one year before, the patient stepped on a board at the edge of the track, fell, and injured the knee. (Previous hyperextension injury three years before.) Immediate pain and swelling ensued. Patient was operated upon elsewhere but no pathologic condition was found. No postoperative support. Two weeks postoperatively the patient kicked a football and the knee became swollen; subsequently, with continued trouble, a palpable mass was noticed, sometimes medially, sometimes laterally. At the second operation in November, 1963, a large osteochondral fragment was removed. The defect in the femoral condyle was represented by a small amount of dishing of the cartilage that was proceeding to complete obliteration. (From O'Donoghue, The Journal of Trauma, Vol. 6, 1966.)

Shearing fractures are the result of a glancing blow almost tangential or parallel to the articular surface. Such a fracture is exemplified by the shearing force of the patella against the lateral femoral condyle as the patella forcibly dislocates across it. The cartilage of the patella may be sheared off (Fig. 61) or the articular cartilage over the femoral condyle may be knocked off with or without a segment of bone (Fig. 66).

Avulsion fractures of the cartilage, often with a shell of bone, in many ways are the most intriguing because of the disability which may result from loss of function of the avulsing agent. A well recognized example is the fracture caused by the traction of the anterior cruciate ligament on the upper end of the tibia (Fig. 67). Similarly, avulsion of the portion of the cartilage by the quadriceps tendon (Fig. 68) or by the medial retinaculum of the patella is frequently seen (Fig. 69). Much less recognized is avulsion of the articular cartilage from the lateral side of the medial femoral condyle at the attachment of the posterior cruciate ligament (Fig. 59). Significantly, this is also a common place for so-called osteochondritis dissecans which is neither a chondritis nor a dissecting lesion.

Although this pathologic condition results from an acute injury, it can readily be seen that each of these types of trauma can under certain circumstances result in the chronic conditions previously mentioned, such as patellar malacia, osteochondritic foreign body and osteochondritis dissecans. Thus a fall on the patella may well cause a stellate type of fracture of the patella with or without compression of the subchondral bone. Early operation makes this abundantly clear (Fig. 60). Delayed observation reveals malacia (Figs. 63 and 70).

Avulsion of the osteochondral fragment by the posterior cruciate ligament is quite obvious if the patient is operated on early (Fig. 59, Case 1). Operation in the chronic stage reveals osteochondritis dissecans (Fig. 59, Case 2). The fragment sheared from the femoral condyle by the dislocating patella is obvious if enough bone goes with it to throw a shadow on a radiograph (Fig. 66). If, on the contrary, a dislocation shears off the undersurface of the patella, so-called patellar malacia may result. If the cartilage alone is sheared off, early surgery reveals the fresh fragment separated from a fresh bleeding bed like coconut meat from its shell. Yet, if this is not surgically treated until chronic

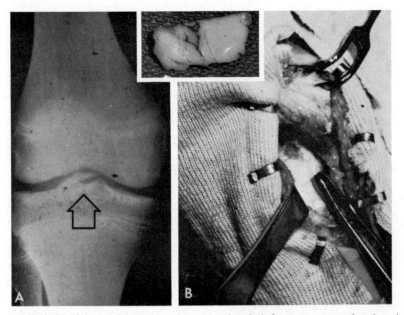

Figure 66. *A,* Twisting injury of knee causing osteochondral fracture, x-ray showing the fragment lodged in the intercondylar notch. *B,* Defect left by the osteochondral fracture of the lateral femoral condyle caused by the subluxating patella as the medial retinaculum ruptured. Inset shows fragment. (From O'Donoghue, The Journal of Trauma, Vol. 6, 1966.)

symptoms supervene, we find a cartilaginous foreign body, often without an obvious defect in the articular cartilage (Fig. 71).

It is difficult to explain osteochondritis dissecans of the femoral condyle as a vascular defect in an area which is so well vascularized. If infarction is the cause of the lesion, why does it not happen in the femoral head, for example,

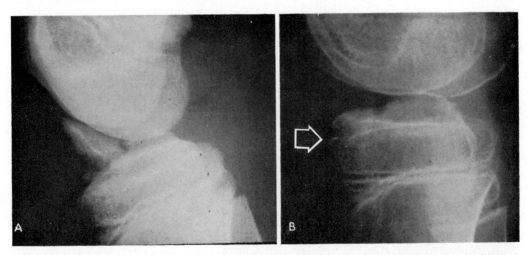

Figure 67. Young girl with injury to the knee from a bicycle accident, six months previously. Marked restriction of both extension and flexion. *A,* Osteochondral fracture caused by the anterior cruciate ligament pulling up the top of the tibia. *B,* Replaced and held by internal fixation through drill holes (arrow). (From O'Donoghue, The Journal of Trauma, Vol. 6, 1966.)

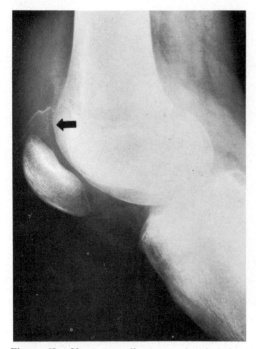

Figure 68. X-ray revealing osteochondral fragment avulsed by the quadriceps tendon. This fragment includes the whole attachment of the quadriceps mechanism. There was substantially more cartilage with the fragment than is indicated by the shell of bone seen in the x-ray picture. (From O'Donoghue, The Journal of Trauma, Vol. 6, 1966.)

where circulation may be regarded as poor, or possibly in the head of the talus or even more likely in the lunate or other carpal bones? We rarely see osteochondritis dissecans in these areas, but we frequently see it where the circulation is very good. The etiology must be trauma and not aseptic necrosis from a primary vascular defect.

The same type of pathologic change may occur in virtually any other location, the exact findings varying according to the nature of the injury. It must be agreed that at least some of the cases which are illustrated here are the direct result of acute trauma. Many others could be shown in which this seems equally acceptable but in which the definitive diagnosis was so late that they were labeled patellar malacia, osteochondritis dissecans, osteochondral foreign bodies and so forth. The patient is entitled to a meticulous examination at the time of his original injury. If at all possible a definite diagnosis should be made before the ideal time for treatment has passed. Most of these cases of osteochondral fractures that are recognized early and treated properly will have an entirely acceptable result. The old concept that hyaline cartilage does not regenerate must be abandoned. I personally have seen many cases in which a large defect from an acute osteochondral fracture has filled in completely. Many cases are seen in which there is a large osteochondral foreign

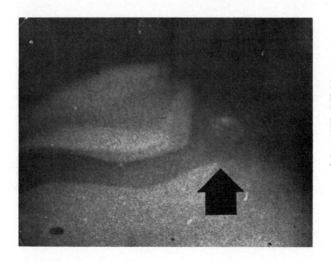

Figure 69. Acute traumatic dislocated patella. Note in the silhouette x-ray the small fragment of the medial border pulled off by avulsion of the quadriceps retinaculum as the patella dislocated. Refer to 406A for technique of x-ray. (From O'Donoghue, The Journal of Trauma, Vol. 6, 1966.)

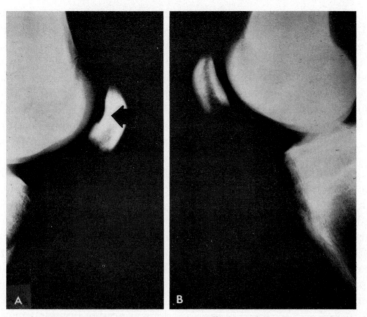

Figure 70. X-ray of a patient with chronic recurring effusion of the knee. *A,* Note the dishing out of the central portion of the patella (arrow). *B,* Normal patella. (From O'Donoghue, The Journal of Trauma, Vol. 6, 1966.)

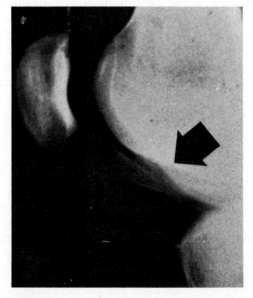

Figure 71. A 28 year old woman who had knee symptoms at age 16 and who has had occasional trouble since. Note the large osteochondritic fragment just below the femoral articular surface (arrow). Careful inspection of all the articular surfaces of the knee failed to reveal any defect from which this fragment was avulsed. The defect had completely filled in during the 12 years. (From O'Donoghue, The Journal of Trauma, Vol. 6, 1966.)

body in the knee without any recognizable defect in the joint cartilage, or with a defect which is essentially obliterated.

Ironically, the more severe injuries are recognized early and treated adequately. Therefore, better results are obtained in these than in the lesser injuries in which the treatment is delayed or inadequate. Thus, the severe injury recognized and treated promptly not only spares the patient the physical, mental and economic trauma of the prolonged period of disability but usually leaves a lesser degree of permanent disability.

DIAGNOSIS

These cases may be quite difficult or even impossible to diagnose early. This certainly should not be used as an excuse not to try. In any case in which the symptoms seem worse than the recognizable findings (i.e., pain under the patella, bloody effusion, tenderness along the condyles of the femur or pain on anterior or posterior stress of the flexed tibia), one should suspect chondral damage. If the patient does not respond to treatment, he should not be called uncooperative or nonconformist. *It is just possible that the treatment is at fault rather than the patient.*

In any acute injury of the joint it behooves us to try to make a definitive diagnosis as soon as possible. A very worthwhile extra dividend may be received from early diagnosis. Thus, if a meniscus rupture is diagnosed promptly and operated at once, it may be possible to recognize associated chondral damage early. Early diagnosis and prompt surgical treatment of an acute dislocation of the patella is the best treatment. Exposure reveals the medial retinaculum to be torn and gaping apart. Unrepaired, it can only heal with redundancy and in many cases with insecurity. Prompt surgical repair obviates this danger. Early surgery may reveal undiagnosable chondral fracture of the patella or femur, which should be treated surgically if treatment is to be successful. The reason for procrastination has often been an unwillingness to accept the responsibility for making a definitive diagnosis and then acting upon it. If you believe that the acute rupture of the meniscus should be treated surgically, how much better it would be to initiate this treatment early and so be able to handle other pathologic conditions in which the treatment must be carried out early if it is to be successful. The percentage of meniscus ruptures that completely heal is not large enough to justify waiting for the second, third or fourth episode before surgical treatment is recommended.

I have urged that the best results can be obtained only by prompt, definitive diagnosis. This may present very serious problems in the acute injury. Of first importance is the fact that the surgeon is cognizant of this injury. If he has a high index of suspicion in cases in which chondral fracture may have occurred, he will be much more likely to make the definitive diagnosis. Careful examination of the patient who presents himself following a fall on the patella, for example, may reveal tenderness around the margin of the patella. There may be evidences of a retinacular tear. Aspiration of the joint may reveal bloody fluid with fat globules. Very careful search of repeated x-rays may give some clue as to the lesion. The fact that these lesions often accompany other injuries to the knee is of great importance. One might hesitate to explore a knee simply on the suspicion of infraction of the patella. On the other hand, if the injury accompanies a retinacular tear, a double dividend may be awarded by permitting early treatment of both lesions. In my practice of early surgical treatment of ligament and meniscus injuries to the knee, I have many times been rewarded by recognition of an associated chondral fracture. Repeated examinations from day to day, not from week to week, and an objective analysis of the positive findings may lead to the proper conclusion. Once reached, the conclusion should be acted upon.

TREATMENT

Once the diagnosis is made, treatment becomes easy. If the patellar retinaculum is torn, it should be repaired. If either cruciate ligament is pulled away, it can be sutured. Not so well defined is the treatment of the chondral fracture. I have not been a proponent of replacement and pinning of the displaced chondral fragment. If it is an osteochondral fragment and is of fairly good size, such as a fragment of the femoral condyle, replacement and internal fixation may indeed result in union. So, too, if the fragment which is pulled off by the anterior cruciate ligament is large, such as a portion of the upper tibia, it may be easily replaced with appropriate suture and firmly held to its bed (Fig. 67). The osteochondral fragment pulled away by the posterior cruciate ligament also may be replaced surgically. If the fragment is small or is mostly cartilage, it should be removed and the ligament repaired to the raw bed. In each of these circumstances, the accompanying lesion demands some period of immobilization so that replacement of the fragment does not entail additional morbidity.

On the other hand, the purely chondral fragment, whether or not it is entirely loose or simply knocked loose and attached in some portion of its surface, poses a different problem. Regeneration of articular cartilage is encouraged by active function. Pinning of the fragment requires not only immobilization but also non-weight-bearing. This is not conducive to cartilage regeneration. My own preference in these instances is to remove the fragment, including all of the margin which is detached from the bone, and to trephine the defect by cutting the cartilage vertical to the articular surface until all of the fragmented or undermined cartilage is removed. This leaves a defect in the cartilage like a pit rather than a saucer.

In acute injury the bed is vascular and should be left alone. The defect should not be saucerized. To taper the cartilage down to the bed simply enlarges the defect. Whether regeneration comes from the bony bed below or whether it grows in from the margin is immaterial, since in either case the defect to be filled will be less in a trephined hole than in a tapered or shaved one. The patient is then encouraged to undertake active function, including weight bearing. Articular cartilage does regenerate. Whether or not it is true hyaline cartilage is beside the point, since it so resembles hyaline cartilage that it cannot be distinguished by observation, palpation, microscopic examination or even by chemical analysis. Certainly, if an acute defect is found in the cartilage, diligent search must be made in the joint to find and remove the fragment.

CHONDRAL FRACTURE

It is not the purpose here to discuss in detail treatment of the chronic chondral or osteochondral fracture. This will be discussed under the specific joint concerned. As has been indicated, these often cannot be distinguished from malacia, from osteochondritis dissecans, from cartilaginous foreign body and so forth. The treatment of each of these may be quite different. I repeat that there is little rationale for shaving of the defect in weight-bearing bone. I frequently do shave the patella, particularly since the lesion is often quite diffuse.

Treatment in the chronic case becomes a matter of salvage. The best judgment must be used, adjusted strictly to the circumstances present. The relatively small, well-defined malacic area should be trephined, not shaved. After trephining, the sclerotic bed should be drilled in order to improve vascularity and to make a more suitable bed in which the new cartilage may develop. Diffuse areas of malacia in the patella, femoral condyle or patellar groove must be shaved until firm cartilage is found, even though bare bone is exposed. If severe enough, patellectomy may be indicated. Patellectomy should be avoided in the young child until clinical trial of other measures is carried out.

In an old avulsion fracture the sclerotic fragment should be removed and the ligament repaired to the freshened bed. I see no purpose in replacing a necrotic fragment. So also, in the old shearing fracture, no attempt should be made to replace the fragment, which at best fits imperfectly into the old sclerotic bed. The fragment should be removed and appropriate treatment applied to the bed. If sclerotic, it should be drilled or curetted; if filled with unorganized debris, it should be curetted; if filled in well with organizing tissue, it should be left alone.

Early treatment is often rewarded by complete recovery. Procrastination might be successful only in the case of a patient without a disabling injury.

OSTEOCHONDRITIS DISSECANS

Osteochondritis dissecans is an articular cartilage involvement occurring most frequently in the knee. There is considerable disagreement concerning the exact etiology; some believe that the condition results from spontaneous ischemic necrosis due to faulty circulation in the epiphyseal vessels, while others believe that it is due to trauma, with a fissure-type chondral fracture down to the subchondral bone. As in so many conditions in which there is disagreement about the exact cause, it is probable that in certain instances more than one factor may be present, and that in others there is a disparate etiology. Thus, it may be that repeated trauma precedes the ischemic necrosis. Or, it may be that the necrosis develops spontaneously, and the actual dislodging of the fragment may be due to trauma superimposed on a pathologic area. It seems probable, however, that localized trauma is the most frequent cause.

In any event, the pathologic condition consists of the separation of a fragment of cartilage from the underlying matrix. This line of separation fills with granulation tissue. The separated fragment necroses because of poor circulation and, in effect, becomes a seques-trum. Since the articular cartilage of this fragment is nourished primarily by synovial fluid, the cartilage does not necrose at this stage but remains intact. In fact, the whole cycle of separation, necrosis, and regeneration may occur without any defect in the articular cartilage, and may terminate in spontaneous healing of the condition. On the other hand, if enough of the fragment is absorbed to permit it to depress into the crater in the epiphyseal bone, fissuring of the cartilage and ultimate separation may occur. It may be that in some cases trauma is the factor that ultimately breaks the fragment loose. So, in some cases the fragment may never separate and spontaneous recovery ensues. In other cases the fragment may become entirely free in the joint and then is a foreign body. The age incidence coincides with the age of active athletics, namely, adolescence and early adulthood. Thus, this condition is frequently seen in athletes. There is no preventive measure of any value.

The condition may be completely asymptomatic and be discovered only by incidental x-rays. More commonly there will be discomfort in the joint, sometimes accompanied by effusion, with symptoms of internal derangement. This may go on until there is actual locking of the joint if the fragment becomes free or if a flap of cartilage turns up and interposes between the articular surfaces. Many patients will present themselves with the complaint of chronic nonspecific joint pain with very few localizing symptoms.

The *management* varies from no treatment to operative excision of the fragment, and will be discussed in detail under the various joint categories. In general it may be said that in the very young, treatment should be conservative, since spontaneous regression will be seen in many cases if the part is protected (Fig. 72). In a non-weight-bearing

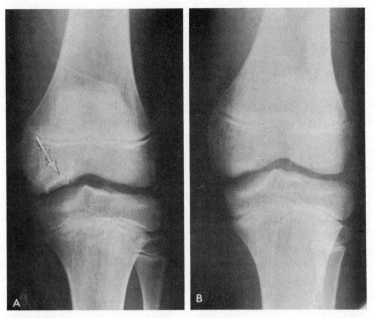

Figure 72.   Osteochondritis dissecans in a 12 year old athlete. *A,* Note the fragment on the medial femoral condyle, not detached. *B,* Five months later the mass is resolving with no treatment.

joint, surgery is less frequently required than in a weight-bearing joint. If the fragment completely separates (Fig. 73) or forms a flap interfering with motion of a joint, surgical treatment is manda-tory and includes removing the fragment and trephining the cartilaginous margins of the crater. Further measures will depend upon the extent and location of the lesion, since function may need to

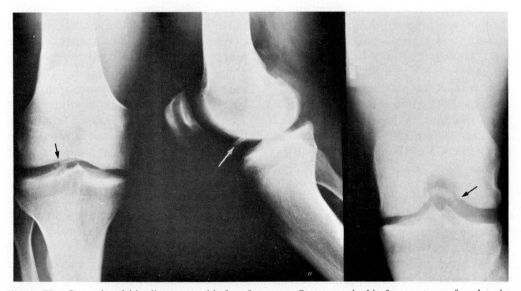

Figure 73.   Osteochondritis dissecans with free fragment. On removal, this fragment was found to be attached to a portion of the posterior cruciate ligament.

be restricted. Drilling of the sclerotic crater may help reconstitution of the cartilage.

MUSCLE CRAMPING

Muscle spasm or cramping is a very frequent complaint in the athlete. I am sure that there are many causes for this condition. I am equally sure that there are many things which are called muscle spasm or cramping that are due to some other pathologic state. Actually, the etiology and the pathologic features seem to be inextricably confused. Many common injuries will cause spasm of the muscle. Some of the more common are a blow to the muscle causing slight infiltration of blood, overstretch of the muscle causing rupture of some of the fibers, and strain by overcontraction of the muscle against resistance. Each of these causes the same type of injury to the muscle-tendon unit.

Frequently the muscle cramp or spasm appears to be an entity in itself. One of the most common and dramatic examples is the severe cramping that occurs in the calf of the apparently normal athlete. While going at full speed he suddenly gets a violent contraction of the calf which pulls the foot down into equinus and causes severe cramping pain. Indeed, this may come on when actual exertion is at a minimum, at least with respect to any overuse or overstretching. There are several causes of this condition, some remediable and some not. There appears to be no doubt that reduction of the quantity of salt by excessive perspiration will cause a condition in which the muscles of the body are quite subject to cramping. Changes in temperature, sudden chilling or even sudden overheating may also be responsible. Dietary considerations are sometimes important. Many of these factors can be obviated in an adequate training program. Such metabolic causes will require more emphasis on prevention than on cure.

In another category are those cases in which there is definite local impairment of circulation to the part, as when the cuff of the pants is too tight around the calf or the calf muscle has been strapped circumferentially in such a way as to interfere with its blood supply. There is no actual pathologic change in the muscle other than rapid build-up of muscle waste products and diminution of oxygen supply. Overfatigue may cause cramping for much the same reasons that constriction does. In this area I think the spasm is basically due to build up of CO_2 and diminution of oxygen, which would indicate that increased oxygenation might help. It has been my observation that individual muscle cramping, not necessarily under violent activity, can often be alleviated by deep breathing. This seems to be further supported by the fact that most of the isolated cramping occurs at night during sleep when oxygen exchange is at a minimum.

Ruling out all these potential causes for cramping, there still remains a group of cases in which there is no specifically recognizable cause for the condition. In most instances the player has had no preliminary symptoms, the muscle jumps into intractable spasm and the player is rendered helpless both by the pain and by the restriction of motion. Examination will elicit nothing other than the contracted muscle. The muscle is not particularly tender. There is no swelling or edema. One should suspect muscle spasm when sudden severe pain occurs in any muscular area of the body. This is particularly prevalent in the neck, in the back, in the hamstrings and calf. The fact that the cramping is common in weight-bearing portions of the anatomy but relatively infrequent in the upper extremities may be of some significance.

Treatment is usually simple and in the majority of instances can be administered by the player himself. His immediate instinct is to apply local pressure to the spastic muscle and to try to force it through a normal range of motion. The player will sit on the ground and grab his calf firmly with one hand while he dorsiflexes his foot with the other—an expedient that is often amazingly effective. The cramp may be released by simple contraction of the opposing muscle so that if there is a cramp in one flank, stretching the muscle by leaning to the opposite side will frequently relieve the tension.

If the player needs help in relaxing his spasm, the same principles apply. Steady, even, firm but atraumatic local pressure will often give dramatic relief. So also will simple stretching of the muscle. The combination of the two appears to be even more effective. One should constantly bear in mind that he is trying to restore only a normal range of motion; he must not overstretch the muscle. In the contracted hamstring, the knee should be extended, but forceful straight leg raising should not be carried out. If the calf is involved, the foot should be pushed up to 90 degrees but not forced into extreme dorsal flexion. For this reason these manipulations should be carefully controlled. Passive manipulation should be applied steadily and smoothly with no jerk or swing. To apply massive force with leverage against a muscle in spasm may result in rupture of the muscle fibers or even avulsion of the tendon, in which case a relatively simple condition is replaced by one much more serious. I know of no place in the treatment of any acute injury where this type of excessive manipulative force is desirable. It certainly is not desirable in the treatment of muscle spasm.

The same thing can be said about massage. Massage directed toward restoring circulation to the muscle is quite acceptable whereas deep kneading or pounding or pummeling of a muscle that is already insufficiently supplied with metabolites can result only in harm. As the muscle spasm relaxes, relatively gentle massage toward the direction of the venous flow may be useful. The muscle may be tapped gently from side to side by the two hands with a rolling manipulation of the muscle between the two palms. Usually this cramp is relatively short-lived, and the player may continue to compete although the condition is quite prone to recur within the immmediate future. If the cramping is more persistent, it will require further treatment. This consists of rest of the part and application of local heat. This can be done by whirlpool baths, warm packs, infrared or diathermy, or in fact any heat modality. Inductive heat appears to be more effective than radiant heat. Massage is valuable in restoring circulation to the muscle.

A patient who has had persistent muscle spasm may have residual soreness and aching in the muscle, and during this period he should avoid forceful activity. A carefully planned regimen of physical therapy with gradually increasing resistive exercises within his tolerance and short of pain-producing stimuli should be carried out. It may well be that these persistent symptoms following cramp are actually due to ruptured muscle fibers with edema and blood infiltration and should be treated as such. The duration of treatment will depend upon the symptoms. We cannot agree that the best treatment for torn muscle fibers with hematoma into the muscles is immediate active use in spite of pain and muscle spasm. Until one is absolutely sure that there has been no damage to the muscle itself in the nature of hemorrhage or edema or separated muscle fibers, there is no place for stretching, massage or active exercise.

PHLEBITIS

Phlebitis is not a common condition in the athlete, at least as a definite clinical entity. There is, of course, a certain amount of phlebitis accompanying contusions, sprains or strains, but this is a secondary local reaction and is quite amenable to the measures taken for relief of the specific injury. In the treatment of any local inflammatory condition one should be on the alert to detect signs of phlebitis. This is particularly pertinent in the lower extremities where the saphenous vein is quite susceptible to inflammation. The symptoms of developing phlebitis may be lost in the symptoms of the original lesion. If the phlebitis is local and of little consequence, rest of the part and support by a snugly fitting elastic bandage may suffice. If it is more generalized and there is considerable febrile reaction, anticoagulant therapy should be instituted. This will require hospitalization. The main factor here is to be on the alert for developing phlebitis so that it can be treated before it becomes a problem.

LYMPHADENITIS AND LYMPHANGITIS

Lymphadenitis and lymphangitis frequently accompany infection and are particularly prevalent following abrasions of the hand and infection around the feet, such as ingrown toenail or severe athlete's foot. The involvement of the lymph system is due to the drainage from the infection. The symptoms are increasing pain in the local lesion followed by appearance of red streaks extending toward the neighboring lymph glands (lymphangitis). If one is familiar with the distribution of the lymph system, he will not expect to find glands at the back of the knee involved in an infection in an area of the foot that drains directly to the groin. These red streaks will have local heat and tenderness but are not particularly painful. Soreness will develop in the regional lymph glands which may become swollen and inflamed (lymphadenitis). Only occasionally will they go on to suppuration.

TREATMENT. The development of lymphadenitis demands more adequate treatment to the local lesion, such as adequate drainage of the infection, elevation of the part and local heat. Antibiotics should be used and one of the broad-spectrum type will usually be adequate. If it is possible to get a culture and determine which antibiotic is most effective, this should be done. This will require 24 to 48 hours and the antibiotic therapy should not be postponed while awaiting a report from the laboratory. If the local lesion is handled well, the secondary involvement of the lymph system will usually promptly subside. Needless to say, active athletics should not be permitted during the period of inflammation, not only to protect the affected player but also to protect his fellows from contamination. This player should not participate in athletics until the condition has entirely subsided and there is no longer inflammation in the glands.

NERVE INJURY

CONTUSION

Fortunately, the nervous system is not too commonly involved in injuries to the athlete because the player is usually in excellent condition with strong muscles to protect the nerves from overstress. In only a few areas of the body are the nerves particularly exposed to trauma, and these will be considered in the discussion of specific areas. The peripheral nerves most frequently involved are the ulnar nerve at the elbow, the peroneal nerve behind the fibular head, the radial nerve in the midarm and the axillary nerve at the shoulder. The injury is usually from a direct blow on the nerve causing a contusion. There is an immediate "shocking" sensation followed by numbness and pain. The condition may be entirely transient. The player may "shake it off" in a few minutes and be none the worse for the experience. If the injury is more severe, there will be persistent aching pain along the distribution of the nerve, the result of swelling and edema and congestion within the nerve and nerve sheath. The treatment of this degree of contusion should depend upon the area involved and the severity of the symptoms. In general, as long as the symptoms are relatively acute, the part should be protected against overuse. By all means the nerve should be protected against further contusion.

In the isolated case there may be paralysis of the muscles supplied by the nerve. This may be immediate due to direct damage to the nerve fibers. In this instance, one should seriously consider whether the nerve may actually have been crushed by the blow. Usually the early symptoms of numbness, aching and pain will be followed by disability of the muscle involved, which may progress to complete loss of function. If the peroneal is involved, there will be a foot drop. If it is the ulnar nerve, there will be weakness and loss of function of the intrinsic muscles of the hand. There may be hypesthesia or sensory loss throughout the sensory distribution of these mixed nerves. As long as this weakness or paralysis continues, the muscle should be supported by cast or brace. Physical therapy should be instituted to encourage return of function in the muscles. Recovery is almost always complete and usually is fairly rapid. The need for further protection after recovery from the paralysis will depend upon the condition of the muscle. The muscle should be protected as long as it is weak. Its strength should be improved by appropriate physical therapy.

STRETCH INJURY

Another type of injury to the nervous system is caused by overstretch of the nerve; for example, overstretching of the peroneal nerve after rupture of the lateral collateral ligaments of the knee. A recent case was seen eight months following an injury in which the patient "sprained" the lateral ligament of the knee. Examination revealed peroneal paralysis with positive Tinel sign just above the head of the fibula. There was instability of the lateral collateral ligament. Exploration revealed a badly scarred peroneal nerve, tightly bound down with scar from torn lateral collateral ligament. The nerve was carefully dissected out with separation of the fibers by neurolysis entirely across the 1½ inch scarred-in area. The lateral collateral ligament was advanced on its femoral attachment. The patient was in splints for eight weeks and wore a dropfoot brace most of the time for one year. At the end of this period he had active but not complete dorsiflexion, with complete recovery from his sensory paralysis except for a little hypesthesia over the top of the foot. His knee was stable. It required three months before he got any return and over a year before it was complete. He is now a college scholarship football player.

In such a case the severity of the ligament injury may screen the nerve condition so that it is not recognized until later. The symptoms will vary with the severity of the injury. If there is a complete avulsion of the nerve, there will be immediate and complete loss of function, whereas if the nerve is stretched but not torn, there will be hemorrhage and shock to the fibers but function will be more slowly and less completely lost. Whenever there has been complete loss of function of a nerve, one must decide whether or not surgical exploration is justified. The examining physician is responsible for the early detection of these injuries. Any statement by the patient about numbness, weakness or loss of motion should be carefully investigated. It is very important to determine the function of the nerve before definitive treatment is undertaken. A classical example is the dislocated elbow. If one discovers some hours, days or even weeks later that there is paralysis of the median nerve, it may be impossible to determine definitely whether this injury was athletic or iatrogenic. It is of particular importance to outline carefully any sensory loss since the diminution or increase of such an area may well be the determining factor in selecting the proper treatment.

TREATMENT. From the surgical standpoint, one should be quite conservative in treatment of an injury to the nerve. In a great majority of these cases gradual recovery will take place as the weeks go by. Such recovery will ordinarily be well advanced at the end of three months if it is likely to be complete. On the other hand, late surgical suture of the nerve may be quite successful and one can afford to delay exploration for a reasonable period of time (three months). Most surgeons agree that if nerve repair is to be done, it should be done within the first three months if at all possible. I should like to repeat that a well regulated, faithfully adhered-to physical therapy program is of extreme importance. This serves to prevent deformity by contracture of the muscles during the period of complete paralysis and serves to build up the strength of the muscles as the nerve function returns.

The subject of nerve involvement in conditions of the neck and spine includes some rather special problems and will be discussed in detail under these headings.

PART III

THE TREATMENT OF INJURIES IN SPECIFIC AREAS

CHAPTER 5

CRANIOCEREBRAL INJURIES DURING ATHLETICS

BY B. J. RUTLEDGE, M.D.

INTRODUCTION

Injuries to the head in sports events account for more fatalities than injuries to any other part of the body. There have been significant changes in the evaluation and management of head injuries since this book was first written over a decade ago.

Football is now the most popular contact sport and close to a million young men are participating in organized football throughout the United States. There has been a renewed impetus in evaluating and investigating head injuries, using the football field as the main research laboratory. During this period of time, changes have been made in the headgear, which for the most part now offers more protection to the player's head; however, lack of unanimity among physicians, coaches and manufacturers concerning helmets still remains prominent. Continuing attention to the modification of face guards is prevalent and important, although there is some expression to do away with these altogether.

With the improvement of the helmet there has been a tendency for players to use their heads as "battering rams," which has resulted in more frequent and serious head and neck injuries. There is and has been a collective effort by neurological and orthopaedic surgeons, as well as by other physicians, to educate coaches, players and officials concerning the dangers of "spearing" or stick tackling. This resulted in the NCAA Rules Committee's action outlawing "spearing" in 1972. Neurological surgeons are increasingly practicing preventive medicine by advising coaches and team physicians of practices that are dangerous to the head and nervous system. It is obvious that neurological and orthopaedic surgeons, team physicians, coaches, officials and manufacturers of sporting goods must work together to lessen the danger of injuries to the head and nervous system in athletic events.

Professional boxing is the only sport in which a player's objective is to render his opponent helpless. A resolution "opposing professional, collegiate

113

and amateur boxing in its present form" was adopted by the Southern Neurosurgical Society in 1970. While professional boxers may receive injuries to the brain, the less adept fighters are injured more frequently and severely. Death usually occurs from severe acute injury to the brain most commonly caused by acceleration and, to a lesser degree, by deceleration of the head. The term "punch drunk" is still the best term for an individual whose symptoms occur from chronic, repetitive insults to the brain.

With increasing participation in noncontact sporting events, there has been a corresponding increase in less serious injuries such as those caused by being struck in the head by a golf club, ball bat or ball, as well as unique injuries from newer sports such as snowmobiling.

The most common cause of death in craniocerebral acceleration injuries is an acute subdural hematoma. Physicians who attend athletes should be taught how to recognize this possibility and neurosurgical facilities must be made available close by. MAST (Military Assistance for Safety and Traffic) helicopter evacuation will enhance the possibility of early surgical intervention in those athletes with signs of increasing intracranial pressure, thereby lessening morbidity and mortality in the coming years. Arteriography is used with increasing frequency to aid in the early diagnosis of surgical lesions created by trauma to the head. In addition, steroids such as dexamethasone and dehydrating agents such as intravenous mannitol are useful in managing severe injuries to the brain. The recent sophistication of measuring blood gases has been a very beneficial adjunct in the treatment of craniocerebral injuries. Last, but not least, the conduct and attitude of individual athletes is of great importance in decreasing the price for participation in contact sports.

PREVENTION OF HEAD INJURIES

It is just as important in the prevention of craniocerebral injuries as it is in the prevention of other injuries that athletes be in excellent physical and mental condition. Preseason health questionnaires and physical examinations are mandatory before beginning practice in contact sports. A clear line of authority must be established by the team physician — he must make the final decision as to a player's ability to participate in his sport. Coaches and instructors must teach participants how to avoid injury. Continued research and early adoption of definite improvements in protective gear, such as helmets and face guards, are necessary. A collective effort is necessary to change the rules in boxing to award the bout to the opponent of any exhausted fighter. A boxer in such a state cannot bring his neck muscles into play and is therefore extremely vulnerable to severe brain injury.

The following conditions should usually disqualify an athlete from participation in contact sports:

1. neurological sequelae from injury to the head or from organic brain disease;

2. uncontrolled episodes of impaired consciousness;

3. temporary paralysis of a limb from any cause;

4. spontaneous subarachnoid hemorrhage;

5. recurring cerebral concussion.

Finally, a player should not re-enter a game after he has been "dinged" (memory affectation after a blow to the head) or after a concussion until he is perfectly normal.

ANATOMY OF THE HEAD

The *scalp* consists of five layers: the hair and skin, the galea, two layers of connective tissue, and the pericranium. The scalp serves as a protective covering for the skull and tends to lessen impact to deeper structures in the cranium.

The *skull* is divided into the cranium and the facial bones. The cranium houses the brain, its coverings, blood and cerebral spinal fluid. The foramen magnum is an opening at the base of the cranium for the passage of the spinal cord. The middle meningeal artery makes an impression in the skull and is of practical clinical significance in craniocerebral injuries, particularly in skull fractures.

The most important of the *brain coverings,* or meninges, is the dura mater, a tough fibrous tissue that serves as the inner lining of the skull and gives protection to the brain. It also provides a firm structure for venous sinuses, which return blood from the brain to the heart. There are two prolongations of the dura mater. One, the falx, divides the cranium into a right and left half; the other, a horizontal portion called the tentorium, separates the base of the brain from the superior portions. The connections from the brain to the spinal cord go through an opening in the tentorium called the incisura.

The middle of the three meninges is the arachnoid; the inner, which is intimately associated with the surface of the brain, is the pia mater. Between the arachnoid and the pia mater is the subarachnoid space, which contains cerebral spinal fluid. This space is traversed by blood vessels.

The brain itself is similar to gelatin in consistency and its average weight is one and one-third pounds. It occupies irregular recesses formed by the cranium and the dura partitions. The falx separates the two large cerebral hemispheres, which are in turn divided into frontal, temporal and occipital lobes. The anterior parts of the frontal and temporal lobes are the frontal and temporal poles, and the posterior portion of the occipital lobe is the occipital pole. The main function of the two cerebral hemispheres is controlling movement of the body, perception of sensation and the higher cerebral functions such as speech, learning, memory and emotion. Each hemisphere controls function in the opposite side of the body.

The cerebral hemispheres are connected with the brain stem, which passes through the incisura of the tentorium down to the level of the foramen magnum at the base of the skull where it becomes the spinal cord. The importance of the brain stem, in addition to transmitting information between the cerebral hemispheres and spinal cord, is control of the vital functions of the body such as blood pressure, heart rate and respiration.

Also located under the tentorium and connected to the brain stem are the two cerebellar hemispheres whose main function is the coordination of movements initiated by the cerebral hemispheres.

Within each cerebral hemisphere is a cavity called a lateral ventricle. The brain stem has two such cavities, the anterior being the third ventricle and that lying near the spinal cord being the fourth ventricle. They are interconnected by small ducts or foramina.

Spinal fluid is found mainly in the lateral ventricles and circulates from there through the third and fourth ventricles. It flows out of the brain through openings in the fourth ventricle, known as the foramen of Magendie and the foramen of Luschka, and then circulates and bathes the brain and spinal cord. The main purpose of spinal fluid is to provide a cushion between the rigid skull and soft brain.

The blood supply to the brain comes from the two carotid arteries and two vertebral arteries. The latter join to form the basilar artery, which then connects with the carotids through smaller branches, forming the circle of Willis at the base of the brain. Venous blood is drained by the internal and external jugular veins.

ASPECTS OF CEREBRAL PHYSIOLOGY ATTENDED BY TRAUMA

CEREBRAL EDEMA

Significant head trauma results in two categories of brain injury. The first is only a transient alteration of brain function without any structural damage, the classic example being concussion. In the other category more serious injury occurs and there is structural damage to the brain coverings or to the brain itself. This damage may result in the development of an expanding mass such as a blood clot within the rigid cranial vault, causing brain compression. Also, serious alterations in cerebral physiology may occur that result in increased pressure on the brain. Either the development of an expanding intracranial mass or a physiological disturbance can result in increased intracranial pressure, which if not relieved promptly will cause permanent brain damage or death.

In structural injuries the brain cells (neurons) usually are damaged to some degree. This alters their physiology in such a way that they accumulate H_2O within themselves: a condition known as *cerebral edema,* which usually takes 24 to 36 hours to develop after an injury. Such an accumulation of mass (in this instance H_2O) within the skull acts in a manner identical with a blood clot and causes increased intracranial pressure.

The brain receives 15 per cent of the body's blood circulation and consumes 25 per cent of its oxygen. Any process impairing the delivery of oxygen to the brain or the removal of carbon dioxide from it results in similar physiological alterations at the cellular level in the brain. Hence, neurons may be damaged and cerebral edema result from anoxia or hypercarbia alone. Causes of poor cerebral oxygenation include obstruction to pulmonary ventilation, such as nose and face injuries, neck injuries, rib fractures with lung collapse, and shock in which blood pressure is too low to adequately perfuse the brain. It should be emphasized that shock is rarely associated with head injuries alone, and when present one should always suspect an associated injury such as a ruptured spleen with intra-abdominal hemorrhage.

The effect of retained carbon dioxide should be elaborated upon. Not only is elevated carbon dioxide directly toxic to nerve cells, producing cerebral edema, but it is also a potent cerebral blood vessel dilator, resulting in the increased flow of blood and fluids to the brain where they accumulate in the injured cells, further elevating intracranial pressure.

A vicious cycle develops in unrelieved cerebral edema. The brain becomes swollen with H_2O, causing elevated intracranial pressure, which compresses and blocks the veins draining blood away from the brain. The result is that more blood is pumped into the brain than can escape through the veins, and intracranial pressure is further elevated. These problems are compounded if a blood clot is also accumulating at the same time from a vessel ruptured at the time of injury.

With severe increased intracranial pressure, blood pressure is elevated, the pulse is slow and there are respiratory changes. When pressure is generalized, such as with edema, decreased consciousness is the most prominent sign. Usually there are no lateralizing signs. In contrast, with an extradural hemorrhage the pupil is dilated and fixed on the ipsilateral side and there is a contralateral hemiparesis. When the brain stem is involved, the temperature regulatory mechanism falters and there is frequently hyperthermia. Decerebrate rigidity is a sign of brain stem dysfunction and is usually bilateral. In this phenomenon the extremities are in extensor rigidity and the upper extremities tend to internal rotation. The rigidity is enhanced by stimulation of the patient, and Babinski's sign is present bilaterally. In increased intracranial pressure caused by chronic subdural hematomas, the pupil is frequently dilated on the side opposite the hematoma owing to compression of the third cranial nerve against the edge of the tentorium.

SKULL FRACTURES

Skull fractures are not common in football. They are more common in sports played on a harder surface and in those utilizing a ball and club. Skull fractures are classified into the following types: (1) closed, or simple, fractures, which do not involve a break in the overlying skin or membranes; and (2) open, or compound, fractures, which involve a tear in the covering adjacent to the fracture.

Linear skull fractures may be sim-ple or compound. Signs of a simple linear fracture are pain, swelling over the fracture line, and discoloration. X-ray studies will reveal a "crack" in the skull. This can be of particular importance if it crosses the groove of the middle meningeal artery, which will be considered in the discussion of extradural hematomas. The simple linear fracture demonstrates that the patient has sustained a physical blow with sufficient force to crack the skull. The fracture itself ordinarily does not require any treatment other than observation in a hospital for 24 hours to be sure that intracranial structures have not been concomitantly damaged. Compound linear skull fractures require early, careful debridement and coverage by appropriate antibiotics.

Depressed skull fractures usually occur when the head is struck by an object such as a golf club and the skull is pushed onto the brain (Fig. 74). These fractures can be compound or simple. When compounded, emergency surgery is indicated for debridement and elevation of bone fragments from the brain. In comminuted fractures I always replace the fragments in the defect, even in a mosaic pattern, if necessary. This is of particular importance in athletes so that they will retain a solid cranium without a skull defect that could require a subsequent cranioplasty with foreign material. Simple depressed fractures can be elevated as elective surgical procedures.

Skull fractures in the bones at the base of the skull cause discoloration around the eyes and nose or over the mastoid and may be accompanied by leakage of cerebral spinal fluid into the ear (otorrhea) or the nose (rhinorrhea). They are not usually visible on x-ray films. This is a special type of compound fracture that should always be managed by a neurological surgeon.

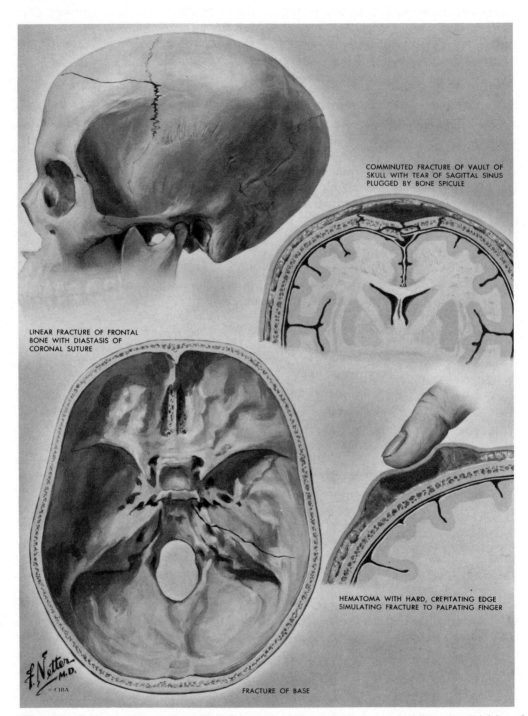

Figure 74. Fractures of the skull. (© Copyright 1953, 1972 CIBA Pharmaceutical Company, Division of CIBA-Geigy Corporation. Reproduced with permission from The CIBA Collection of Medical Illustrations by Frank H. Netter, M.D. All rights reserved.)

CEREBRAL CONCUSSION

Concussion is a syndrome in which there is an immediate impairment of neural function following a blow to the head. This deficit is usually noticeable in the degree of consciousness but may also involve memory, visual disturbances or equilibrium problems. In third degree concussions there is unconsciousness for more than five minutes and moderate retrograde amnesia. No treatment is required because there is no permanent deficit, although a decision does have to be made concerning a participant's return to play after such an injury. Multiple concussive episodes may result in permanent sequelae, and individuals reflecting this pattern need to be evaluated by a neurological surgeon to determine whether they should continue in athletics. Multiple concussive blows to the head, as those received in boxing, can result in a combination of symptoms from involvement of the pyramidal, extrapyramidal and cerebellar pathways. The common symptoms are slurred speech, dull face, slowness of movement and mentality, and tremor. Slang terms to describe an individual with such symptoms are punch drunk, goofy, slap happy, stumblebum and slugnutty.

CEREBRAL CONTUSION

Cerebral contusion is a bruising of the brain. When a small area of the brain is involved it is difficult to distinguish from a concussion and no permanent effects occur. In more severe contusions, cerebral edema with brain swelling results in increased intracranial pressure. If a generalized contusion with bruising of the brain stem occurs, decerebrate rigidity follows and the patient may die or have a permanent deficit after a long illness. The usual treatment is medical to reduce increased intracranial pressure with good oxygenation, dexamethasone and mannitol, along with the usual supportive nursing care. Diagnostic studies such as angiography and echoencephalography are utilized to help determine whether surgical intervention may be warranted. A decrease in the level of consciousness is the single most important sign in determining the need for surgery. Subtemporal decompression can be a lifesaving procedure for a patient with this condition.

EXTRADURAL HEMATOMA

This hemorrhage usually results when a fracture tears the middle meningeal artery (Fig. 75). Typically the patient is unconscious for a short period of time and then returns to normal. Drowsiness and headache ensue an hour or more later, followed by vomiting, dilation of the ipsilateral pupil and contralateral hemiparesis. Time is of the essence at this point because if the pressure is not relieved, respiration decreases, both pupils dilate, decerebrate rigidity occurs, and finally respiratory paralysis and death result. Surgical treatment is mandatory. In the emergency room, if necessary, a burr hole is placed on the side of the dilated pupil. After evacuation of some of the blood clot, a craniectomy is done and the remaining clot removed; bleeding is then controlled. Recovery should be complete if the clot is removed before there is bilateral brain stem compression.

ACUTE SUBDURAL HEMATOMA

This entity is the most frequent cause of death from trauma in contact sports. The patient usually remains unconscious following the injury and

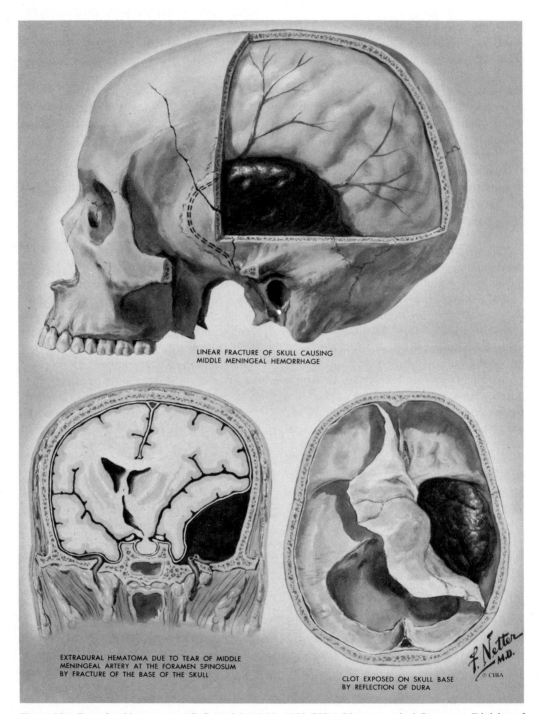

LINEAR FRACTURE OF SKULL CAUSING
MIDDLE MENINGEAL HEMORRHAGE

EXTRADURAL HEMATOMA DUE TO TEAR OF MIDDLE
MENINGEAL ARTERY AT THE FORAMEN SPINOSUM
BY FRACTURE OF THE BASE OF THE SKULL

CLOT EXPOSED ON SKULL BASE
BY REFLECTION OF DURA

Figure 75. Extradural hematoma. (© Copyright 1953, 1972 CIBA Pharmaceutical Company, Division of CIBA-Geigy Corporation. Reproduced with permission from The CIBA Collection of Medical Illustrations by Frank H. Netter, M.D. All rights reserved.)

shows signs of rapidly increasing intracranial pressure. This condition is usually caused by contracoup movement with contusion and laceration of the brain and tearing of vessels. The mortality rate is extremely high and many patients succumb without the benefit of neurosurgical consultation or surgery. The treatment is appropriate craniotomy with removal of the blood clot and control of hemorrhage with coagulation, metal clips, suturing, gel foam and/or surgicel. In those patients who do survive, morbidity is severe.

CHRONIC SUBDURAL HEMATOMA

Fortunately in my practice I have not had any patients with acute subdural hematomas from participation in football. I have had several patients with chronic subdural hematomas with complete recovery in all instances (Fig. 76). One boy was playing for his coach-father and he continued to play football the following year against my advice.

Chronic subdural hematomas are always caused by trauma. Usually the trauma to the head is considered insignificant and is sometimes forgotten completely. The pathophysiologic manifestation is bleeding in the subdural space from a torn bridging vein from the brain to the superior sagittal sinus. The subdural space is developed by the blood from a potential space from which absorption does not occur. In about a week a neomembrane surrounds the blood and the hematoma gradually increases in size by osmosis through a semipermeable membrane and by further bleeding from stretched, small vessels.

Symptoms are initially mild to nonexistent and, if present, usually disappear in a few days. A patient harboring a chronic, subdural hematoma will feel normal for several weeks and then will complain of headache. The headache becomes more severe and is unrelenting. Other symptoms include loss of appetite and vomiting, drowsiness, personality change, blurred vision and gait disturbance. Approximately 50 per cent of patients have bilateral hematomas; 40 per cent have papilledema. The diagnosis may be confirmed by brain scan. Arteriograms will show the hematoma in 95 per cent of the cases.

Treatment is removal of the hematoma through trephine openings in the skull. Occasionally a large osteoplastic flap is warranted. These patients are prone to have temporary convulsions following surgery and should be treated with intravenous sodium Dilantin. The symptoms disappear quickly following surgery and recovery is complete. I do not recommend that athletes continue to participate in contact sports after having a subdural hematoma.

INTRACEREBRAL HEMATOMA

This condition is rare in athletic trauma. Since the symptoms progress slowly, diagnostic studies such as brain scans, EEGs and angiograms are more important in determining the management of these cases. Causes other than trauma have to be considered and ruled out. Intracerebral hematomas may be treated medically or surgically; results of treatment vary.

COMBINED INTRACRANIAL INJURIES

I recently had a patient who was involved in an auto racing accident. He was reported to be confused immediately following the accident and was conscious when I saw him about three hours later. He had some tenderness on

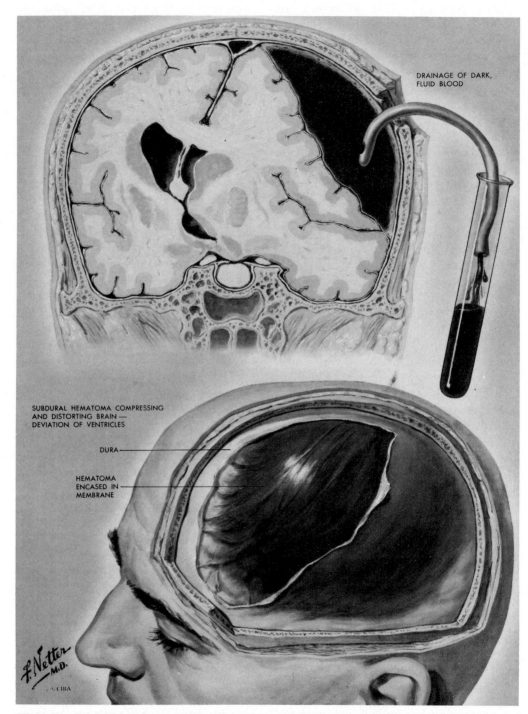

Figure 76. Subdural hematoma. (© Copyright 1953, 1972 CIBA Pharmaceutical Company, Division of CIBA-Geigy Corporation. Reproduced with permission from The CIBA Collection of Medical Illustrations by Frank H. Netter, M.D. All rights reserved.)

the left side of his head and was dysphasic, but otherwise he had no complaints, was alert and had no other abnormalities.

A skull series revealed a linear fracture across the groove of the left middle meningeal artery. He was therefore admitted to the Intensive Care Unit of the Oklahoma Neurological Surgery Institute and Allied Sciences for observation.

The following morning he was the same neurologically. About 4:00 A.M. on the third day I was called and told that he was very somnolent. When I examined him he had a dilated, fixed pupil on the left side and was semicomatose. His respirations were full at the rate of eight per minute, his pulse was 56 and his blood pressure had risen to 190/110. He also had a slight weakness of the right extremities and a positive Babinski sign on the right. A left carotid arteriogram was immediately obtained, which showed elevation of the middle cerebral artery such as that seen with an intracerebral hematoma; the angiogram also revealed a subdural hematoma.

The patient was taken to the operating room and a perforator and burr opening revealed an extradural hematoma. A subtemporal decompression was performed and the hematoma was evacuated. The dura was discolored and when it was opened a large subdural hematoma and a swollen, contused temporal lobe were revealed. It was necessary to do an osteoplastic flap to remove all of the "currant jelly–like" subdural hematoma. A portion of the contused and softened temporal lobe was also removed.

On the following morning the patient appeared as he did on the day of his admission. He was discharged from the hospital in six days and was asymptomatic at the time of my examination one month later.

DIAGNOSIS AND EMERGENCY TREATMENT OF HEAD INJURIES

Any blow to the head is potentially serious and should be so considered. Coaches, teammates and trainers may receive the first warning of an injury to the head by watching the game itself and the individual.

The first thing to do for a player with a suspected head injury is to render lifesaving measures such as establishing an airway and maintaining blood circulation. Closed heart massage or defibrillation, a recent innovation, may be necessary. The player should not be moved.

A bolt cutter should be available for rapid removal of the face guard; headgear should not be removed except for a specific reason, since concomitant neck injuries are always suspected in players who sustain injuries to the head. Next a thorough, unhurried examination should be made. After the general examination, the head should be palpated and a brief neurological examination should be made, including examination of the pupils and movement of facial muscles and extremities. A decision must then be made as to the method of moving the patient. If there is any suggestion of a neck injury, such as pain or tenderness in the neck or weakness in the extremities, great care should be taken to keep the patient's head in a neutral position while moving him to a firm stretcher where his head can be kept immobilized to avoid further injury. Any player who is unconscious, if only for a few minutes, must leave the field of play.

A decision must be made on the playing field as to who should be sent to the hospital for further evaluation and tests. In general, only the "ding" or concussion lasting a minute or two with rapid recovery of all senses should be allowed to pass without further examination. All other injuries, including those with possible neck injuries, should rapidly be taken to a hospital with neurosurgical facilities.

At the hospital, x-ray films of the skull should be obtained. Cervical spine films should usually be obtained, since head and neck injuries are frequently associated and a comatose patient will be unable to complain of neck pain.

All concussions lasting more than five minutes or those associated with posttraumatic amnesia should be admitted for observation for the development of symptoms of increased intracranial pressures. Likewise linear skull fractures without neurological deficit should be observed for 24 hours, especially if the fracture line crosses the middle meningeal artery groove or venous sinus.

All other injuries demand neurosurgical consultation. The neurosurgeon can usually decide on the basis of history and neurological examination whether the patient can be managed medically or if he will require surgery. If there are any doubts, further studies may be necessary. These include echoencephalography, which detects shifts of normal midline structures caused by mass lesions, and cerebral angiography, which more accurately defines intracranial masses by outlines of intracranial blood vessels. Brain scans and EEGs are useful in chronic and subacute conditions. If the patient's condition is deteriorating rapidly, there is not time for these studies and the patient must be taken to surgery immediately for diagnosis and treatment.

MEDICAL MANAGEMENT OF HEAD INJURIES

The patient's vital signs, pupils and ability to move extremities should be recorded every hour to detect signs of developing increased intracranial pressure. The head should be elevated 30 degrees to assist venous drainage of the brain. The airway must be kept clear to prevent hypoxia or hypercarbia by turning the patient from side to side frequently and by nasopharyngeal suctioning. Tracheostomy may be necessary if indicated by measurement of the patient's blood oxygen and carbon dioxide. Because of cerebral edema, dexamethasone, a steroid, is frequently given intravenously to stabilize cell membranes and to help prevent the accumulation of fluid. Mild dehydration is also useful in treating cerebral edema; therefore, the patient's intake of fluids is restricted and 20 per cent mannitol may be given intravenously to further dehydrate the brain. Since the patient's level of consciousness is the most sensitive clinical indication of intracranial pressure, sedation is avoided. For analgesia codeine is preferred because of its minimal sedative effects and because it does not change pupillary signs as morphine derivatives can.

SURGICAL MANAGEMENT OF HEAD INJURIES

The surgical treatment of head injuries has been discussed largely under the specific conditions. Usually Decadron and mannitol are used preoperatively in all conditions. Decadron is usually continued in decreasing doses for several days postoperatively, depending on the patient's condition. Mannitol may be continued if postoperative cerebral edema is a problem. Usually this subsides in five to seven days. Uncontrollable cerebral edema may require a decompressive procedure involving removal of a portion of the cranial vault to allow the swollen brain to expand. Some medical centers place devices between the skull and brain at the time of surgery to monitor exact intracranial pressure and help determine the best therapy.

REHABILITATION

The importance of rehabilitation has long been recognized in sports injuries. Emphasis has been placed on athletes' returning to active participation in sports; trainers have been the stalwarts in this cause. Although this approach is important in head injuries, serious brain injuries require a prolonged, sophisticated team approach to return the patient to a normal active life and, if possible, to continued athletic endeavors. Sequelae from brain injuries are very complex and can cause mental deficiency, sensory or motor aphasia, pain, paralysis, sensory loss, disturbance of balance, and incontinence of the bladder and bowel. One or more of these symptoms can tax the energy of teammates, coaches, relatives, trainers and physicians.

In addition to the need for many medical specialists, paramedical personnel such as speech therapists, psychologists, physical therapists and visiting nurses are important. Most communities do not have the necessary medical talent to deal with and rehabilitate players suffering from severe head injuries. Initially, these individuals should be in a general hospital with an active neuro-surgery service and ancillary programs for rehabilitation. Fortunately, prolonged symptoms from brain injury are not as common in athletic trauma as those following a spinal cord injury. However, when they do occur, there are a few cities in the United States that have excellent rehabilitative facilities and those should be utilized by athletes suffering from neurological deficit to aid in their total and effective recovery. Every coach and team physician should be familiar with the nearest appropriate rehabilitation center.

REFERENCES

Anderson, B. D., Kraus, J. F., and Mueller, C. R.: The effectiveness of a special ice hockey helmet to reduce head injuries in college intramural hockey. Med. Sci. Sports. 2:162–164, 1970.

Beedle, C. W., Kovacic, C. R., and Moon, D. W.: Peak head acceleration of athletes during competition — football. Med. Sci. Sports. 3:44–50, 1971.

Karleen, C. I.: Snowmobiling with associated maxillofacial injuries. Minn. Med. 56:975–979, 1973.

Lavine, S. A.: Field diagnosis of athletic injuries. Md. State Med. J. 20:45–47, 1971.

Lynch, S., and Yarnell, P. R.: The "ding": amnestic states in football trauma. Neurology. 23:196–197, 1973.

Norrell, H.: The neurosurgeon's responsibility in the prevention of sports injuries. Clin. Neurosurg. 19:208–219, 1972.

Schneider, R. C.: Head and Neck Injuries in Football. Baltimore, Williams and Wilkins Co., 1973.

Unterharnscheidt, F. J.: Head injury after boxing. Scand. J. Rehabil. Med. 4:77–84. 1972.

CHAPTER 6

INJURIES OF THE FACE

ANATOMICAL CONSIDERATIONS

A brief discussion of some of the anatomical characteristics of the face is pertinent since they relate specifically to the type of injury to be expected and the treatment recommended. Practically the entire face is subcutaneous. The skin extending from the hair line above to the neck below is stretched over subcutaneous bone with relatively few areas protected by any intervening structure. In the upper face, the hard bone of the skull is separated from the skin only by the very thin muscles of the scalp and the aponeurosis connecting these muscles. The bony structures of this portion of the face are entirely immobile and serve as protection for the brain. At the supraorbital margins, the layers of the cranium separate to form the frontal sinus, which may be of almost any size. The characteristic "beetling brow" does not necessarily imply any change in contour of the cranial cavity but rather a large frontal sinus. This portion of the face is essentially part of the skull. Moving laterally from the midline in front, one finds the temporal fossae

filled with the fanlike temporal muscles. The muscle layer here is considerably thicker than directly in front. The supraorbital nerves pass out of the orbital cavity through the supraorbital foramen at the junction of the inner and middle thirds of the superior orbital margin and pass subcutaneously up over the forehead. The essential injury in this area is contusion and its complications rather than strain or sprain.

The central portion of the face, that is, the area between the supraorbital ridges and the bottom of the superior maxilla, presents a complicated maze of anatomical structures, some of which will be considered in more detail later in the description of injuries to the various organs. The facial bones, which in the infant are separated by suture lines, become fused relatively early, but the very irregular suture lines persist and may well be confused with fracture lines. The orbit, for example, is a complete bony socket, open only anteriorly and posteriorly, yet is made up of five or six different bones fitted together as in a jigsaw puzzle. The central portion of the face also has no motion between its bony structures. However, it is involved in motion of the lower jaw, since many of the muscles attached to the lower jaw have their origin on the fixed bones of the face. The lower portion of the face, the mandibular portion, consists of the horseshoe-shaped mandible, which has bony contact with the rest of the skull only at the temporal articulations and the teeth.

Injuries to the face are not nearly so frequent now as they have been in the past. The football headgear and the various other helmets worn serve to protect not only the skull but also the upper portion of the face. With the addition of a bar of some type extending across the front of the face, the incidence of injuries to the supraorbital ridge, the zygomatic process, the malar bone, the nose, the teeth and jaw has been greatly reduced. Almost all of the professional and university teams now require some sort of facial protection. Many of the high school and junior schools are rapidly following suit (see Chapter 2, Prevention of Injuries). I will not attempt in this section to give the detailed treatment of each of the areas of the face but rather will discuss those features of injuries that are likely to fall under the aegis of the one treating athletic injuries.

LACERATION OF THE FACE

The broad expanse of facial skin with underlying subcutaneous bone is subject to contusion, abrasion and laceration more than any other type of injury. The abrasion and laceration should be treated as elsewhere. One should bear in mind, however, that an intervening aponeurotic layer is present between the skin and bone on the forehead. It is important in laceration of the *forehead* or of the *scalp* to determine whether the underlying muscle or galea has been damaged. Each laceration should be carefully cleaned and the wound margins separated sufficiently to explore the depths of the wound. There is no substitute for irrigation with copious quantities of clean water. This is not necessarily sterile water. Running water from the tap of the city water system is adequate and is always available. If it is possible to hook up a tube or hose the procedure is simplified. Under hospital conditions it is better to use sterile saline. It should be emphasized that it is the force of the flowing water that cleans out the contaminants. If nothing else is available, an ordinary shower may be utilized in the preliminary cleansing.

Usually in athletics the wound is through the skin only and is in the nature of a crushing, tearing injury rather than a direct cut. Such a wound extends deep enough to expose but not damage the galea. It should be thoroughly cleansed and hemostasis secured either by direct pressure or by injection of the skin edges with procaine plus epinephrine. The use of procaine is advisable in any event, since it will make the repair of the wound much less painful. Once the skin edges are anesthetized they can be retracted gently and the area underneath investigated. Since the skin over the forehead is quite loose, the defect in the underlying structures may be some distance above or below the split in the skin itself. The skin can be readily shifted and with a small curved forceps any underlying defect can be explored. If there is a defect in the galea, careful palpation will determine whether or not this extends downward to include the skull. Only after careful exploration of the wound should the skin be closed. Here, as anywhere in the face, it is extremely important to appose the skin edges accurately. Whether you are a believer in multiple, very small sutures or favor fewer but more widely spaced ones, the end result will depend greatly upon how accurately the edges of the skin are apposed. The skin cannot accommodate for overlapping or a vertical shift of its edges and a troublesome and unsightly ridge will remain if the original suture is sloppy. If the galea has been damaged and the wound can be thoroughly cleansed, the galea can be closed with one or two interrupted sutures. The wound should be carefully inspected daily for any accumulation of fluid under the skin or under the galea. This is a relatively silent area from the standpoint of sensitivity and a tremendous abscess may develop with relatively few symptoms. The abscess may spread under the skin or under the galea over the whole top of the head. Athletic participation may be permitted after a laceration of the area is carefully protected by a contact pad. A special foam rubber pad in the football helmet may be necessary. In other sports an appropriate protective pad may be molded to form a cup over the involved area.

Laceration of the *eyebrow* is a relatively common injury and requires the same treatment as indicated above. If the laceration is in the region of the supraorbital nerve, this nerve may be severed. In such an instance repair of the nerve should be carried out to avoid subsequent troublesome anesthesia, tenderness or itching on this side of the forehead.

In the *central portion* of the face laceration is also quite frequent and here again one must determine carefully whether or not there is damage to the underlying structures. This is quite obvious in lacerations about the eye. Lacerations about the face require meticulous handling and one must condemn the prevalent custom of rushing the player to the dressing room where someone places several stitches to close the wound with scant reference to either

asepsis or accurate apposition. The emergency is not that great. If it is absolutely necessary for the player to compete throughout the remainder of the game, a suitable pad should be applied as a temporary expedient, with the definite understanding that a complete repair will be done at the earliest possible moment. Although this course is not recommended, it certainly is better than to accept a less than perfect apposition of the wound edges. The definitive treatment should be carried out directly after the completion of the game and not the next day. If a delay of a few hours is unavoidable, the application of pressure and cold to the wound will help to control the swelling. By the next day it will be virtually impossible to carry out actual plastic closure of the laceration. Ideally, the suture should be done at once. It will never be as easy again. If the laceration is at all extensive it is preferable to anesthetize the wound edges, preferably by infiltration of procaine plus epinephrine as indicated above. It is particularly important that laceration of the *eyelids* receive very accurate closure in an effort to match up the skin creases. This is even more important if the laceration crosses the skin creases, since an irregular scar will disfigure the eyelid and interfere with its motion.

So also laceration through the *alae of the nose* should be carefully closed, great care being taken to secure accurate apposition of the edges of the nostril. Similarly, laceration involving the *ear* requires accurate repositioning of the skin. In fact, there is no area of the face where meticulous handling is not essential. It is extremely distressing to have a scar across the face with one edge of the skin higher than the other. This is disfiguring in the female and is very distressing to the male, since it interferes with shaving. It also is often a source of unsightly ingrown hairs.

CONTUSION OF THE FACE

By far the most common injury to the face is contusion. This may involve damage to the skin when it is caught between the hard, underlying bone and the force of the blow. The skin over the face is loose and an area of areolar tissue is present between it and the underlying structures. In the forehead there is an areolar space between the skin and the galea or the frontalis, offering ample room for local swelling with hematoma formation. A blow to the forehead is likely to be followed immediately by extensive swelling, which may be diffuse, having the shape of an egg transected on its long axis, or local with simply a rounded area of local swelling. One should assure himself that there is no serious underlying pathologic condition by close attention to the general symptoms of the patient as well as by local and general physical examination. Immediate application of cold and pressure will minimize the local swelling and may prevent to a great extent the infiltration of blood. It is debatable whether or not the local swelling should be aspirated. Very frequently the swelling is more in the nature of bloody edema than hematoma, and in such an instance aspiration will be unrewarding. Only when the area feels distinctly fluctuant is aspiration indicated to expedite recovery. After the area is aspirated under careful aseptic precautions, it should be infiltrated with hyaluronidase, then cold and pressure applied. The latter can be done quite simply by a circumferential wrap around the head. If it causes distressing headache after a few hours, it is too tight and will need to be released and rewrapped. The ordinary elastic bandage makes a very adequate pressure bandage. If there are no complications, there is no contraindication to athletic participation following such a contusion.

COMPLICATIONS OF CONTUSION

Injury to the Brain

The most critical complication of contusion of the forehead is injury to the brain, and this has been discussed previously (Chapter 5). I believe it should be emphasized here, however, that if the patient has actually been knocked unconscious by such a blow, he should be kept under very careful observation for at least 12 hours and resumption of athletic competition should not be permitted within that time. This is because of the danger of delayed intracranial hemorrhage or edema.

Fracture of the Skull

If the blow was so forceful as to fracture the skull, the patient should be immediately removed to a hospital and kept under constant observation. The most important consideration here is damage to the brain, and this should take precedence over any attempt at correction of the deformity. There may be a fracture of the frontal bone, which will involve the frontal sinus and not actually break into the cranial cavity. In such a case the deformity is usually minimal and requires no treatment. If the whole anterior wall of the frontal sinus is collapsed, advice should be sought from a competent otolaryngologist to determine whether or not the fragment should be elevated.

Supraorbital Nerve Damage

Contusion of the supraorbital ridge may cause damage to the supraorbital nerve as it passes over the ridge in the subcutaneous tissue. Expectant treatment is usually adopted here because in contusion the nerve is rarely severed and complete recovery follows. This is particularly true since this is a sensory nerve and tends to regenerate quite promptly.

INJURY IN THE VICINITY OF THE EAR

Injury to the external ear is not common in amateur athletics. Professional prizefighters are frequently injured in this area, but in the amateur ranks the athlete usually wears a protective pad. In football the ear is protected by the helmet.

In the simple contusion in which the ear is smashed against the mastoid, prompt care may often prevent seriously deforming sequelae. The ear should be carefully examined. Any hemorrhage between the perichondrium and cartilage should be aspirated under most aseptic conditions. If early hemorrhage is not present, an ice pack should be used to reduce the local edema. If edema persists and there appears to be fluid in the soft tissues that irons out the wrinkles and crevices of the ear, one might seriously consider release of the pressure of this fluid by multiple small incisions. These should be made under the most aseptic precautions, since infection in this area may be very serious.

A chronic infection may well supervene when contamination develops as a complication of the treatment of contusion and hematoma or when the initial injury breaks the skin. This causes local swelling and edema but has little or no systemic reaction. When the cartilage is involved, there may be either dissecting infection along the perichondrium or an aseptic necrosis of the cartilage. This type of infection is very difficult to manage and the team physician would do well to seek specialized care from the plastic surgeon.

The resulting scar from contusion with infiltration of blood through the soft tissues results in some thickening of subcutaneous tissue and perichondrium

so that each subsequent injury is more serious than the previous one, and the final result is the well-known cauliflower ear, which defies any very definitive treatment. Careful release of tissue tension by pressure bandage and application of ice are excellent preventive measures.

A laceration of the ear may occur from a sharp instrument. Much more common is the avulsion in which the ear is partially torn away. Such an injury occurs when the ear is forcibly pulled forward and the skin fold between the scalp and the ear is split. As the ear falls back into its normal position, this split may be completely concealed and infection may supervene because of contamination of the wound. Given a history of such an injury, a careful inspection of the ear should be made. If there is a laceration it should be carefully cleansed and sutured. Any tear in the external ear itself must be meticulously apposed, particularly if the auricular cartilage is torn; otherwise, an unsightly notch will appear at the suture line.

Injury to the *internal ear* is not frequent. The possible exception is the ruptured ear drum. The history of blow across the side of the head with pain, slight hemorrhage from the ear and a feeling of fullness in the ear demands investigation of the drum. These ruptures of the drum usually heal spontaneously, but in the young athlete, if there is any question at all as to damage of the drum or inner or middle ear, the service of a competent otologist should be provided. Perhaps the most dangerous sequela is infection.

INJURY IN THE VICINITY OF THE EYE
BY C. P. WILKINSON, M.D.

The eye and its surrounding structures are occasionally seriously injured in athletic competition. Although severe injuries of the lids and the globe should be managed by an ophthalmologist, most such cases are initially seen by the team physician, and the importance of a routine examination of the eye in any case in which trauma has occurred in or around the orbit cannot be overemphasized. The team physician is not expected to handle severe ocular injuries, but it is quite important that he develop an awareness of the types of injuries that can occur as well as a practical knowledge of their management.

Orbit. The orbit is constructed to give protection to the eye. The supraorbital ridge above, the infraorbital margin below, the malar bone on the temporal side, and the nasal bone on the inside all serve to form a recess protecting the eye from a blow due to large objects.

A direct blow to the anterior orbit is typically followed by the rapid passage of serum and blood into the soft tissues of the lids, frequently resulting in their closure. Hemorrhage can also occur more posteriorly in the orbit, and swelling in this area will usually result in a significant degree of proptosis and ophthalmoplegia. In addition there may be subcutaneous or subconjunctival emphysema from fractures of sinuses. Focal anesthesia of the skin may occur if the nerves supplying such areas are damaged by fractures of the bones upon which they lie. The immediate concern of the primary physician should be to rule out severe intraocular trauma. The eyelids must be separated, utilizing lid retractors if necessary. (These can usually be more easily used if an anesthetic drop is first placed between the lids and on the cornea.) Movement of the eye should be observed both to assess the function of the respective eye muscles and to view more effectively the conjunctiva and sclera. Severe limitation of movement in any direction may be due to a blow-out fracture of the orbit or to neuromuscular damage, and

this finding should prompt referral to an ophthalmologist, as should severe ocular trauma of any kind. The lids should be carefully examined for lacerations. Any question regarding facial fractures should be followed up with X-ray studies. (It should be noted that routine films frequently do not detect orbital blow-out fractures.) If one is satisfied that there is no underlying ocular complication, he should promptly treat the patient. The most important measure in this early stage is an adequate ice pack. This should consist of crushed ice folded in a soft cloth such as a towel rather than an ice bag. The ice bag is heavy and cumbersome, and it is generally poorly tolerated by the patient. It should be noted that if the patient has an intraocular injury, an ice pack or any other device increasing pressure upon the eye should *not* be applied to the lids.

Lids. As in the case of orbital trauma, the first step in caring for an injury of the lid is to carefully examine the eye itself. The general management of lid trauma is the same as for lacerations and avulsions elsewhere. Lacerations of the lid involving the lid margin or severe avulsions of the lid should prompt referral to an ophthalmologist or plastic surgeon. Of special importance are injuries to the lacrimal apparatus. Any laceration near the medial canthus should prompt a detailed examination of the puncta and canaliculi leading into the lacrimal sac, and any laceration extending through these structures should be referred to an ophthalmologist for meticulous repair.

Globe. The cornea is the most exposed portion of the eye, and the most common eye injury in sports is abrasion of the cornea by either a fingernail or a rough foreign body. A patient typically complains of significant pain and a foreign body sensation, even when the offending agent is no longer present. A drop of a topical anesthetic will temporarily make the patient quite comfortable in most cases. The cornea should be inspected with a bright light using oblique illumination. If no foreign body is seen on the cornea, the upper lid should be everted and the patient instructed to look down. Frequently a foreign body will lie on tarsal conjunctiva. Foreign bodies in both of these locations can frequently be easily removed with a moist cotton applicator following the instillation of a topical anesthetic drop. If no foreign body is found and no corneal abrasion noted, commercially available fluorescein dye may be instilled into the eye to outline the area of epithelial damage. Corneal abrasions are usually managed with mydriatic drops, antibiotic drops, and patching. Mild abrasions usually heal quite quickly. If any doubt exists about the severity of the injury, ophthalmologic consultation is necessary.

For a rupture or laceration of either the cornea or the sclera, prompt consultation must be obtained. As noted previously, it is extremely important for the team physician to be aware of these possibilities in any case in which severe blunt trauma has occurred around the eye. Once detected, such eyes should no longer be manipulated. Corneal lacerations frequently are complicated by incarceration of iris, which distorts the pupil. Similarly, anterior scleral lacerations or ruptures are frequently complicated by uveal prolapse, and a very dark tissue is typically observed between the edges of the white scleral wound.

Blunt trauma to either the cornea or sclera frequently results in the presence of intraocular hemorrhage, and the term hyphema refers to blood in the anterior chamber. This is quite frequently associated with other severe intraocular injuries, and the detection of any blood in the anterior chamber or vitreous cavity should result in the referral of the pa-

tient to an ophthalmologist. Blunt trauma to the eye is generally followed by inflammation of the iris and ciliary body. Such eyes frequently exhibit either a dilation or constriction of the pupil, which may persist for days or even permanently.

Other Injuries Affecting The Eye. Mild injuries to the eye may cause varying amounts of irritation associated with mild changes in vision and lacrimation, and transient diplopia may occur after apparently minimal head injuries. Any of the symptoms that do not quickly clear should lead to an ophthalmologic consultation.

INJURY IN THE VICINITY OF THE NOSE

Contusion of the nose presents many fascinating aspects, as has been recorded in song and story. However, it is not particularly funny to the recipient of the blow. Here again, careful attention to the possible complicating factors is most important. If the patient is seen before swelling occurs, a very adequate examination can be made digitally from the nasal bone to the infraorbital margin. A simple speculum and a flashlight will enable one to examine the inside of the nose fairly well in the early stages. Careful observation of the face may also reveal telltale deformity, particularly lateral deviation of the nose. I think it is of some advantage to have the patient look at himself in the mirror and also for the doctor to study the patient's physiognomy in the mirror. A tangential view of the nose is extremely important. With the patient lying supine the doctor can look across the forehead, down the bridge of the nose to the tip and observe a deviation that may not have been noticed otherwise. Palpation of the two nasal bones between the fingers will be rewarding, since one can outline the

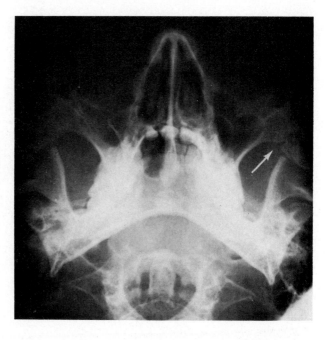

Figure 77. Fracture of zygomatic arch and malar bone bilaterally. Note the good view of the nasal arch. (For technique of x-ray, see Fig. 78.)

exact area of pain on pressure. This may have some significance particularly if the pain is at the junction of the nasal bones with the frontal process or at their junction with each other in the midline. Careful palpation may determine a difference in the angle of the ridge of the nose. One side may seem flat and the other bulging. Sometimes actual crepitation can be felt. All this is much more effective if done early. In the later stages, swelling is very likely to be unilateral or at least worse on one side than the other, and one will be convinced there is gross deformity of the nose when there is simply unilaterally increased swelling. X-ray study, while important, may be quite unsatisfactory. Tangential x-ray studies of the nose may reveal variation of the angle of the bones with each other or possibly a defect or fracture line (Figs. 77 and 78). Again, one must be very wary not to interpret a suture line as a fracture line.

If there appears to be a fracture of the nose, the patient should be referred promptly to a surgeon skilled in such

cases. It will be his responsibility to decide upon the proper time for reduction of the fracture. It is unwise for the untrained physician to attempt reduction of the displaced nasal bones. The nose is an extremely prominent feature and may deviate from normal if the correction is imperfect. This crooked proboscis may haunt the unwary. Additionally, the internal mechanism of the nose with the intricate arrangement of the septum and various turbinates requires especial skill to prevent persistent intranasal symptoms.

Bleeding from the nose is a very common accompaniment of a blow, owing to the extremely copious blood supply of the nasal mucosa. Fortunately, bleeding from the nose is usually readily controlled without resorting to any major procedure. The patient should hold himself upright if possible rather than lie down or hold the head low. The nasal area should be covered with cold cloths or ice to constrict the vessels. Under ordinary circumstances if the patient is kept quiet and semierect

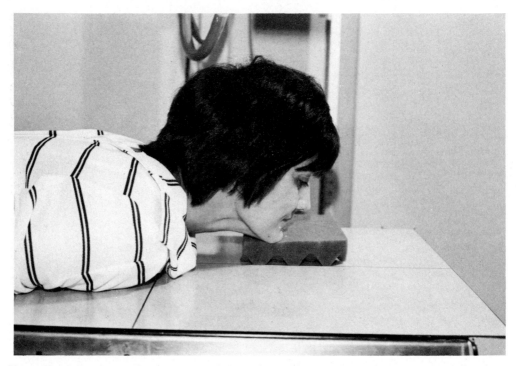

Figure 78. Exaggerated Water's position. The nasal arch. the zygomatic arches and malar bones are well visualized in this variation of the routine Water's position. Place the patient's head so that a line from the external auditory meatus to the symphysis menti is perpendicular to the table. The chin may need to be elevated by a sponge to assume this angle. Center cassette to outer canthi, and the central ray perpendicular to the cassette.

and if cold cloths or ice is applied, the bleeding should stop promptly. If the bleeding is profuse and not easily arrested, careful packing of the anterior nares may reach the area of bleeding and control it. A tampon soaked in thrombin will be of help. It should be emphasized that the packing should not be forced deep into the nose or placed under pressure. Pressure is not required with this type of pack. If it becomes necessary to pack the posterior nares, the equipment of the emergency room and the skill of one accustomed to working in this area are required.

Nasal packing should not be left in place for a long time, since it may force an infection backward through the cribriform plate and cause dangerous meningitis. Because the trauma of removing the pack will sometimes reinitiate the bleeding, various measures have been suggested to permit its easy removal. The pack may be inserted within a very thin film of rubber, such as a condom, packing the rubber ahead of the gauze so as to make a finger-like pouch. Vaseline gauze may be used. However, this method does lessen the effectiveness of the pack, and gauze directly against the area, particularly if impregnated with thrombin, will be much more effective.

INJURY IN THE VICINITY OF THE MALAR BONE AND SUPERIOR MAXILLA

Injuries to the malar bones, zygoma and orbit used to be extremely common in football, particularly from the opponent's helmet or knee. The almost universal use of the face bar has very materially reduced this type of injury so that where we used to see many fractured zygomas, orbits and noses, we seldom see them anymore—another evidence that we are constantly striving to handle injuries by prevention rather than by treatment. This is true for the most part and is particularly documented by the use of the face bar and the mouthpiece.

Contusion over the malar bones or superior maxilla extending back to the zygomatic arch may well cause a fracture in this area (Figs. 77 to 80). Fracture of the malar bone extends into the maxillary sinus. So too, on frequent occasions, does fracture of the superior maxilla, and then it should be considered to be an open fracture. A blow of sufficient severity will justify investigation to determine whether or not a fracture exists. Here again, as in the case of the nose and orbit, early examination is extremely important, since the next day

the face will simply be a mass of tense, swollen edematous skin that prevents any pretense of adequate physical examination. Since the maxilla is important for attachment of the upper teeth, and the zygoma and malar bone are concerned with protection, and since all these bones are related with the orbit, the teeth and the mandible, careful attempt should be made to evaluate adequately any deformity. The maxillofacial surgeon should be consulted in case of serious injury. Expectant treatment should be carried out while awaiting consultation, since it is important to control the swelling as much as possible.

Contusion around the mouth may cause damage to the teeth, and this is usually accompanied by laceration of the lip. One should examine the inside of the lip, since there may be an extensive laceration here that does not extend

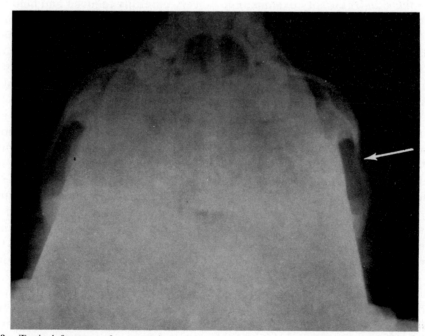

Figure 79. Typical fracture of zygomatic arch on the right. Note normal arch on the left. (For technique of x-ray, see Fig. 80.)

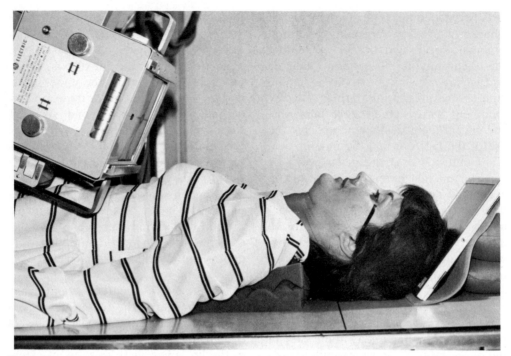

Figure 80. Zygomatic arches. Both zygomas may be shown on one cassette in a position that is comfortably assumed by the injured patient. With the patient supine on the table, elevate the shoulders with sandbags so the chin can be elevated. Align a cassette at a 30 to 45 degree angle at the vertex of the head. The central ray should bisect the orbitomeatal line at an angle of 120 degrees to the cassette.

through the skin. A cursory examination of the teeth may fail to reveal the entire damage. A tooth that in breaking has included a portion of the alveolar process may not appear to be loose or broken. Direct pressure over each tooth will usually determine whether or not the attachment of that tooth is damaged. In many cases if a tooth is broken with a portion of the alveolar process, healing will occur if it is properly replaced and held, whereas if it is overlooked, a subsequent blow, although relatively minor, may knock the tooth completely out. Careful examination is the watchword here. A massive fracture of the face is uncommon in ordinary sports and if it occurs it should be readily recognized. The injury most likely to be overlooked is the one that seems relatively inconsequential.

A fractured alveolar process that includes one or more teeth should be very carefully reduced and held reduced by interdental wiring. In some instances simply wiring the upper teeth to a molded arch wire will be adequate. In others it may be necessary to wire the two jaws together. A good deal of expensive dental reparative work may be avoided by adequate early care in these cases. It is important to remember that any open wound about the mouth is subject to infection. Although the patient may be relatively immune to his own organisms, one cannot assume this to be the case. Any fracture of the alveolar process, into the sinus, into the nose or into the mouth should be considered an open fracture. Antibiotics are recommended and prompt attention must be given to any developing abscess. This applies to the lower as well as the upper jaw. For prevention of injury to the teeth, the molded mouthpiece is extremely effective. It should be required equipment. The day when an athlete is identified by having lost his upper front teeth should be in the past.

INJURY IN THE VICINITY OF THE LOWER JAW

Dislocation of the Temporomandibular Joint. Such injuries are infrequent in the athlete who is not subject to the forces that ordinarily cause them. In the ordinary process of mastication, the condyle of the mandible swings forward out of the cotyloid fossa and subluxates each time the mouth is opened. The force that causes dislocation is one that forces the mandible to open wider than its normal range on either or both sides. Dislocation may occur as the result of yawning, at which time the jaw is actively opened beyond its normal capacity and the condyle slips forward in front of the fossa and locks in this position. Conceivably it could be caused by forcible opening of the mouth, but the immediate response of muscular resistance to this motion will usually prevent the dislocation. The dislocation usually occurs at a time when the muscles that pull the teeth into occlusion are relaxed in a synergistic manner as the muscles that open the jaw contract. An attempt to open the mouth widely, as to bite a large apple or to insert a billiard ball, may result in dislocation and locking of the temporomandibular joint. Once the condyle slips forward and locks, muscle spasm occurs and contraction of the masseter and temporals firmly locks the jaw in the dislocated position. This may be a habitual condition and result much as any habitual dislocation either from an abnormally relaxed joint or from stretching the capsule by repeated episodes of dislocation.

The dislocated jaw can be readily reduced if the patient can be made to relax. Before an attempt is made at reduction, the patient should be relaxed somewhat by sedation. In a cooperative patient, the operator's thumbs may be inserted onto the posterior inferior molars while the index fingers are locked under the point of the chin. Pressure downward on the thumb will unlock the condyles and rotatory pressure forward on the fingers will reduce the forward displacement. If the patient cannot relax, a light anesthetic may be necessary and will make the reduction easy. Forcible traumatic manipulation is neither necessary nor advisable.

If this has been the first episode, the jaw should be prevented from opening widely for a considerable period of time. Preliminary treatment by a Barton's bandage (Fig. 84) for a week or ten days will usually be adequate if the patient is cooperative enough to avoid overopenings of the jaw as in yawning. In recurrent habitual dislocation there probably is little value in temporary immobilization. I have seen many cases of habitual dislocation that were extremely distressing, particularly because of an almost irresistible impulse to yawn and so cause a recurrence. These cases have been relieved by wiring the teeth in apposition for four to six weeks. Threatening to wire the teeth together has in many instances been effective.

Fracture of the Mandible. The mandible is much more susceptible to damage than is the superior maxilla or the temporomandibular joint. Since fracture of the mandible is usually caused by a direct blow, a contusion may be the first thing that calls attention to the injury. Any contusion involving the mandible should be carefully examined. The entire inferior margin of the mandible is subcutaneous and by palpating carefully along the subcutaneous border one can determine areas of tenderness, areas of local swelling or any irregularity of this margin. If the injury is major, the fracture of the mandible may be quite obvious. The jaw will hang open, the lips may be badly swollen. There will be hemorrhage in the mouth where the gum is torn as the jaw fragments separate. These cases are readily diagnosed. Of greater difficulty is the case with little or minimal displacement. After careful observation and palpation the patient should be asked to open and close his mouth and to appose his teeth. Since most athletes with these injuries are young individuals, they usually have a complete set of molars. These should properly occlude without discomfort if there is no displacement. This is the best single test of the accuracy of reduction of any deformity following fracture. It is not advisable to attempt to produce motion at the fracture site. If motion is observed, however, it is quite obvious that a fracture is present. Roentgenographic examination in both anteroposterior and lateral planes should be made and should be carefully interpreted.

Fracture of the tooth-bearing area of the mandible is more readily deter-mined than is fracture posteriorly where it may cross through the angle of the jaw (Fig. 81), through the condyle or through the condylar neck (Figs. 82 and 83). Here again, careful palpation is important. Have the patient open and close his jaw and observe whether or not the chin swings to one side or the other. Palpate the condyle as it comes forward out of the glenoid. Both of these signs are valuable. If the teeth appose properly and there is some question as to whether or not the jaw has been broken, a supportive bandage such as Barton's bandage (Fig. 84) should be applied to the mandible to hold it to the maxilla until a more detailed examination is made. If the mandibular fracture is undisplaced or can be readily reduced, interdental wiring to fasten the upper and lower teeth firmly together should be carried out. If perfect reduction cannot be obtained and one cannot be assured of perfect occlusion, consultation should be sought as early as possible. If there is any question about the occlusion, the patient's dentist may be

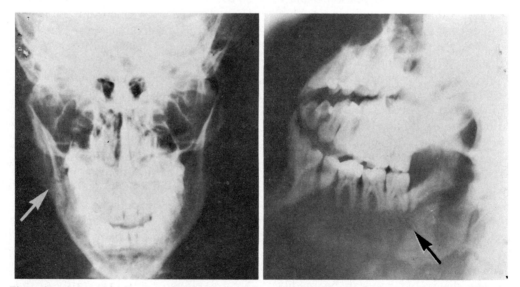

Figure 81. Incomplete fracture of angle of mandible on the left. This should be treated by immobilization of the jaw with interdental wiring.

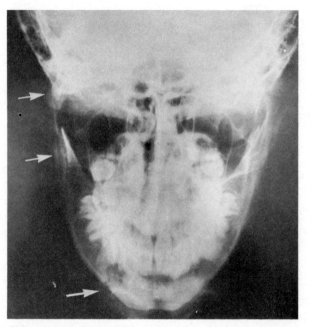

Figure 82. Fracture of the neck of the condyle on the right with fracture through the mandible on the same side. Whenever one fracture is shown in the mandible, search carefully for the second.

able to provide a valuable hint as to any change in the position of the jaw. Frequently malocclusion predates the injury, so it is wise to consult with the patient and with his parents to determine whether or not the patient previously had an overbite, underbite or irregular occlusion. I well recall spending

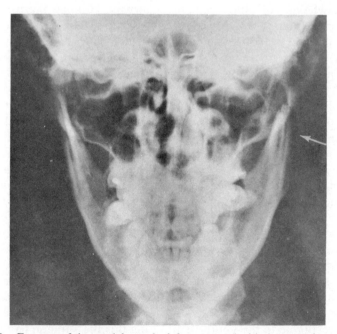

Figure 83. Fracture of the condyle on the left, compared with the normal on the right.

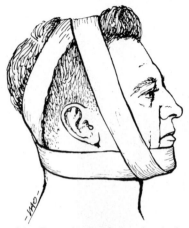

Figure 84. Barton's bandage. A single turn. Many more turns make a firm, compact dressing.

an inordinate amount of time one humid Sunday morning in an attempt to get good occlusion in a man who had been more than slightly inebriated the night before. His truculence had been rewarded by a blow to the chin. In confiding to his wife that we were unable to get good occlusion, she examined his mouth and said it had never been better than that. This proved to be the case. A little foreknowledge of this patient would have prevented a good deal of needless, painful and arduous manipulation.

The management of the patient with his teeth wired together can be difficult, particularly if he is a young and impatient athlete. Actually it is more difficult when his teeth fit well than when they do not, since it is easier for him to eat through the interstices of the teeth if they do not fit perfectly or if one is knocked out. We do not recommend knocking out a tooth to permit eating, however. It is important that the patient have adequate caloric and vitamin intake during the period when he cannot chew. Rich soups, whipped potatoes and gravy, and ground meat can be handled quite well. These will be very much more acceptable to the youth than

a constant diet of malted milks and sweet drinks.

INTERRUPTION OF AIRWAY

One of the unusual complications of fracture of the face that occurs particularly in reference to the mandible, but may also occur in the maxilla, is interruption of the airway. This complication is, of course, first in order of importance in any injury, taking priority over hemorrhage, contamination, unconsciousness or any other complication. The patient cannot long survive without adequate respiration. Occasionally in fractures of the superior maxilla, edema may be severe enough in the back of the soft palate and in the throat to seriously interfere with respiration. It is the rule for nasal obstruction to occur in almost all of these injuries, hence breathing must be through the mouth. Swelling of the back of the tongue that presses the tongue against the pharynx is a very real hazard. Whoever is to care for the person with this type of injury should be warned of the urgency of an adequate airway. Holding the tongue forward by insertion of an anesthetist's airway is of value.

In fracture of the lower jaw, hemorrhage from the external maxillary artery may cause sufficient swelling at the base of the tongue and front of the neck to seriously interfere with breathing. While this is not common, it is extremely distressing when it occurs. At Children's Memorial Hospital a case of fracture of the mandible was accompanied by considerable bleeding. It was felt permissible to proceed with reduction of the fracture and apposition of the teeth by interdental wiring. In subsequent hours these measures compounded the problem rather than improved it. The swelling increased and a tracheotomy was necessary to permit breathing. Following this the surgeon had to tie off the carotid before the hemorrhage could be adequately controlled. It follows that any fracture of the mandible should be carefully observed and not left unattended until the critical period is past, that is, for 12 to 24 hours.

PENETRATING INJURIES

Occasionally there may be an injury to the face by a penetrating sharp object and the complications of such an injury, particularly injury to the eye, demand immediate hospitalization and definitive care. An injury to the *mouth* with damage to hard or soft palate or with severe intraoral bleeding may be easily overlooked. In case of any suspected penetrating wound, the patient should be questioned as to the nature of the injury and carefully examined to determine the depth of penetration and any possible damage to the underlying structures. Another area of the face that is rather frequently injured is the *tongue*. The most common injury of the tongue occurs when it is caught between the upper and lower teeth as the teeth are forcibly apposed in response to some external force. This is a painful injury but usually is not severe. If the laceration goes completely through the tongue, it should be carefully sutured, apposing the edges exactly. Overlapping of the edges will give troublesome irregularity, which may require the service of a plastic surgeon at a later date.

It should be evident that the importance of this chapter could be greatly minimized by mandatory mouthpieces and mandatory face guards. It has been my observation over the years that these facial injuries have been reduced very drastically, and I attribute most of this to prevention by protection. The basis of adequate protection is a well-fitted helmet to which face bars can be attached. Many times the young athlete is impatient of anything that smacks of undue protection. It should be recalled that while he may be extremely smart, he has not yet developed much common sense and so it is necessary to think for him by strict requirements concerning the mouthpiece and the face bars. In the university programs fractures of the malar bone, zygoma and nose used to occur frequently, and, along with knocked out teeth, were in fact among the most common injuries in sports. These have been essentially eliminated from football by teams that insist on wearing of the mouthpiece and the face bars.

CHAPTER 7

INJURIES OF THE SHOULDER GIRDLE

In contrast to the pelvis, which is a solid bony ring that provides great stability for transmitting the body weight from the trunk to the lower extremities, the shoulder girdle is a very loosely constructed, highly mobile mechanism of bones, muscles and ligaments designed to give great mobility to the upper extremity with only sufficient stability to provide a proper foundation for the muscular activity of the upper extremity (Fig. 85). The skeletal connection of the shoulder girdle to the trunk is extremely tenuous and consists only of the relatively insecure articulation of the inner end of the clavicle against the sternum and the first rib (Fig. 86). I will discuss only those details of anatomy that are needed to orient the reader in regard to the various areas of injury, since a full anatomical study of this region would of necessity be voluminous.

Briefly, then, the *clavicle* acts as a strut or crane arm to prevent the

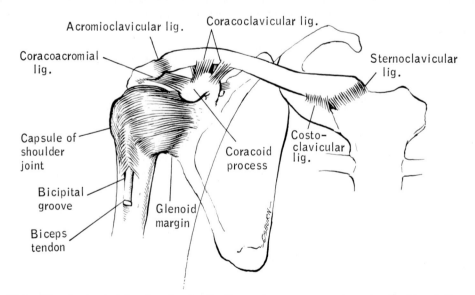

Figure 85. Anatomical drawing showing the ligamentous structures about the shoulder girdle.

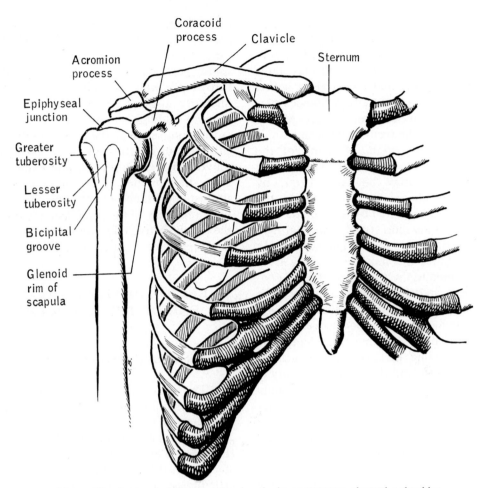

Figure 86.   Anatomical drawing showing the bony structure about the shoulder.

shoulder from dropping forward across the chest. It is a rigid long bone with its inner end apposed to the sternum and its outer end apposed to the acromial process of the scapula. Thus it maintains a constant distance between the upper end of the arm and the midline of the chest. The shoulder may move forward, backward, upward or downward, but so long as the clavicle maintains its integrity the shoulder will not approximate the sternum. Thus, it may be seen that the clavicle has a vital role in shoulder function. The various muscles and ligaments about the thorax and neck tend to stabilize the clavicle in this posi-

tion. Its function is well illustrated by the forward displacement of the shoulder that results when the clavicle is completely broken.

The *scapula* is a broad membranous bone designed primarily for muscle attachment (Figs. 86 and 127). It has no bony connection to the thorax. Its concave undersurface lies over the muscles of the posterolateral thoracic cage. On motions of the arm and shoulder, the scapula glides over the muscles of the chest wall through a wide range of motion, which may be inward, outward, upward, downward, rotatory or any combination of these movements. Its range of motion is subject to the limitations of the clavicular strut and the excursion of the various muscles that control its motion. These muscles have both synergistic and antagonistic action which under normal circumstances permits very smooth movement of the scapula over the trunk. The scapula also serves as the origin of many of the muscles that move the arm. This motion of the arm may be carried out by various mechanisms. For example, the scapula may be fixed by synergistic contraction of antagonists, and the arm then moves in relation to the rigid scapula. In this instance the muscles running from the scapula to the trunk are in tonic contraction, and the muscles running from the scapula and trunk to the upper extremity move the upper extremity on this firm base. On the other hand, the muscles fixing the arm to the scapula may be fixed, and the upper extremity is then moved by gliding of the scapula over the chest wall. Obviously, neither of these situations exists in the pure state under ordinary circumstances. Usually the movement is a synchronous one of the upper arm on the scapula and the scapula on the trunk. This makes for extremely smooth and coordinated action and permits precise motions of the upper extremity where controlled mobility is a good deal more important than stability. One of the early signs of a lesion about the shoulder girdle is a disturbance of this coordinated movement. Various clues may be obtained as to the character of the lesion by careful study of the motion of the arm and shoulder girdle, noting any disturbance of scapulohumeral rhythm.

There follows a discussion of various injuries to the shoulder in relation to specific areas. It should always be borne in mind, however, that the shoulder is an extremely complex mechanism and that anything affecting one portion is bound to have an effect on the other components of the girdle. This is particularly pertinent because of the function of the upper extremities and more particularly in relation to the throwing arm. Conditions of the shoulder girdle have been the ruin of many a budding star whose major forte is throwing, such as the baseball pitcher, the football quarterback, the basketball player, the tennis player, and even the horseshoe pitcher. Rehabilitation is of utmost importance and ofttimes the complete recovery of function depends upon the rehabilitative effort applied to the injured part (see Chapter 22).

REGION OF THE STERNAL END OF THE CLAVICLE

ANATOMICAL CONSIDERATIONS

The integrity of the sternoclavicular joint is maintained by the ligamentous structures that bind the inner end of the clavicle to the sternum and the first rib (Fig. 87). There is little inherent bony stability in this articulation. Indeed, the articulation is notably insecure. The inner end of the clavicle resting against the oblique outer angle of the manubrium is in contact with not more than one-half of the surface area of the end of the clavicle. It is secured by the *sternoclavicular* ligament, a circumferential band of capsular tissue passing from the head of the clavicle to the sternum. This ligament serves to hold the clavicle against the sternum rather than to hold it down. The major structure holding the inner end of the clavicle down is the *costoclavicular* ligament. This is a broad band arising on the proximal one-fourth of the inferior margin of the clavicle and extending in an oblique manner downward and inward to attach to the first rib. This ligament is analogous to the coracoclavicular ligament at the outer

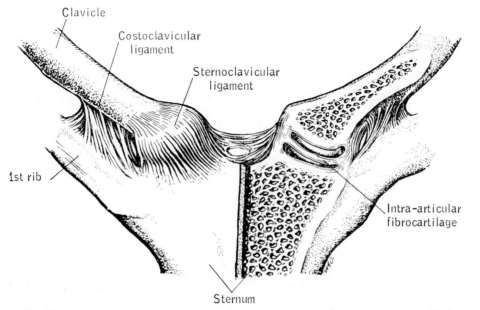

Figure 87. Detail of inner end of the clavicle showing (left) the sternoclavicular area with ligaments intact, (right) cross section. (Redrawn from Spalteholz, Hand Atlas of Anatomy, published by J. B. Lippincott Co.)

end of the clavicle. These two ligaments together prevent the clavicle from displacing upward at either end.

It seems strange that this joint is not injured more frequently, considering that it does have rotatory motion and has little anatomical security.

CONTUSION

Contusion in this area is not frequent since the athlete has been trained to protect the area of the anterior part of the neck and chest by tucking his chin down. In football the shoulder pads protect the area fairly adequately. Contusion here is treated as elsewhere. Disability is slight unless hemorrhage is extensive.

SPRAIN

The most common injury to the sternoclavicular joint is sprain (Fig. 88, *A*). The force applied to cause this injury is one which thrusts the shoulder sharply forward. As the shoulder girdle moves forward and inward, force is applied along the long axis of the clavicle, and the clavicle may be disrupted anywhere along its length. These forces on reaching the sternoclavicular joint will tend to impel the inner end of the clavicle medially, upward and forward. The leverage may be such that it is medially, upward and backward. In either instance the major strain will be upon the costoclavicular ligament. If this gives way, the inner end of the clavicle slips upward and medially as the sternoclavicular ligament gives way. If the force is arrested after minimal damage, the result is a mild (first degree) sprain of these ligaments. Stronger application of the force may rupture the sternoclavicular capsular ligaments while the costoclavicular ligaments remain relatively intact. In this case the inner end of the clavicle may snap in front of or behind the sternum and be held firmly in position by the intact costoclavicular ligament (Fig. 88, *B*). The treatment of this

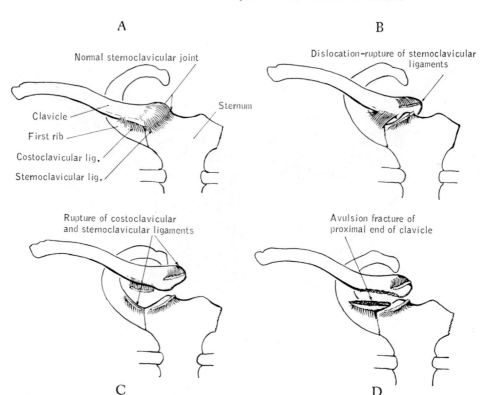

Figure 88. *A,* Normal sternoclavicular joint. *B,* Dislocation with rupture of sternoclavicular ligaments. The inner end of the clavicle is caught behind the sternum. *C,* Similar injury with rupture of both the costo-clavicular and sternoclavicular ligament with the end of the clavicle free. *D,* Avulsion fracture of proximal end of clavicle with rupture of sternoclavicular ligament.

latter condition may be relatively simple if recognized early. Simple traction applied to the shoulder to pull it backward and outward with simultaneous direct pressure on the inner end of the clavicle will usually snap the bone back into place. If the costoclavicular ligament is intact, a simple yoke or sling may be adequate for fixation.

If the driving force continues and the costoclavicular ligament is torn, dislocation or subluxation of the inner end of the clavicle takes place, causing severe (third degree) sprain. In this instance the proximal end of the clavicle is much more free and may ride upward over the sternum toward the midline (Fig. 88, *C*). Another modification of the same type of injury consists of a

fracture-dislocation in which some part of the inferior portion of the proximal end of the clavicle remains fixed by the ligament, whereas the upper portion of the clavicle breaks away and dislocates. This undisplaced fragment may include the whole costoclavicular attachment as well as the inferior portion of the head (Fig. 88, *D*). In this instance treatment is much more favorable, since open reduction and fixation of the main portion of the clavicle to the undetached inferior segment is relatively simple. Careful internal fixation should result in complete recovery (Fig. 89). Even if treatment for this condition is delayed, it remains much more favorable because there is a firm base to which to attach the displaced portion of the clavicle. In this instance open operation and fixation should be recommended at any time and any stage of the injury (see Figs. 90, 91, and 92).

The *treatment* of a mild or moderate (first or second degree) sprain is the treatment of sprain in other areas. The local treatment is application of cold, then heat, compression, local injection and protection. Protection consists of immobilization of the shoulder or application of a figure 8 yoke, which tends to hold the shoulder girdle backward, combined with adhesive strapping of the local area. Strapping of the inner end of the clavicle is ineffective, since it does not prevent the motion that causes stress on the ligament.

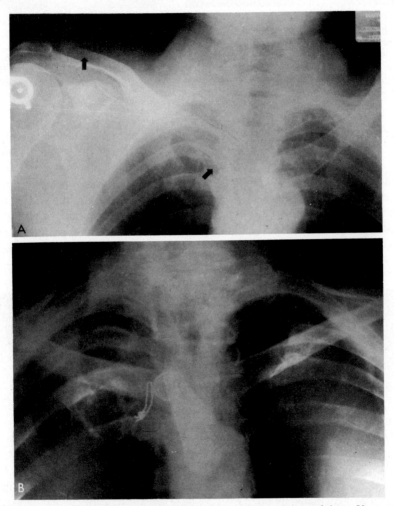

Figure 89. This patient was struck by a car and examined two weeks post-injury. X-rays were taken, but no fracture was found. His complaint was that he couldn't lift the right arm, and it was painful at the inner end of the collarbone; it hurt to turn his head, with pain in the chest. Examination revealed marked prominence of the inner end of the right clavicle, the clavicle set forward on the sternum. *A,* X-ray showing the inner end of the clavicle was anterior and superior to the sternum. Under anesthetic this was not reducible. Open operation showed the mass of healing debris beneath the clavicular head. On cleaning this out there was found to be a gutter of bone, which consisted of the section of inferior cortex of the clavicle as shown in Figure 88*D. B,* This was reduced and held by fixation wires, one through the sternum and one through the clavicular fragment. Good recovery.

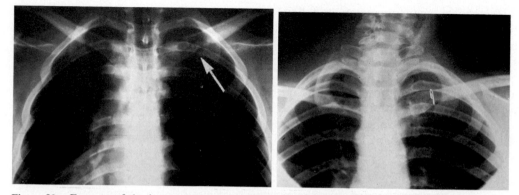

Figure 90. Fracture of the inner end of the clavicle on the right (arrow). Clinically the patient, a boy, appeared to have sternoclavicular dislocation. His injury, which was actually a fracture-dislocation, consisted of approximately the upper one-third of the inner end of the clavicle together with the shaft breaking off from the lower two-thirds, which remained attached to the sternum and to the first rib. Repair was readily made by suture to the undisplaced fragment, which simplified the whole procedure. The displacement was primarily forward and therefore was not well revealed in the film. The x-rays are posteroanterior views.

DISLOCATION

If the ligament tear is complete (third degree) and the inner end of the clavicle dislocates, prompt reduction and operative repair of the ligaments will give very good results. Unfortu-nately, the condition is usually not recognized in its early stages and chronic upward displacement remains (Fig 93). This delay in diagnosis is contributed to by the fact that the deformity is not dramatic and that local swelling will obscure observation or palpation of the displacement. Added to this is the problem

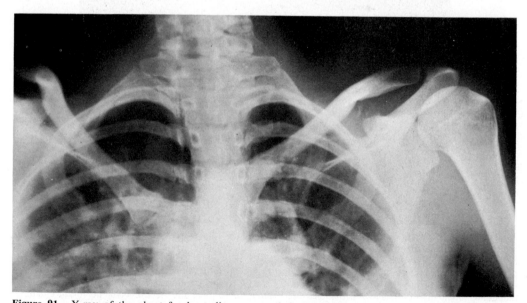

Figure 91. X-ray of the chest for lung disease revealed abnormality of the sternum. Clinical examination then revealed dislocation of the inner end of the clavicle, riding above and behind the sternum (left). (For technique of x-ray, see Fig. 92.)

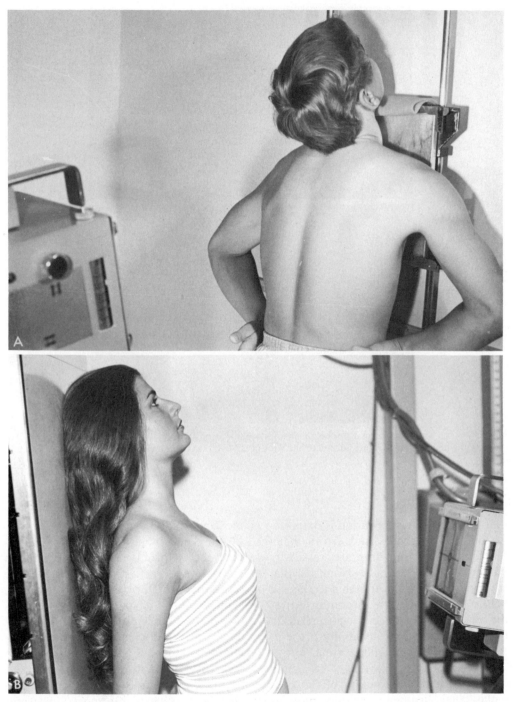

Figure 92. Dislocation of the inner end of the clavicle. Radiographs of sternoclavicular articulations made in routine positions are frequently difficult to interpret. The view in Figure 91 was obtained by a routine examination for apices of the lungs. *A,* With the patient in a posteroanterior position for lungs, shoulders depressed and touching the cassette, the central ray should be directed 10 to 15 degrees to the head and centered to the third thoracic vertebra. *B,* The patient may be more comfortable in an anteroposterior position. In this view the patient should stand slightly away from the table in order to lean back in a slightly lordotic position. The shoulders should be depressed and touching the table. The central ray should be directed to the sternoclavicular joints at a 15 to 20 degree cephalad angle. Note: Technical factors for ribs or cervical spine give better visualization.

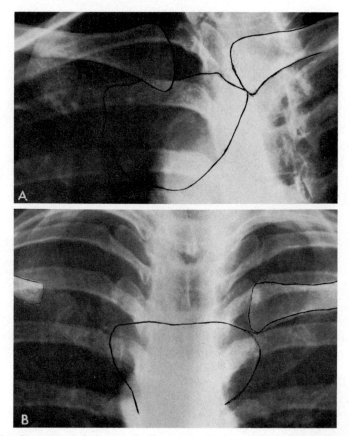

Figure 93. *A,* Showing original displacement of sternal end of clavicle. *B,* Removal of sternal end. Too much of the bone has been removed, since the major portion of the costoclavicular attachment has been lost.

that good x-ray visualization is extremely difficult to obtain, and errors in interpretation of the films are relatively common (Fig. 92). The result is that several weeks will often have elapsed before persistence of discomfort after the swelling has subsided calls attention to the deformity and instability present. At this time it is difficult to treat.

TREATMENT. Various measures designed for reconstruction of the costoclavicular ligament are not particularly successful, certainly not to the point where athletic participation should be encouraged after the procedure. It is unwise to fuse this joint because motion in the sternoclavicular joint occurs in almost any motion of the shoulder girdle. Usually one must be reconciled to accept the deformity and advise enough restriction of activity to minimize the discomfort. At this time local measures, such as corticoid injections, are palliative only. This is not to say that operative reconstruction should never be attempted. However, we usually reserve reconstruction for those cases marked by disabling pain as a result of the displacement. One of the most successful procedures to relieve pain in frank dislocation is resection of the inner end of the clavicle proximal to the costoclavicular attachment (Figs. 94 and 95). If the costoclavicular ligament is torn or redundant, an attempt should be made to reconstruct it.

REGION OF THE CLAVICULAR SHAFT

CONTUSION

The portion of the clavicle lying between the coracoclavicular ligament attachment, which coincides with the beginning of the distal flat portion of the clavicle, and the proximal expansion leading to the sternoclavicular joint is designated as the shaft of the clavicle. Since the clavicular shaft is subcutaneous, it is subject to contusion, the skin and periosteum over the clavicle being impinged between the hard bone and the striking object. The injury is ordinarily readily recognizable because of local swelling. Hematoma formation may occur, but it is not common in this area. Infiltration of blood into the skin and subcutaneous tissue usually occurs. Following a severe contusion, the possibility of an injury to the underlying bone must always be considered. This can be settled fairly well by physical examination since fracture of the clavicle usually will result in considerable pain on any attempt to move the shoulder, whereas simple contusion will not be painful on motion. Later, when there is diffuse swelling and blood infiltration, there may be pain on motion and the exact diagnosis will be more difficult. In case of doubt, x-ray will help to confirm the diagnosis.

There is nothing out of the ordinary about the *treatment* of contusion in this area. The usual measures are local injection, compression, cold and, later, heat. Simple contusion will require relatively little immobilization of the shoulder, and by proper padding athletic participation may be continued. Continuation of pain on use of the shoulder should arouse suspicion of a greater in-

jury, and x-ray 10 to 14 days subsequent to the injury will often show a fracture even though early films have been negative. Incomplete fractures may be revealed by early callus formation or by signs of absorption at the fracture line.

FRACTURE

Fracture of the clavicle is a frequent athletic injury. It is much more likely to occur in the preadolescent or adolescent youngster than in the adult (Fig. 96). In the adult, ligament injury at either the inner or outer end of the clavicle is more likely to occur than in the youngster. A detailed description of the various types of fracture of the clavicle will not be given here, but a few generalities peculiar to athletic injury will be stated.

TREATMENT. One of the most common injuries in childhood is fracture of the shaft of the clavicle. The bone is subcutaneous, and it is fully exposed anteriorly as it arches forward. A direct blow against the outer point of the shoulder jams the shoulder inward. At this age the most vulnerable area in the clavicle is the shaft. Because of the forward bowing, the end-to-end stress increases the arc, and at some point the anterosuperior cortex of the bone gives away. As the bone bows forward, it angulates at the fracture site (Fig. 98). In most cases the fracture of the anterior cortex permits the elastic posteroinferior cortex to bend. The result is a greenstick fracture with or without angulation, but always with good apposition. Further stress may complete the fracture, and loss of apposition occurs (Fig. 97). Torsion force does not ordinarily fracture the shaft. A direct blow may cause a fracture, but this is much more likely after adolescence when the bone becomes more brittle. One must be particularly wary of the greenstick

Text continued on page 156

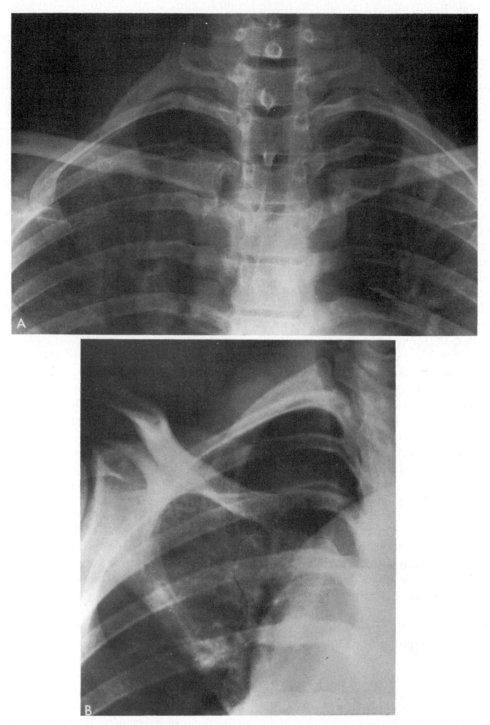

Figure 94. This 19 year old boy had a recurrent dislocation of the inner end of the right clavicle, two years' duration. He was a champion swimmer and had increasing trouble with his back stroke. *A*, Standard anteroposterior view not specific for dislocation. *B*, The oblique view shows the gross dislocation superoposterior, as in Figure 88*C*.

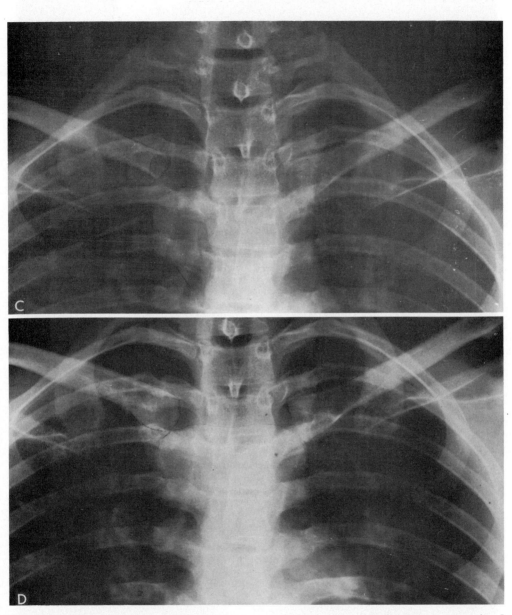

Figure 94 *Continued.* *C*, After resection of the inner end of the clavicle. *D*, One year postoperative. In this young person the inner end of the clavicle has regenerated with minimal displacement. He has no complaint of the shoulder and is swimming without difficulty.

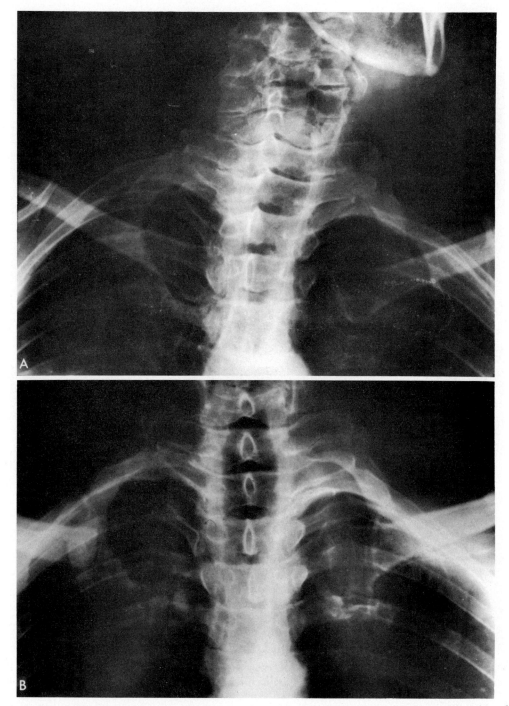

Figure 95. *A,* Wrestling injury one year before, diagnosed by an orthopaedic surgeon as dislocation of the inner end of the clavicle without definitive treatment. The patient had persistent pain localized in the sternoclavicular joint and reconstruction was not feasible this long post-injury. *B,* Resection of the inner end of the clavicle was carried out. The acute pain was somewhat relieved in the sternoclavicular area, but the patient still had gross complaint in the cervical spine, the glenohumeral joint, and the acromio-clavicular joint.

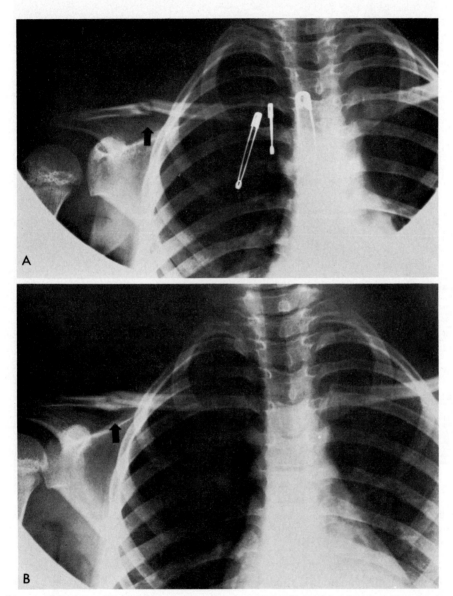

Figure 96. *A*, Eight year old child with complete fracture of the shaft of the clavicle with upward angulation and offset held in yoke (arrow). *B*, Note modeling, which developed during a two month interval.

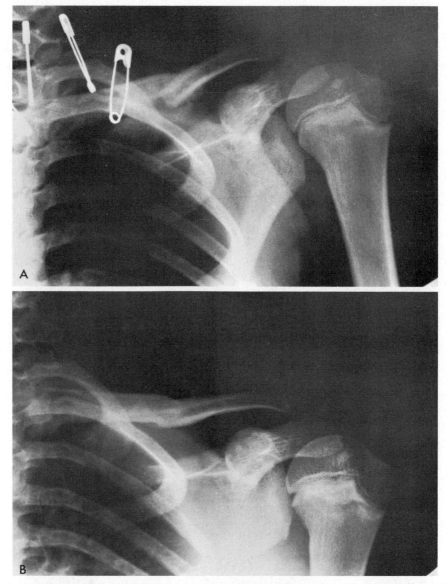

Figure 97. *A,* Twelve year old child held in yoke, with overriding and angulation. Massive callus has developed beneath clavicle. *B,* Note modeling and disappearance of excessive callus.

fracture without displacement, since unprotected it may progress into a fracture with angulation or even with complete displacement.

In the young patient with a painful injury of the shoulder that is causing tenderness directly over the shaft of the clavicle, one should suspect greenstick fracture without displacement (Fig. 98).

Early x-rays may be negative, and the first convincing signs of a fracture may be palpable callus formation which later (10 to 14 days) may show up in the repeat x-rays. One should always obtain a vertical view of the clavicle as well as the standard anteroposterior view (Fig. 100). If there is any doubt, the child should wear a yoke to hold the shoulder

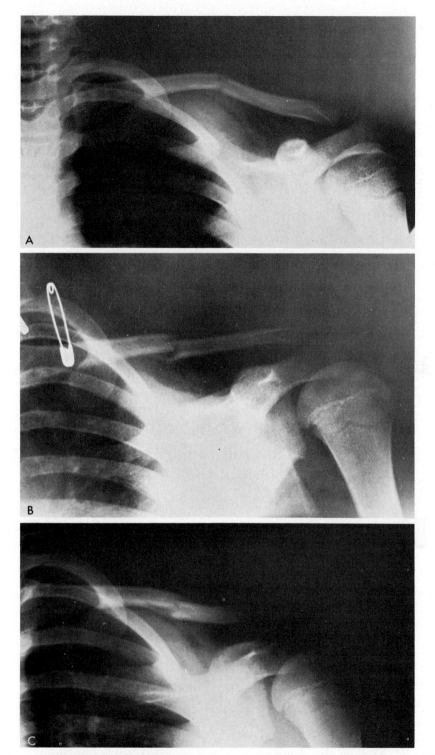

Figure 98. *A*, Child, age 10, with greenstick fracture of the clavicle. Excessive upward and forward angulation was manipulated to break the greenstick. *B*, Position in yoke. *C*, Union at six weeks. Note modeling.

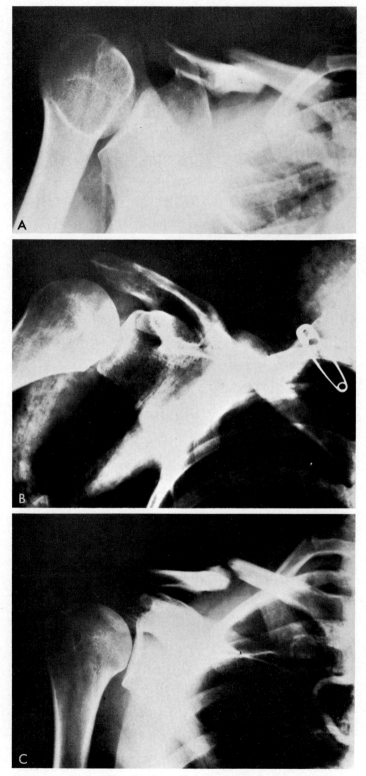

Figure 99. *See legend on the opposite page.*

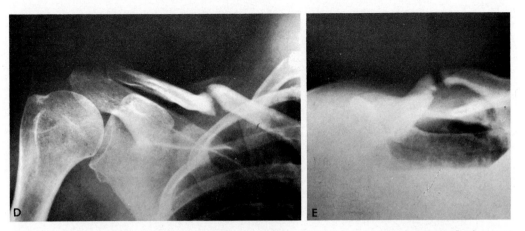

Figure 99. Young adult with an oblique fracture middle third of the clavicle with butterfly fragment. *A*, Original anteroposterior view. *B*, Position in yoke. *C*, One week post-injury. *D* and *E*, Eighteen months post-injury, essentially same position as original, with nonunion; anteroposterior and vertical views. (See Fig. 100 for technique of this vertical view.)

back, or at least a sling. My own preference is for an elastic yoke made of stockinet in which cotton or soft felt pads have been placed.

The fracture of the clavicle in a child (male up to 12, female up to 10) is relatively easy to treat. Open operation is seldom, if ever, indicated in a child of this age; however, the fracture should not be ignored. Without deformity a simple yoke will suffice. In children, considerable deformity will be corrected by modeling, so that the fracture which is offset or angulated, or both, may terminate with a normal appearing bone. True enough, the youngster has great compensatory capacity and one may accept positions that would be intolerable in the adult. This should not be taken as an excuse for sloppy care, and every effort should be made to restore the alignment and length of the clavicle to normal even though this requires anesthesia. The fracture will not ordinarily require open reduction, since it is not necessary to have end-to-end apposition so long as length is reasonably well maintained. It should be emphasized that these statements apply to children and that the term "children"

refers to bone age rather than to chronological age. The 13 year old girl with a fractured clavicle should be treated as an adult since her bone growth may well be completed. The husky 6 foot boy of 14 may have bones quite comparable to the average male of 16 or 17. One only deludes himself if he expects compensatory correction of a deformity in a person whose bone growth is relatively complete (Figs. 99 and 100). I have no hesitation in advising open reduction of a fractured clavicle in a teenager if he is approaching the end of his growth period.

It should also be pointed out that an athlete does have certain important characteristics. In the first place, he is healthy and strong. In the second place, his skeletal structures must be restored to normal if possible. In the third place, healing time is vitally important. These factors must be considered in selecting the method of treatment of fracture of the shaft of the clavicle. My own preference in athletes of high school age or over is open reduction, with internal fixation by intramedullary pinning which is later removed (Fig. 101). This permits early mobility of the shoulder and pre-

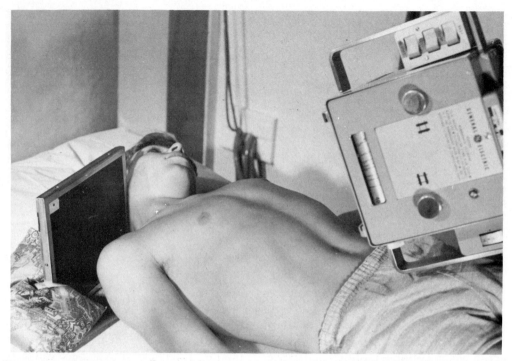

Figure 100. Frequently malposition or nonunion of the clavicle can best be determined by a vertical view of the clavicle (axial projection). With the patient in a supine position, elevate shoulders about 5 centimeters. Turn the patient's head to the unaffected side as far as possible. Place a cassette in a vertical position at the top of the shoulder, pressing it into the neck in order to view as much of the clavicle as possible. Depress the shoulders and pull the arms downward. Tilt the tube so the central ray is as horizontal as possible as it bisects the clavicle. Extreme expiration helps to depress the chest. If the fracture is medial, also angle the tube outward about 10 or 15 degrees.

vents atrophy of muscle and stiffness of the joints. It does demand the ultimate in surgical technique and asepsis. One must have available a strong, healthy patient; intact, uninfected skin; a qualified anesthetist; a first class surgical facility; proper tools; and last but not least a capable surgeon. Lacking any one of these, conservative treatment is preferable.

On occasion comminution at the fracture site will make it advisable to support the intramedullary rod by wire sutures looped around the fragment. The wire sutures alone are usually not secure enough to permit the free use of the arm that is possible with the intramedullary rod (Fig. 102). In any event, the arm should be immobilized in a sling with a swathe (Fig. 103) for at least a

couple of weeks to permit the local reaction to subside. The patient is encouraged to wear the sling alone for another two weeks and given permission to take it off ad lib. He should wear the sling while carrying out ordinary activities.

REGION OF THE OUTER END OF THE CLAVICLE

ANATOMICAL CONSIDERATIONS

At the outer end of the clavicle an ingenious arrangement of bone and ligament promotes stability between the clavicle and scapula and prevents the clavicle from displacing upward but at the same time permits a wide range of motion of the upper extremity (Fig. 85). The outer end of the clavicle butts against the anteromedial aspect of the acromion and is firmly bound to the acromion by the *acromioclavicular* ligaments (capsular ligaments). A wedge-shaped fibrocartilaginous articular disc formed by a thickening of the anterosuperior part of the capsular ligament extends downward into the joint. It lies between the upper portion of the outer end of the clavicle and the acromion. This is sometimes referred to as the semilunar cartilage of the shoulder. The top of the shoulder presents a U-shaped bony subcutaneous surface, the anterior

wing of the "U" beginning as the flat outer end of the clavicle, crossing the acromioclavicular joint and extending to the flat anterior process of the acromion which makes the bottom of the "U," directed laterally. The posterior wing of the "U" is the spine of the scapula which extends from the acromion transversely across the broadest portion of the scapula to blend into its vertebral border. This whole bony "U" is subcutaneous (Fig. 104).

The acromioclavicular ligaments surround the joint but run in an almost horizontal direction in the anatomical position so that they are well designed

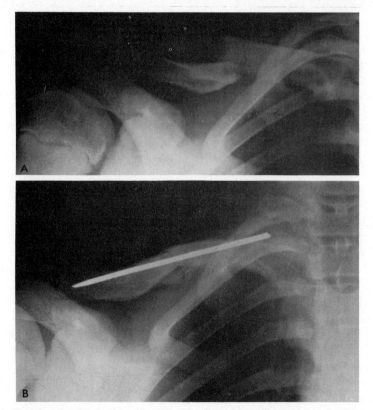

Figure 101. *A,* Showing the fracture proximal to the coracoclavicular ligaments. Note particularly the upward riding of the proximal fragment and the normal relationship between the distal fragment and the scapula. It is virtually impossible to reduce and hold this fracture without internal fixation, since the shoulder tends to fall downward and the proximal fragment to ride upward.

B, In this case fixation was intramedullary with the partially threaded pin left protruding under the skin proximally. This permits better motion of the shoulder than if the pin protrudes distally. The pin is removed after union is complete. The open epiphysis of the humerus indicates that the patient is an adolescent. Nonetheless, open reduction was indicated.

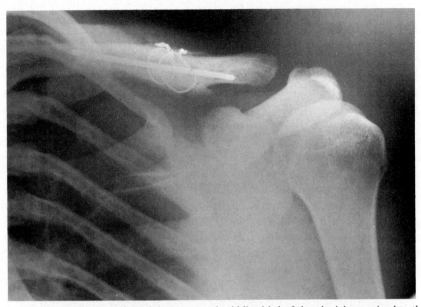

Figure 102. Fracture at the junction of the outer and middle third of the clavicle proximal to the coraco-clavicular ligament, held by intramedullary wire fixation. Comminuted butterfly fragments were held by two stainless steel wire loops. There was no damage to the ligaments of the shoulder.

to prevent distraction of the two bones but are poorly designed to prevent upward displacement of the clavicle on the acromion. The ligaments between the clavicle and the coracoid process of the scapula make up for this deficiency. The coracoid process extends forward from the scapula much like a pointing finger crooked slightly laterally. It lies directly underneath the clavicle, being separated from it by approximately 1.2 cm. The long axes of the two bones are at right angles. The ligaments arising along the superior surface of the coracoid twist approximately 90 degrees to attach along the undersurface of the clavicle as a broad, flat band with different divisions, the trapezoid attaching most distally, the conoid proximally. Actually, these divisions are usually indistinguishable after an injury. These ligaments have a much more vertical course than the acromioclavicular ligaments and effectively hold the clavicle down to the scapula.

From the anterior portion of the coracoid the *coraco-acromial* ligament extends upward and laterally to attach to the top of the acromion in front. This ligament plays no part in acromioclavicular stability but actually serves to reinforce the glenohumeral joint in front. The section of the clavicle from the conoid portion of the coracoclavicular ligament to its distal end is called the *interligamentary* portion. In this region it is a broad, flat bone with no medullary canal. Proximal to this the clavicle becomes rounded and takes on the typical characteristics of a long bone. The upper surfaces of the clavicle and the acromion together with the spine of the scapula form the superior portion of the shoulder and are subcutaneous.

CONTUSION

The top of the shoulder is frequently contused. Because of the subcutaneous character of the bone there is often a subperiosteal hematoma and even more frequently rather severe damage to the skin. Contusion here is

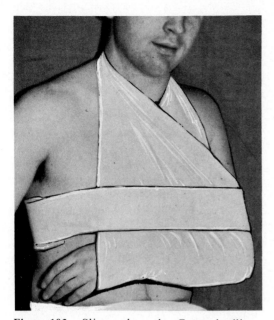

Figure 103. Sling and swathe. General utility dressing for shoulder fixation. This does not give adequate support for acromioclavicular sprain or dislocation. It is ideal for more moderate injuries, for postoperative care, and the like. Note the hand is supported in the triangular sling, yet is free for movement of the elbow and utilization of the fingers. The circular adhesive strip is double thickness and is placed over gauze to avoid irritating the skin of the chest wall. This circular swathe limits external rotation and abduction to any desired amount, depending upon its tightness.

treated as in other areas. The major problem is to determine whether or not there is more serious injury to the underlying structures. One should locate accurately the area of contusion and by careful examination determine whether or not there is involvement of the acromioclavicular joint. In such a case the contusion may be entirely incidental.

STRAIN

Since the deltoid muscle attachment encompasses the entire outer clavicle and the acromion, strain may be a problem. However, contusion of the deltoid is much more common than strain. The deltoid has a broad attachment without any particularly well-localized area of stress. If muscle tendon injury occurs, it is usually in the muscle belly. The most common site of this in the whole deltoid mechanism is at the attachment of the deltoid muscle to the shaft of the humerus.

Treatment should be that of muscle strain elsewhere, i.e., rest, heat, protec-

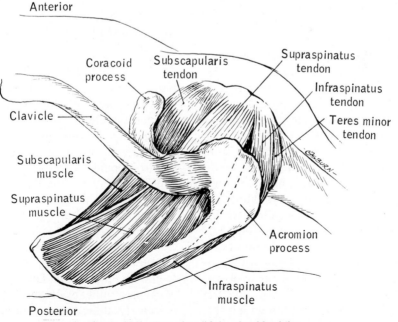

Figure 104. Top view of the shoulder joint.

tion, and gradual resumption of active motion with no passive stretching. Complete rupture of a segment of the deltoid is unusual in the athlete.

Occasionally the deltoid may be subject to chronic strain in the throwing arm and may require treatment. This is much more common around the glenohumeral joint, in the biceps, in the rotator cuff, or in the attachment of the triceps to the glenoid. This will be discussed in relation to the glenohumeral areas.

SPRAIN-SUBLUXATION-DISLOCATION

Since there is no "built-in" bony stability between the acromion and clavicle, it follows that the entire integrity of this joint is maintained by ligamentous support. A sprain of these ligaments is caused by anything that forces the acromioclavicular joint through a range of motion beyond its normal capacity. Normally this joint has but little excursion. The acromioclavicular ligaments completely surrounding the joint permit only a certain degree of rocking motion but allow no actual flexion or extension.

Various forces may cause injury to the acromioclavicular joint. The most common is a downward blow against the outer end of the shoulder driving the acromion downward, the clavicle remaining upward. Another is traction on the arm pulling the shoulder away from the chest wall and causing true lateral displacement of the acromion. Neither of these, however, can adequately account for the instances of injury to this area caused by falling on the outstretched arm or on the point of the elbow. The football player is well protected by shoulder pads from a downward blow against the top of the shoulder. The sport most commonly involved in this type of force is polo,

where the horseman falls and lands on the unprotected point of the shoulder. I believe the mechanism causing the majority of these injuries in football is falling on the outstretched hand or flexed elbow with the arm flexed forward 90 degrees and in a neutral lateral position. In this position the humerus drives against the glenoid and acromion, pushing them forcibly backward, and the clavicle remains forward so that stress is applied to the acromioclavicular and also the coracoclavicular ligaments. This same mechanism could well cause an isolated injury to the acromioclavicular ligament by rotation of the scapula to permit the acromion to move backward while the coracoid either remains in normal relationship with the clavicle or actually rotates forward. As these various forces occur, stress is applied to the acromioclavicular ligament which permits a certain amount of upward displacement of the outer end of the clavicle. The tension is then taken on the coracoclavicular ligaments. Either of these may be injured to a variable degree.

Mild (First Degree) Ligament Sprain

In a mild sprain the force is contained before any real damage is done. There is slight tearing of the fibers of the acromioclavicular or coracoclavicular ligament. In this case there is little or no disability of the shoulder. There is localized pain over the area of injury. This pain may be directly over the acromioclavicular joint or may be medial to the acromioclavicular joint just in front of the clavicle in the sulcus between the clavicle and the coracoid. In the well-muscled individual this may be difficult to elicit by palpation. The differentiation between a mild sprain and a contusion is extremely difficult since a mild sprain does not entail any hypermobility, and indeed, ordinary motions of the shoulder girdle will elicit no pain.

Treatment here is relatively unimportant and actually treatment of contusion and sprain may be quite similar, that is, local injection into the tender area, cold followed by heat, and the use of padding to protect from a blow rather than to restrict motion.

Moderate (Second Degree) Ligament Sprain

In a moderate sprain of these ligaments we predicate relatively severe damage to the fibers of the ligament and in this case the symptoms will be more pronounced. Since there has been tearing of some of the ligament fibers, there will be pain on forced motion of the shoulder even though there is no actual hypermobility of the clavicle on the acromion. In such a case we do not expect the clavicle to be riding high. There will be pain, swelling and tenderness, with the pain increased by an attempt to separate the acromion and clavicle by pulling on the arm. There is also pain on depressing the acromion in relation to the clavicle by pulling straight down on the arm with the arm against the side. This case can be distinguished from contusion by the severity of the symptoms and their aggravation when the ligament is placed under stress. Within a short time there will be local swelling at the joint that may simulate upward displacement of the clavicle.

Treatment of a moderate sprain of the acromioclavicular or coracoclavicular ligaments should be local and general. Local treatment is the same as for mild sprain; i.e., local injection of procaine plus hyaluronidase, application of cold followed by heat, pressure dressing in case of swelling. Protective treatment here is all-important, since it is vital to prevent subsequent injury. One must visualize that a definite portion of the ligament is torn or avulsed and that the remaining portion is substantially weakened. If athletic participation is permitted in contact sports, the next blow may well complete the tear.

It is important that the arm be strapped to the side in such a way as to push the arm upward and the clavicle downward. This can be done by various methods. One of the simplest and best for this type of injury is as follows. With the arm at the side and the elbow flexed to 90 degrees, the midpoint of a long strip of 3 inch tape is placed under the forearm about 2 inches distal to the elbow and carried forward up over the shoulder proximal to the acromioclavicular joint and then down the back, crossing toward the opposite side. The posterior portion of the long strip should go up the back of the arm, cross over the shoulder from back to front, then diagonally across the chest again medial to the acromioclavicular joint (Fig. 105, *A*). The dressing is completed by a circumferential strip of protective tape placed around the arm and the chest to hold the arm to the side (Fig. 105, *B*). These are the key straps of the dressing. The dressing is made more comfortable by suspending the forearm loosely in a choker-type sling made of elastic stockinet around the wrist and behind the neck (Fig. 105, *C*). Additional adhesive strapping can be applied for compression directly over the shoulder if desirable. The principle of this support is that, as the weight of the forearm and hand drops distally, the lever fulcrum is at the broad band of the tape under the proximal forearm, and the short posterior arm of the lever tends to thrust the humerus upward as the hand drops downward. There are obviously many modifications of this type of support, and any one that effectively holds the clavicle down and the arm up is satisfactory (Fig. 106).

This type of support is continued a minimum of six weeks in order to per-

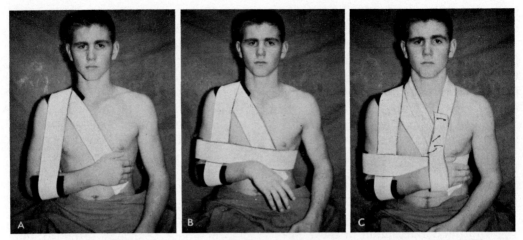

Figure 105.   Strapping to support the acromioclavicular joint in acromioclavicular sprain. *A,* The vertical strip which holds the humerus upward and the clavicle downward. Note particularly the length of the strip, since it extends from the waist line in the back to the waist line in front as a single strip. Note the leverage action as the hand and forearm drop downward at the waist, the short lever of the inner end of the ulna pushing the humerus upward.

B, The application of a tape swathe to hold the elbow to the side. This strip should not be tight. Before this strip is applied, a powdered ABD pad is placed in the axilla.

C, Choker sling of stockinet is added. This sling is loose and may be changed from the hand to the wrist or eliminated altogether as the patient wishes. Some of the details to note are the felt pads (here used with blue felt for contrast) to protect the skin at the pressure areas. There are also the felt pads within the stockinet behind the neck and under the hand.

mit the ligaments to unite and become relatively strong. It should be borne in mind that the simple force of the weight of the arm hanging at the side may be sufficient to distract the ligament ends. A period of rehabilitation will be required in order to mobilize the shoulder and improve the muscle tone in the upper extremity before participation in sports is advisable. (See Fig. 161.) Such a plan carefully followed will result in complete recovery from a rather severe injury, whereas if continued function is permitted the ligaments will gradually stretch and result in a loose acromioclavicular joint which is subject to either chronic disability or repeated injury.

Severe (Third Degree) Ligament Sprain (Subluxation-Dislocation)

Severe (third degree) ligament sprain is one in which one or more of the ligaments have been completely torn. It can be classified roughly into two categories: (1) complete tear of the acromioclavicular ligament with the coracoclavicular ligament intact and (2) a complete tear of the coracoclavicular and acromioclavicular ligaments.

Severe (Third Degree) Sprain of the Acromioclavicular Ligament.   It is possible for a complete tear of the acromioclavicular ligament to occur along with an incomplete tear of the coracoclavicular ligament. The force applied here is downward on the acromion and usually has an outward component so that the acromion is forced outward and downward away from the clavicle. This causes rupture of the horizontal fibers extending from the clavicle to the acromion. The resulting symptoms depend to some extent on the degree of injury to the coracoclavicular ligaments. If this is slight and largely of the distal component, the symptoms will be those of moderate sprain, that is, local pain, swelling, and tenderness in the acromio-clavicular joint. There will be pain on any effort to distract this joint or on downward pull on the arm or on manipulation of the shoulder toward wide abduction. There will frequently be a mild degree of instability between the outer end of the clavicle and acromion, with the clavicle appearing to be slightly higher than the acromion. The space between the clavicle and acromion may well be widened in comparison to the normal or to the opposite shoulder. There will not be extensive upward riding of the clavicle in relation to the acromion. This cannot take place with intact coracoclavicular ligaments. One may visualize that there has been complete rupture of some of the fibers of the

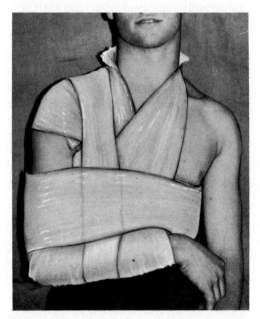

Figure 106. Modification of dressing shown in Figure 105, which we often use postoperatively. In this instance the initial application is the pressure dressing over the wound and top of the shoulder using Elastoplast. The second step is the application of a triangular sling carefully pinned around the elbow. Step 3 is the application of a swathe around the body to hold the arm to the side. The dressing is stabilized then by the vertical strip applied as in Figure 105, only over the dressing rather than over the skin.

acromioclavicular ligament but that the scapula has rotated downward rather than displaced downward. The coracoclavicular ligament is still effective in holding the clavicle in its normal position in relation to the acromion.

TREATMENT. Treatment of this type of acromioclavicular injury taxes the best judgment. Far too often the injury is treated by the so-called conservative method, with resulting chronic relaxation of the acromioclavicular joint, arthritic changes and disability that may later require surgery eventuating in less than a complete recovery. On the other hand, one hesitates to perform an open repair in the absence of upward displacement of the clavicle. Local treatment consists of the usual measures: aspiration, injection, cold then heat. The subluxation should be reduced by downward pressure on the clavicle and upward pressure on the arm. The temptation then is to maintain this reduction by external fixation, and this is usually done by the method previously described (Fig. 105). That this is often ineffectual is indicated by the wide variety of methods suggested as improvements, i.e., support in a plaster jacket with straps over the clavicle in order to hold it down and various other lever actions designed to hold the acromion and clavicle together. In the final analysis I think internal fixation is probably desirable in the majority of cases in the young athlete. If one can obtain complete reduction manually, it indicates that there is no interposing tissue between the two bones. It is justifiable then to attempt skeletal fixation by pins across the acromion and the joint into the clavicle, without open reduction. Proper positioning of the pins is extremely difficult and this method is not for the uninitiated. However, the operator who has repeatedly inserted these pins at open reduction may be able to place two pins in a position adequate to hold the bones together. This is much easier to do under television control. Since it is important to prevent distraction of the acromion from the clavicle as well as to hold the clavicle down, a smooth pin with 1 inch overlay screw thread at one end is desirable.

Complete Rupture of the Acromioclavicular and Coracoclavicular Ligaments. The second type of third degree sprain presumes a complete rupture of both the acromioclavicular and coracoclavicular ligaments (Fig. 107). In this injury there is more swelling, more tenderness, and pain is elicited on any manipulation of the shoulder. The characteristic finding, however, is marked upward riding of the outer end of the clavicle in relation to the scapula (Fig. 108). This may be quite obvious in clinical examination of the patient. If the patient is examined sitting up and if swelling is not severe, the outer end of the clavicle can be felt and seen pushing

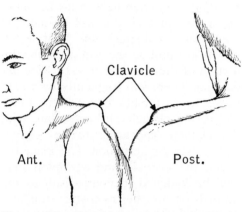

Figure 108. Sketch shows dramatically the upward displacement of the outer end of the clavicle in complete acromioclavicular dislocation. (From DePalma, Fractures and Dislocations—An Atlas, Vol. 1, p. 227.)

up under the skin while the acromion remains downward. This finding may be completely obscured when the patient is lying supine, but when he stands (Figs. 109 and 110), particularly with some weight in the hand, it becomes quite obvious. Comparable pictures of the two shoulders in the standing position will reveal the displacement. In this instance the displacement of the clavicle is primarily upward, whereas in the other type of subluxation the acromion pulls away from the outer end of the clavicle rather than downward. However, both types of displacement may well be present.

TREATMENT.   Although this dislocation is usually readily reduced, it is virtually impossible to hold reduction in a manner that will allow primary repair of the torn ligaments at their normal length. When one recalls the pathologic changes this is apparent. In order for the clavicle to displace upward, the distance between the clavicle and coracoid must be increased (Fig. 107). The coracoclavicular and acromioclavicular ligaments are avulsed or torn, and unless the clavicle is held in the anatomical position until healing is complete, subluxation will inevitably recur and a pain-

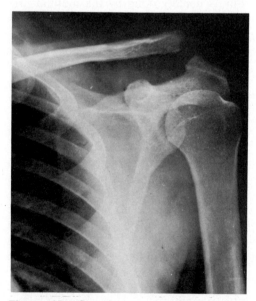

Figure 107. Complete acromioclavicular dislocation with obvious tearing of both coracoclavicular and acromioclavicular ligaments. Note particularly the wide space between the coracoid and clavicle with the clavicle riding high above the acromion. The x-ray was made with the patient standing but with no weight.

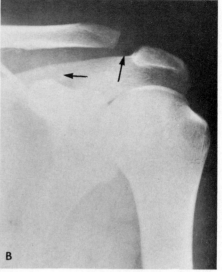

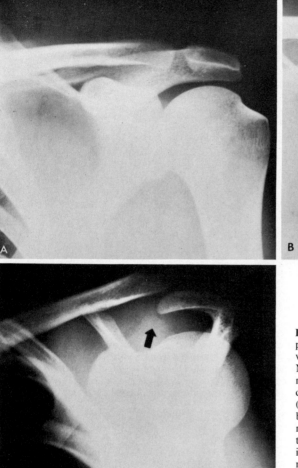

Figure 109. *A*, With the patient supine, no dislocation is noted. *B*, Standing with 4 pounds suspended from the wrist. Note particularly the widening at the acromioclavicular joint (1) and also difference in distance between the clavicle and coracoid (2). This is not as dramatic as Figure 107, but comparison with the supine position makes it quite obvious. *C*, Lateral view of the acromioclavicular joint made as shown in Figure 110, showing the complete separation.

ful, weak shoulder may be the result. For this reason it is my opinion that in the athlete a complete tear of these ligaments should be treated by surgical repair.

Again, we are faced with two alternatives. Once surgery has been decided upon, one must resolve whether the operation should be designed merely to hold the clavicle in position or to repair the torn ligaments as well. It is my belief that if one is going to go to the trouble to do an open operation to fix the clavicle in position, he should take advantage of this opportunity to appose and suture the torn ends of the coracoclavicular ligaments. In the ordinary case this can readily be accomplished, because after the skin is divided and the outer end of the clavicle is freed from its muscle attachments, the outer end may readily be displaced upward. Ready access can be had to the area of the injury between the clavicle and coracoid, and in most instances sutures can be placed in the coracoclavicular ligaments

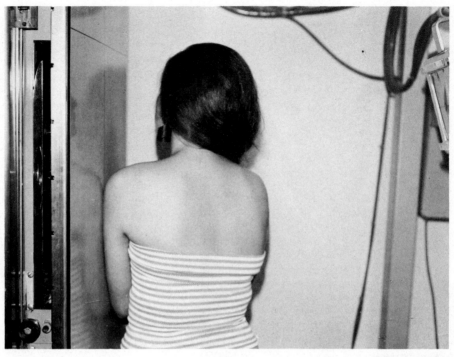

Figure 110. To demonstrate the separation shown in Figure 109*C*, a lateral projection may be made. Instruct the patient to place the hand of the affected arm under the opposite axilla, allowing the injured shoulder to hang as relaxed as possible. The acromioclavicular joint should be positioned to the center of the table. The unaffected side should be rotated about 45 degrees away from the table. The tube is angled downward 20 to 25 degrees and the central ray is directed to the acromioclavicular joint. The cassette should be centered to the central ray.

while the clavicle is displaced upward and can be tied after replacement of the clavicle and fixation in its normal position.

Of vital importance is firm fixation of the clavicle to the scapula. This can be done by various methods, depending upon the choice of the surgeon. Basically the methods of fixation are either by transfixion of the acromion and clavicle or by fixation of the clavicle to the coracoid, or by both. A good method for fixing the clavicle to the acromion is the use of transfixion pins, preferably threaded in part, passing through the acromion, across the joint and into the clavicle. It is necessary to use two pins, since one may not give sufficient fixation (Fig. 111). If this is done, no fixation is needed between the coracoid and

the clavicle other than the ligament repair.

Other methods of holding the coracoid and clavicle together are the lag (Bosworth) screw which transfixes the clavicle (Fig. 112) and extends into the coracoid, or suture around the coracoid and clavicle with fascia, braided silk or wire. There are some disadvantages in each method. Previously I have expressed a preference for double pin fixation across the acromioclavicular joint. Because of the many complications resulting from this method of fixation, my present choice is the use of a Bosworth screw. Since it is necessary to expose the coracoid process to repair the coracoclavicular ligaments, the insertion of the screw is somewhat simplified. However, it is a technical exercise and may at times be quite frustrating. It is of absolute importance that the thread of the screw engage completely through the coracoid or else the fixation will be lost (Fig. 113). A few hints as to this method: The Bosworth screw is specifically designed to permit up and down motion of the clavicle on the neck of the screw. Therefore, the hole in the clavicle should be slightly larger than the shaft of the screw. It must not be unduly large or the screw head may erode through it more readily. Since the coracoid process has no specific function in regard to its position, there is naturally a great deal of variation between individuals in the exact course of the coracoid. This points out the validity of my statement that exposure of the coracoid helps, because you can actually have the coracoid exposed and be sure that the screw fixation penetrates through both cortices. After this screw is placed, you should be able to move the clavicle up and down on the screw a millimeter or so. My reason for adopting this

method is that this does permit relatively rapid resumption of activity, although it would be wise to protect the shoulder against football for eight weeks. I have, however, permitted an occasional college athlete to return to play after carefully explaining to him the risk of damage. So far none of them has broken the screw, although in two instances the screw was slightly bent. I would like to emphasize here again that any type of nonabsorbable fixation should be removed after eight or ten weeks, when one must assume that the ligament has united.

After threaded pin fixation is completed, the acromioclavicular ligament should be carefully repaired. Strong internal fixation permits rapid mobilization of the shoulder joint and so shortens the period of disability. It is advisable for the arm to be held in a sling for several weeks. This will permit active motion but protects against unguarded activity. Any type of metallic internal fixation should be removed

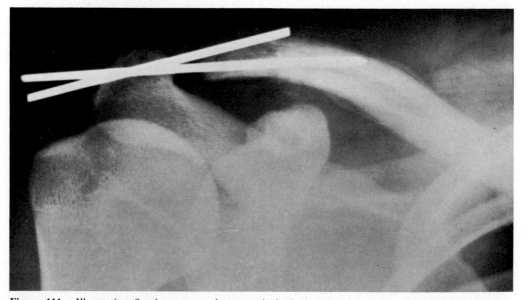

Figure 111. Illustrating fixation across the acromioclavicular joint with two partially threaded pins. This is an old case as indicated by the calcification about the clavicle, and it was felt advisable to resect 1 cm. of the outer end of the clavicle. Wider resection than this is neither necessary nor desirable. Note the close approximation of the clavicle and coracoid. These pins should be removed after 8 to 10 weeks.

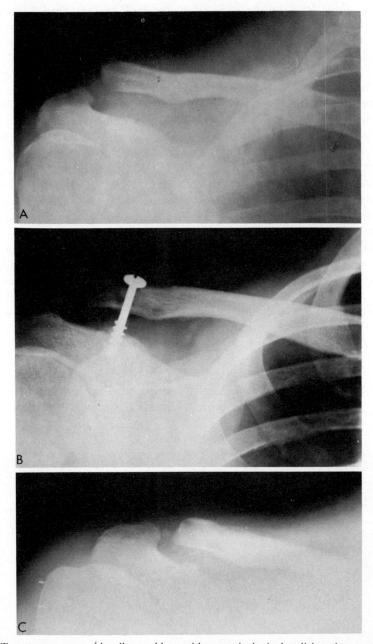

Figure 112. Twenty-two year old college athlete with acromioclavicular dislocation on the right side. *A*, X-ray shows marked upward dislocation of the clavicle with separation between the clavicle and the acromion. The patient was treated elsewhere in a Kenny Howard sling for six weeks but the deformity persisted. I saw him three months post-injury, at which time the outer end of the clavicle was resected. Reconstruction of the acromioclavicular ligament by the conjoined tendon of the biceps and coracobrachialis. Half of this tendon was dissected free, reflected upward and fastened to the outer end of the clavicle through drill holes. This was also supported by the clavicular acromial ligament, which was detached from the acromion, left attached to the coracoid process and fastened to the clavicle. Position was secured with Bosworth screw. *B*, X-ray six weeks postoperative shows the Bosworth screw holding in position. *C*, X-ray three months postoperative following removal of the Bosworth screw. Position is secure although there is considerable reaction around the joint. He is playing basketball with no complaint of the shoulder.

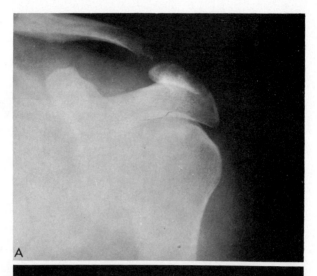

Figure 113. This 22 year old male dislocated his coracoclavicular joint 10 days before being examined. He is a Judo instructor and unable to use his shoulder. Examination revealed upward riding of the outer end of the clavicle with instability, tenderness, and pain on abduction. *A,* X-ray shows the wide separation at the coracoclavicular level. Note the degenerative change at the outer end of the clavicle just two weeks post-injury. *B,* Open reduction and repair of the coracoclavicular ligaments carried out with resection of the distal tip of the clavicle. The Bosworth screw is holding the clavicle reduced. *C,* Five months later after removal of the screw. Note some regeneration of the outer end of the clavicle and no upward displacement.

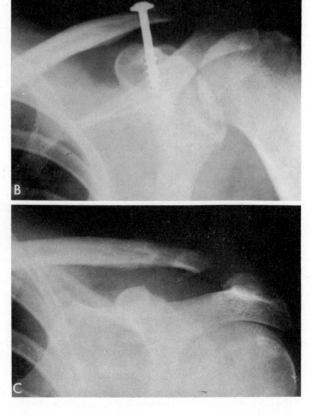

after eight weeks. This includes the Bosworth screw, which may work loose and break; the circumferential suture or wire, which may erode through the clavicle (Fig. 114); and the transfixion pins, which, after a certain period, may migrate (Fig. 115). Following successful repair with a good functional result, the patient may resume unlimited activity. It is wise for him to wear particularly

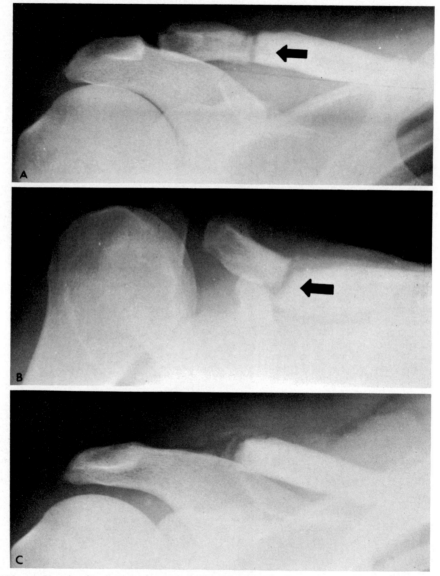

Figure 114. *A*, Showing fixation of outer end clavicle by braided silk through drill hole in clavicle (arrow). This is a late postoperative picture and is suggestive of erosion of the suture. *B*, Complete erosion through the clavicle with pathological fracture (arrow). *C*, After removal of the outer end of the clavicle. Some disability persists.

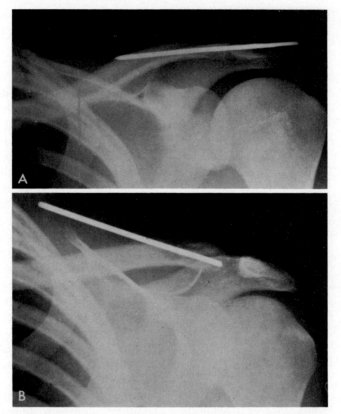

Figure 115. *A*, Acromioclavicular joint fixed by single nonthreaded pin. *B*, Migration of this pin — fortunately after healing of the ligaments. This could have been prevented by having a portion of the pin threaded. It is inadvisable to have the threaded part of the pin across the joint because it may break through the threaded area. Migration can also be prevented by bending the end of the pin.

well-designed shoulder pads after such an injury. However, the best the shoulder pad can do is to protect the shoulder against a direct blow. It has no effect on forces that are transmitted through the arm.

CHRONIC LESIONS OF THE ACROMIOCLAVICULAR JOINT

A chronic irritative lesion of the acromioclavicular joint can be the consequence of repeated injuries which cause the acromion and clavicle to impinge forcibly (Fig. 116). Repeated minor sprains of the capsular ligament that result in thickening of the ligament

and local swelling in the joint are another cause of this condition. It may go on to calcific or osseous deposits within the ligament or joint. Since calcific deposits are basically degenerative and osseous deposits are basically reparative, ossification of the coracoclavicular ligament does not seem to impair its function. I have seen many cases with what appears to be complete ossification of the ligament, yet completely asymptomatic. I would strongly urge against removal of an osseous deposit in the ligament, since this may substantially weaken the ligament. There may be involvement of the intra-articular fibrocartilage, even with ossification or fragmentation of the cartilage (Fig. 117). The result is pain and

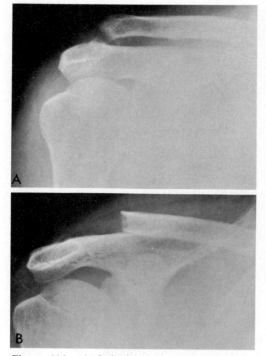

Figure 116. *A,* Irritative lesion. Degenerative changes and chronic arthritis from dislocation of the clavicle upward, although the space between the coracoid and clavicle seems quite narrow. *B,* Shows resection of the outer end of the clavicle distal to the coracoclavicular ligaments. Note upward displacement of the clavicle, which persists owing to elongation of the coracoid ligament.

tenderness elicited particularly by abduction of the arm, as this movement forces the acromion and clavicle together.

TREATMENT. This condition is basically a traumatic arthritis and may be treated as such by local heat, rest, injection of a long-acting local anesthetic and a corticoid preparation. It may be quite distressing because it is magnified by athletic activity such as throwing, falling on the outstretched hand or in fact any forceful activity of the shoulder girdle. If it does not respond adequately to nonsurgical treatment, surgery is justified. At this time the fibrocartilaginous disc should be removed and the joint carefully inspected. If there are definite irreversible changes in the articular cartilage, it is wise to resect 1/2 or 3/4 inch of the outer end of the clavicle (Figs. 118 and 119). Care should be taken to stay distal to the coracoclavicular ligament. This usually will give excellent results with good function of the shoulder, although sometimes there is persistent pain or tenderness. Recognizable weakness may persist.

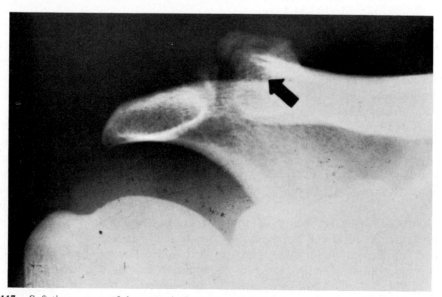

Figure 117. Soft tissue x-ray of the acromioclavicular joint showing ossification of the capsule and cartilage (arrow).

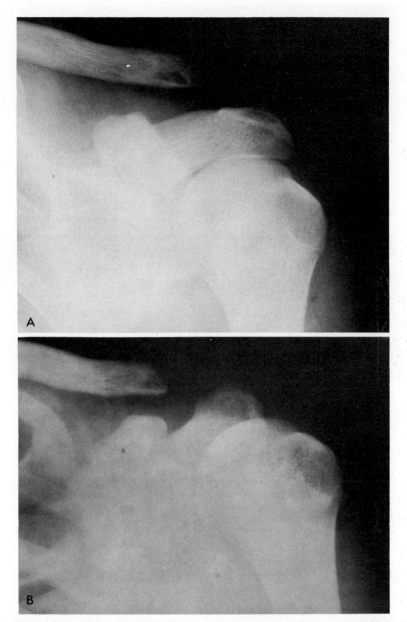

Figure 118. This 16 year old boy has had chronic acromioclavicular dislocation for the last two years following a football injury. After three weeks with his arm at his side he was operated on elsewhere, a screw was put in the shoulder, and the arm was bound down for four weeks. After the screw was removed his symptoms recurred and the knot recurred on the shoulder. He had a second reconstruction with the screw being removed at 10 weeks. Two months later it began to bother him again with pain at night, pain on lifting and a feeling of something slipping in the shoulder. My examination two years post-injury revealed a painful shoulder at the outer end of the clavicle with upward riding. Pain particularly on abduction. *A*, X-ray shows upward riding of the clavicle with separation between the coracoid and the clavicle. Preoperative diagnosis: Degenerative arthritis with instability. At surgery the large, thick scar was excised. The acromioclavicular ligament was divided lineally and 1 cm. of the distal end of the clavicle was removed, since the outer end of the clavicle impinged on the acromion from pressure, especially in abduction of the arm. *B*, Postoperative x-ray shows no evidence of reossification. No upward riding of the clavicle. No complaints.

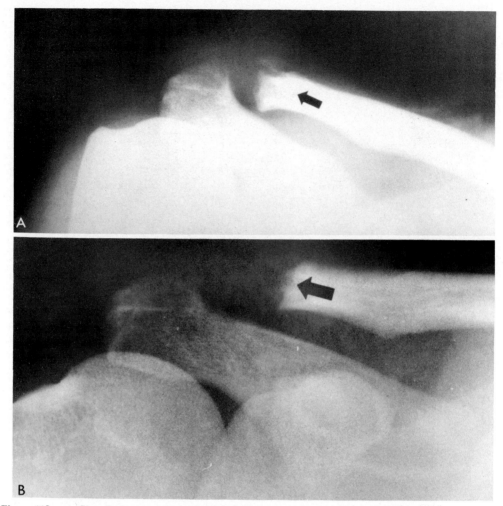

Figure 119. *A,* Chronic degenerative arthritis with production of bone around the clavicle. *B,* Illustrating resection of the outer end of the clavicle, two months postoperative.

FRACTURE

By "outer end of the clavicle" I am referring to that area distal to the coracoclavicular ligaments. This part of the clavicle is a broad, flat bone without a distinct medullary canal. The forces likely to cause a fracture of the clavicle in this area may be the same as those causing ligament injury. As the acromion is driven downward in relation to the clavicle, the coracoclavicular as well as the acromioclavicular ligaments may remain intact and the bone will break proximal

to the coracoclavicular ligaments. This will be a fracture of the shaft of the clavicle (Fig. 101), usually in the outer part of the middle third of the bone. In this instance the distal fragment will remain in normal relationship to the scapula while the proximal fragment rides upward. Whereas this fracture is not actually one of the outer end of the clavicle, it does require mention here since it is virtually impossible to reduce and hold without some form of internal fixation. In the previous discussion of dislocation of the outer end of the clavi-

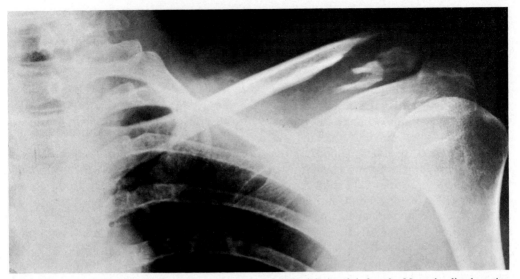

Figure 120. Comminuted fracture of the outer end of the clavicle in adult female. Note the distal portion is fragmented and remains intact to the acromion, whereas the proximal just rides upward. There must be rupture of the coracoclavicular ligament.

cle, mention was made of the difficulty of holding the clavicle down in spite of the fact that its entire length is intact for the application of direct pressure downward. When the fracture is just proximal to the coracoclavicular ligaments, the sharp distal end of the proximal fragment not only is short but lies close to the neck and is not amenable to fixation by direct pressure. This type of fracture is best treated by intramedullary fixation following open reduction. To some extent these same principles apply to

any fracture of the middle third of the clavicle, but they are particularly pertinent as the ligamentous area is approached.

Another combination of forces may cause the fracture to be distal (Figs. 120 and 121) to the coracoclavicular ligaments and so be an *interligamentary* fracture. In this instance, as the acromion is driven downward the acromioclavicular ligaments remain intact, but the coracoclavicular ligaments rupture. The fracture occurs within the flat distal

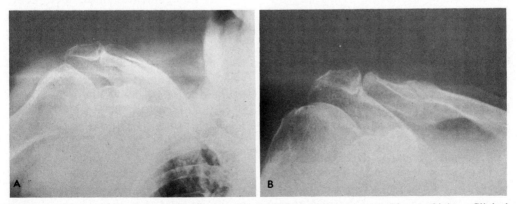

Figure 121. *A,* Anteroposterior view of outer end of the clavicle showing no evidence of injury. Clinical diagnosis of fracture led to vertical x-ray *B,* which revealed interligamentary fracture of the clavicle.

portion of the clavicle. The distal fragment accompanies the acromion and is displaced downward; the proximal fragment displaces upward. The important consideration in this fracture, as compared to the one previously described, is that in the first instance the coracoclavicular ligaments remain intact and so the outer end of the clavicle remains securely fastened to the scapula. After reduction or internal fixation of the two fragments the acromioclavicular area is secure. In the instance under consideration the coracoclavicular ligaments are ruptured and fixation of the clavicle to the scapula is impaired.

This type of injury also requires open reduction, at which time the coracoclavicular ligaments should be sutured. The fracture line may be at any level between the two ligaments. If the distal fragment is small and involves only the outer 1 inch of the clavicle, it is preferable to remove the fragment, repair the coracoclavicular ligaments and thus shorten the healing period and diminish the probability of pain at the acromioclavicular joint following recovery. This is particularly pertinent if a comminuted fracture involves the articular portion of the outer end of the clavicle. In many instances a small fragment will remain attached to the acromioclavicular ligament. This should by all means be removed. The surgeon must rely upon his good judgment as to whether in a given case it would be better to obtain bony fixation or to remove the fragments. As a rule of thumb, one might say that if he can obtain adequate surgical repair of the coracoclavicular ligaments there will be less necessity for bony union between the two fragments, and thus the distal fragment might well be removed. Similarly, if the distal fragment is small or comminuted, bony security between the two fragments is not readily obtainable anyway, and these fragments would be best removed. On

the contrary, if ligament repair seems insecure, the additional security of bony union in order to take advantage of the stability of the acromioclavicular ligament is important and one would prefer to leave the fragment in.

Interligamentary fractures may also be the result of a direct blow. In such a case the fracture line may be of any character. It may be comminuted, oblique, spiral or transverse, but is most frequently either oblique from above, downward and inward, or comminuted. Since both the acromioclavicular and coracoclavicular ligaments are intact, any extensive degree of displacement is unusual in this fracture by direct blow. Treatment is primarily supportive. A three-inch loop of tape is passed beneath the flexed elbow and then crossed over the outer end of the clavicle. Felt pads should be placed over the top of the shoulder to give some degree of downward pressure. The arm should be in a sling (Fig. 105).

It will thus be seen that from the standpoint of treatment it is quite important to distinguish between an interligamentary fracture by direct trauma of the bone and one caused by disrupting forces applied indirectly. In those caused by direct trauma, treatment requires only a relatively short period of external fixation, whereas in the other types with ligament damage open reduction is the treatment of choice. If open reduction for some reason cannot be carried out, then the same type of fixation should be used as was mentioned in relation to dislocations of the outer end of the clavicle, namely, the type of support that is designed to push the humerus upward and the clavicle downward (Fig. 105).

Rehabilitation is extremely important in these injuries (see Fig. 161), and it will proceed much faster if there is good internal fixation of the bones. Needless to say, athletic competition should not be permitted until healing is complete. In the case of torn ligaments this will require eight weeks; in case of fractures the period depends upon the progress of healing as checked by x-ray examination.

It should be remembered in any discussion of injuries about the shoulder that the ligament attachments in tearing away may include a fragment of bone, the so-called *avulsion* fractures. These should be treated basically as a ligament injury. For example, the coracoid may be pulled off by the coracoclavicular ligament (Figs. 122 and 179), the small fragment of the proximal end of the clavicle may be torn off by the sternoclavicular ligament, or a segment of the acromion or distal end of the clavicle may be avulsed by the acromioclavicular ligament. In each instance the treatment is basically that of ligament injury. In the majority of instances it is advisable to remove the fragment unless it is

large enough to allow its fixation to the parent bone, in which case the additional stability gained by the fragment may be of considerable value. This is particularly pertinent at the inner end of the clavicle where it is difficult to hold the clavicle down by ordinary suture through the ligament, and the firmly fixed proximal fragment may be utilized to fasten the clavicle down.

Fracture of the Acromion

Many of the same forces that fracture the outer end of the clavicle may also fracture the acromial process. By far the most frequent force is direct trauma, which simply breaks off the end of the bone at any point distal to its attachment to the body of the scapula through the spine of the scapula. These fractures are usually without gross displacement and usually require little treatment in themselves. It is important

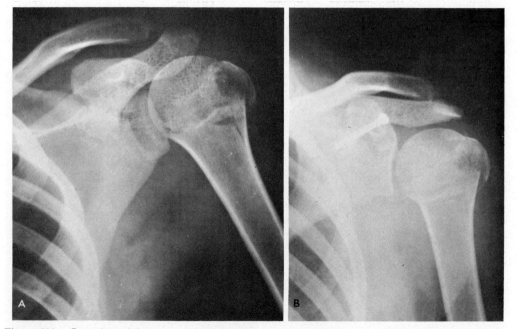

Figure 122. Comminuted fracture of the surgical neck of the humerus and greater tuberosity without displacement. Note, however, avulsion fracture of the coracoid process, which was pulled off by the conjoined tendon of the short head of the biceps, the coracobrachialis, and the pectoralis minor muscles. This was reduced and held by screw fixation, the whole shoulder then being treated by sling only. (Also see Fig. 179.)

to recognize such a fracture. A fracture without displacement may not be well visualized in the ordinary x-ray view, and it may be necessary to take a vertical view through the distal end of the acromion to show it (Figs. 123, 124 and 125). If there is any question, repeated x-ray pictures are important. Many of these cases will be diagnosed as a contusion, and the fracture is recognized only after the "contusion" has failed to heal within a reasonable period of time.

TREATMENT. In the unusual case in which there is nonunion of the fracture of the acromion, the distal fragment can generally be removed without serious disability to the shoulder if the deltoid muscle is sutured to the remaining bone. Indeed, if the acute fracture involves as little as ½ inch of the distal end of the acromion, the best treatment will be excision of the fragment, since healing will be much more rapid and with much less likelihood of any residual complication.

Occasionally the acromion may be fractured by indirect force caused by upward dislocation of the humerus against the acromial process (Fig. 126). This usually is a major injury and will require specialized treatment. Frequently open reduction is necessary because of the probability of soft tissue interposition preventing reduction of the dislocation. More frequently the force will cause subluxation only. The fracture will be incomplete. Again treatment is dependent on recognition of the injury and requires some degree of protection of the arm against wide abduction. If displacement is gross, open reduction is advisable. At operation the fragment may be removed if small. If it is larger, open reduction and threaded wire fixation may be carried out.

REGION OF THE BODY OF THE SCAPULA

CONTUSION

The only area of the scapula that is commonly subject to contusion is its spine from the vertebral border to the

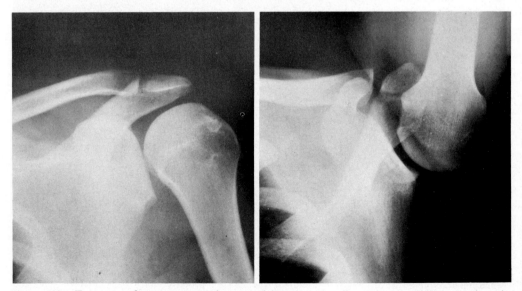

Figure 123. Transverse fracture across the acromial process by direct downward force against the acromion; *A*, Note anteroposterior view is negative. *B*, Vertical view shows fracture clearly. (See Fig. 125 for technique of x-ray.)

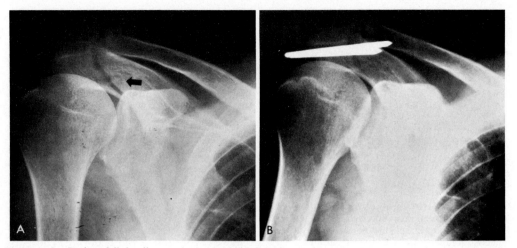

Figure 124. Patient fell, landing on the back of his shoulder. *A,* Note the oblique fracture of the acromion with some displacement. *B,* After internal fixation because of instability of the fragment, which involved the acromioclavicular joint. (See Fig. 125 for technique of x-ray.)

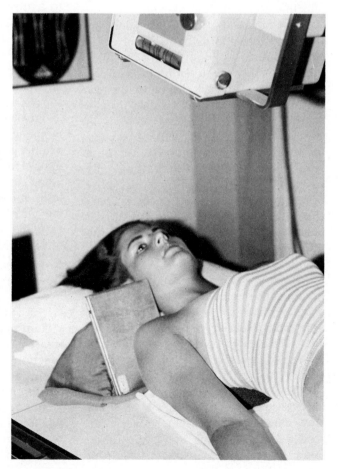

Figure 125. Positioning for acromion. Several views are often necessary to demonstrate fractures of the acromion. View *A* in Figure 124 is obtained by placing the patient supine on the table. A cassette angled about 10 degrees should be supported at the top of the shoulder. Supinate the elbow and depress the shoulder. With the tube angled about 10 degrees cephalad, direct the central ray to the acromioclavicular joint. View *B* of Figure 123 is a projection similar to a standard AP of the shoulder, except the arm is elevated above the head to rotate the acromion posteriorly. A lateral view of the scapula (Fig. 131*B*) with the body also rotated slightly to bring the acromion into view, or an axillary view of the shoulder may be necessary.

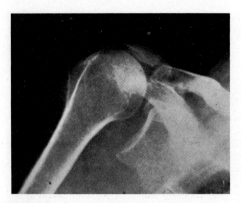

Figure 126. Dislocation of the glenohumeral joint with fractured acromion. It is unusual to get this picture, since the dislocation is usually spontaneously reduced and the severity of injury may well be overlooked. (From McLaughlin, Trauma, p. 263.)

tip of the acromion. This area is entirely subcutaneous and the skin may be severely contused between the underlying bone and the external blow. There may be a contusion of the bone. The diagnosis is readily made on the basis of the local reaction to the lesion with tenderness directly along the bone, usually sharply localized. Ordinary motions of the shoulder or scapula will not be painful in simple contusion. In case of a severe injury, x-ray visualization may be necessary to eliminate the possibility of a fracture of the spine of the scapula (Fig. 131). It may be necessary to get tangential views in order to visualize the fracture line. In contact sports such as football, this area is very adequately protected by shoulder pads and so is infrequently hurt. *Treatment* is the application of cold, then heat, local injection and protective padding. With adequate padding, no interruption of participation in competitive sports need be expected from this type of injury.

The muscles overlying the scapula may be subject to contusion by a direct blow catching the muscle between the hard underlying bone and the striking force. This may be distinguished from other injuries by the localization of the tenderness plus pain on active contraction or passive stretching of the involved muscle. *Treatment* consists of cold, followed by heat, local injection and rest. It is unusual for ossification to occur following contusion of the muscles about the scapula.

STRAIN

The area of the scapula is quite subject to strain since the entire bone serves for the origin or insertion of many muscles (see p. 142). In many instances extremely powerful muscles may attach throughout a relatively small area (Fig. 127). Thus, it may be possible for the powerful latissimus dorsi muscle to avulse its attachment from the inferior angle. This may cause avulsion of the bone but more commonly results in a simple strain with rupture of some of the fibers at their attachment to the bone. A similar injury may occur at the superior angle of the scapula where the levator scapulae and rhomboideus minor may be subject to the same type of injury. Less frequently there may be injury in the region of the trapezius along the spine of the scapula or of the teres minor or triceps. Similarly, there may be damage to the rhomboideus major at its attachment along the vertebral border.

Acute Strain

All of these injuries are caused by violent muscle action and for this reason treatment must provide restriction of function of the muscle involved. In an acute injury *treatment* consists of local application of cold followed later by heat, injection of a local anesthetic plus hyaluronidase into the hematoma, and restriction of function of the muscle that has been damaged. The last can be carried out by placing the arm in a sling, which moderately restricts the activity of the arm. If the injury is severe, athletic competition is interdicted. Healing usually takes place without major definitive treatment. However, if a detectable fragment of bone is avulsed through an appreciable distance, one should seriously consider early removal of the fragment of bone and suture of the muscle to the fracture bed. While this may seem a little radical in a situation in which spontaneous healing will probably take place, one must bear in mind that these situations involving actual separation of an avulsed fragment of bone frequently lead to nonunion with persistent pain. The athlete may better accept surgical treatment entailing a few weeks of early complete disability, but offering the opportunity for more complete recovery, rather than months or years of disability of a lower grade. This is particularly pertinent when one considers that the best nonsurgical treatment also should entail complete rest.

Chronic Strain

These same areas in the scapula may be involved in chronic irritative lesions with chronic strain of the various muscle attachments. In this situation ordinary function of the muscle is

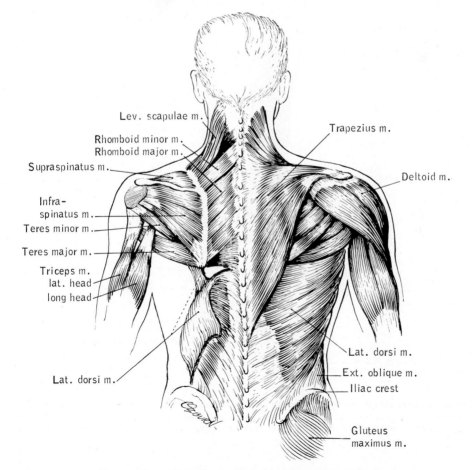

Figure 127. *A*, Muscle attachments about the shoulder.

Illustration and legend continued on the following page.

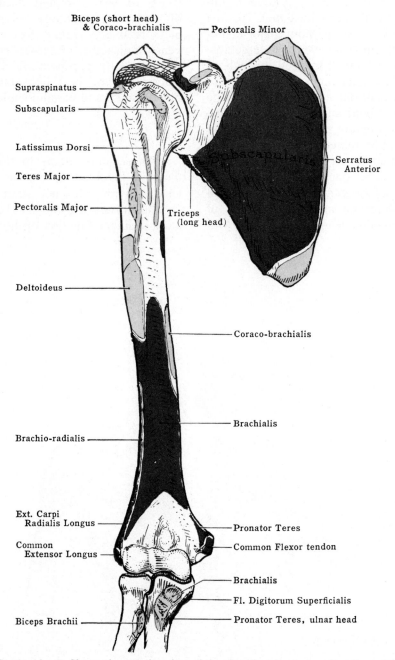

Figure 127 *Continued.* *B*, Shows the anterior view of the shoulder clearly revealing the multiple muscle attachments of the scapula. The whole undersurface of the scapula is occupied by the subscapularis while the serrati muscles attach along the vertebral border. The biceps and pectoralis minor attach to the coracoid.

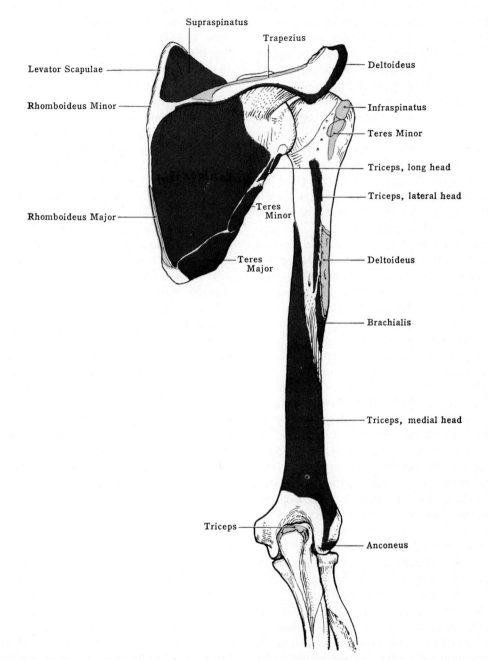

Figure 127 *Continued.* *C,* In the dorsal view it is even more significant noting the spinatae, the supra above and the infra below the spine, the trapezius on the spine and the deltoid on the spine. Along the border are the teres major, the teres minor and the triceps. Stability of the shoulder is increased by attachment of the rotator cuff muscles to the humeral head and also between the subscapularis by the pectoralis major coming across and attaching to the humerus without a specific scapular attachment. (*B* and *C* reproduced by permission from: J. B. Grant. An Atlas of Anatomy. Sixth Ed. © 1972, The Williams and Wilkins Company, Baltimore.)

usually pain-free. Violent exercise, particularly against resistance, causes recurrence of the symptoms of pain, muscle spasm and restriction of motion. This is the same type of chronic strain that may occur at the attachment of the tendo Achilles or at the epicondyles of the elbow or in the hamstrings. *Treatment* may be extremely discouraging since resumption of forceful activity will often cause recurrence of symptoms. Fortunately, this is uncommon around the scapula as opposed to the glenohumeral joint. A period of complete rest may be rewarding if continued over a long enough period. This may be supplemented by two or three injections of local anesthetic plus a corticoid preparation. Careful! Great care must be used that function is actually restricted to that tolerated by the muscle without increasing the irritation.

In the type of case just described, the general plan of treatment would be as follows: Every effort is made to pinpoint exactly the location of the lesion. This area is then injected with a local anesthetic. If this completely relieves the pain during the effective period of the anesthetic, one may feel confident that he has reached the area involved and may then proceed with local injection of a corticoid preparation. Following these measures, local inductive heat, as by diathermy, microtherm or ultrasound, should be utilized once or twice daily for 20 minutes. The injection may actually increase the pain immediately after the effect of the anesthetic is lost. There then may be 12 to 36 hours of acute exacerbation of pain, oftentimes to the extent that sedation is required. The pain and other symptoms should then gradually subside until marked improvement is obtained. If this improvement persists for several days but the symptoms then gradually recur, the injection should be repeated before the symptoms become too severe again.

This may be done several times so long as gradual overall improvement is taking place. A course of treatment consists of four to six injections beginning one week apart (no oftener) and progressing to ten days to two weeks to three weeks apart. As activity is resumed, great care should be used that rehabilitation progresses below the level of irritative activity. Several months of pain-free activity should elapse before violent exercise of the involved muscle is permitted.

This recommendation for treatment of the chronic condition should not be extrapolated into treatment for an acute strain. There is no indication for the use of any corticoid in the acute injury. Also we are discussing here muscle strain, not tendon. A good basic principle is that corticoid should never be injected into a tendon itself, although it may be proper to inject it into the tendon sheath or peritendinous tissue. The danger of penetration of the tendon itself should be very well recognized. One may get some idea as to whether or not it is in the tendon because of the resistance to injection, since the tendon is a dense structure and ordinarily does not accept local injection without considerable pressure which may, indeed, increase the necrosis by pressure.

BURSITIS

There are many bursae around the body of the scapula (Fig. 128), since bursae are found in any area where friction would otherwise develop between layers of tissue. One can readily appreciate their frequency in this area of excessive motion between the various muscles attaching to the scapula. Probably the most constant bursa, except those in direct relationship to the glenohumeral joint, is that one lying between the body of the scapula and the muscles of the chest wall. This bursa is not

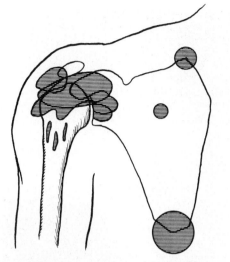

Figure 128.   Showing the multitude of bursae around the shoulder, particularly around the glenohumeral joint. (Redrawn from Codman.)

frequently described anatomically and may indeed develop as a result of irritation between the scapula and the muscles following some type of injury. A bursa may be high up under the supraspinous portion of the scapula or may be lower lying beneath the infraspinous part. Symptoms of bursitis in this area are related particularly to motion of the scapula against the chest wall, so that approximating the scapulae posteriorly or crossing the arm across the chest anteriorly will elicit pain and frequently, when this motion is carried out under tension, crepitation.

Treatment of this condition is by rest, heat and local injection. The general plan should be to determine as accurately as possible the exact location of the bursa involved. In subscapular bursitis, since the scapula overlies the bursa, it may be quite difficult to actually localize this area. It is easier to get a needle into the area under the scapula with the scapula rotated forward. The test of the accuracy of the localization of injection is the prompt relief of pain, which continues while the local anesthetic is effective. For this reason it is important to use a long-acting local anesthetic. After each location is injected, one should wait a few minutes to see if the symptoms are relieved. By this means it may be possible to spot the exact area of the inflammation. This area should then be injected with a long-acting local anesthetic in which has been mixed a corticoid preparation. Immediate relief should ensue. If it does not, the procedure may not be successful. The patient should be warned that the pain may be more severe for 12 to 36 hours. If after this preliminary period he gets complete relief and then the symptoms begin to recur, the injection should be repeated within another seven to ten days. This series may be continued three to five times at gradually increasing intervals. More injections than this probably will not be effective and may actually cause damage.

FRACTURE

Fracture of the body of the scapula is not a common athletic injury because of the protection given the bone by overlying and underlying cushions of muscle. Usually, only a violent force will cause fracture. Mention was made earlier of avulsion injury and fracture of the spine of the scapula. The body of the scapula can be fractured by muscle contraction but this is extremely unusual. Symptoms will be those of a severe contusion and the diagnosis must be made by x-ray.

TREATMENT.   Reduction of a fracture of the body of the scapula (Figs. 129 to 133) is rarely necessary. In fact, it is virtually impossible to reduce the fragments short of open operation. Since the body of the scapula is primarily for muscle attachments, the only indication for internal fixation of the fragments would be their actual overlapping with a resulting roughness of the undersurface

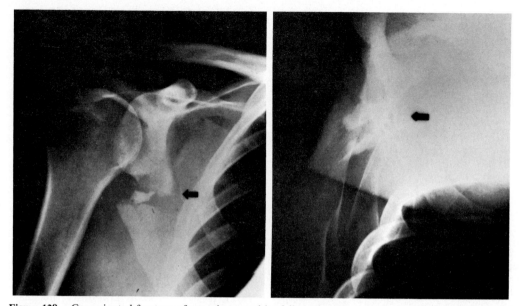

Figure 129. Comminuted fracture of scapula caused by fall on the outer aspect of the shoulder. Humeral head drove against the glenoid, fracturing the neck with comminuted fracture lines extending throughout the body of the scapula. No treatment is required other than support.

of the bone, extreme enough to interfere with motion of the scapula over the chest wall. This rarely occurs and I have never seen it as a result of athletic injury.

Treatment, therefore, is local, consisting of aspiration and hyaluronidase injection (not a corticoid) of the hema-toma, early cold followed by heat, and protection against extremes of motion. It is probably advisable to use a firm compression bandage from 24 to 48 hours, strapping the scapula snugly against the chest wall. The arm is then placed in a sling (Fig. 106). This retentive dressing should be removed after 7

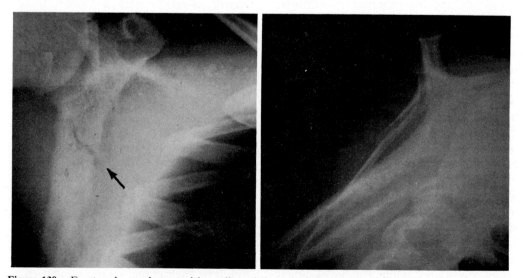

Figure 130. Fractured scapula caused by a direct fall on the blade of the scapula. Comminuted fracture without displacement. (For x-ray positioning of AP and lateral views, see Fig. 131.)

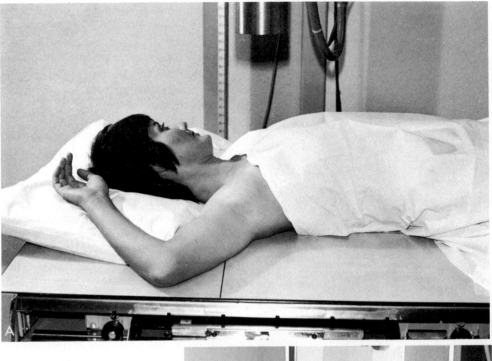

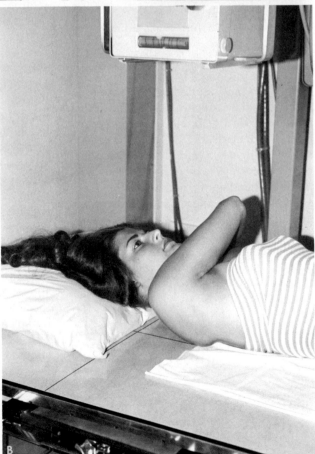

Figure 131. *A*, Body of the scapula. Position the patient in a supine position with the affected scapula in the center of the table. Abduct the arm, pulling the scapula away from the body. Supinate the forearm and immobilize if necessary. Direct the central ray to the center of the scapula. Exposure should be made at full expiration. *B*, Lateral projection of scapula. Position the patient as for the AP projection in view *A* except that the affected arm should be drawn across the chest as far as possible. Adjust the position of the arm until the scapula is drawn away from the rib cage and can be felt at right angles to the table. The central ray should be directed to the center of the scapula and center of the cassette. Frequently, positioning for a lateral of the dorsal spine will show a good lateral projection of the scapula.

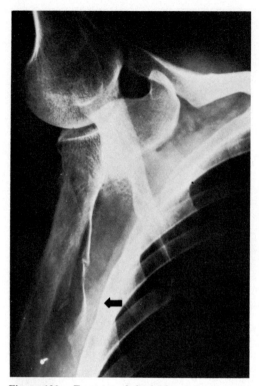

Figure 132. Fracture of the body of the scapula revealed by radiograph made with the arm in wide abduction.

to 14 days and motion of the shoulder and scapula encouraged within the limits of pain. It should be emphasized that it is inadvisable to immobilize the shoulder for more than a few days. The protective sling which is utilized will permit pendulum exercises which should gradually increase both in range and frequency as the pain and tenderness subside. Active function will return promptly, but it may be many months before forceful use of the extremity is pain-free.

REGION OF THE SHOULDER JOINT (GLENOHUMERAL JOINT)

ANATOMICAL CONSIDERATIONS

The functional anatomy of the shoulder joint defies brief description.

The student is referred to the classic book *The Shoulder* by E. A. Codman, whose narrative description of the functional motion of the shoulder joint in 1934 has not been improved upon. Only a few essentials of functional anatomy can be touched upon here.

The shoulder is an extremely complex joint owing to the fact that not only the glenohumeral joint itself but the structures making up the foundation for the glenohumeral joint are extremely mobile, so that many of the muscles and indeed even the ligaments may have separate functions under different circumstances. In describing motions of the shoulder, one had best proceed from the base of the anatomical position with the arm at the side, the palm against the thigh and the scapula snugly against the chest wall. Because of the complexity of motion of the shoulder it has become desirable to have some sort of standard that can be universally adopted to describe the motions of the shoulder. This study was carried out by the American Orthopaedic Association and shown in their *Manual of Orthopaedic Surgery* as illustrated in Figure 134. Note the base line is the anatomical position. In Part I of these illustrations it should be understood that with the patient supine or standing with the arm at the side, palm against the thigh, the shoulder is in neutral position and all motion of the shoulder relates to this position. This will clarify the semantics of the description of restriction of motion. Structurally, the joint is a modified ball and socket without bony stability. Whereas the acetabulum is designed to give maximum stability to the hip and yet maintain some degree of motion, the shoulder joint sacrifices stability for extreme mobility.

The glenohumeral joint itself consists of a small, shallow, saucer-like structure on the neck of the scapula (glenoid fossa) (Fig. 86) and the head of the humerus. The humeral head rests against the glenoid and is so much larger than the glenoid that the latter serves not so much as a receptacle for the head as it does as a base against which the head may be stabilized in its circumduction motions. The capsule of the joint is somewhat redundant but is reinforced in front by capsular thickenings which give some degree of stability anteriorly. These bands, which consist of the superior, medial and inferior glenohumeral ligaments, are tight when the humerus is placed in external rotation and abduction. It can be appreciated that, from the

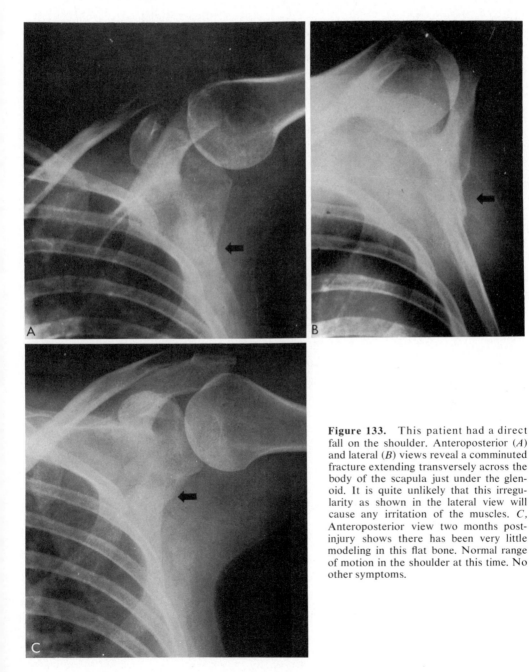

Figure 133. This patient had a direct fall on the shoulder. Anteroposterior (*A*) and lateral (*B*) views reveal a comminuted fracture extending transversely across the body of the scapula just under the glenoid. It is quite unlikely that this irregularity as shown in the lateral view will cause any irritation of the muscles. *C*, Anteroposterior view two months postinjury shows there has been very little modeling in this flat bone. Normal range of motion in the shoulder at this time. No other symptoms.

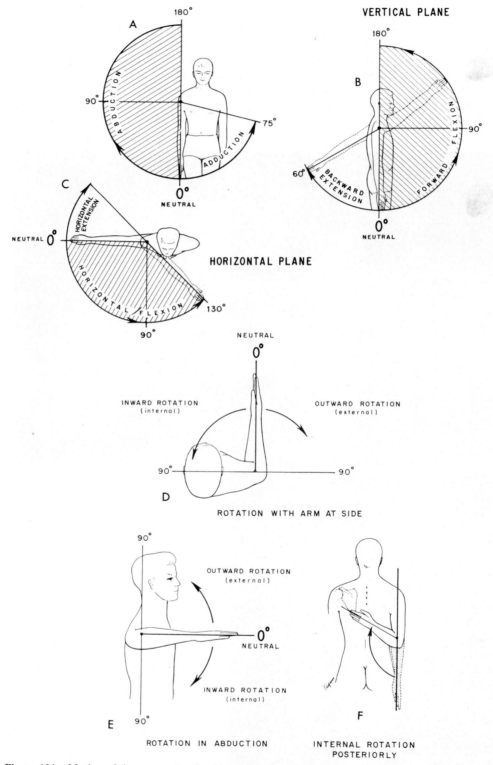

Figure 134.   Motion of the arm at the shoulder. (American Orthopaedic Association's Manual of Orthopaedic Surgery.)

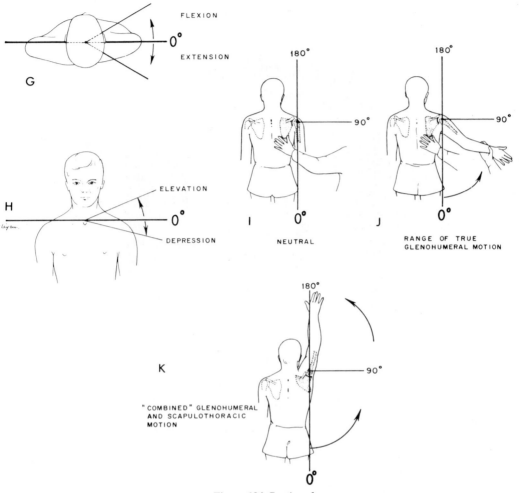

FLEXION

0°

EXTENSION

G

180°

90°

0°

NEUTRAL

I

180°

90°

0°

RANGE OF TRUE
GLENOHUMERAL MOTION

J

ELEVATION

0°

DEPRESSION

H

K

180°

90°

0°

"COMBINED" GLENOHUMERAL
AND SCAPULOTHORACIC
MOTION

Figure 134 *Continued.*

standpoint of ligament stability, they are not sufficient to hold the head against the glenoid but simply tend to prevent anterior displacement as the head rotates into abduction-external rotation.

These deficiencies in ligament structure are counterbalanced by the muscles of the rotator cuff (Fig. 135). These muscles pass from the scapula anteriorly, superiorly and posteriorly over the humeral head, attaching around the periphery of the head to the greater tuberosity. Together they form sort of a hood (Fig. 104). By a tonic contraction of these muscles the head is supported snugly against the glenoid (Fig. 136).

The various tendons of the rotator cuff are indistinguishable as they reach their attachments, and they form a continuous cuff around the neck of the humerus. In addition to these muscles, namely, the supraspinatus, infraspinatus and teres minor, anterior support is given by the extremely strong subscapularis tendon which passes directly in front of the humeral head in the anatomical position, covering approximately its inferior two-thirds (Fig. 137, *B*). These muscles acting individually cause rotation of the humeral head, the exact rotation depending upon the position from which the movement starts. From the

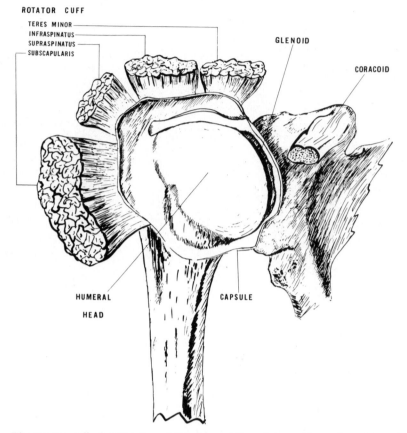

Figure 135. The rotator cuff, showing the relationships of the rotator cuff muscles with each other and with the capsules of the joint and the long head of the biceps which traverses between the subscapularis and supraspinatus. (Redrawn from Codman.)

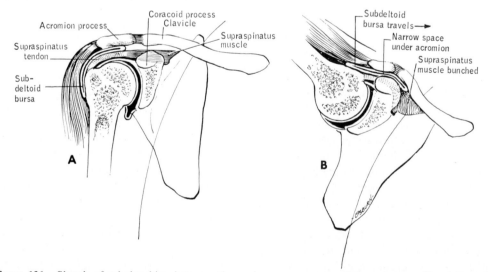

Figure 136. Sketch of relationships between the various components of the rotator cuff and the subacromial bursa. Note that the bursa underlies the acromion and the deltoid with more of it under the deltoid with the arm at the side.

A, Relationships with the arm at the side. *B*, With the arm widely abducted, showing "travel" of the bursa. Also narrow space for rotator cuff as it passes under acromion.

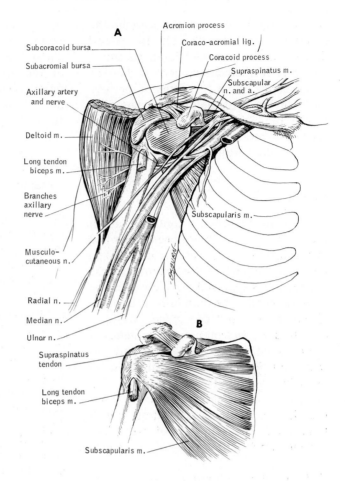

A

Acromion process
Coraco-acromial lig.
Coracoid process
Subcoracoid bursa
Supraspinatus m.
Subacromial bursa
Subscapular n. and a.
Axillary artery and nerve
Deltoid m.
Long tendon biceps m.
Branches axillary nerve
Subscapularis m.
Musculo-cutaneous n.
Radial n.
Median n.
B
Ulnar n.
Supraspinatus tendon
Long tendon biceps m.
Subscapularis m.

Figure 137. Anatomical drawings of anterior region of shoulder with the anterior muscles removed.

A, With the subscapularis in situ showing the nerve supply to the deltoid muscle by the circumflex (axillary) nerve passing behind the humerus. Also, the relationships of the bursae.

B, Detail of the subscapularis and supraspinatus with the overlying structures removed. Note tendon of the long head of the biceps passing into the tunnel to become intracapsular.

anatomical position the subscapularis is an internal rotator. In a similar manner the teres minor supports the shoulder posteriorly and acts as an external rotator from the anatomical position.

While one is likely to think of the main function of the rotator cuff as being abduction and rotation of the arm, a more essential function is that of holding the humeral head against the glenoid to permit abduction of the arm by the deltoid and other muscles without subluxation of the humeral head downward, since the socket of the glenoid is not sufficient to maintain stability (Fig. 136). Without the suspending action of the rotator cuff muscles, the head of the humerus would subluxate inferiorly as

the arm is abducted. To further complicate the picture of the tendons situated about the shoulder, the long head of the biceps passes through the bicipital groove, or tunnel, in front of the humeral head to pass over the head of the humerus, becoming intracapsular and finally reaching its attachment at the top of the glenoid (Fig. 137).

This entire layer of muscle and tendon lies beneath the acromion. The more superficial covering of the shoulder joint consists of the bony acromial process, which is reinforced in front by the coraco-acromial ligament to act as a roof over the medial part of the humeral head. The lateral continuation of this roof is the deltoid muscle, which arises along the spine of the scapula, the acromion and the clavicle to extend down over the shoulder joint. Its fibers converge to their attachment at the deltoid tubercle about two-fifths of the way down the shaft of the humerus laterally. It can be seen that the shoulder joint proper is protected from external violence by the acromion and the deltoid.

CONTUSION

The most common contusion about the shoulder has already been described in the discussion of the acromion. The deltoid is subject to contusion, lying as it does in its exposed position over the humeral head. The deltoid is a thick resilient muscle and can stand considerable trauma. In competitive athletics it is protected well by shoulder pads so that contusion here is not common even in major trauma. The *treatment* is that of contusion anywhere else: cold, compression, heat, local aspiration, injection, rest. The duration of treatment depends upon the severity of the injury.

Axillary Nerve Damage

As the result of contusion over the front of the shoulder there may be damage to the axillary nerve. This nerve comes off the brachial plexus as a branch of the posterior cord at about the level of the coracoid process, leaves the posterior cord at a rather acute angle, and proceeds sharply laterally and a little forward before it swings backward and continues laterally behind the shaft of the humerus. A direct blow striking just between the coracoid and the head of the humerus may contuse this nerve (Fig. 137).

The principal symptom of axillary nerve damage is a severe, numbing pain in the arm that causes the player to feel that the arm is useless. He may believe that his shoulder has been broken or

that his arm has been "numbed." Examination at this time will reveal hypesthesia and reluctant function of the muscles of the upper arm. This rapidly disappears. Notable also is the inability to abduct the arm actively in the early stages. In a simple contusion this promptly clears, and sometimes within a few minutes or at the most a few hours active function will reappear. Recovery is often so rapid that the player is able to return to the same game after a brief period of rest. In this instance one can visualize that the nerve has received a sufficient blow to cause temporary numbness, as when the ulnar nerve receives a blow at the elbow.

In the occasional case there will be persistent paralysis of the deltoid with an area of hypesthesia in the sensory distribution of the axillary nerve. If the patient is examined early, the findings will be basically negative, that is, there is no true paralysis of the hand or sensory loss, but the arm feels "asleep." There will usually be tenderness deep in front of the shoulder just lateral to the coracoid process. If the symptoms persist 24 to 48 hours, the pattern of loss of function of the axillary nerve becomes clearer. Much more frequently there will be a period of apparent complete recovery with only occasional aching pain. This is followed by the onset of loss of function of the deltoid and development of anesthesia in the sensory distribution.

TREATMENT. In the case marked by continuous and severe loss of function of the axillary nerve from the time of the accident, one is hard put to decide whether to recommend early exploration of the nerve or to wait for return of function. As a general rule, a period of watchful waiting is justified, the exact time depending upon the completeness of the loss or signs of possible recovery and function.

In the case that develops gradually

over several weeks, we may visualize a contusion and hematoma, with scar formation about the nerve that finally becomes constrictive. This lesion is usually incomplete, but weakness in the deltoid and loss of strength of abduction may be extremely distressing to the athlete. In many instances he is unable to raise his arm over his head. In other instances a complete paralysis of the nerve follows. I believe that if there is progressively increasing loss, exploration should not be delayed. In any event, I see little reason to wait beyond three months unless there is in the meantime some sign of improvement. During this period physical therapeutic measures are of great value in maintaining the muscle tone, and electrical stimulation of the deltoid is permissible on a professionally controlled basis. Care should be taken to prevent contracture of the shoulder with shortening of the adductors, with the result that the arm cannot be passively elevated.

At operation the axillary nerve should be exposed through the anterior incision if the blow has been frontal. By an approach along the deltopectoral interval and with reflection of the deltoid laterally, the brachial plexus may be exposed medial to the coracoid, the incision extending up under the clavicle. Access to this area is markedly facilitated by detaching the distal 1 inch of the coracoid and reflecting the biceps, coracobrachialis and pectoralis minor. The plexus can now be examined from the clavicle to the superior axillary fold.

Nerve operations in this area, and, in fact, in any other, require special technique and are not for the occasional surgeon. One practical approach to the problem is combined surgery by the orthopaedist and neurosurgeon. This is an area frequently entered by the orthopaedist during shoulder reconstruction. He may be better prepared for the exposure, whereas the exact decision as to

what to do with the nerve may require the specialized knowledge of the neurosurgeon. The author has participated in several such cases with good success. One patient had a neuroma just distal to the separation of the axillary nerve from the posterior cord. This was resected, the nerve was repaired, and good function returned. The player went on to a stellar career as a football player with no restriction of abduction of the shoulder. Two recent cases revealed rather minimal findings at operation, but there were definite adhesions about the nerve that caused it to assume a more acute angle as it left the cord. This was aggravated by certain positions of the arm. In this instance the injury responded well to simple neurolysis and freeing of the adhesions. Several months may be needed for complete recovery.

It should be emphasized that the great majority of these cases are transient and probably of little true significance. Their recurrence may be avoided by an adjustment of the shoulder pad to protect this area a little more adequately. I believe the shoulder pad itself may often be the offender. As the arm is thrown up sharply and the shoulder pad comes forward its narrow edge is driven against the front of the shoulder, penetrates the sulcus between the muscles and reaches the nerve.

STRAIN

While contusion is a relatively minor problem about the shoulder, strain is an extremely major one. There may be some damage to the muscle or musculotendinous structures in any muscle that attaches at the shoulder. Since these muscles are many and the forces to which they are subject are legion, it is difficult to encompass this whole subject in a few short paragraphs.

The injury may be anything from a

mild (first degree) strain with some inflammation to complete avulsion of the tendon (third degree) or of the tendon plus a fragment of bone. The symptoms will be similar but will vary considerably in degree. So, too, there is considerable difference between the type of symptoms in an acute (third degree) and a chronic strain. These differences have been discussed at some length elsewhere (see p. 62).

Some grouping of the muscles involved will aid in the understanding of the pathologic changes present. The major internal rotators of the humerus are the subscapularis attaching to the lesser tuberosity, the latissimus dorsi and the teres major inserting into the internal lip of the intertubercular (bicipital) groove, and the pectoralis major inserting at the outer lip of the intertubercular groove. Injuries to these attachments will be caused by forceful external rotation of the humerus against the resistance of these muscles or on active internal rotation of the humerus by their violent contraction. These muscles are opposed in external rotation by the muscles of the rotator cuff, particularly the infraspinatus, supraspinatus and teres minor. Both internal and external rotation are supported by the anterior and posterior fibers of the deltoid respectively.

The symptoms of an injury to these muscles are local tenderness at the site of their insertion, with pain elicited by active contraction or by passive stretching of the muscle involved. Thus, in an injury to the subscapularis, internal rotation of the arm against resistance or external rotation of the arm passively should cause pain in the same area, namely, over the lesser tuberosity.

Adduction of the arm is also carried out by many muscles. The internal and external rotators acting synchronously serve to adduct the arm against the chest wall. However, injury to the adductors of the arm is infrequent without some rotational component, so that ordinarily adduction and internal rotation or adduction and external rotation will be the forces involved. The injury will probably be confined to either the internal or external rotators rather than to both.

In abduction of the shoulder the muscles of the rotator cuff fix the humerus against the glenoid and the deltoid raises the arm from the side (Fig. 138). True enough, the supraspinatus muscles have an abduction component, but this is with a very short lever, and much more important than their ability to initiate abduction of the arm is their stabilization of the humeral head.

Lesions of the Rotator Cuff

Rotator cuff lesions are common in the adult, their frequency becoming greater as age advances. They are initiated by degenerative change in the tendons of the rotator cuff (Fig. 138). In the athlete such lesions are probably due mainly to attrition as the cuff passes under the acromial process. The isolated rupture of a portion of the cuff is an incident in the degenerative process and not the result of acute ligament or tendon rupture as in the case of the characteristic avulsions of the athlete. While in the adult so-called "subdeltoid bursitis" is usually a sign of degenerative change in the rotator cuff, true bursitis occurs in the young athlete caused by a friction between the two walls of the subdeltoid bursa as they are impinged between the acromion and the cuff. This will be described later. The occasional case of calcification seen in the young athlete is probably in the bursa itself.

I do not recall having seen an acute rupture of the rotator cuff in the athlete unless it was accompanied by dislocation of the shoulder. Classic rotator cuff

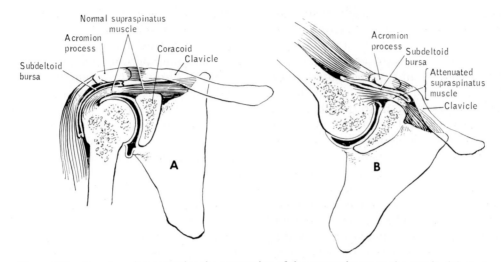

Figure 138. Drawings demonstrating the attenuation of the supraspinatus as the arm is abducted.

rupture, or supraspinatus rupture, is usually the result of active abduction of the arm against resistance and is not often a major injury. On the other hand, the acute rupture of the cuff seen in the combination of strain, sprain, subluxation and dislocation is due to a passive force with the humeral head forcibly jammed against the components of the cuff or with the elements of the cuff ruptured as the head dislocates and slips downward in relation to the glenoid.

The rotator mechanism is subject to strain in the forceful motion of the shoulder in throwing or in tackling or wrestling. In such an injury the tenderness will be along the greater tuberosity and the pain will be in the shoulder or at the deltoid insertion. It may or may not be localized, depending upon the promptness of examination, since the pain very rapidly becomes diffuse. There may be considerable difficulty in determining just what muscle action causes pain in the tendons of the rotator cuff, and this condition is readily confused with subacromial bursitis. Actually, abduction of the shoulder, particularly against some resistance, will usually cause pain. If this strain is accompanied by some swelling and inflam-

matory reaction over the tendon, it may well cause symptoms of accompanying bursitis.

Strain and Tenosynovitis of the Long Head of the Biceps

Another tendon quite subject to strain at the shoulder is the long head of the biceps (Fig. 137). This tendon passes through the tunnel formed by the intertubercular groove plus a thick fibrous roof, so that the tendon is in effect in a sheath throughout an area of 1 to 2 inches in front of the humeral shaft. It passes through the groove, becomes intracapsular and traverses the shoulder to attach on the superior lip of the glenoid above the humeral head. Motion of the shoulder with the elbow fixed, particularly in extension, causes this tendon to slide up and down forcibly through the groove. It may be subject to strain at its attachment to the glenoid but is more likely to develop tenosynovitis where it passes through the tunnel. The irritation of constant motion increases the inflammatory reaction until the tendon slides reluctantly through the tunnel and finally may cease to slide altogether. This tenosynovitis of the biceps tendon is extremely distressing from the standpoint of function of the shoulder since, with the restriction of motion and pain, many of the motions of the shoulder joint become quite limited. This is particularly true of abduction and external rotation, so that rotation at the glenohumeral joint becomes virtually impossible. Snap extension of the elbow increases this pain.

This condition may be diagnosed by localization of tenderness along the bicipital groove and by pain on rotation of the shoulder. The location of the tenderness moves with the humeral head as it rotates. There is pain on active contraction or passive stretching of the biceps with its distal attachment fixed. A test for this motion is to extend the elbow and posteriorly flex the arm at the shoulder. This causes the tendon to slide through the groove. So also, active function by pulling the arm forward across the chest with the forearm extended and with resistance against the hand will cause pain. In checking this motion one should be sure that the scapula does not simply rotate forward and so simulate glenohumeral motion whereas the motion is actually between the scapula and the chest wall.

Treatment of this condition is by local measures. The extremity should be put at rest. The tender area should be injected with local anesthetic and inductive heat utilized to reduce inflammatory reaction. If the condition is relatively chronic, injection of corticoid will often be quite effective. The same precaution should be used here as mentioned elsewhere. The injection should not be into the tendon but into the bicipital tunnel. Injection of the tendon may well cause degenerative changes and accelerate rupture. The same serial injections that are used in similar conditions elsewhere are effective here.

If the condition is intractable and does not respond to local treatment, surgical treatment may be highly successful (see Surgical Technique, p. 204). In this instance the shoulder is approached anteriorly, the bicipital groove is opened throughout its length, and the tendon is dislocated from the groove and detached from its glenoid attachment so that it no longer crosses the shoulder joint. It may then be replaced into the bicipital groove and sutured snugly.

Tenosynovitis in the bicipital groove may go on to complete adherence of the tendon. This interdicts any extensive range of motion of the shoulder and one of two things occurs. Either the shoulder motion is restricted or the biceps ruptures proximal to the groove. In many instances there will be restriction of motion and then a sudden painful snap, after which it is noted that the shoulder motion is less restricted. This condition is not frequent in athletic injuries since it usually predicates some pre-existing degenerative change in the tendon itself. If it occurs it usually demands surgical treatment with removal of the remaining portion of the tendon from the glenohumeral joint and fixation of the proximal stump to the groove.

Acute Rupture of the Long Head of the Biceps Tendon

Acute rupture of the biceps tendon (Fig. 139) occurs as a result of forceful contraction of the biceps muscle or of forceful movement of the arm with the biceps muscle contracted. The injury may be avulsion of the tendon from the muscle belly or the tendon may rupture anywhere along its course or be pulled free from its attachment to the glenoid. The history is of immediate, sharp pain followed by tenderness along the course of the long head of the biceps. Diagnosis is made by having the patient contract the biceps with the arm abducted and externally rotated with the elbow at

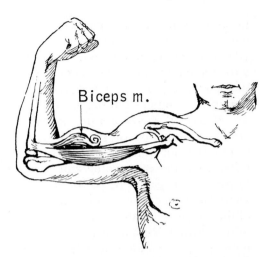

Figure 139. Showing biceps lesion; biceps bunching. Long head of biceps has given way, permitting the muscle to retract toward the elbow.

90 degrees (Fig. 139). If the tear is complete it will be noted that the muscle belly moves away from the rupture.

If acute rupture is diagnosed, the *treatment* is surgical. No attempt should be made to restore the attachment to the glenoid. The long head of the biceps should be fastened into the bicipital groove (see Surgical Technique, p. 204). Prompt recovery follows surgical treatment. Unrepaired rupture usually results in some weakness of the arm and frequently in pain, depending upon the location of the tear.

Subluxation of the Biceps Tendon

Another traumatic condition about the tendon of the biceps is a rupture or stretching of the fascial covering of the bicipital groove that permits the tendon to subluxate from the groove. This may occur as an acute injury. The predisposing factor for this condition is a congenitally shallow bicipital groove. The intertubercular groove not only may be shallow but may be broader than normal, which permits the tendon to flatten out and slide back and forth within the groove itself (Figs. 140, 141 and 142). The patient complains of a snap anteriorly in the shoulder with pain fol-

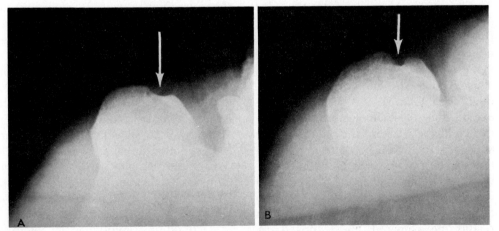

Figure 140. *A*, Young lady with recurrent attacks of severe shoulder pain. Careful history elicited the fact that each attack started with a snap in front of the shoulder. Her findings were that of bicipital tendinitis during an attack. Between attacks she was completely relieved. Rotation of the arm at 90 degree abduction caused extreme pain. Her diffuse shoulder tenderness was localized at the bicipital groove. At surgery the shallow groove was noted with a redundant roof so that the tendon could slide out of the groove. The glenoid attachment of the biceps tendon was transferred to the bicipital groove with relief of symptoms.

B, A normal bicipital tunnel for comparison. (See Fig. 141 for technique of x-ray in positioning for bicipital tunnel.)

lowed by residual soreness along the bicipital groove elicited by the same motions that cause pain on tenosynovitis. Indeed, it may be indistinguishable from tenosynovitis. In the muscular athlete it may be difficult to palpate the subluxating tendon. If the condition becomes chronic as the result of a defect of the roof of the groove with redundant tissue, a chronic synovitis usually occurs. On motion of the shoulder there is painful snapping as the tendon slips back and forth out of the groove, particularly on rotation of the arm. This condition also should be treated by surgical fixation of the tendon into the groove after detaching the tendon from the glenoid.

SURGICAL TECHNIQUE. The surgical technique for transference of the long head of the biceps into the bicipital groove is as follows: The shoulder is approached anteriorly with the arm draped free to permit manipulation. It is not necessary to reflect the anterior one-third of the deltoid from the clavicle. By palpation locate the raphe between the anterior and middle thirds of the deltoid. The longitudinal incision from the edge of the acromion extends distally along this raphe for about 3 inches. The fibers of the deltoid can be separated along this line with but little trauma. This exposes the roof of the subacromial bursa. Care should be taken not to extend this dissection more than $2\frac{1}{2}$ inches distally from the edge of the acromion lest there be damage done to the axillary nerve which extends forward on the deep surface of the deltoid to supply its anterior one-third. By rotation of the arm the bicipital groove can readily be palpated and exposed. A silver probe should be passed up along the tendon from below the bicipital groove through the groove. This will give some indication as to the degree of constriction present. The roof of the tunnel is now split along the tendon up to the insertion of the rotator cuff. This will expose the pathologic condition, which might be constrictive tenosynovitis, fraying of the tendon, adhesions to the tendon sheath or possibly dislocation of the tendon from the groove.

If any of the aforesaid conditions are present, the tendon should be transferred. Incision in the tunnel is extended proximally and the rotator cuff incised to permit a finger to be passed into the joint. The finger passes along the tendon of the biceps to its attachment to the rim of the glenoid. With a long scissors or a tenotome the tendon is detached as near as possible to its attachment to the glenoid. The tendon is then pulled down into the wound and may be securely sutured into the bicipital groove using drill holes along the margin of the groove as necessary. Exploration of the joint is carried out through the split in the rotator cuff to reveal any disease of the articular cartilage on the humeral head. If this is present and needs treatment, the incision through the rotator cuff may be extended to permit more thorough exploration of the joint. The rotator cuff is then carefully repaired, inverting the knot into the substance of the cuff. Suitable wound closure using intracutaneous wire suture is carried out.

Postoperatively a sling and swathe are applied to the shoulder, and pendulum exercises, limited in range, may be initiated almost from the beginning (Fig. 161). After two weeks the stitches are removed and the sling is replaced without the swathe, and activity of the arm is increased. At the end of four weeks all fixation should be removed and rehabilitative exercises continued.

Conditions involving the bicipital tendon and bicipital groove are particularly pertinent to the athlete, since many sports involve the throwing motion of the arm. This includes the baseball pitcher, the football quarterback, the batter and the tennis player.

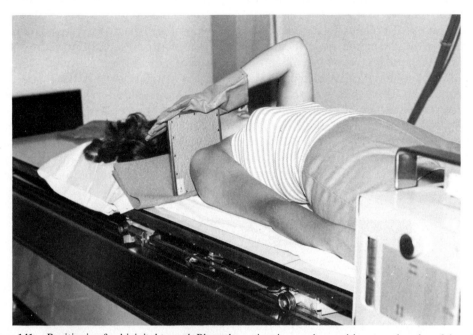

Figure 141. Positioning for bicipital tunnel. Place the patient in a supine position near the edge of the table. Extend the arm, palm up, alongside the body. Place a cassette above the shoulder in a vertical position. Adjust the tube in a horizontal position slightly external to the elbow so that the central ray may be directed along the shaft of the humerus through the groove. Palpation of the groove will aid in determining the angulation of the tube, usually 20 degrees medially.

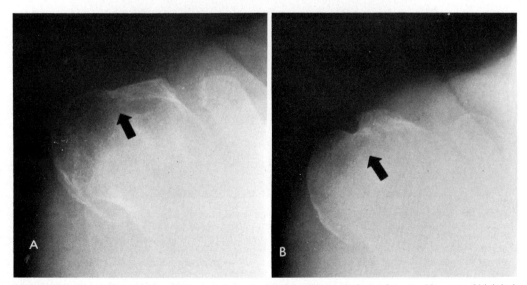

Figure 142. Old avulsion injury of lesser tuberosity by the subscapularis tendon. *A*, Absence of bicipital groove (arrow). *B*, Normal groove for comparison (arrow).

This motion is particularly inhibited by bicipital tendon problems. It is especially pertinent to recognize this since correction of the defect, whether it be an adhesive tenosynovitis, fraying out of the tendon, subluxation or dislocation of the tendon, is the same, namely, transference of the attachment of the biceps tendon from the top of the glenoid into the bicipital tunnel (Fig. 143). Following this, the long head of the biceps is no longer involved in shoulder motion and

recovery can be very prompt and complete. This condition has characteristic symptoms; hence, the diagnosis can be quite secure, often confirmed by x-rays profiling the bicipital tunnel. The remedy is a relatively nontraumatic operation that removes the biceps tendon from the shoulder and fastens it into the bicipital groove. To take the young athlete who can no longer throw and by a procedure of short morbidity permit him to throw without inhibition is very grati-

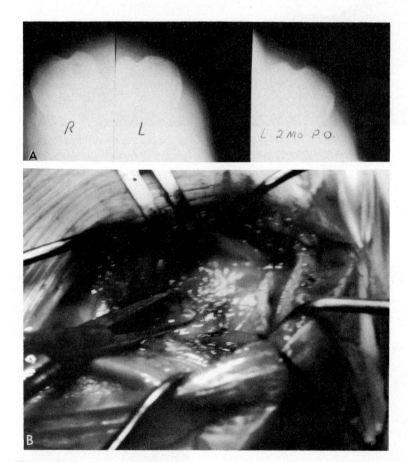

Figure 143.   This professional baseball player had increasing trouble with the left shoulder all through the season. He is left-handed. Finally, by the end of the season he could no longer pitch. He feels something "roll over" in his shoulder if he throws. Examination revealed pain over the anterior shoulder and the bicipital groove, traveling with the groove on rotation of the arm. A snap was noted when the arm moved from external rotation to internal rotation. *A,* Shows relatively normal groove on the left as compared with the right. Note, however, the angle is distinctly more acute than average (60 to 75 degrees). This shows a little more clearly in the postoperative view (upper right). *B,* The deltoid splitting incision with the bicipital tendon retracted to the left. The extreme width of the tunnel is seen by the span of the Kelly forceps across the incision. The tendon was removed from its attachment and sutured into the groove. He returned to baseball pitching.

fying to both the patient and physician. I urge definitive diagnosis of shoulder lesions in the young athlete.

BURSITIS

Acute Subacromial (Subdeltoid) Bursitis

The major bursae about the shoulder are the subacromial, the subcoracoid and the subscapular (Fig. 137). The subacromial bursa lies underneath the acromial process and extends out under the deltoid muscle to lie between the acromial process and deltoid and the humeral head and the rotator cuff. The bursa is separate and distinct from the glenohumeral joint and has no connection with it. It permits the tendons surrounding the humeral head to slide freely under the acromial process (Fig. 136). This bursa is frequently involved in injuries about the shoulder since any irritative lesion involving the rotator cuff will cause inflammatory reaction within the bursa, so that the symptoms of bursitis may well obscure the primary lesion. Subacromial bursitis may be caused by excessive friction between

the cuff and the acromion. As the irritation increases the thickness of the bursal lining, the pressure increases, and the rolled-up synovium may form a fold that will at first snap as it slips under the glenoid (Fig. 144). Later it may check abduction at the point of impingement. The condition may also be caused by a direct blow over the shoulder which causes an inflammatory reaction that is aggravated by further motion. Primary subacromial bursitis is not common in the athlete. The bursitis is usually a secondary reaction, so it behooves one to search for the primary lesion before instigating treatment.

Symptoms of acute subacromial bursitis are pain on motion of the shoulder, particularly abduction, tenderness over the tuberosity just distal to the acromial process, and pain on rotation of the shoulder, particularly internal rotation. Rotation forces the inflamed walls of the bursa into tight approximation, so that manipulation of the arm into wide abduction, as in the throwing motion or reaching behind the back, will elicit major pain.

TREATMENT. Acute bursitis is treated by rest and local heat using wet packs, radiant lamp or diathermy. It will

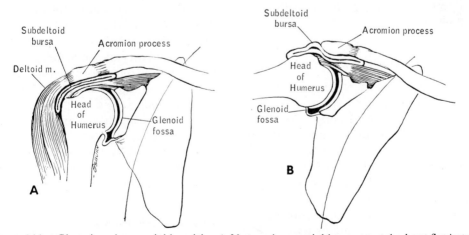

Figure 144. Chronic subacromial bursitis. *A*, Note subacromial bursa stretched out flat between acromion and deltoid above and rotator cuff and humoral head below. *B*, On abduction of the arm the thickened bursal wall cannot slide under acromion and so "bunches up" and checks motion.

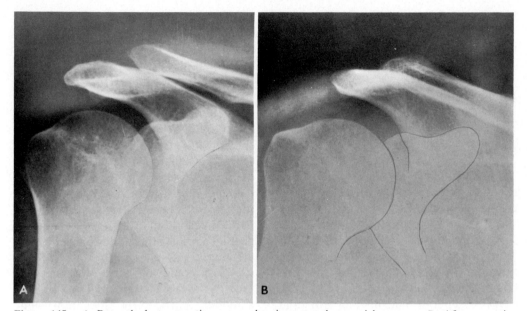

Figure 145. *A*, Retouched preoperative x-ray showing normal acromial process. *B*, After resection of the distal portion of the acromion which delays the impingement of the bursa under the acromial margin.

usually subside fairly rapidly. The condition is particularly annoying to the athlete and almost inevitably he will start active use of the shoulder before the inflammation has subsided. This results in renewed irritation of the bursa. It should be emphasized that comprehensive treatment of acute bursitis will prevent repeated recurrence of the acute bursitis or a resultant chronic synovitis, adhesions and a chronic subacromial bursitis.

Chronic Subacromial Bursitis

Chronic subacromial bursitis causes subacute or recurrent pain around the subacromial bursa. This may be due to chronic inflammation within the bursa itself but is much more likely to be due to irregularity of the bursal walls caused by adhesion between the two layers of the bursa or by irregularity and thickening of the rotator cuff which may be the result of a minor tear of the tendons. Symptoms of such a condition are pain on extremes of motion, particularly abduction, crepitation on rotation

and occasionally "snapping" of the shoulder when the roll of thickened synovium at the edge of the acromion finally snaps beneath it with a palpable painful click (Fig. 144).

In chronic bursitis the *treatment* is injection into the bursa of a local anesthetic and a corticoid in serial fashion (see p. 84). If this fails, surgical intervention should be carried out. The surgeon should be warned against excising the walls of the bursa if roughened surfaces are left to rub together. In case of an irregularity of the distal portion of the acromion, this portion may be excised. Indeed, up to 1 inch of the acromion may be excised in the presence of irreversible irregularity of the rotator cuff, with little resultant disability (Fig. 145). Occasionally the coraco-acromial ligament may be involved and it too should be excised if necessary.

Subscapularis Bursitis

The subscapularis bursa is a further extension of the sac surrounding the subscapularis tendon (Fig. 136). It usually has a direct connection with the joint. True bursitis here is not frequent. Usually there is more complicated involvement of the glenohumeral joint itself. There may, however, be a separate *subcoracoid* bursa that is a further extension of this same sac. Pain and tenderness in the area of the coracoid aggravated by external rotation of the arm against resistance or active internal rotation should make one suspect involvement in this area. Local treatment is of value. Physical therapy and local injection will usually give good relief.

Any of these bursae can give rise to prolonged disability. This is particularly true if the athlete is unwilling to rest the shoulder for a sufficient time to permit the inflammation to subside. Too early resumption of activity leads inevitably to recurrence of symptoms. Every time the symptoms recur they are more resistant to treatment. Finally irreversible disability ensues.

SPRAIN

It has been noted previously that the ligaments or capsule contribute but little to the stability of the shoulder joint. The shoulder is pressed into the glenoid by the rotator cuff, which consists of tendons. There is but little inherent stability of the shoulder owing to the capsular ligaments. As a result, the only sprain which commonly occurs in the glenohumeral joint is that occurring from external rotation–abduction of the shoulder. As the shoulder is abducted and externally rotated, tension is placed upon the anterior capsule with its ligament reinforcements (Fig. 146, *A*). The head tends to slide forward against the coraco-acromial ligament and against the capsule inferior to it. The coraco-acromial ligament, being an extremely strong structure, forces the head downward and tension is exerted on the anterior capsule and the capsular ligaments. As the abduction–external rotation force continues (as with the arm in the overhand throwing position), the capsular ligament may tear partially or completely (Fig. 146, *B*). This may occur at the attachment of the capsule along the labrum of the glenoid or indeed anywhere in the anterior capsule. If the tear is incomplete the shoulder does not subluxate or dislocate. The motion is arrested short of dislocation.

DIAGNOSIS.   One of the symptoms

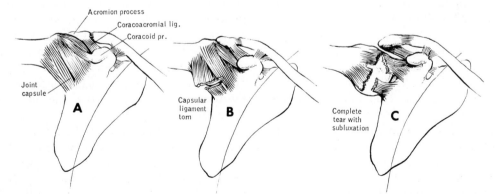

Figure 146.   Various degrees of sprain of the shoulder caused by abduction – external rotation. *A*, Normal abduction – external rotation showing the anterior inferior portion of the capsule taut. *B*, Forced external rotation combined with posterior flexion causes capsular tear – moderate (second degree). *C*, Continuation of this motion rotates the anterior and inferior fibers to be superior and anterior, respectively. The head emerges through the rent in the capsule and will dislocate if the movement continues – severe (third degree).

of such a condition is pain at the time of the injury. The player will usually relate that his arm was forced backward and upward. For example, in an attempt to tackle another player as he runs by, the arm is carried forcibly backward and externally rotated (see Fig. 171). The pain is promptly relieved as the arm is placed at the side and there may be relatively little discomfort as long as the arm remains in this relaxed position. If the sprain is more severe there will be aching pain, which is particularly aggravated by external rotation of the humerus. The player prefers to hold the arm to his side.

On examination there will be resistance to external rotation–abduction and pain on this motion. Marked muscle spasm of the adductors and internal rotators is stimulated by any attempt to externally rotate or abduct the arm. This motion will be more or less restricted depending upon the severity of the injury. On palpation there is tenderness in front of the shoulder joint, not along the bicipital groove but medial to it, and down to the anterior portion of the humeral head and glenoid. This area may be difficult to palpate in the muscular athlete. Owing to the multiplicity of structures subject to injury in this area it may be extremely difficult to differentiate the condition from such things as a strain of the subscapularis attachment, strain of the rotator cuff and involvement of the pectoralis major, all of which give similar symptoms.

Since the treatment is basically the same for all of these conditions, the exact diagnosis may not be essential. However, there is one distinguishing characteristic. With a sprain of the ligament there should be no pain on active adduction or internal rotation of the shoulder within certain limits such as would be elicited with strain of the rotators or adductors. This is true particularly if the patient is examined early.

The injury may be mild (first degree), moderate (second degree) or severe (third degree). This depends upon the point at which the abnormal motion of the shoulder is arrested. Since the shoulder capsule is well relaxed with the arm at the side and internally rotated, it is usually considered that rest in this position with a sling and swathe (Fig. 103) will be adequate, since the tendency is for the fibers of the torn capsule to fold together. It is, however, vitally important to know how severe the tear is in order to regulate the period of protection and the degree of activity to be permitted.

If the sprain is mild and the shoulder has not subluxated, it may only be necessary to prevent abduction and external rotation for a few days. If the lesion has been more extensive (moderate) and the head was partially subluxated, a longer period is necessary. It should be two weeks in a sling and swathe followed by restraining strap in order to prevent abduction and external rotation (Fig. 147). The protection should be continued for six to eight weeks even if the patient is entirely symptom-free. If the sprain has been severe and the capsule completely torn and the head dislocated with or without spontaneous reduction, it is much more important to prolong the immobilization. In athletes most recurrent dislocations are caused by faulty healing of the ligaments so that redundancy of the ligament is present. This is usually caused by too early stress before the fibers have actually healed. In this severe sprain the immobilization should be by sling and swathe for four weeks and after this the restraining strap for three or four months. Only in this way is there a reasonable chance that the ligaments and capsule may heal short enough to prevent recurrent slipping.

TREATMENT. Since in sprain the capsule is completely relaxed with the

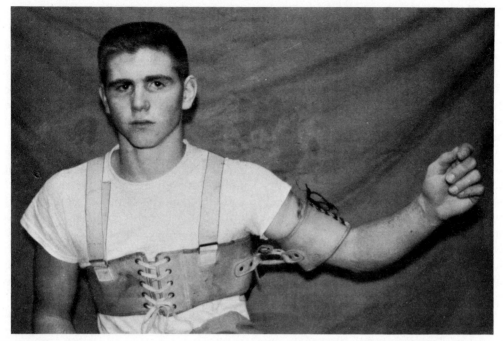

Figure 147. Type of chain restraint popular with football players. Note the heavy leather strap around the chest not tight enough to interfere with respiration, and the wide leather band around the arm. In most instances now the chain between the two bands is replaced by a leather strap as indicated here. This does not prevent external rotation but does check abduction to some degree, depending upon the tightness of the connecting strap.

arm in adduction and internal rotation, it is not necessary to immobilize the shoulder completely. Treatment should be by sling preferably worn under the shirt so that the arm is supported at the side and external rotation and abduction are prevented. A simple swathe over the chest and around the arm will accomplish the same result (Fig. 103). The patient should be instructed that any active use of the hand and forearm that does not cause discomfort is desirable. If the sprain is severe, four weeks of protection in a sling are necessary. In a less severe case (second degree), the wearing of a simple restraining chain (Fig. 147) may permit active participation in sports. A belt is placed around the chest, another around the arm, and the two are connected by a strap or chain of a length suitable to restrict abduction at the desired angle. This treatment is based on the fact that strain is not applied to this torn structure until the arm is in wide abduction and external rotation.

SUBLUXATION

Anterior Subluxation

Subluxation of the shoulder is caused by the same basic mechanism that causes a sprain. This is particularly true of the anterior-inferior subluxation, which is the most frequent type of athletic injury to the shoulder. As the arm comes up into external rotation—abduction, the superior portion of the rotator cuff becomes posterior whereas the anterior-inferior ligaments become anterior. In this position the humeral head is thrust forcibly against the glenohumeral ligaments in front, using the rotator cuff as a sling around which the head rotates against the anterior capsule (Fig. 146, C). This causes a tearing of the anterior capsule, and if this tearing is relatively complete the humeral head will actually subluxate forward and ride over the rim of the glenoid. The force being arrested, the movement reverses and the head promptly slips back into its normal position without ever having completely dislocated from the glenoid. It can readily be seen that this type of subluxation is actually a third degree sprain that has caused disruption of the anterior capsule, since in a normal shoulder the head cannot slide over the glenoid rim without loss of integrity of some portion of the shoulder capsule. In the young adult this is almost always the anterior thickening of the capsule.

SYMPTOMS. The history is important in this condition. The history is of the arm being thrown up into external rotation and abduction and the feeling that the shoulder is slipping out of position, accompanied by severe pain in the anterior portion of the joint. Immediate relief is obtained as the arm slips back into neutral position, and there may be very little discomfort so long as the arm is supported at the side. The symptoms will be identical to those of a second degree sprain, only more severe. Any attempt at abduction–external rotation will cause muscle spasm and pain, and in many cases the feeling of imminent dislocation. The patient will often volunteer the statement that his shoulder has been out of joint and slipped back in. Indeed, it is often impossible to determine whether the injury has been a subluxation or a spontaneously reduced dislocation.

TREATMENT. Treatment is based on the assumption that there is actual structural damage to the shoulder. I cannot overemphasize the importance of adequate treatment for subluxation or spontaneously reduced dislocation

of the shoulder. This condition frequently occurs in the shoulder predisposed toward dislocation with flattening of the glenoid or a defect in the humeral head. It also occurs in an anatomically normal joint. If the torn ligaments are protected in the relaxed position there is every expectation that they will heal completely without undue lengthening. If constant irritation and stretching are permitted, the ligaments will heal not only with overlength but with scar rather than ligament structure, and potential weakness remains. This invites recurrence of subluxation, finally dislocation and often recurrent dislocation. External rotation–abduction of the arm must not be permitted during the healing period.

The treatment is basically the same as that for second degree sprain, namely, fixation of the arm at the side in a sling with the arm enclosed in either the shirt or a circumferential swathe (Fig. 103). Meddlesome manipulation of the shoulder to determine the progress of the repair is to be condemned. Ligament structures heal slowly and the initial anastomosis between the torn ligament ends is extremely insecure. One single motion in external rotation–abduction will be enough to disrupt the infant union and successive motions constantly separate the edges. The patient, the coach and indeed the physician must restrain their curiosity as to the progress of this repair and assume that short of three weeks there is no union and that it takes six weeks for union to be secure even under favorable circumstances. Careful treatment of this initial lesion may result in complete recovery. Unwise manipulation may result in a recurrent condition of the shoulder.

Inferior Subluxation

Whereas the common subluxation of the shoulder is anterior, there is another type of subluxation of the humeral head that should be mentioned although it is not common in the athlete. I refer to the inferior subluxation in which the humeral head actually hangs out of the glenoid, the head riding over the inferior rim. This is, of course, a frequent occurrence in paralytic conditions of the shoulder and as a result of overheavy traction by a hanging cast. As such it is readily explained by the antecedent history and is not particularly related to athletic injuries. It is possible, however, to have acute subluxation of the shoulder as a result of injury to the rotator cuff. It is to be recalled that the rotator cuff suspends the head against the glenoid by the tonic action of the rotator muscles (Figs. 135 and 136). A rupture of any one of these muscles, as for example the supraspinatus or teres minor, will not result in any actual subluxation of the humeral head. However, if the whole rotator cuff is avulsed, the suspensory action of the cuff is lost and the humerus can be held in proper position only by strong contraction of the deltoid and other extrinsic muscles of the

shoulder. This is a major injury and may have extremely distressing sequelae.

The writer recalls a recent case in which a young adult fell from a truck; his glove caught on the sideboard and his fall was sharply arrested by his arm extending directly upward. The sudden suspension on his relaxed arm resulted in extreme pain and disability in the shoulder. His early examination and treatment were unfortunately superficial, consisting of application of a sling for a couple of weeks and then encouragement to return to work. At the time this patient was examined nine weeks after his injury he wore a very snug sling with pressure under his elbow. He was extremely apprehensive on removal of the sling and when he was persuaded to permit his extrinsic muscles to relax he had pain in the shoulder and the feeling that the shoulder had slipped out of place. Examination revealed a definite interval between the acromion and the head and it was possible to slip the head in and out of the shoulder joint inferiorly. This finding was confirmed by both examination and x-ray (Fig. 148).

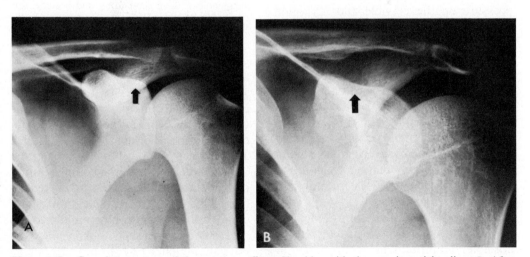

Figure 148. Complete rupture of the rotator cuff. *A,* Shoulder with the arm in a tight sling. *B,* After removal of the sling and with no added weight, note wide separation between the acromion and the head with the head hanging downward over the glenoid rim.

This patient was extremely apprehensive because he had learned that whenever he would relax the shoulder the head would fall out of joint. It would not actually dislocate but would subluxate inferiorly.

This patient's *treatment* was by open operation, at which time the whole rotator cuff was found to be detached and the whole area scarred in with resultant increase in length of the rotator cuff tendons. In the operation the entire cuff was pulled downward like a hood over the tuberosity and sutured there. This gave an extremely stable shoulder immediately. Snug support was continued eight weeks to prevent re-stress. The result was complete stability of the shoulder but considerable restriction of motion, which could be attributed to the long immobilization—nine weeks preoperative, six weeks postoperative.

Admittedly this was an unusual injury, but I believe it could have been diagnosed early by careful history and physical examination supported by x-ray. For this degree of subluxation I do not believe nonsurgical treatment is appropriate. However, if nonsurgical treatment is elected, the arm should be supported at the side with downward pressure on the clavicle and acromion and upward pressure on the humerus in an effort to induce the rotator cuff to resume its normal position. The inadequacy of this becomes apparent when it is recognized that this is a tendon avulsion and that the tone of the involved muscles, particularly as they go into spasm with the injury, will inevitably pull the tendon away from its attachment. The primary treatment should be surgical with repair of the rotator cuff down to the humerus.

A sprain or subluxation of the humeral head inferiorly *by abduction* is possible, but infrequent. At the height of abduction the humeral head levers against the tip of the acromion and the posterior portion of the head drives

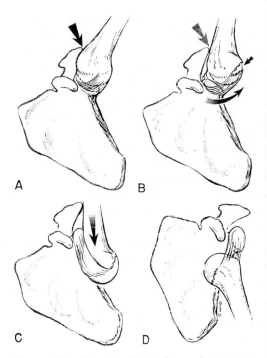

Figure 149. Drawing illustrating various stages in the inferior sprain-subluxation-dislocation of the shoulder. *A*, Arm in complete abduction with the scapula rotated, the tuberosity serving as a fulcrum for the acromion; stress is applied to the inferior glenohumeral ligaments. *B*, The force continues, the ligaments rupture, the head subluxates. *C*, As the force continues further the head goes into typical position of luxatio erecta and completely dislocates. The inferior capsule is completely torn. *D*, After the arm drops back toward the anatomical position the head remains subglenoid or may slip further and become subcoracoid. (From DePalma, Surgery of the Shoulder, J. B. Lippincott Co.)

against the structures inferiorly (Fig. 149, *A*). This results in tearing of the capsule and ligament, and if the tear is complete the humeral head may ride out on the inferior glenoid rim (Fig. 149, *B*). This is an extremely severe injury, and if the force continues a complete inferior dislocation of the humerus results (Fig. 149, *C*). If the dislocation is not complete, the arm drops promptly to the side and is resolutely held in place by the patient, since he feels any attempt to abduct it will cause it to slip out of place. The history of the type of injury plus the fact that the tenderness is deep in the axilla up against the inferior portion of the humeral head will serve as a key to the diagnosis. Active abduction per se is not painful, because if there is any strain on the internal structures, muscle spasm will force the arm to the side before the movement is extensive enough to be painful.

Treatment is by sling with the arm at the side. Since only complete abduction will put strain on this redundant inferior capsule, athletic participation may be allowed in a few weeks, provided that abduction of the arm is prevented. The degree of restriction of abduction necessary can be determined by steadily abducting the arm to the point where pain is elicited. Abduction beyond this point should be prevented by suitable apparatus. The familiar chain restraint, with a wide band around the chest, a band around the arm and the two connected with a chain or strap is adequate (Fig. 147).

Posterior Subluxation

Posterior subluxation of the shoulder, meaning an incomplete posterior dislocation, presumably may occur (Figs. 150 and 151). The forces involved usually are direct backward thrust of the humerus with the arm forward flexed. This drives the head posteriorly from beneath the acromion. The posterior portion of the rotator cuff is in this instance damaged and the humeral head slides posteriorly. Owing to the muscular character of the posterior structures, the subluxation is immediately reduced spontaneously and in my opinion its diagnosis with any degree of certainty is virtually impossible. The symptoms are those of strain of the posterior structures, pain on reproduction of the force causing dislocation so that with the humerus flexed forward and pushed backward there is a feeling of discomfort, and pain posteriorly in the shoulder. Attempts to internally rotate and flex the arm across the chest will also elicit pain. On examination tenderness is posterior and about the humeral head; indeed, the symptoms are identical with those of strain or partial avulsion of the external rotators of the shoulder.

TREATMENT. Treatment is by immobilization with the arm at the side. Ordinary internal rotation to the extent

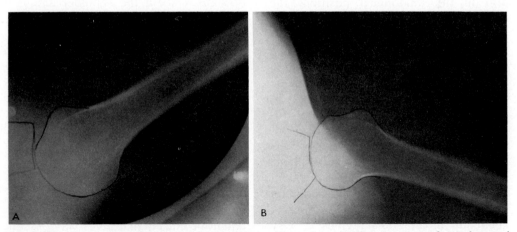

Figure 150. Posterior subluxation of the shoulder, axillary view. *A,* The arm swung forward toward the midline. As the head rotates it slips out of the glenoid posteriorly. This required posterior reconstruction of the capsule. *B,* The horizontal position. (See Fig. 151 for positioning of patient for x-ray.)

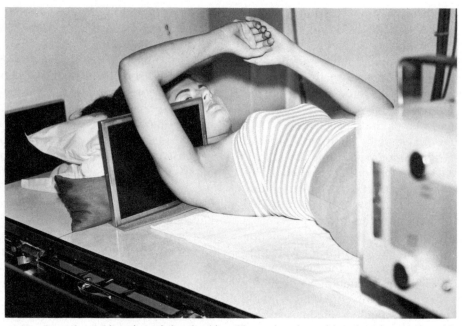

Figure 151. Posterior subluxation of the shoulder. The patient is positioned supine on the table with the shoulders elevated by a pad. The arm is positioned as for an axillary view except that it is brought up and rotated toward the midline. The cassette is supported in a vertical position behind the shoulder. The central ray is directed horizontally to the head of the humerus. The tube usually needs to be rotated medially about 10 degrees.

of placing the forearm across the chest is not interdicted, particularly if it is not painful. If this results in painful strain posteriorly, the arm may be immobilized at the side in a plaster spica with the arm in the anatomical position, the elbow flexed to 90 degrees and the forearm extended directly forward—a position similar to that used in certain fractures about the elbow. The duration of immobilization will depend upon the degree of symptoms and the amount of damage. The shoulder should be protected for about six weeks. It is an unusual force that causes this injury and is not likely to be recurrent. This explains the more rapid rehabilitation in this condition than in anterior subluxation where the position of external rotation–abduction in athletic activities is very frequent and so needs to be guarded against for a longer time.

DISLOCATION

Anterior Dislocation

Dislocation of the shoulder follows the loss of function of the restraining structures about the shoulder and is a result of the same mechanism that causes the subluxations described previously. By far the most common type of dislocation of the shoulder in young individuals of athletic age is the anterior-inferior (Fig. 152, A). This is pure dislocation, unaccompanied by fracture, in young individuals. As age advances, the ligaments become firmer and the bone less strong, so the dislocation may be accompanied by avulsion fracture rather than a tear of the ligament. In the young athlete it is almost always the ligament or muscle that gives way. As the arm is forced into abduction and external rotation, the humeral head is thrust

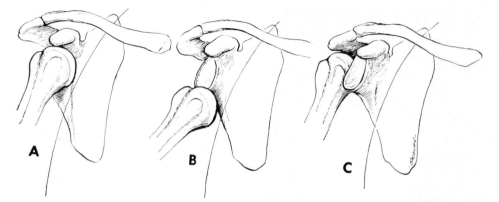

Figure 152. Dislocations of the shoulder. *A*, Typical subcoracoid dislocation. *B*, Subglenoid dislocation. *C*, Posterior dislocation.

against the anterior portion of the gleno-humeral joint, the coraco-acromial ligament serves to force it downward and it then emerges anteriorly and inferiorly into the redundant area of the capsule, which is protected by the glenohumeral ligaments (Fig. 85). These give way when they are torn from the glenoid labrum or because of avulsion of the labrum or actual disruption of the ligaments. The head of the humerus slips over the glenoid rim, immediately slides forward to lodge between the rim of the glenoid and coracoid process, and the arm drops toward the side but not against it. This is the classic dislocation of the shoulder in young persons (Figs. 153 and 154). The damage to the liga-

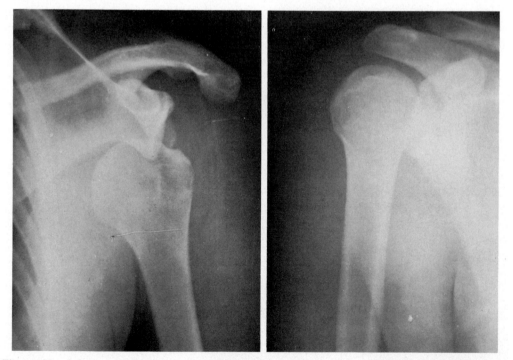

Figure 153. Subcoracoid dislocation of shoulder. In this case the head may well have displaced inferiorly and then swung around to antero-inferior and so subglenoid. Note head is proximal to inferior glenoid rim and caught between glenoid and coracoid process.

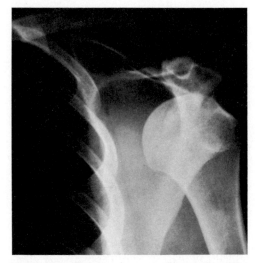

Figure 154. Twenty-six year old wrestler. The arm was forcibly jerked, dislocating the shoulder anteriorly. Anterior-posterior view illustrating subcoracoid dislocation.

ment may be a transverse tear across the capsule, and in addition the capsular reinforcements known as the glenohumeral ligaments may split with one passing above the humeral head and one below it. In some instances they actually grasp the humeral head in such a way as to impede reduction.

SYMPTOMS. While the diagnosis of the dislocated shoulder by appearance alone may be difficult in an extremely well-muscled or heavy individual, it is usually easy. The acromion is prominent with a definite defect below it rather than the usual rounding out of the deltoid muscle (Fig. 155). The arm tends to be held away from the side and rotated slightly externally, so that it is virtually impossible to move the forearm across the chest or abdomen in front of the body or to bring the elbow to the side. On examination the defect below the acromion is, in early cases, readily palpable, and the roundness of the humeral head as it rests against the coracoid is also readily felt anteriorly. An attempt to manipulate the arm or to force the elbow to the side causes pain. The patient will usually permit some increase in abduction and external rotation but will resist adduction and internal rotation. At the time of this examination a careful neurological examination should be made, since an injury to the brachial plexus occurs quite often in dislocation of the shoulder. Neuro-

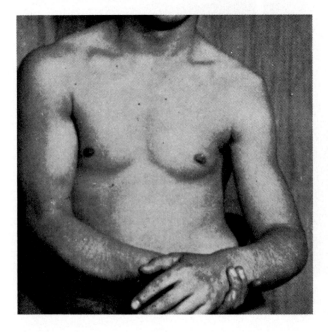

Figure 155. Photograph of subcoracoid dislocation of the shoulder. Note the prominent acromion, the arm held away from the side, the flat deltoid. (From McLaughlin, Trauma, p. 246.)

logical examination to determine the integrity of the nerves should be done before an attempt is made at reduction. If this is not done one may wonder whether a neurological deficit discovered later was caused by the injury itself or by the trauma of the reduction.

TREATMENT. Dislocation of the shoulder is an acute emergency and should be reduced as soon as adequate facilities are available. On occasion it may readily be reduced directly after the injury before pain and muscle spasm have developed. However, this is not to be attempted by the uninitiated since irreparable damage may be done to the bone or capsule and particularly to the nerve structures about the shoulder by unwise manipulation. Under no circumstances should force be used. The major obstacle to reduction is general spasm of the muscles about the shoulder, so that the humeral head is firmly fixed against the coracoid and under the glen-oid rim. Any attempt to move it from this position will only increase the spasm. I cannot too severely condemn forcible manipulation of the shoulder, which not only will not accomplish the purpose of the reduction but simply will increase spastic fixation.

The first prerequisite for reduction of the dislocation is complete relaxation of the shoulder. This may be possible without general anesthesia, but once the dislocation has persisted beyond the first few minutes it becomes extremely difficult to obtain relaxation short of use of a general anesthetic. This is particularly true in the athlete who is very muscular, extremely apprehensive and at the age where he has not yet developed sufficient equanimity to permit voluntary relaxation of these painful structures.

If the doctor sees the player at the time of his injury and is skilled in manipulation of the shoulder, he may attempt immediate reduction on the field without anesthesia. This is accomplished by laying the patient flat on his back on the ground, grasping his arm securely either by the wrist or with the elbow flexed and exerting direct traction distally. The traction should be gentle and not accompanied by any attempt at lateral motion (Fig. 156). In certain instances the humeral head will slip quietly into position. The time-honored method of placing the foot in the axilla is fraught with danger. Its only justification is to permit the operator to steady himself, not to permit him to use excessive force or traction. The unshod foot should be used and great care taken not to put direct pressure against the humeral head (Fig. 157); rather, the foot should be against the chest wall. Care-

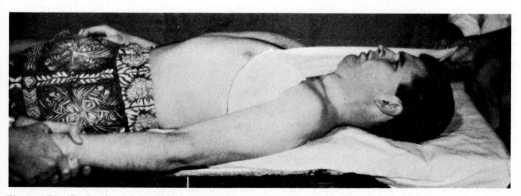

Figure 156. Reduction of the dislocated shoulder by steady, even pull on the arm in the supine position. The padded strap through the axilla is for mild countertraction and is often not necessary. This may be with or without anesthesia.

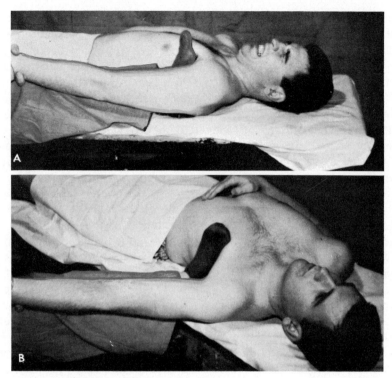

Figure 157. *A,* The improper method. Note the foot is directly in the axilla, impinging the brachial plexus against the dislocated humeral head while the arm is levered over the foot. This can cause serious damage to the brachial plexus and is quite painful. *B,* The proper position with the foot against the axillary wall for pressure while steady, even traction is made at about a 45 degree angle.

less use of the foot in the axilla may well result in damage to the structures of the brachial plexus, since they may be tightly caught against the humeral head.

If, after a reasonable trial of traction (60 seconds), the head does not reduce, the attempt should be abandoned. The player should be taken from the field to a place suitable for more adequate treatment. Preferably he should be taken promptly to the infirmary or hospital, and x-rays should be made of the shoulder to confirm the diagnosis and to reveal any accompanying bony abnormalities. Even if the dislocation is promptly reduced by traction, x-ray study should be made to eliminate the possibility of accompanying bony injury.

After the x-ray is made, a second

and more comprehensive effort may be made to obtain reduction by simple traction. Detailed description of the various methods of reduction is not appropriate here, but a few deserve mention. The simplest one is to exert traction directly on the line of the trunk or possibly in slight abduction, with the patient flat on his back (Fig. 156). It must be emphasized that this traction must be pain-free or it will not accomplish its purpose. In another method the patient lies prone on the table with the involved arm hanging over the edge either with or without a weight suspended from the wrist (Fig. 158). Similar reduction may be carried out with the patient sitting, the arm hanging over the suitably padded back of a chair (Fig. 159). In all instances care must be taken that there is no pressure on the axillary structures. If these methods do not suffice for reduction, the patient should be given an anesthetic and an extremely atraumatic reduction carried out, preferably by traction as in Figure 156. If this fails, reduction may be accomplished by the Kocher maneuver (Fig. 160) or by whatever careful manipulation will bring the head into proper relation with the glenoid. I cannot overemphasize the importance of atraumatic, careful, gentle manipulation. Force is not required to reduce the dislocated shoulder. Relaxation is imperative either with or without general anesthesia. Following reduction, x-ray examination should be made to confirm the position and again check for possible bony abnormalities or injuries.

Attendant fractures about the shoulder are not common in this age group. However, they may occur and as such will require definitive treatment. Avulsion of the greater or lesser tuber-

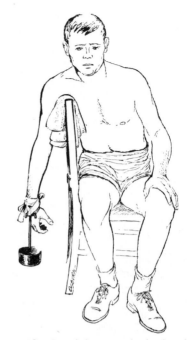

Figure 159. Pendulant method of reduction without anesthesia. Note the pad in the axilla, the weight suspended from the wrist, not grasped by the hand. This method is not as safe or as satisfactory as the method shown in Figure 158.

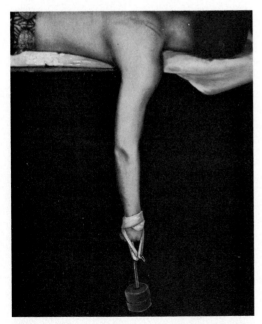

Figure 158. Pendulant method of reduction without anesthesia. The weight must be suspended by the wrist, not grasped by the hand, since complete relaxation is essential. The shoulder should swing free and the patient should be comfortable or else he will not relax.

osity, fracture of the glenoid, fracture of the acromion, and involvement of the biceps tendon are complications that will demand the best care of the skilled orthopaedist. If the shoulder does not readily and completely reduce, repeated attempts at manipulation are not justified and open reduction should be done.

The occasional damage to the nerves that accompanies injury to the brachial plexus may be the cause of considerable concern. Competent neurosurgical consultation is advisable in such cases of nerve injury. Ordinary watchful waiting will be the treatment of choice, anticipating a gradual return of function since this damage is usually peripheral — a contusion to the nerve, which will probably recover promptly. If recovery does not occur, exploration of the nerve is advisable, and considerable judgment is required to determine the best time for it. Since recovery will occur in many cases without explora-

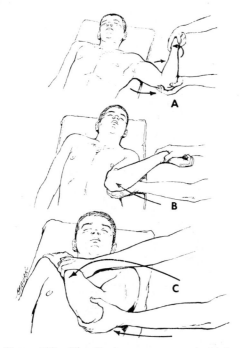

Figure 160. The Kocher maneuver. *A*, Abduction–external rotation. *B*, Adduction–external rotation. *C*, The completed maneuver with internal rotation of the adducted arm. Complete relaxation is essential for this maneuver to be effective. It cannot be successfully carried out if the patient resists, either consciously or unconsciously.

tion, this avenue is usually postponed several months. Once the indications are clear, however, it should be recommended and carried out without delay.

Following successful reduction, the after-treatment consists of immobilization of the arm in a sling providing support under the elbow, with an added swathe around the chest in order to prevent abduction of the arm (Fig. 106). It should be emphasized that for an acute complete dislocation to occur there must be serious damage to the ligaments and capsule of the joint. Thus, continued immobilization is required until they attain some degree of healing in direct apposition. The arm should be held in a sling for a minimum of three weeks and then mobilized only within the limits of pain. Active participation in sports without protection should not be permitted in less than six weeks. I fear that this regimen is usually not carried out, since in most cases following reduction the player usually recovers promptly and within two weeks his arm feels very good to him. Overoptimism may persuade him to participate, whereupon the dislocation promptly recurs. The patient should be encouraged to exercise within the limits of pain and the restriction of his dressing (Fig. 161). After three weeks of immobilization, rehabilitative measures may be stepped up sharply, particularly active motion against resistance to develop the muscles of the shoulder. Even during the time the arm is suspended in a sling and swathe, active use of the hand and the forearm and tonic contraction of the muscles about the upper arm and shoulder will permit the player to keep his arm in relatively good condition. It is extremely important that the musculature of the shoulder be in good condition before unprotected use of the arm is permitted, since so much of the stability of the shoulder depends upon the strength of the muscles involved.

One need not fear restriction of motion as the result of immobilization of the arm at the side in this age group, although in the elderly this is an ever present danger.

Posterior Dislocation

Posterior dislocation of the shoulder is uncommon as an athletic injury. However, I have seen many late cases and the majority of them were unrecognized primarily. The cause is a direct driving force against the lower end of the humerus with the arm flexed forward. This force transmitted up the arm drives the head out posteriorly. No gross deformity of the shoulder is evident. The patient resists any motion of the shoulder, and upon careful palpation less fullness of the humeral head in front and some increased fullness behind are felt. There is increased prominence of the coracoid. This is readily determined only very early, since within a short time swelling about the shoulder from this extremely disabling injury will screen any visible physical findings. Motion of the shoulder is sharply re-stricted by muscle spasm. X-ray exami-nation is extremely important but diffi-cult to interpret. In the late cases I have seen, x-rays had uniformly been taken but were as uniformly misinterpreted. The pertinent finding in the x-ray, as noted by comparison with the opposite shoulder, is not any actual displacement

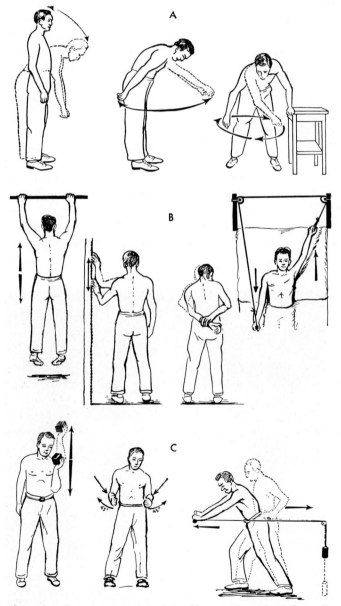

Figure 161. Typical exercises for reconstruction of shoulder muscles. (From Cave, Fractures and Other Injuries. Year Book Publishers.)

of the humeral head backward but an overlapping of the head of the humerus and glenoid (Fig. 162). This overlapping is not possible in a straight anteroposterior view of the normal shoulder, but it is extremely easy to overlook in any case. It indicates that the humeral head is posterior to and slightly medial to its normal position, so that the convexity of the humeral head does not fit against the concavity of the glenoid but appears medial to it (Figs. 162 and 163).

Special x-ray views in posterior dislocation are often necessary. The axillary view (Fig. 163), if possible technically, is especially useful. Other views at various angles can be composed by a roentgenologist and should be useful if uncertainty persists.

TREATMENT. If seen early, reduction of the dislocation is done by traction forward and pressure forward on the humeral head (Fig. 164). The head usually will slip into place with an audible click. If the patient is seen later an anesthetic may be required. If he is seen very late the dislocation may be impossible to reduce nonsurgically. It is frequently accompanied by fracture of the posterior portion of the glenoid, which may include as much as half of the entire glenoid. If this fragment does not replace into good position, surgical resection or internal fixation should be carried out. If the dislocation is seen late and is accompanied by this fracture, it is necessary at open reduction to remove the fragment and to replace by suture the capsule to the remaining rim. If the fragment is large, it should be replaced and supported by a bone graft.

Inferior Dislocation

Inferior dislocation of the shoulder occurs as the arm is forced into straight abduction. As the lateral part of the neck of the humerus impinges against the acromion, the head is forced lat-

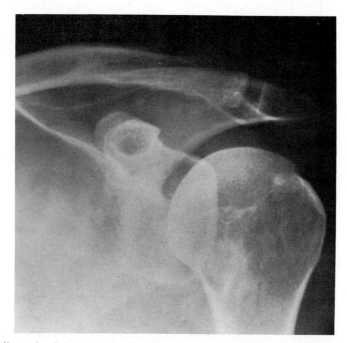

Figure 162. Radiograph of the shoulder showing posterior dislocation. To a casual glance no lesion is apparent. Careful inspection will reveal the head of the humerus medial to the glenoid convexity.

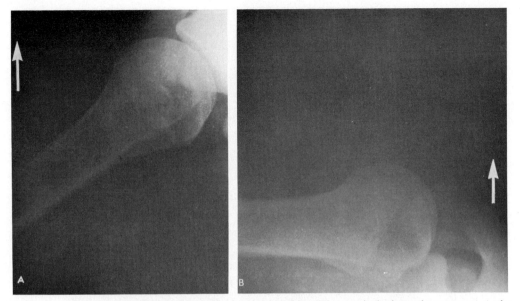

Figure 163. Recurrent posterior dislocation of the shoulder. The vertical views demonstrate *A*, the position with the head in the glenoid; *B*, with it dislocated posteriorly. Arrow indicates posterior direction.

erally against the inferior portion of the capsule and the capsular ligaments (Fig. 149). As the ligaments rupture or tear away from the lower glenoid margin, the humeral head displaces laterally and slips downward over the inferior lip of the glenoid. As the arm is lowered to the side, the head slides anteriorly and the dislocation becomes a subcoracoid dislocation (Figs. 149, *D,* and 153). The significance of this series of events is that the dislocation may be particularly resistant to any type of manipulative reduction other than straight traction. Indeed, many of the cases which reduce readily by straight traction in the long axis of the body may well be those in which the head has come out almost directly inferiorly. At the time of the examination it may be impossible to determine whether or not the head has come primarily forward or has gone directly inferiorly. Careful x-ray study should be made to determine the exact position of the head and whether there has been bony damage.

If the straight abduction force continues and the arm is forced over the head toward the midline of the body, a much more serious injury occurs. The humeral head is literally stripped of its attachments so that the capsule and rotator cuff have completely lost their integrity. In this instance the head locks in a position under the glenoid with the shaft of the humerus pointing directly upward, so that the arm is held high over the head (*luxatio erecta*) (Fig. 165). This does not often occur as the result of an athletic injury. It is an extremely major injury. It is likely to be accompanied by nerve damage and will probably demand surgical intervention even if primary reduction can be obtained. In such an instance, repair of the rotator cuff may be indicated. This may well have been the injury to which I referred on page 213 of this chapter. In such a case there will be so much damage to the whole mechanism that the humeral head actually hangs out of the glenoid. At the time of the reduction of luxatio erecta, extreme care should be taken to avoid forceful manipulation,

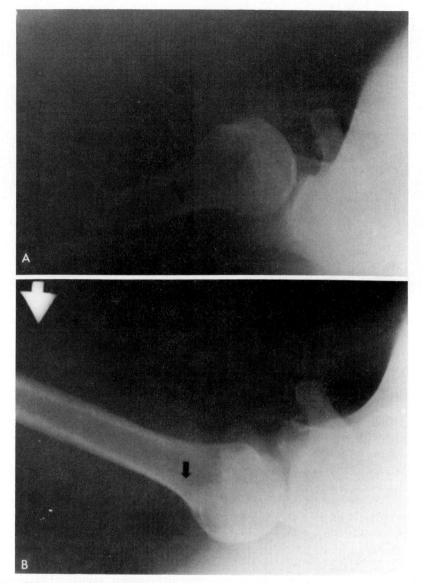

Figure 164. This 22 year old college athlete injured his shoulder at age 16 playing football and has had constant trouble with the right shoulder since. He soon was able to slip it in and out of the socket. *A,* Shows normal relationship of the glenoid on forward pressure. *B,* Shows it displaced out of the glenoid posteriorly on backward pressure. This was treated by posterior reconstruction. At two years postoperative he still feels some instability of the shoulder but it doesn't bother him.

since it may well add to the damage to the muscles, blood vessels and nerves. Under no circumstances should forcible reduction be attempted without anesthesia and under no circumstances should any force be used in repositioning the arm with the patient anesthetized.

Recurrent Dislocation

By far the most common recurrent dislocation of the shoulder is anterior dislocation. This occurs basically in two categories: first, a recurrent dislocation as the result of repeated episodes of

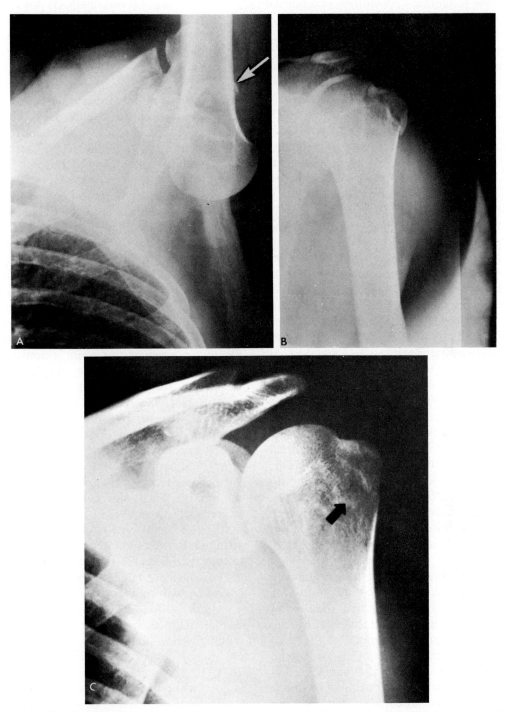

Figure 165. *A,* Case of luxatio erecta. Arrow indicates avulsed tuberosity indicating the severe disruption of the rotator cuff. It is extremely unusual to get an x-ray in this position, since ordinarily the arm drops back to the side and the dislocation becomes subcoracoid. *B,* Following open reduction, internal fixation of the rotator cuff which was found to be completely avulsed off the humerus. *C,* One year later, excellent function. (Courtesy, Dr. Sam Moore.)

acute traumatic dislocations in a normal shoulder, and second, a recurrent dislocation as the result of congenital deviations about the glenohumeral joint. It is of some importance to distinguish between these two conditions, since the latter condition is likely to be bilateral and will demand surgical correction. If the deformity is severe enough, athletic competition should be interdicted until satisfactory stability has been obtained.

The first variety, namely, that occurring because of repeated trauma, is usually the result of an acute injury untreated or inadequately treated at the time of the first dislocation. There seems to be little difference in the recurrence of dislocation whether or not immobilization has been respected. Because of extremely high (75 to 80 per cent) recurrence, perhaps the acute dislocation should be treated surgically. The capsule fails to heal or heals too long and the next dislocation tears it a little bit more. With each successive dislocation less force will be required for the dislocation and it reduces more easily. Finally the condition develops where the shoulder dislocates by simple abduction–external rotation without actual trauma. This type of case is readily amenable to surgical treatment. In some instances it may be improved by a long period of immobilization, provided there have not been too many episodes of displacement. If, for example, it is the third episode and the shoulder has previously been inadequately immobilized, one might be justified in putting the arm at rest at the side for eight weeks, hoping that union and shortening of the ligament will occur. If this fails and if the recurrent episodes of subluxation or dislocation interfere with necessary activity, operative reconstruction of the shoulder can be carried out very successfully. I have operated upon many dislocations in this category and have rarely seen recurrence in an athlete.

There are various methods for reconstruction of the recurrent anterior dislocation of the shoulder. Many of these methods seem to be entirely successful. My own preference is for a modification of the Putti-Platt procedure including meticulous repair of whatever lesion is found in the shoulder joint. The essence of this method is to reinforce the anterior capsule by the very massive subscapularis tendon. I think this will be entirely adequate in most cases; however, since exposure is quite good at this point, the detached labrum should be trimmed away leaving no cartilaginous bodies. If the capsule and periosteum are stripped off the anterior margin of the glenoid, they should be replaced and fastened through drill holes to the glenoid rim. If there is a large Bankhart type of pouch, this should be eliminated by plication of the capsule. My reason for recommending this more extensive procedure is that many recurrent dislocations in the shoulder of the athlete are, in fact, dislocations of a normal shoulder. Hence, if a normal shoulder succumbs to dislocation under the forces applied to it by the athlete, my aim would be to make the shoulder even stronger, anteriorly, than it was prior to the injury. This may entail 10 to 15 degrees of restriction of external rotation, but I have not found this any obstruction to the function of the shoulder, except, perhaps, for the baseball pitcher. Personally, I have not had this problem even with pitchers.

In the second category, that of congenital malformations of the shoulder, reconstruction may be necessary and may be wholly successful (Figs. 166 and 167). In these cases dislocations may occur without any serious trauma. Study of the opposite shoulder should always be made.

Recurrent *posterior* dislocation of the shoulder is not frequently encountered, since the primary condition itself

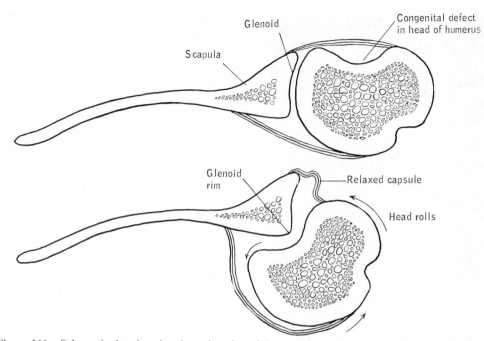

Figure 166. Schematic drawing showing relaxation of the capsule as the glenoid rim drops into the congenital notch in the humeral head. This relaxation permits the head to slip out of the glenohumeral joint. (H. Osmond Clark, Journal of Bone & Joint Surgery, Vol. 30-B.)

is infrequent. I have personally seen more unreduced than recurrent posterior dislocations. One of the latter was in a swimmer who had the feeling his arm would subluxate at a certain point of his back stroke to the extent that it interfered markedly in the success of his swimming. Examination in these cases usually will not elicit pain and it is infrequently possible to demonstrate the subluxation clinically. One may depend almost entirely on the story of the patient that he has the feeling that the shoulder slips out posteriorly. Note carefully the position of the arm at which the head tends to slip. Often the history of falling on the outstretched arm or falling on the elbow with the arm forward will be a guide. In the case of the aforementioned swimmer the arm was repaired posteriorly. A defect in the posterior capsule was found and we were able to plicate it with good support. He went on to be a champion Olympic swimmer with complete recov-

ery from his instability. A procedure similar to the Putti-Platt in front may be carried out using the infra spinatus muscle-tendon to prevent posterior displacement of the head.

Recent studies have indicated more and more that there is a very great tendency for acute subcoracoid dislocation of the shoulder to recur. Some series put it as high as 85 per cent. According to these series, it has not really made much difference just what the primary treatment was. Whereas in my discussion above I blamed inadequate primary care for recurrent dislocation, many of these studies seem to indicate that it does not really make that much difference. Our experience has shown us in other situations that when ligaments are torn, acute surgical repair is the best way to obtain normal function. Combining discouraging high percentages of recurrences after primary dislocations with the demonstrated fact that torn ligaments heal best by putting their liga-

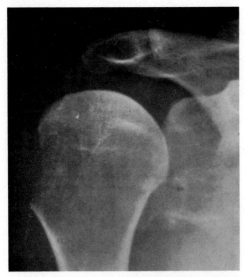

Figure 167. X-ray showing congenital defect in the humeral head. As the flat portion of the head is opposed to the glenoid, the diameter of the head is markedly shortened and the capsule relaxed, predisposing to dislocation.

ment ends together, the question immediately arises, Why not do a primary surgical repair on an acute dislocation? I do not know of any of my colleagues who subscribe to this method or who really have even tried it; but we have gradually evolved into knowing that ankle dislocations need to have ligament repairs, acromioclavicular dislocations do better with ligament repairs, certainly sternoclavicular dislocations do better with ligament repairs, so I think there might be a valid case made for recommending early operation with a reconstructive type repair in the acute case in order to avoid two long periods of morbidity—the first one at the acute injury, then the intervening morbidity when it keeps slipping out of place, and finally the morbidity involved in the reconstruction. My prediction would be that in the relatively near future this procedure may become an accepted policy. Certainly it is not accepted at the present time, and I repeat I know of

no one who actually recommends this, including myself.

FRACTURE

Fractures about the upper end of the humerus are not common in athletes, and those that do occur are often the result of a dislocation of the shoulder, a frequent injury in this age group.

Avulsion Fracture

This uncommon type of fracture in athletes occurs about the glenohumeral area as a result of the traction of a tendon or ligament on a bony process, as in dislocation of the shoulder, which accounts for the majority of cases. The most frequent of the avulsion fractures involves the greater tuberosity.

Avulsion of the Greater Tuberosity. In anterior dislocation of the shoulder, as the arm rotates up and out and the humeral head slips forward, the extremely strong pull of the muscles of the rotator cuff may fix the tuberosity in situ. This results in separation of the tuberosity from the shaft. This may occur as an avulsion of the rotator cuff, an avulsion of a thin shell of bone, or an avulsion of the entire tuberosity (Fig. 168). The symptoms will be those of a severe injury to the shoulder. The dislocation may or may not have been spontaneously reduced, but the player will usually relate that his shoulder has slipped out of the joint. It may have been reduced by a spectator or fellow player, or possibly the player's own motion will have reduced it spontaneously.

If the shoulder is dislocated, great care should be taken in the x-ray interpretation of the film made before and after reduction to rule out such a fracture. If spontaneous reduction has occurred, careful palpation will reveal tenderness over the greater tuberosity. There will be pain on an attempt to actively abduct or to externally rotate the arm. Given these findings, careful x-ray study should be made with the head in various positions of rotation, since in some positions the fracture may seem to be reduced and in others it may appear to be displaced. The fracture in the tuberosity may be visualized well in some cases and poorly in others (Figs. 169 and 170).

TREATMENT. If the fracture is an incomplete one and if the tuberosity remains in place in all positions of the humeral head, treatment may be nonsurgical. Simple immobilization of the arm in a sling will usually suffice. If this does not serve to relieve the pain, the addition of a swathe around the chest may do it. There is no need for a plaster spica in the ordinary case. If there is persistent displacement in any position of the humeral head, surgical intervention is desirable. While healing in malposition may be acceptable in older people with sedentary habits, deformity of the head is not well tolerated by a person who has to use the arm in violent exercise, such as throwing or swinging a tennis racket or many of the other things required of the athlete. The tuberosity can be readily exposed by a muscle-splitting operation through the upper portion of the anterior third of the deltoid and fixation should be by suture, staple, screw or whatever method seems best. If the entire tuberosity is detached,

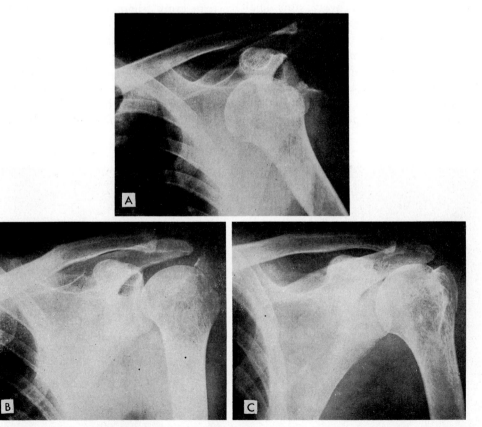

Figure 168. Residual displacement of tuberosity fragment. *A*, Original dislocation. *B*, Following reduction by simple traction. *C*, Following cuff repair and reattachment of the tuberosity fragment. Result was excellent. (From McLaughlin, Trauma, p. 252.)

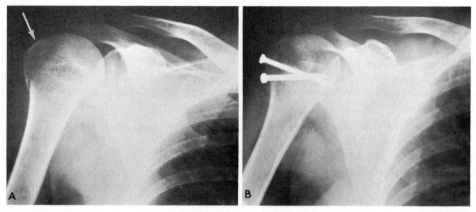

Figure 169. *A*, Radiograph showing avulsion of the greater tuberosity of the humerus. It does not reveal the displacement well, but careful study will indicate that the top of the fragment is well above the rim of the head, whereas in the reduction film it is replaced below the margin of the head. *B*, Postreduction film.

it should be replaced and held by internal fixation (Fig. 169, *B*). If a shell of bone has been torn away, this shell should be surgically excised and the tendon repaired to the avulsed bed. If extremely secure internal fixation of the fragment is not obtainable, removal of the fragment is advisable.

Following repair, rehabilitation will depend somewhat upon the security of the fixation. If fixation is very secure, either by a screw or a staple through a firm bony fragment or by adequate suture of the tendon through drill holes, motion can be started just as soon as the operative reaction subsides, provided it does not include active abduction of the arm. If the arm is abducted against gravity, the humeral head is forced against the glenoid and the rotator cuff takes up

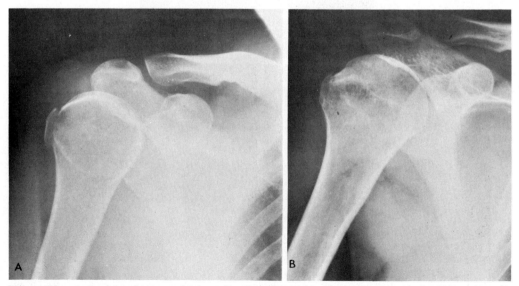

Figure 170. *A*, Avulsion fracture of tuberosity, the tuberosity remaining near its situs and not elevated. *B*, Nonsurgical treatment permitted solid union.

its function of suspending the head to prevent the slipping downward due to the leverage of the deltoid. This puts unusual stress on the tuberosity and must not be permitted. Pendulum movements against gravity, however, are acceptable on the first day (Fig. 161). Such active abduction-contraction with the arm at the side does not have the leverage disadvantage of abduction against gravity. It may be permitted up to 45 degrees and should not be against resistance until union is progressing well.

Avulsion of the Lesser Tuberosity. The subscapularis muscle, which is attached to the lesser tuberosity, is a very massive muscle and is a strong adductor and internal rotator of the arm. Violent external rotation and abduction of the arm against the resistance of the subscapularis may cause rupture of the subscapularis tendon or avulsion of the tuberosity. The history will usually be of violent and rapid external rotation of the arm, as in attempting to tackle a player as he is going by (Fig. 171). The symptoms will be identical to those of sprain of the subscapularis tendon, with tenderness at the lesser tuberosity. There is pain on active internal rotation and on passive external rotation and/or abduction of the arm. Diagnosis of avulsion fracture must be made by x-ray. Here again one should try to determine whether the avulsion is complete or incomplete. It is necessary to take pictures in various positions of the arm and at various angles of the tube in order to demonstrate that the tuberosity is indeed firmly fixed in all positions. If it is separated, it will be pulled medially toward the coracoid. This is most readily demonstrated by x-ray with the arm abducted. The tunnel view along the bicipital groove may be quite enlightening. Figure 171*B* illustrates the end result of unrecognized or incomplete avulsion of the lesser tuberosity.

TREATMENT. Definitive treatment of this avulsion fracture is necessary in the young athlete. If separation of the fragment in any position of the humeral head can be demonstrated, surgical repair should be carried out. The same principles of fixation are used as noted above (greater tuberosity). If the fragment is large, it may be secured by metallic fixation. If it is small, it should be removed and the tendon repaired to the bone. The latter procedure is probably the method of choice since it expedites the recovery. The approach is made by using the first stage of the Putti-Platt or Magnuson shoulder reconstruction. This approach is along the deltopectoral groove. The anterior one-third of deltoid attachment is reflected from the clavicle, after which the injured area is readily available. Following repair the arm should be immobilized at the side in a sling with a swathe around the chest. The duration of immobilization will depend upon the degree of fixation obtained. Four weeks should be the minimum and throughout this period active rehabilitation of the arm may be carried out short of abduction or external rotation.

Fracture by Direct Violence

In the young athlete the humeral head, which is strong and resilient at this age, is not frequently broken by direct trauma. If fracture does occur, it is a stellate fracture usually without displacement and hence very difficult to recognize. In fact, it may be recognized only by repeat films after two weeks, which show absorption around the fissures. The history is of a direct blow, as in a fall on the shoulder or by a blunt object directly against the humeral head. The cartilage of the humeral head is somewhat less resilient than the other joints, but there is no doubt that a direct blow to the head may cause chondral fracture with either fissuring of the carti-

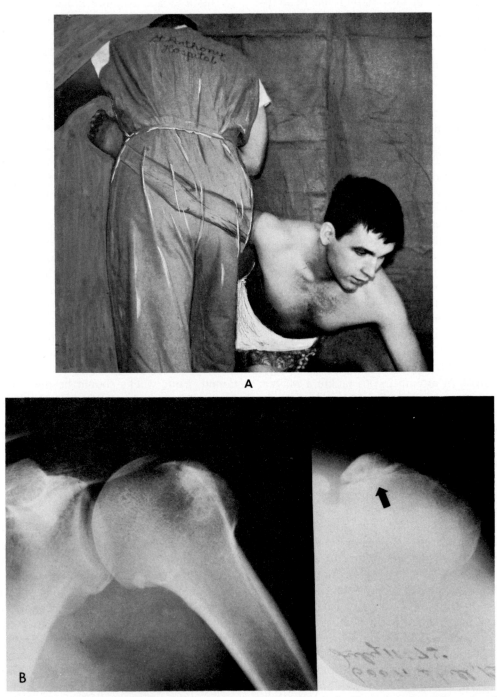

Figure 171. *A,* Typical position causing avulsion of the subscapularis. The arm is forcefully externally rotated but not widely abducted. *B,* This patient injured his arm several years ago and received no treatment. He is now asymptomatic except for slight restriction of external rotation. *Left,* external rotation view shows a large lesser tuberosity. This is much more specific in the tunnel view, *right.* Note the tremendous overgrowth of the lesser tuberosity with nonunion of the fracture. (For technique of tunnel view, see Fig. 141.)

lage or the actual dislodging of the fragments of cartilage. Fracture of the subchondral bone may lead to later chondromalacia of the bone or osteochondritis dissecans. None of these injuries is particularly disabling when it involves the head of the humerus. This is not a weight-bearing joint and there is a relatively small proportion of the head in contact with the glenoid at any one time. A little irregularity is well tolerated. By the time the fracture is recognized, the necessity for any immobilization will probably be past, since the only immobilization indicated would be to suspend the arm in a sling and encourage motion within the limits of pain. In certain cases the humeral head may be pushed in much as one collapses one side of a ping-pong ball and probably by the same cause, that is, direct trauma over a relatively localized area. This may be caused by driving the ball of the humerus against the posterior lip of the glenoid or conceivably against the acromion.

This condition will have the same symptoms as contusion of the shoulder but they are more severe. Pain is out of proportion to that of ordinary contusion of the deltoid. Careful x-ray study with the head rotated in various positions will reveal the defect (Fig. 172). A posterior defect in such a position that the posterior edge of the glenoid may drop into it as the arm is abducted and externally rotated will predispose toward dislocation in identically the same manner as a congenital defect does.

TREATMENT. We have in at least one instance been able to reduce this deformity by drilling through the humeral head from the opposite side and actually pushing the cartilage upward by gently passing a punch through a drill hole made at the opposite side of the head. The defect was then packed with cancellous bone (Fig. 172). If the defect does not appear to be too severe, expec-tant treatment may be carried out, and if subluxation occurs, anterior plication may be done as in the repair of recurrent dislocation of the shoulder.

Fracture by Indirect Violence

This type of fracture is not common as a result of athletic endeavor, but occasionally fractures through the surgical neck of the humerus will occur instead of a dislocation of the shoulder. In the adolescent this fracture may be through the proximal epiphysis (Fig. 173). In such a case the history of a violent injury followed by severe pain, localized swelling and tenderness together with resistance to any motion of the glenohumeral joint will suggest this serious injury. If the fracture is complete, x-ray will definitely confirm the diagnosis and appropriate measures can be carried out for treatment (Fig. 174). It should be borne in mind that if the injury involves epiphyses, it is advisable to get as good reduction as may be obtained by atraumatic manipulation. If atraumatic closed manipulation is unsatisfactory, open surgery should be carried out.

The chief diagnostic problem will arise with the incomplete fracture in which the displacement is slight. Here again x-ray will be confirmatory and treatment should be of the nonmeddlesome variety. It will be adequate to apply a sling with the arm to the side and to permit pendulant and pain-free movement from the beginning or at least as soon as the immediate reaction has subsided. Many weeks and months of rehabilitation may be spared if motion is initiated early in these shoulder injuries.

Fracture of the Glenoid

Avulsion Fracture. Avulsion fracture of the lip of the glenoid may occur in combination with a complete or an incomplete dislocation of the shoulder ei-

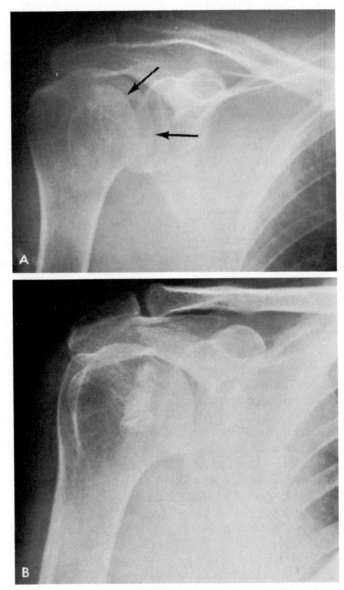

Figure 172. *A,* X-ray of the humeral head following "contusion." Careful study will reveal two lines of periphery of the head, indicating a large segment of it has been displaced (arrows). *B,* The displacement reduced and bone-bank bone packed into the defect. This is done by drilling a hole through the opposite side of the head. The fragment was driven back in position by an impactor.

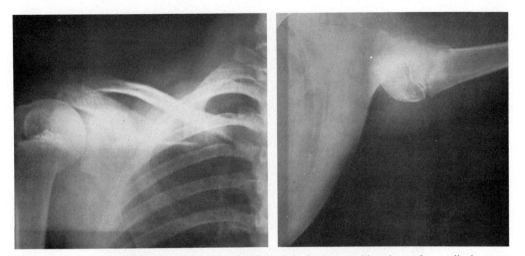

Figure 173. Fracture adjacent to proximal epiphysis of the humerus with only moderate displacement. Treatment by simple sling and swathe fixation.

ther anteriorly, posteriorly or inferiorly. In these instances the rim of the glenoid is avulsed by the capsular attachment rather than broken off by the humeral head, since the humeral head is round

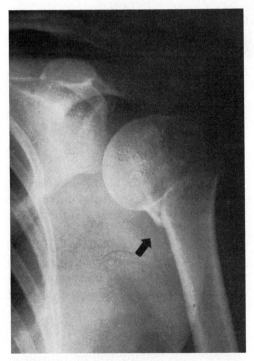

Figure 174. Fracture of the surgical neck of the humerus without displacement (arrow). Treated by sling without the necessity for cast.

and traverses the same arch as the glenoid. As the head slides over the glenoid rim, the capsule becomes very taut and may break off a fragment of bone rather than separate the capsule. Thus, the anterior dislocation will pull off the antero-inferior margin (Fig. 175), the posterior dislocation, the posterior margin (Fig. 176), and the straight inferior dislocation (luxatio erecta), the inferior margin of the glenoid. The clinical pathologic change is not so much fracture of the glenoid as a capsular tear. In most instances nonsurgical treatment will suffice and either bony or firm fibrous union will result. It is unusual for a single injury to cause enough relaxation of the ligament or capsule to cause recurrent dislocation, but repeated injuries may well do so, each one requiring less trauma than the one before. If so, appropriate measures for the recurrent dislocation are in order. A reconstruction operation may be the answer if athletics are to be continued.

In the spontaneously reduced dislocation in which at the time of the examination the shoulder is in normal position, these glenoid marginal fractures will give good insight into the degree of trauma. What may appear to be a simple

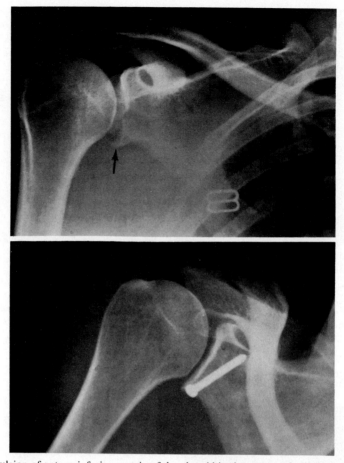

Figure 175. Avulsion of antero-inferior margin of the glenoid in the course of a dislocation of the shoulder which was spontaneously reduced. Since the fragment was large it was treated by open reduction and internal fixation.

sprain or contusion may be revealed as a spontaneously reduced dislocation with attendant damage to the capsule.

Another type of avulsion fracture about the glenoid that is peculiar to athletes is avulsion of a piece of bone by the triceps attachment along the inferior rim of the glenoid. Symptomatically there is pain on active stretching of the triceps muscle, and palpable tenderness along the inferior rim of the glenoid will usually be present. The fragment is difficult to visualize in the x-ray and may appear more as an area of calcification than as an avulsed fragment, particularly if the injury is recurrent in type

(Fig. 177). Ordinarily, firm fibrous union will bind the fragment of the glenoid and there will be no residual symptoms. In the occasional case there will be pain on forcible use of the triceps. This is particularly likely in one who has to throw hard or use the arm in violent overhand motion as in tennis. In this case removal of the fragment of bone and re-suture of the tendon to the bed will result in relief of symptoms.

Following the acute injury a period of rest with local heat followed by active physical therapy will be of help in rehabilitation. It must be remembered that too early resumption of the violent

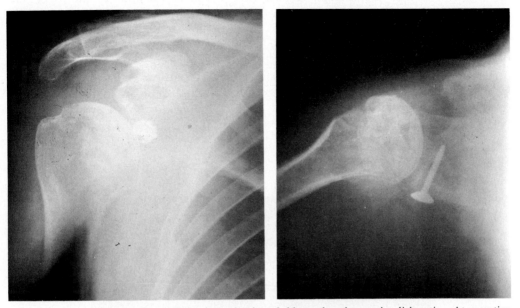

Figure 176.   Postoperative picture following reduction of old unreduced posterior dislocation. At operation the posterior margin of the glenoid was found to be displaced posteriorly.

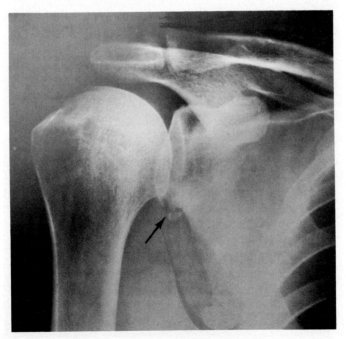

Figure 177.   Fragmentation and calcification of the inferior lip of the glenoid following injury. This may have been from incomplete dislocation or from pull of the triceps tendon.

activity that caused the original lesion will cause prompt recurrence. This accounts for the extremely poor results from treating shoulder lesions of this type in a baseball pitcher. Any change in his throwing habits will usually result in loss of effectiveness and he soon resumes the same type of strain that hurt him in the first place.

Chronic irritation of the triceps attachment in this area may cause a deposition of calcium, which may be quite diffuse. It may be impossible in a chronic case to distinguish between the primary avulsion of a portion of the glenoid and deposits of calcium within the tendon of the triceps (Fig. 178). Since the treatment is identical, namely,

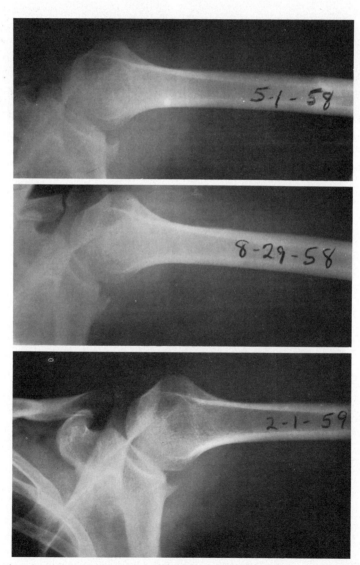

Figure 178. Series showing progress of calcification in the vicinity of the lower lip of the glenoid. This may well have been a partial avulsion of the triceps tendon with calcification and the resultant hematoma. (Rex Diveley, M.D., Baseball Shoulder, J.A.M.A., Nov. 21, 1959.)

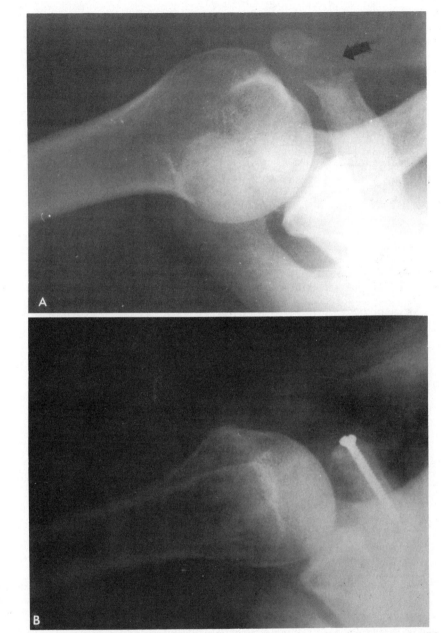

Figure 179.   Professional football quarterback whose left arm was struck while coming forcibly forward as he was tackling an interceptor. Severe pain and loss of function in the shoulder. Unable to throw. *A*, X-ray reveals an avulsion of the tip of the coracoid with some separation of the fragments. At surgery the tendons involved were found to be the coracobrachialis, the biceps, and a small portion of the pectoralis minor. *B*, The coracoid fragment was replaced and held with a screw. He had a good and uneventful recovery and was back playing the same season.

SHOULDER SERIES

Subluxations — Dislocations

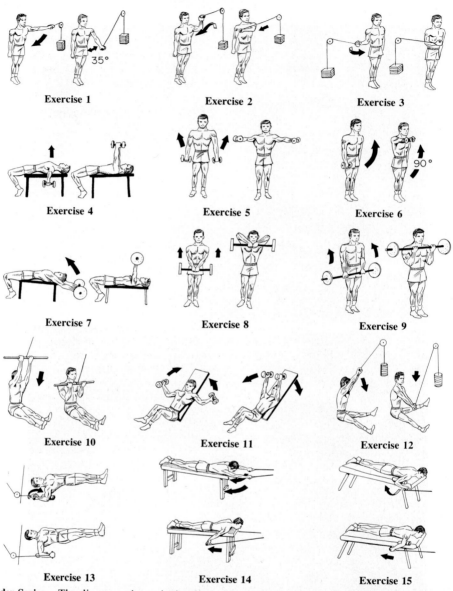

Exercise 1 Exercise 2 Exercise 3

Exercise 4 Exercise 5 Exercise 6

Exercise 7 Exercise 8 Exercise 9

Exercise 10 Exercise 11 Exercise 12

Exercise 13 Exercise 14 Exercise 15

Shoulder Series. The diagrams above depict the series of exercises utilized by West Point cadets following shoulder subluxation, dislocation or surgery. This exercise program is modified as demanded by range of motion of the injured shoulder, and is instituted when range of motion in external rotation and abduction is about 75 per cent of normal.

It should be specifically noted that this is a total upper body reconditioning program with all major muscle groups being challenged. A low weight, low repetition work-out is begun, and the cadet is progressed on individual events as tolerated. Some exercises, particularly 3, 7 and 13, will be very difficult for some subluxators or dislocators if they have not had surgery.

It is felt that by employing the above program, re-injury of the involved shoulder or new injury to an adjacent part has been minimized. The above program will take at least 40 minutes even if done by the most aggressive athlete. The cadet is returned to full unrestricted activity when upper body performance is approximately symmetrical.

The exercises contained in the diagrams of the West Point shoulder reconditioning program represent the evolution of rehabilitation spanning many years and many individuals. The West Point Orthopaedic Service, Physical Therapy Department and Office of Physical Education have all contributed to the program now in use.

242

physical therapy leading up to final surgical excision if it fails, the exact diagnosis probably is not too important.

Fracture by Direct Blow. The same force applied to the lateral side of the shoulder which may break the humeral head may also fracture the glenoid. This is a stellate fracture and in the athlete is usually without displacement. Gross displacement of the glenoid requires violent trauma. No treatment is necessary other than protection of the arm during the acute period by the application of a sling. The glenoid will tolerate a great degree of deformity with deep fissures in its surface without material interference with the function of the shoulder, since weight bearing is not involved.

A fracture of the glenoid may be caused by falling on the flexed elbow. In this case the humeral head may be driven forward or backward in such a way as to knock off a large portion of the anterior or posterior portion of the glenoid. In either case, if there is gross displacement of the anterior lip of more than 1 centimeter, the best treatment will be surgical replacement of the fragment (Fig. 175). If the posterior one-third of the glenoid is broken off, posterior subluxation or recurrent dislocation is likely to occur (Fig. 176). This deformity of the glenoid is easily corrected in a fresh fracture but is extremely difficult to correct following recurrent posterior dislocation. In the athlete such a fracture should be treated surgically using a posterior approach similar to that employed in recurrent posterior dislocation of the shoulder. When the rim of the glenoid is readily visualized extracapsularly, internal fixation may be utilized to restore the buttress. Similarly, in rupture of an anterior fragment that consists of as much as one-fourth of the glenoid, surgical repair should be carried out early.

Stellate fractures that simply enlarge the glenoid or increase its concavity will usually cause no disability.

Avulsion of the Coracoid Process

An injury that occasionally occurs in the shoulder is an avulsion of a portion of the coracoid process by the conjoined tendon of the biceps and coracobrachialis and to a lesser extent the pectoralis minor. As with any avulsion of a tendon, it is more favorable for repair than rupture of the tendon or rupture of the muscle-tendon junction. The proper procedure in avulsion of the coracoid is to expose the coracoid process and, if the fragment is intact and long enough to accept the screw firmly, to replace the process and hold it with a screw. If the fragment is too small, the tendon can be sutured through drill holes to the coracoid, although this is not quite as favorable a type of fixation. The coracoid can be readily exposed by the lower end of the incision used for reconstruction of the shoulder. It is not necessary as a rule to remove any of the deltoid from the clavicle. It can be retracted, exposing the area adequately. One may expect complete recovery following this type of injury and successful fixation (Fig. 179).

REHABILITATION

Rehabilitation is of extreme importance in any condition involving the upper extremity, perhaps more important than in any other area of the body. The reader is urged to carefully study the section on rehabilitation in Chapter 22. West Point Military Academy has an unusually fine program of rehabilitation as exemplified by the exercise diagrams shown on page 242 which the staff use and hand out to injured cadets. They have kindly consented to their inclusion in this book.

CHAPTER 8

INJURIES OF THE UPPER ARM

This chapter will deal with the area between the shoulder and elbow joints and will not include discussion of either joint. *Anatomically* the arm consists of a single long bone relatively circular in cross section which is completely surrounded by muscles along which various vessels and nerves traverse from the shoulder to the lower arm. Injuries to this area are those peculiar to this anatomical type and are similar to those of the thigh.

CONTUSION

There is little subcutaneous bone in the upper arm, since in all locations the skin is separated from the bone by an intervening layer or layers of muscle. This single exception is at the distal attachment of the deltoid to the lateral humerus. *Contusion of the skin,* therefore, is likely to be relatively benign and asymptomatic and to require little treatment. The structures lying between the skin and the bone, however, are quite subject to injury by contusion.

Contusion of Muscle

A direct blow over the biceps muscle in the front of the arm may well

result in a contusion and hematoma of this muscle. However, this injury is neither frequent nor often disabling because of the thick muscle pad and the relatively smooth bone. Similarly, a direct blow over the triceps at the back of the arm may result in a painful, tender muscle but is not apt to present major complications.

In the presence of a contusion of the muscle, whatever its location, our first consideration is to rule out complications such as hemorrhage, nerve damage and fracture of the underlying bone. If there is any suspicion of fracture an x-ray should be made. Careful examination of the muscle and tests of its function will usually reveal whether or not there has been a major rupture of the muscle fibers.

In the absence of any major complication, *treatment* will vary depending upon the symptoms. If there is painful dysfunction I recommend the early application of a cold pack. The arm should be wrapped snugly with sheet wadding, followed by an elastic bandage extending from the fingers to the axilla. Over this is applied the ice packs, which are held on by a second elastic bandage so that the ice pack can be changed at regular intervals without disturbing the pressure on the arm from the underlying elastic bandage. This way it is not necessary to stop the cold treatment by changing the dressing as the ice packs warm up. More pressure should be applied in the vicinity of the contused area. The arm is then placed in a sling to put the involved muscle at rest. If the symptoms persist after 48 hours, the cold pack may be replaced by the application of local heat, using an electric pad, inductive heat or hot packs. Within a few days after the most acute symptoms subside, pain-free activity may be permitted. The whirlpool bath is a useful adjunct at this stage. The patient should be advised to use the arm strictly within the limits of pain. There is no place for massage or passive motion in the early treatment of a muscular contusion. Rehabilitation may progress parallel to the subsidence of symptoms. In this situation, as in so many others in the athlete, too early and too extensive use of the involved muscle will only prolong the disability—a fact that needs repeated emphasis. Should a hematoma develop it is treated by aspiration, local injection and pressure bandage.

Contusion of Tendon and Bones (Blocker's Exostosis)

An injury of unusual significance is a *contusion of the middle third of the arm in the vicinity of, and actually just over, the attachment of the deltoid muscle on the lateral aspect of the humerus.* In this area the bone approximates the skin quite closely, particularly in the sulcus between the anterior distal portion of the deltoid and the belly of the biceps. This coincides with the area most frequently struck by the blocker as he throws his arm up to check the impetus of the charging, opposing player. A direct blow by the hard headgear and, more particularly, repeated blows in this area will result in contusion of the tendon of the deltoid and of the periosteum

of the humerus where the deltoid inserts. Adding to the vulnerability of this particular area is the fact that the anterior edge of the shoulder pad usually extends to about this level, and the edge of the pad itself may well contribute to the damage rather than protect the area. The hemorrhage that occurs ordinarily is not extensive and, indeed, is not enough to be palpable as a hematoma. If this condition is recognized early, it can be treated by adequate protection with a simple fiberboard pad, which prevents recurrence of injury. Suitable measures such as local injection into the bruised area and early cold followed by heat will usually give prompt relief of the early lesion.

If the condition progresses and becomes chronic, a painful *periostitis* and *fibrositis* may develop. This is manifested by extreme tenderness just lateral to the belly of the biceps at the deltoid insertion. Treatment is by protection against further blows and local injection of a long-acting anesthetic and a corticoid preparation. Frequently dramatic improvement will result following such an injection. There is a definite tendency toward recurrence, however, and once this painful condition has developed, the player should be instructed to wear a suitable contact pad. This must be firmly fastened to the arm so that the pad itself does not slip around and cause further irritation.

As a further sequence of this same condition, there is often spur formation along the bone (Fig. 180). This is not a true myositis ossificans but rather an irritative *exostosis* that arises from the bone and has all the characteristics of bone. It is not infiltrated through the muscle as is myositis ossificans. This exostosis extends anterolaterally, usually with a relatively sharp edge. It may become quite disabling owing to the pain of a direct blow. Once it reaches this stage it is not easily pro-

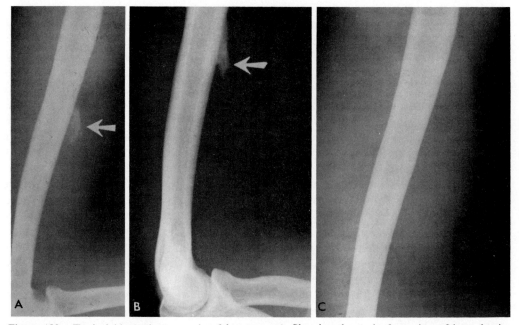

Figure 180. Typical blocker's exostosis of humerus. *A,* Showing the early formation of bone having the appearance of myositis ossificans. Immature nature of the growth is indicated by irregular margins and relatively light deposit. *B,* The mature growth now appears as an exostosis firmly attached to the humerus with mature bone. *C,* Some months after removal. This mass did not recur because it was allowed to mature before it was disturbed surgically.

tected by a pad. The treatment of this condition is surgical excision, but it is extremely important that the growth be entirely mature before its removal is considered. The majority of these cases do not advance to this degree, and if they are asymptomatic no treatment is indicated. The growth actually may appear and regress spontaneously (Fig. 181). If the mass is surgically removed during the formative stage, it will recur. The author recently had a case in which the original lesion seemed quite mature and was surgically removed before examination here. In a very few weeks there was development of a second exostosis above the level of the old lesion (Fig. 182). Although the main mass of bone seemed mature, there was still a portion of it in the formative stage and the surgery simply triggered the formation of another spur. For a more complete discussion of myositis ossificans

and exostosis, see the general discussion in Chapter 4, page 50 and the more specific discussion in Chapter 17, page 506. Whereas in myositis ossificans of the quadriceps active use appears to be the aggravating factor, in the described condition in the arm the exciting factor is repeated contusion. The patient can usually use his arm very well if he avoids a direct blow. The muscles themselves are not primarily involved, since the mass usually lies in the plane between the deltoid and the biceps.

Contusion of the Radial Nerve

As the radial nerve leaves the posterior cord and passes down the arm, it passes in a spiral fashion from superomedial to inferolateral along the muscular spiral groove of the humerus. The nerve here is in closer relationship to

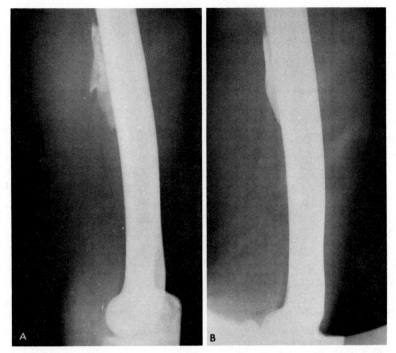

Figure 181. *A,* Exostosis in front of the humerus two months after injury. The patient was advised that the growth was immature and should not be disturbed. *B,* Five months later the mass has regressed, matured and is asymptomatic.

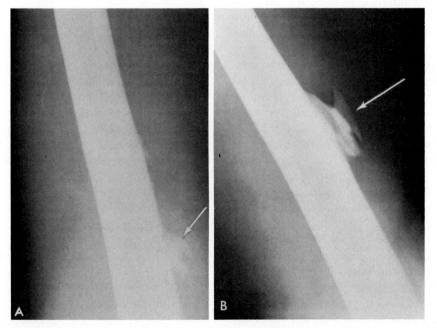

Figure 182. Exostosis in front of humerus. *A,* The original lesion, matured, which was removed with no recurrence locally. *B,* Subsequent recurrence at a higher level without intervening injury.

the bone but is covered by the bellies of the triceps muscle. As it swings laterally just above the lateral epicondylar ridge, it becomes much more subcutaneous and is quite liable to contusion. A direct blow on the posterolateral arm may cause a serious lesion of the nerve. Usually it is accompanied by a shocking, tingling sensation extending to the radial portion of the hand, and the hand is "numbed."

There is no specific early *treatment* for this condition other than that for contusion anywhere, i.e., early cold followed by heat and protection. If there is an actual radial palsy, suitable splinting should be applied to the wrist and hand to overcome the wrist drop and loss of extension of the fingers and thumb. Usually the involvement is not complete. Sensation may be impaired in the radial distribution, but it is almost always present to some extent. Indeed, there may be complete motor loss with complete retention of sensation. Paresthesias are common. In such a case, early surgery is not advisable, but if the condition continues for three or four months without definite signs of improvement in voluntary motion, surgical intervention is indicated.

Usually the condition is one of constriction and edema, rather than actual severance of the fibers, and may be relieved by appropriate neurolysis. At operation the nerve is carefully exposed and traced through the contused area. If it is bound down to the humerus or is caught in scar, it must be freed by meticulous atraumatic dissection. Any constrictions of the sheath are released. If the constriction is not too mature, the sheath may be expanded by injecting saline into it and forcing the column of saline past the constriction. After the nerve is entirely free, an effort should be made to suture the muscle layers so as to place an intervening muscle layer between the nerve and the bone. This con-

dition is not frequent but is extremely distressing when it does occur.

STRAIN

Acute Strain

The muscles of the arm are subject to acute strain in excessive muscular activity. This strain may vary from a mild (first degree) irritation of the tendon or muscle to a complete (third degree) rupture. The tendinous strains will be discussed in conjunction with the adjacent joints. It may be difficult in some instances to distinguish between contusion of the muscle and acute strain or partial rupture. Indeed, frequently, the two may be simultaneous. That is, while the muscle is under a rather severe strain, it may receive a direct blow and the fibers may rupture. Clinically some distinction can be made between acute strain or muscle rupture and contusion, because in strain function of the part is likely to be more painful than palpation, whereas in contusion the reverse is usually true. If a strain is suspected, for example in the biceps, the muscle should be carefully checked throughout its length and the exact area of tenderness to palpation determined. Palpation may also determine whether or not there is a defect in the muscle or some change in its shape. A test of function, particularly against resistance, will usually reveal a localizing point of pain, tenderness or separation.

Proper *treatment* should be instituted according to the findings. In strain it is extremely important that the muscle be protected from overuse or overstretch. It is therefore more vital to protect the arm in a sling or even a splint than it is to treat the condition locally. Optimum treatment is cold pack, later heat, compression and protection by splinting. As the acute symptoms subside, a more definitive diagnosis may be made and subsequent treatment determined. That is, if there appears to be a major defect in the muscle (severe), more extensive treatment will be required than if the strain is mild. If it can be determined that there is an actual rupture of the muscle or musculotendinous junction (severe), surgical repair should definitely be recommended. Since surgical repair is most successful if done early, the importance of an early definitive diagnosis is apparent. The muscle most frequently damaged in the upper arm is the biceps, not only because it is more subject to a direct blow, but also because the blow frequently will occur while the biceps is in strong contraction.

If the rupture is at the musculotendinous junction, the same symptoms may be present as with rupture of the tendon, except that the tenderness will be in the muscle rather than over the tendon. Tests for configuration of the biceps with the muscle in contraction may give a definite lead as to the completeness of the rupture (see Fig. 139, page 203). If this condition is to be treated nonsurgically or if the rupture is not complete, splinting should be continued at least three weeks and should be followed by a sling that will restrict extension at the elbow. The patient should be cautioned not to contract the biceps against resistance. In the vast majority of the cases the rupture will be incomplete. The intact portion of the muscle protects the injured area and holds the torn fibers in relatively good apposition.

Chronic Strain

Chronic strain is much more likely to occur in a tendon and will be considered in our discussion of the adjacent joints. There may be a chronic strain of the musculotendinous junction or in the muscle itself, which is evidenced by pain on overuse — either repetitive overuse or a single massive effort. This will differ from acute strain in that there will be no local signs of hemorrhage, swelling or separation of the muscle or tendon fibers. Instead, there is a feeling of strain on forced activity, followed by stiffness and spasm of the muscle after a period of rest. The patient may go to sleep at night with only moderate soreness and awake in the morning with muscle spasm, stiffness and pain, much more severe than it had been the night before. The situation may develop in the baseball pitcher or the weight lifter or the javelin thrower.

The only real solution to this problem is rest and avoidance of the type of activity that caused the condition in the first place. This is quite disrupting to the young athlete, and he frequently returns to his activity too soon and has prompt recurrence of his trouble. *Treatment,* therefore, should be local injection, local heat, protection against excessive use but not immobilization. Function should be encouraged, but it should remain strictly within the limits of comfort. Since it is not necessary to use the upper extremity for weight bearing, the requisite inactivity can usually be accomplished without special apparatus. A sling may be required to remind the youth that strenuous activity is interdicted. The patient should be given a clear understanding of the rationale of the treatment. If this is comprehended, a high degree of cooperation can be expected. The physician interested in the treatment of athletes should inform himself as to the anatomical characteristics of the muscles involved in the function of the arm and be prepared to guide the patient in the selection of those activities which he may continue and those which he should abandon. This is particularly pertinent as rehabilitation progresses and it becomes necessary to permit greater activity. If the strain is the result of a particular activity, as for example, baseball pitching, it may be found that the patient can tolerate some other field position before he can return to pitching, since a somewhat different muscle activity is demanded of the pitcher than of the infielder, for example. So also, the pole vaulter might be permitted to participate in the hurdles or the high jump much sooner than he could his pole vaulting.

FRACTURE

Fracture of the humerus may occur but is not a common injury in athletic competition. In any injury that seems to be severe, x-ray examination should be made. In the shaft of the humerus the x-ray leaves little doubt as to whether or not there is a fracture. Fracture almost always causes some interference with function. The exception may be the greenstick fracture in the younger individual where the bone may be broken but the fragments are not disrupted. This can also be readily determined by x-ray visualization.

As with any injury in athletes, the goal of *treatment* must be complete recovery. One is, therefore, more justified in adopting definitive treatment than he would be in an older person. If a treatment can be utilized that will permit rehabilitation at a relatively early stage, this of course should be considered. Rehabilitation should be instituted as promptly as possible, but participation in sports must not be allowed until the fracture is entirely healed and the muscles restored to normal size and tone. With an injury to the arm, it is usually entirely feasible to continue conditioning of the rest of the body and, indeed, of many portions of the arm itself during the actual healing period of the injury.

CHAPTER 9

INJURIES OF THE ELBOW

ANATOMICAL CONSIDERATIONS

The elbow is a complicated joint consisting of three different articulations, those between the ulna and humerus, the radius and humerus and the radius and ulna. While functionally it is primarily a hinge joint and so has motion in flexion and extension, it also participates in the rotatory motions of the forearm through the articulations of the radial head with the ulna and with the lower end of the humerus. The olecranon and coronoid processes of the ulna form a deep socket (the olecranon fossa) which encircles the trochlea of the lower end of the humerus and provides a very stable joint. This joint permits only flexion and extension. The ulna does not rotate. On the other hand, the upper end of the radius makes a very unstable connection with the lower end of the humerus, the button-like head of the radius having a shallow depression with the same arc of curvature as the transverse arc of the capitellum of the humerus. On flexion and extension the head of the radius travels from the front to the back of the capitellum by simple gliding action. On rotation of the forearm the button of the radial head rotates through the shallow socket on

the side of the ulna while its proximal end simply turns on the capitellum.

The integrity of the relationship between the head of the radius and the ulna and humerus depends entirely upon ligaments (Fig. 183). The radioulnar articulation is stabilized by the annular (orbicular) ligament, which holds the head and the neck of the radius firmly against the radial fossa of the ulna. The stability of the radius and the lower end of the humerus is largely capsular in character, there being no collateral ligament extending from the outer side of the humerus to the head of the radius. A lateral ligament extends from the lateral epicondyle to a very firm connection with the annular ligament. Thus, the lateral integrity of this joint also depends upon the continuity of the annular ligament of the radius. On the medial side there are very strong ligaments extending from the medial epicondyle down to the medial surface of the coronoid and downward and backward to attach to the whole length of the olecranon from its proximal tip to the base of the coronoid process. The anterior part of this ligament is cordlike, whereas the posterior part is shaped like a fan with the handle attached to the humerus. With the elbow in extension the anterior portion of the ligament becomes very tight while

251

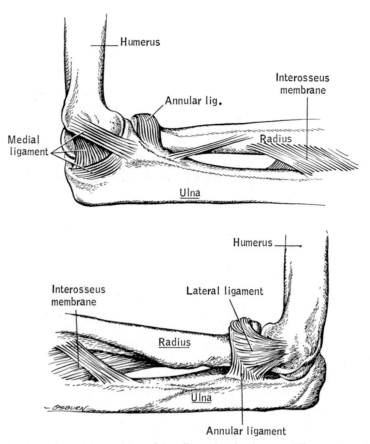

Figure 183. Medial and lateral views of the elbow showing bony and ligamentous structures.

with the elbow in flexion the posterior part of the fan is tight. The capsule of the joint is relatively relaxed. There is no check ligament as such. Extension of the elbow is prevented as the olecranon process impinges against the olecranon fossa of the humerus. Flexion is checked by pressure of the muscles of the forearm and arm or by the coronoid process against the humerus. Rotation of the forearm is entirely dependent upon a smooth radial head with its outer circumference intact.

CONTUSION

There are several areas of subcutaneous bone at the elbow. The entire olecranon is subcutaneous as are the medial and lateral epicondyles and the supracondylar ridges. As might be expected in these circumstances, contusion to the elbow is a common injury. Falling on the flexed elbow crushes the skin against the hard bone of the olecranon and may result in severe contusion and abrasion or even laceration over the point of the elbow. Since this area is relatively insensitive, the injury is not especially painful; indeed, it may be overlooked. The area of the lateral condyle and the radial head, however, is quite sensitive, and a painful bruise here may follow a direct blow to the side of the elbow—the medial side less often because of its protected position. In contusion of any of these areas care should be taken to determine whether there are other lesions. In cases of doubt x-ray examination is indicated.

In the uncomplicated contusion, *treatment* will depend upon the degree of injury. Often none is required. If there is an accompanying hematoma, it should be aspirated and local injection with hyaluronidase may be carried out. The area is then wrapped in sheet wadding with the elbow as near a right angle as is comfortable to the patient. A snug elastic bandage is wrapped over the arm from wrist to axilla. In the early stages cold should be applied by ice pack. After 48 hours heat may be used if symptoms persist. A sling should be worn if an elastic bandage is used, otherwise flexion and extension of the elbow against the tight bandage will simply aggravate the contusion.

Periosteal irritation may develop as a result of a direct blow over the subcutaneous bone. In this instance the bone remains tender and is very sensitive to pressure. This condition responds well to local injection of a long-acting anesthetic and protection by adequate padding. A corticoid may be injected only if the condition is chronic.

Contusion on the back of the arm over the triceps tendon may cause tenosynovitis in the area with resulting pain, particularly on forced passive flexion of the elbow. As a rule this is not severe enough to cause impairment of triceps function. The usual measures prevail. Heat, rest and injection usually give prompt relief.

Contusion of the Ulnar Nerve

Contusion of the ulnar nerve is quite frequent because of its anatomic position at the elbow. As it traverses the inner side of the arm, it passes behind the medial condyle through a tunnel, the floor of which is made up of the ulnar groove of the humerus, the roof being a rather loose fibrous sheath. As the arm flexes and extends, the nerve slides up and down in the ulnar groove. In this region the nerve is subcutaneous and lies directly on the bone. Hence, a direct blow may damage the nerve to a greater or lesser extent, depending upon the strength and direction of the force applied. The so-called "crazy bone" should have been named the "crazy nerve" although certainly the bone does participate in the etiology of the syndrome. A direct blow causes immediate severe pain with a shocking sensation extending down to the ring and little fingers. This paresthesia is usually transient, disappearing after a few minutes or several hours depending upon the severity of the injury.

Under ordinary circumstances no permanent injury results from ulnar nerve contusion, but occasionally there may be late sequelae. If the injury was sufficient to cause bleeding into the nerve, adhesions may form within the nerve trunk itself, resulting in the development of ulnar palsy. The same effect may occur if the irritation is external to the nerve and there is constriction within the groove. In either event the nerve fibers are constricted, lose their elasticity and a progressively increasing ulnar palsy results. The symptoms of delayed palsy consist of gradually increasing numbness along the ulnar distribution of the forearm and hand. This includes the ulnar side of the lower forearm, the little finger, half of the ring finger and the fourth and fifth rays of the hand. The pain is ordinarily much more severe in the hand than at the elbow, although both may be quite painful. As the loss of nerve function continues there will be marked atrophy of the intrinsic muscles of the hand. It should be recalled that a great majority of the intrinsic muscles of the hand are supplied by the ulnar nerve. One of the early symptoms is inability to adduct the little finger so as to place it against the ring finger. The metacarpal shafts will become more prominent because of intrinsic muscle atrophy. Contracture of the fingers will result as the condition progresses and typical deformity occurs.

Definitive *treatment* in the early stages of ulnar palsy will usually prevent permanent disability. The condition is not amenable to local injection and similar measures. If there is a definite palsy and the nerve appears to be constricted, treatment should be surgical. The skin is incised along the course of the nerve, which is then freed from the groove. Neurolysis is carried out to release the sheath, and the nerve is transposed forward to pass in front of the condyle rather than behind it. If this operation has not been delayed too long, very good recovery can be expected.

STRAIN

Muscle-tendon strain about the elbow is quite frequent owing to the extremely forceful action required at the elbow joint in many sports. The powerful triceps muscle attaching to the olecranon is subject to strain anywhere from its attachment on the olecranon to the musculotendinous junction. The symptoms are tenderness over the involved area, pain on forceful extension of the forearm against resistance and pain on complete passive flexion of the elbow. There may well be local heat if the condition is acute enough, although this is not a diagnostic sign. Forceful active extension of the arm as in throwing will aggravate the condition.

Another common area of strain is in the biceps where it attaches below the neck of the radius. The biceps has a firm tendinous attachment to the radius and through the bicipital aponeurosis (lacertus fibrosus) to the fascia of the forearm. Strain may occur anywhere in

this complex and indeed may be severe enough to tear the lacertus or to avulse the biceps from the radius. The signs of tendon rupture may be somewhat obscured, particularly if the radial attachment pulls off and the lacertus remains intact or if the lacertus pulls off and the radial attachment remains intact. Under these circumstances the shortening and bunching of the biceps that is so characteristic may not be present (Fig. 139, page 203). If there is complete rupture of the radial attachment it should be replaced surgically. This is true whether the attachment is torn from the muscle, torn in its substance or pulled off the bone. It is not necessary to repair the lacertus in the case of an independent injury. In fact, the lacertus is very infrequently torn since there is a certain amount of elasticity to its lateral attachment.

There may also be strain about the brachialis near its attachment to the ulna or of the anconeus or indeed of any of the muscles about the elbow. The symptoms will be those of disturbance of function of the particular muscle involved.

Another very frequent area of strain is on the medial or lateral epicondyle of the humerus. Overuse, particularly in throwing, may well cause irritation of the muscle fibers at their attachment with partial rupture of the fibers and hemorrhage. This results in an epicondylitis if not treated promptly. The early symptoms of the condition are tenderness, perhaps local swelling and pain on use of these muscles in forcibly gripping or forcibly pronating or supinating the forearm, as the case may be. Gripping will cause pain whether it be medial or lateral, since in gripping the extensors and flexors both contract. Treatment of the acute injury is by local injection with a long-acting local anesthetic. Particularly important are immobilization and protection from function. Any painful function should be interdicted. If the third degree sprain occurs, there may actually be an avulsion of the muscles on either epicondyle (see Avulsion Fracture, p. 273).

Tennis Elbow

A type of condition about the elbow that is quite common in athletes, particularly in part-time athletes, is the so-called tennis elbow. Tennis elbow is one of those diagnoses similar to shin splints or belly ache. In this instance the name comes from the location. It has no relation to the type of injury. There are at least four distinct, different conditions that present themselves and are commonly called tennis elbow. Physical examination will usually distinguish between them. On the other hand the history is very likely to be the same, that is, some unusual exertion involving a grip of the hand with lateral play of the wrist. The name "tennis elbow" derives from the fact that it frequently happens in someone who plays tennis before becoming well conditioned. There is pain in the lateral side of the elbow, sometimes on the medial side of the elbow, aggravated by gripping and rotating. In the days antedating the vacuum sweeper it was also called "rug beater's elbow." There are various other adjectives to describe the condition in relation to the activities that ordinarily involve lateral movement of the wrist, as in tennis playing, beating a rug or using a hammer; even overuse such as shaking hands at a reception can bring on the symptoms. This will be described in detail under Epicondylitis below.

The various conditions on the lateral side which may be labeled tennis elbow are (1) true epicondylitis of the extensor supinator aponeurotic attachment to the lateral epicondyle; (2) radial ulnar synovitis marked by development of a pannus of synovium between the radius and ulna; (3) strain in the aponeurosis itself often directly over the radial head; and (4) radial humeral bursitis. It can be seen from the close proximity of the epicondyle and of the radial humeral joint and the supinator aponeurosis how they could be confused. Often, indeed, they are caused by the same condition, namely, overuse of the mechanism. On the medial side of the elbow, ulnar neuritis will sometimes be classified as tennis elbow although this also is readily distinguishable from medial epicondylitis. I urge discarding the term tennis elbow in favor of a more definitive diagnosis.

Epicondylitis

A type of involvement that is peculiar to the elbow develops along the medial and lateral epicondyles. The extensor-supinator muscles arise along the lateral epicondyle and the flexor-pronator muscles arise along the medial epicondyle, where they have an aponeurotic attachment. Either by contusion of the area or more commonly by strain, an irritation develops at the attachment of the aponeurosis to the bone that is quite characteristic. There is pain along the epicondyle which is aggravated by gripping. The pain extends down the corresponding group of the muscles, either medially or laterally, sometimes as far as the wrist. In the normal mechanism of clenching the fist, one of the first phases of action is strong contraction of the carpal extensors in order to fix the wrist. If this did not occur the wrist would go into flexion and an ineffective fist result. This is exemplified by the hand in which there is radial paralysis. One is unable to make a fist, not because he cannot flex the fingers but because he cannot stabilize the wrist. So when the hand grasps an object, tension is placed on both the flexors and extensors of the wrist. Hence, gripping will cause pain whether the involvement is medial or lateral. On examination there is tenderness localized to the epicondyle or upward along the supracondylar ridge for a short distance. The tenderness may also extend down over the radial head, but in the true epicondylitis the acute tenderness is directly on the epicondyle.

This condition may be extremely aggravating particularly since it will often be chronic and recurrent and is increased by many activities of the forearm and hand. *Treatment* demands rest, and in the severe case a splint that fixes the wrist in slight dorsiflexion and the elbow at 90 degrees may be needed. Local heat by diathermy, electric pad or whirlpool is useful. Dramatic results are often obtained by local injection, my preference being a long-acting local anesthetic plus a corticoid preparation. The needle should be inserted directly into the area of involvement with multiple puncture points. The anesthetic is injected until the tenderness is entirely relieved, after which the corticoid is injected into the same area. Following such an injection the pain may be much more severe for 12 to 24 hours but then subsides, and the symptoms gradually improve until by the end of a few days they may be entirely gone. Should the symptoms then recur, a second or even a third or fourth injection may be necessary to obtain permanent relief. Throughout this period the patient must avoid the activities that caused the trouble. This frequently poses a problem since the activity that caused the condition may be an integral part of the regimen of this particular patient. Thus a pole vaulter may be unable to grasp his pole, a javelin player may be unable to snap his wrist or the baseball pitcher may have trouble gripping the ball or in sharply extending his elbow to throw. Hand shaking may be the offending activity and the resulting disability has been known to interfere with the activities of public figures. If nonsurgical measures fail, the condition can ordinarily be relieved by detaching the muscles from the epicondyle and smoothing the bone, thus eliminating the irritated area and permitting the muscle to heal.

While epicondylitis may follow a relatively acute strain, it more often results from a chronic degenerative change by attrition of the aponeurotic fibers at the elbow. This occurs in certain types of athletics such as baseball pitching, but it is not common in ordinary athletic pursuits, the acute sprain being the more likely cause. If there is degenerative change, there may be calcification or even spur formation over the epicondyle. The patients present themselves complaining of an aching pain on the outer or inner side of the elbow which is made more severe by active use of the forearm and hand.

This type of epicondylitis may seriously interfere with athletic competition, not so much because of pain at the elbow but because of restriction of use of the hand. The tender point should be protected by a contact pad. The patient should be warned to avoid gripping. Since this is extremely difficult in most sports, it may be necessary to forbid participation for a period of several weeks. Another measure to avoid recurrence of this distressing condition is rehabilitation of the muscles involved. Most of us agree that tennis elbow is a result of overstress from overuse, and it is axiomatic that overuse is very much more likely to occur in the ill-conditioned muscle. Rehabilitative exercises for the wrist and hand (see p. 804) will be extremely productive in preventing recurrence of the condition and increasing endurance of the forearm and hand.

So, the term tennis elbow is not entirely restricted to epicondylitis. Other conditions grouped under this category are radial head capsulitis and radiohumeral bursitis, each of which is discussed in the following sections.

SPRAIN

Since the elbow is a stable joint, ligament injury here is relatively uncommon. It is virtually impossible to sprain the elbow by excess flexion. In excessive extension, on the other hand, as the olecranon impinges against the back of the humerus, the continuing force pulls the coronoid away from the trochlea of the humerus. This results in injury to the anterior portion of the collateral ligaments, particularly on the medial side. This injury may vary from a partial tear of little significance (first degree) to complete rupture (third degree) of the ligaments and capsule. As the force stops short of complete rupture the elbow flexes, the tension is relaxed and there is no feeling of instability at the elbow joint because of its inherent bony stability and because of the fact that it does not require the degree of stability for weight bearing that is necessary at the knee.

The patient with such an injury will present himself with a history of hyperextension of the elbow and severe pain on the medial and sometimes the lateral side of the elbow which is relieved by flexion, so that he ordinarily will have his hand tucked into his shirt or his thumb hooked over his belt to prevent elbow extension. The symptoms at the time of the examination vary directly according to the severity of injury. Pain is not ordinarily a prominent factor. There will be localized tenderness at the site of the tear, either along the ulna on the medial side or along the epicondyle. There may also be pain along the lateral collateral ligaments at the site of the tear. Any attempt to extend the arm causes pain, and motion is stopped short of complete

extension by muscle spasm. I have never seen a case in an athlete in which I could demonstrate excess motion indicating a complete tear without complete dislocation.

The collateral ligaments may also be sprained by lateral motion. Forced abduction of the extended arm will damage the medial ligaments. Forced adduction will damage the lateral. Here again, instability is extremely infrequent, and I find it very difficult to determine whether or not the rupture is complete unless there has been a complete dislocation of the elbow. A "sprain fracture" due to avulsion of the ligament with a fragment of bone may be revealed by x-ray examination. Symptoms in the case of lateral stresses will be localized to the one side with the same findings as those for hyperextension, that is, tenderness along the site of the tear, local swelling and pain on attempt to reproduce the causative force.

Treatment of such a sprain is relatively simple. In the acute stage cold followed by heat and a protective sling will be adequate. Use of the extremity should be restricted for the first few days, but unless the injury is quite symptomatic a splint is not necessary. As the acute symptoms subside, more motion may be permitted but always within the limits of pain for at least four weeks. At this time active, unprotected function should be encouraged.

DISLOCATION

As the hyperextension force at the elbow continues, the olecranon remains fixed in the olecranon fossa, extension of the arm levers the coronoid completely around the trochlea, and the lower end of the humerus slides forward and downward to lodge against the anterior ulnar shaft distal to the coronoid (Fig. 184). At the same time the capi-

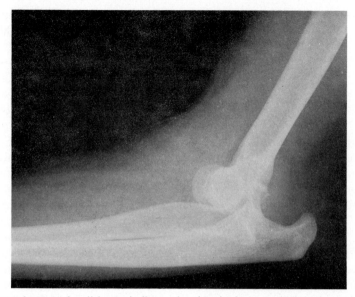

Figure 184. Lateral x-ray of a dislocated elbow, showing the lower end of the humerus resting on the ulna in front of the coronoid. Note fragmentation of the coronoid.

tellum, by virtue of rupture of the lateral collateral or annular ligaments, slides forward and downward so that it rests on the radial neck. There may be a lateral component of this dislocation, so that the coronoid of the ulna may lie behind the capitellum rather than the trochlea (Fig. 185), in which instance the radial head is displaced laterally and does not appose the humerus.

Dislocation of the elbow cannot occur without rupture of the collateral liga-

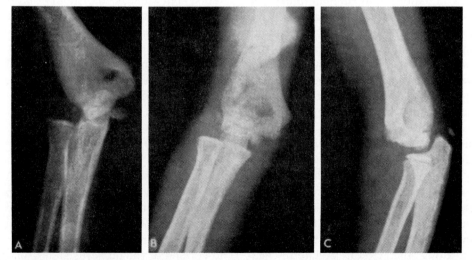

Figure 185. A fracture-dislocation of the elbow in a child. *A*, Anteroposterior view before reduction. Note lateral displacement of the forearm in relation to arm. The medial epicondylar epiphysis is displaced with the ulna. *B*, Anteroposterior view after reduction. Note epicondylar epiphysis caught in joint. Also note the lateral displacement. *C*, Lateral view after reduction. Note epicondyle in joint. This must be surgically removed from the joint and fixed to the medial condyle.

ments. In many instances the force is relieved before this dislocation becomes complete and the elbow components slip back into their normal relationship. This subluxation, or spontaneously reduced dislocation, presumably has occurred whenever complete rupture of both collateral ligaments is diagnosed. The dislocated elbow has a rather typical deformity with the olecranon prominent posteriorly and with the forearm extended beyond a right angle. If the dislocation remains unreduced, immediate, extensive swelling occurs, rapidly obliterating the bony landmarks about the elbow.

The most pressing requirement on examination of such a patient is to determine the circulatory capacity to the hand, since circulatory changes rapidly become irreversible. One should carefully determine the presence or absence of the radial pulse. Careful attention should be given to the capillary circulation of the nail beds. A second requirement is investigation of nerve function. The median is the nerve most likely to be involved as it is caught on the end of the humerus as the bone slides forward. Interference with the nerve supply should be carefully determined. It is extremely important to record any neurological change *before* an attempt at reduction is made or else one may never know whether the nerve damage was immediate and was caused by the dislocation or if it was caused by the trauma of reduction or developed later because of swelling and edema.

TREATMENT. A dislocated elbow is a surgical emergency. The result obtained from treatment of such an injury depends to a great extent upon the length of time the dislocation has been unreduced. If the arm is seen immediately after the injury (for instance on the playing field), one should take the time to investigate the circulation of the hand and to make a rough evaluation of the nerve supply. At this time, while the arm is numb and swelling has not taken place, it may be possible to reduce the deformity at once and without anesthesia. This must be done by the gentlest means, since forceful manipulation not only will increase the muscle spasm and prevent reduction but may also cause severe damage to the nerve or blood supply, which may have been spared at the time of injury. If the forearm is displaced laterally, usually to the radial side, the upper arm should be steadied by the doctor with one hand while with the other he grasps the forearm just below the elbow. By gentle manipulation the lateral deformity is usually easily corrected. Once this is accomplished the right arm of the operator must be shifted to grasp the wrist and steady, even traction applied along the long axis of the forearm as the elbow gradually moves toward extension. If this causes pain and spasm the attempt should be discontinued. If the patient can relax his muscles the elbow may slip easily into position. This may be facilitated by slight hyperextension of the forearm, which permits the coronoid to slide under the trochlea, whereupon the dislocation will be reduced as the forearm is gently flexed. If the emergency reduction is not successful or if the patient is not seen immediately, he should be moved to the nearest place where there are proper facilities for x-ray and anesthesia. X-ray examination before the reduction is highly desirable. This not only will provide some idea as to the exact location of the bones but also will demonstrate any accompanying fractures (see Figs. 185, 188 and 189).

Fractures frequently accompany dislocation of the elbow, the most common being those of the epicondyles, the coronoid and the radial head. The fractures are of either the avulsion or leverage type, and may greatly complicate the treatment of the dislocated elbow. The coronoid may be injured as it passes under the humerus by combination of muscle pull and direct impingement, the significance being that there may be avulsion of the anterior capsular ligaments and also of a portion of the brachialis attachment. Similarly the epicondyle may be avulsed by pull of the flexors or extensors. The medial epicondylar epiphysis is most frequently pulled off, since it is the last epiphysis at the elbow to close. It may well be avulsed and the small button epiphysis be overlooked in its displaced position (Fig. 185). Many of these fractures require open reduction. If for any reason open reduction of the fracture must be delayed beyond an hour, the dislocation should be reduced at once — under anesthesia if necessary. It is extremely important that the dislocation be reduced at the earliest possible moment even if a second anesthetic will be required for later surgical replacement of a fragment. Prompt reduction of the dislocation will prevent excessive swelling in the soft tissues, excessive and long-continued stretching of the nerves or blood vessels and other serious complications. The elbow invariably should be x-rayed following reduction *before application of a splint* (Fig. 185). I wish to emphasize this point, since it is very difficult to visualize by x-ray a small displaced fragment about the elbow through a plaster splint. If there is any doubt at all as to the relationship of the epicondyles or coronoid or radial head, similar x-rays should be made on the normal elbow in a similar position and the two films carefully compared.

Following reduction of the dislocation one should again painstakingly assess the circulation of the hand. If possible the elbow should be splinted at 90 degrees (Fig. 186). The circulation should again be evaluated in this position both before and after the application of the splint. Similarly, a check of nerve function should be carried out, although

this must await recovery from the anesthetic. It should be done at the earliest possible moment, since it is extremely important to know at what stage nerve symptoms develop. The decision as to the method of management of the nerve injury may depend wholly upon this knowledge. If there is sudden complete loss of function of the nerve at the time of the accident early repair is indicated, whereas if the onset is gradual a more conservative attitude should be adopted. If the circulation is not intact with the elbow at 90 degrees, the elbow should be extended to that position at which the circulation is satisfactory.

If there is evidence of arterial spasm with a white hand and absent radial pulse, an emergency situation exists that calls for immediate measures to restore the arterial circulation. A stellate ganglion block should be accomplished. Vasodilator drugs should be given. Cold may be applied to the opposite hand. If such measures do not restore the arterial pulsation, the arm should be opened in the antecubital area and the artery identified and examined. Appropriate measures to restore circulation, such as stripping the artery if it is in spasm, repair, graft or ligation if it is lacerated, are then carried out. These measures must not be delayed until irreversible changes take place in the hand. The hand is extremely vulnerable to circulatory disturbance. Simple loss of radial pulse does not mean arterial insufficiency. Loss of the pulse must be accompanied by signs of actual ischemia of the hand in order to justify exploration of the artery.

The duration of immobilization depends somewhat upon the degree of reaction in the elbow. Immobilization should be by anterior and posterior plaster splints and not by a solid cast (Fig. 186). There must be no constriction in the antecubital space. By the use of anterior-posterior splints the degree of ten-

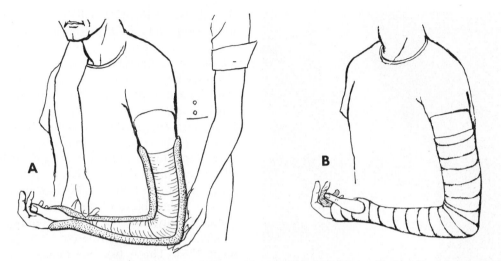

Figure 186. The anterior and posterior splint. *A*, Plaster splints carefully molded to the arm over sheet wadding. *B*, The dressing completed by application of gauze bandage.

sion in the forearm tissues can be assessed readily by palpation along the sides of the splint. The splints may be loosened if necessary and tightened as the swelling subsides. No attempt should be made to mobilize the arm until the swelling is well under control. If the case has been seen early and reduction carried out promptly, there probably will not be excessive post reduction swelling. In such a case the arm should be immobilized in double splints for two weeks. At the end of two weeks if no pain and swelling are present in the elbow the anterior splint is removed and the posterior one continued. The posterior splint will permit a few degrees of flexion and extension and is worn for one more week, a total of three weeks. The arm is then placed in a sling which is to be worn another week. At the end of this time (four weeks) unrestricted active use of the arm can be permitted. Passive stretching has little place in the rehabilitation of the elbow. There will be marked stiffness of the elbow following dislocation, but motion should be complete after several months if meddlesome passive stretching is avoided.

Rehabilitation commences immediately by use of the fingers and thumb, by setting the muscles of the forearm and by setting the muscles of the upper arm, all within the limits of pain. As the course of treatment progresses to the use of the posterior splint alone, active flexion and extension of the elbow are permissible, since this splint will "hinge" at the elbow. When the splint comes off, active use is encouraged, again within the limits of pain. Not before six weeks should strenuous motions be carried out. Any attempt to forcibly extend the elbow by passive stretching tends to delay the healing, to increase the inflammatory reaction around the elbow and to encourage bony deposits. These deposits are not in the muscle as in the case of a myositis ossificans, but are infiltrated throughout the capsule and ligaments of the joint (Fig. 187). Gravity is of great benefit in restoring extension, and it may be acceptable to add to the effect of gravity by a lead wristlet (a pound or two). Little is gained by carrying a heavy weight, at least in the first six to eight weeks. A dislocated elbow is a serious injury and

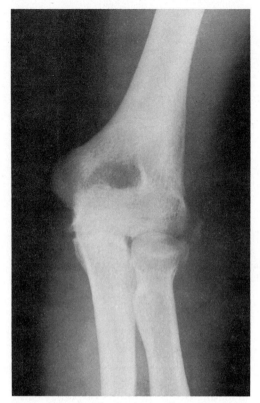

Figure 187.   Ossification in the elbow capsule following dislocation.

the elbow, ossification will surround the joint completely, causing serious disability. This tendency toward ossification should be recognized. Prompt care and rigorous management tend to minimize the deposit. Adequate immobilization during the acute stage directly after the injury encourages absorption of the extravasated blood and minimizes ossification. Repeated manipulation at intervals of several days with resultant irritation tends to increase the ossification. Later in the rehabilitation any attempt at forceful motion of the elbow stimulates ossification in the capsule (see Fig. 206, page 277). These osseous deposits are not myositis ossificans, since they do not occur in the muscle. *Once the condition begins, treatment consists of immobilization and protection rather than manipulation.* Nothing is gained by trying to prevent stiffness by manipulation once ossification is present. The temptation to remove the bone surgically should be resisted for many months. It may ultimately be advisable to attempt excision of some ossific plaques, but any attempt to do this before the deposit is entirely mature and completely stable will only result in increased ossification. Indeed, it may recur in any event.

will require prolonged aftercare. It should result in little or no permanent disability in the young athlete.

Ossification of the capsule of the elbow occurs not only with frank dislocation but with many lesser injuries of the ligament and capsule, since this area is particularly prone to ossification. This often results in serious restriction of motion of the joint. The most vulnerable areas are around the coronoid process of the ulna in the anterior capsule, and the olecranon process of the ulna in the posterior capsule. Any ossification of either of these areas seriously restricts motion of the elbow. Ossification may also occur as a plaque of bone along the collateral ligaments where it not only restricts motion but may be quite painful on function. Occasionally, following dislocation or fracture-dislocation about

FRACTURE–DISLOCATION

As has been noted above, fractures frequently accompany elbow dislocations. This is particularly true of those epiphyses that have not entirely closed. It is very common for the medial epicondylar epiphysis to be pulled off.

Epicondyles

The epicondyles serve for the attachment not only of the collateral ligaments of the elbow but also of strong muscles. All of these attachments are put under great stress during dislocation

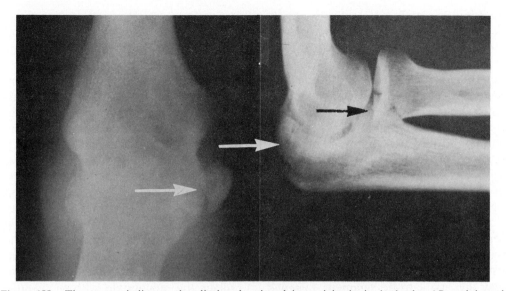

Figure 188. The arrow indicates the displaced epicondylar epiphysis in both the AP and lateral views. Note the fracture of the radial head without displacement (black arrow), which does not require treatment.

of the humerus, whether this dislocation is straight forward or has a lateral component. The bones carrying attachments of muscles are likely to be grossly displaced if the fracture is complete (Fig. 188). Reduction of the elbow may catch the fragment within the joint (Fig. 185), and this may actually prevent complete reduction. X-ray examination as soon as possible after reduction of the dislocated elbow is imperative, whether or not one was made before the reduction (Fig. 189). An avulsed condyle should be replaced surgically, even when the

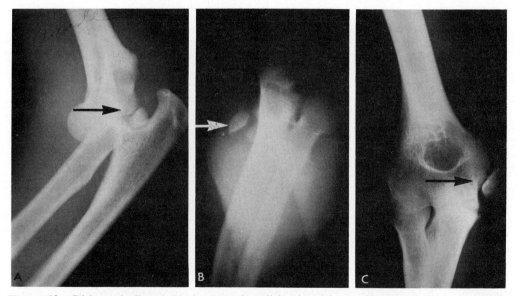

Figure 189. Dislocated elbow with fracture of medial epicondyle. *A*, Showing dislocation with displacement of condyle into the joint (arrow). *B, C,* Showing reduction with poor position of the epicondyle (arrows).

avulsion is simply of a muscle attachment with a small splinter of bone (Figs. 190 and 191), since firm fixation of this attachment will permit much more rapid motion and complete rehabilitation. The detached epicondyle tends to rotate because of the pull on its periphery, so that it frequently presents its cortical surface toward the humerus and the fractured surface toward the skin (Fig. 192). Nonunion is quite common and growth disturbance inevitable when this occurs and is untreated (Fig. 193).

At operation the muscle or ligament attachment is carefully replaced with or without the fragment of bone. If the fragment is small it is better removed and the aponeurotic ligament fastened to the raw bone of the humerus. A larger fragment may be held in place by nail or screw or other suitable internal fixation (Figs. 190 and 192). Rehabilitative measures can proceed at about the same rate as if there had been no fracture once internal fixation is secure. Any internal fixation should be removed after four to six weeks, particularly if it crosses the epiphyseal cartilage.

Ulnar Nerve Injury

The ulnar nerve is usually not injured in a posterior dislocation of the elbow. However, in a fracture involving the medial epicondyle, ulnar nerve injury occurs with some frequency. This emphasizes the importance of careful evaluation of nerve function prior to any manipulation or surgery. If there is evidence of ulnar nerve damage, the nerve should be carefully examined at the time of the operation on the medial epicondyle. If there appears to be a possibility of its future involvement in scar, it should be transposed forward. On the other hand, if there is no sign of ulnar damage, it may be quite possible to replace the epicondyle without disturbing the nerve. The surgeon must always be conscious of the nerve so that it is not inadvertently damaged by either the instruments or the internal fixation. Hence, it is desirable to locate the nerve early and to be sure of its integrity at the termination of the operation before the wound is closed.

Following operation the function of the nerve should be determined at the

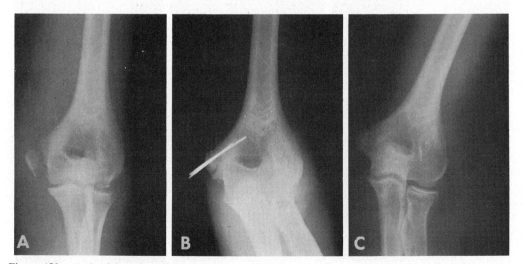

Figure 190. *A*, Avulsion of medial epicondyle. *B*, Replacement of condyle, held with nail, *C*, Late x-ray shows firm union.

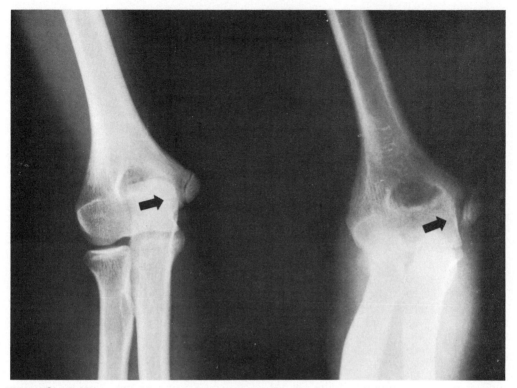

Figure 191. Injury to the elbow of a 13 year old girl while doing a handspring. *A*, Original x-ray showed no fracture, although there was much tenderness around the medial epicondyle. *B*, Two weeks later: separation of the epicondyle with some downward slipping.

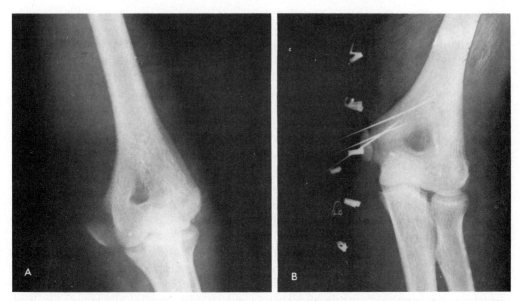

Figure 192. *A*, Avulsion fracture of medial epicondyle with 90 degree rotation of the fragment. *B*, The fragment reduced and held with multiple Kirschner wires.

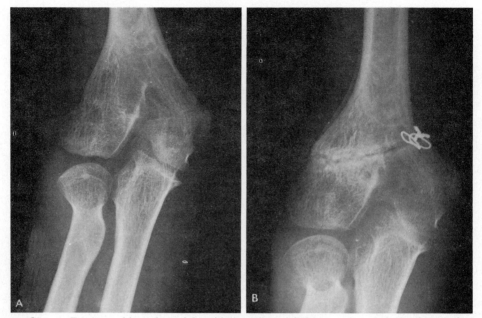

Figure 193. *A,* Fracture of lateral condyle with growth retardation, causing marked cubitus valgus. *B,* Correction by osteotomy.

earliest possible moment. If this is not done one may, upon the discovery of an ulnar palsy several days later, be unable to determine whether it was caused by a gradual constriction of later scar formation or by actual injury at operation. This may have a great deal of prognostic importance. If the involvement is evident immediately after surgery and was not apparent preoperatively, one should seriously consider reopening the wound for examination of the nerve. This is particularly true if the loss of function is complete. On the other hand, if the onset is gradual after a day or two, immediate attention must be given to relieve any possible pressure. If the splint is tight, release it. If the pressure is from internal tension, the splints should be removed and the elbow gently extended to whatever degree is necessary to relieve the tension. Late paresthesia or anesthesia is another problem, and a great deal of judgment is required in determining the proper measure and the proper timing. If the condition is pro-

gressive, one must decide whether surgical treatment is necessary. If the nerve is to be transposed, it must be done before permanent changes occur in the nerve.

Coronoid Process

The coronoid may be broken off at the time of dislocation of the elbow (Figs. 194 and 195). If the fragment is small but somewhat displaced, it is best removed. If it comprises the major portion of the coronoid, its replacement may be necessary. This is a difficult procedure and should be postponed until the swelling of the elbow has subsided.

Radial Head

At the time of dislocation of the elbow, the radial head is forcibly driven against the lower end of the humerus and is frequently damaged. Indeed, many complete fractures of the radial head have probably been accompanied by dislocation of the ulna that has reduced spontaneously. Treatment of a complete fracture of the radial head is almost always surgical, since it is necessary that the head be undistorted if normal rotation of the forearm is to be expected. Therefore, following a dislocation, the head should be carefully examined by x-ray (Fig. 194). A fragment that involves less than one-fourth of the entire circumference of the radial head, particularly if it is on the lateral aspect of the head, may be removed and the remaining intact head left in situ. One will often discover, however, that there is also a comminuted fracture of the remaining portion of the head as well as the small segment. These fractures are not avulsion fractures, since there is nothing attached to the rim of the radial head. They are caused by direct force; hence, there may be extensive chondral damage which does not show on the film. There also may be damage to the cartilage of the capitellum of the humerus (Fig. 196). These factors present another argument for early surgery in fracture of the radial head in order that the nature of the lesion can be determined and proper measures undertaken.

If there is a complete fracture of the radial head, particularly if it is comminuted in type, the head should be removed and the annular ligament carefully repaired if it has been disrupted (Fig. 197). Most fractures through the radial neck in adults should also be treated by excision of the radial head. Fractures occurring in children before the upper radial epiphysis has closed should never be treated by excision of the head, because of the disability following growth disturbances and radial shortening. In these cases the head should carefully be replaced by open reduction if manipulation fails, if there is angulation over 30 degrees or if there is any lateral displacement.

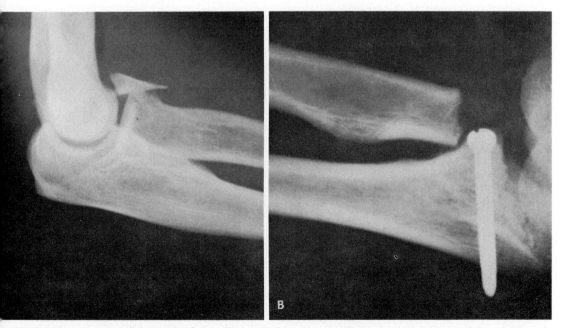

Figure 194. Fracture-dislocation of the elbow. *A*, Fracture of radial head and fracture of the ulnar coronoid, with displacement. *B*, Resection of the radial head, replacement of the ulnar coronoid and fixation by screw. Good stable elbow with no restriction of flexion extension resulted.

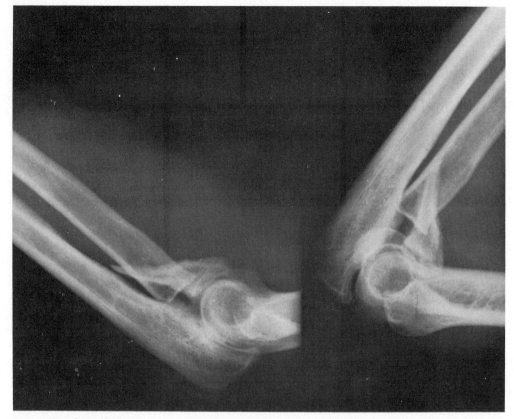

Figure 195. Case similar to Figure 194. Fracture-dislocation of the elbow with fracture of the radial head and the coronoid. X-rays made 15 months postoperatively, at which time the radial head was removed. Failure to replace the coronoid resulted in complete block in flexion at 115 degrees and in extension at 35 degrees. Patient has traumatic arthritis of the elbow which increases his disability.

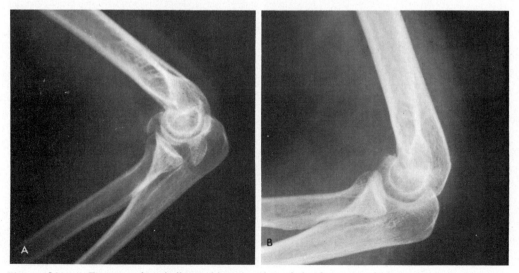

Figure 196. *A*, Fracture of capitellum with separation of the fragments. This is the same force that might break the radial head. *B*, Following open reduction with removal of small fragments and replacement of major fragments. Excellent function.

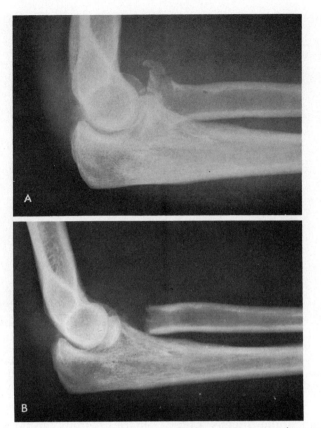

Figure 197. Fracture of the radial head. *A*, The comminution. *B*, Treatment by resection of the head.

Olecranon

Almost all dislocations of the elbow are posterior. That is, the forearm moves posteriorly in relationship to the arm (Figs. 184 and 189). This frequently has the lateral component indicated above. A true anterior dislocation of the elbow is virtually impossible without fracture of either the olecranon or the lower humerus. Anterior fracture-dislocation is a very serious injury usually resulting from force applied directly on the back of the flexed elbow (Figs. 198 and 199). The olecranon breaks, the triceps attachment holds the proximal fragments posteriorly, the lateral ligament gives way and the humerus moves backward and downward into the fracture line. This same force may cause a fracture of the trochlea of the humerus or indeed of the entire distal end of the humerus. As the ole-

cranon is driven into the distal end of the humerus it may act as a wedge and cause a condylar or T fracture. The radial head is not usually fractured in either of these instances, since the forces applied do not put stress on it.

This injury must be treated surgically in order to obtain accurate replacement and firm internal fixation of the fragments. The exact type of fixation depends upon the pathological conditions. If the fragment is a single large block, it may be held very well with a long intramedullary screw or pin. If the fragments are more comminuted, a small plate may be needed. Some of the fragments or, indeed, all of the fragments may be removed with suture of the triceps tendon to the remaining olecranon (Fig. 200). One may remove a surprising amount of the olecranon process and not materially impair function of the elbow if the triceps is care-

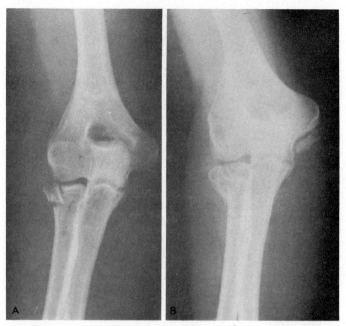

Figure 198. Fracture-dislocation of elbow. *A*, The dislocation was reduced and the radial fragments allowed to remain. *B*, Subsequent picture shows good healing of the radial head but with deformity and restriction of rotation, ossification of the medial capsule with restriction of flexion and extension, and pain. Radial head resection would have permitted earlier motion and better rehabilitation. The radial head should now be removed, but the ultimate result will not compare with that of early surgery.

fully repaired, since the triceps sling gives sufficient stability. The elbow will tolerate considerably more roughness of the olecranon than the knee will of the patella because weight bearing is not involved. Open reduction following these injuries permits careful inspection of the cartilage, not only of the olecranon fossa but also of the humerus. The chondral fragments can be removed and the cartilage smoothed out with gratifying results.

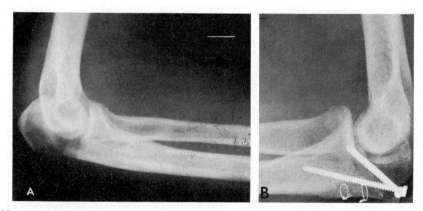

Figure 199. *A*, Fractured olecranon at its base. This will require long intramedullary screw or pin for firm fixation. Treatment refused. Result—traumatic arthritis of the elbow with restriction of motion and pain. Fibrous union of the fragment. *B*, Case similar to *A*. A fractured olecranon but with fractured coronoid. Note oblique screw transfixing olecranon and coronoid, with longitudinal screw extending into the shaft. It is probably better to use a longer screw in the shaft, but in a young individual good purchase can often be obtained without using an intramedullary nail or screw.

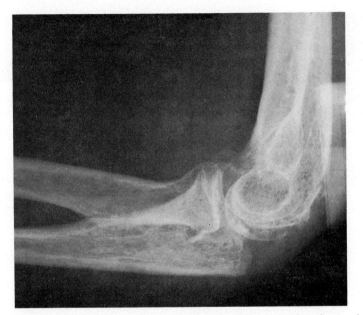

Figure 200. Fracture of olecranon after excision of broken tip and repair of tendon to olecranon. Excellent functional result.

The following steps are imperative in the treatment of complete dislocation of the elbow:

1. One must evaluate the circulation of the hand first.

2. The nerve function of the hand must be determined before manipulation.

3. Reduction must be completely atraumatic.

4. Careful x-ray study should be made after reduction *before* the splint is applied.

5. Appropriate treatment must be instituted for accompanying fractures about the elbow.

6. The elbow must be immobilized by plaster splints. It is not sufficient to simply use a sling.

7. Early forceful passive stretching of the elbow must *not* be carried out.

8. Patient, active rehabilitation will usually result in normal function.

FRACTURE

A complete discussion of fracture of the elbow, which is a large subject

indeed, is not necessary here, the reader being referred to the many excellent standard texts on treatment of fractures. However, there are certain peculiarities in the management of athletes with fracture about the elbow that should be emphasized.

A fracture of the elbow in a growing child is an extremely serious injury. The anatomical structure of the elbow is such that in children a supracondylar fracture, like a dislocation, may cause irreparable damage to the vessels, which may catch over the end of the bone with resulting impairment of the circulation. The fascia of the forearm is relatively inelastic and subject to intense pressure by swelling, which may result in irreparable damage to the forearm and hand (Fig. 201). Anyone who has seen or treated a case of Volkmann's contracture (Fig. 202) knows what a catastrophe it is. Of particular significance is the acute ischemia resulting from arterial spasm. This is contrasted sharply with the swelling of the hand resulting from venous congestion. The hand is cold, white and feels numb. There is no capillary pulse. This is an

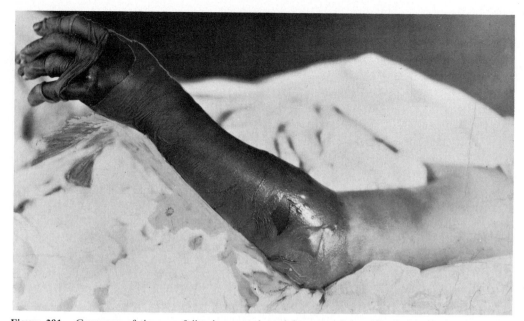

Figure 201. Gangrene of the arm following a neglected fracture of the elbow. Amputation just below the shoulder was necessary.

extreme emergency, and much more serious than ordinary congestion and swelling. It probably will not be relieved by ordinary measures such as straightening the elbow. It is obvious that any gross displacement at the fracture site should be completely reduced, particularly if there is anterior displacement. However, this condition may not be relieved by simple release of the pressure.

This syndrome demands immediate

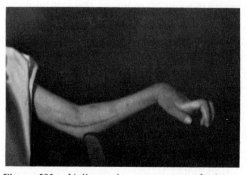

Figure 202. Volkmann's contracture—final result. This is an essentially useless arm and hand despite yeoman efforts at rehabilitation, including extensive surgery.

stellate ganglion block and immersion of the opposite hand in alternate ice and hot water. If such measures do not result in prompt restoration of circulation, the artery should be explored by incision in the antecubital fossa. The artery must be inspected, and if caught on a bony fragment, must be released. Oftentimes the artery is free but in spasm. Stripping of this artery will often relieve the spasm and restore circulation. If the artery is lacerated or severed, it must be repaired, replaced or ligated. Simple ligation will often relieve spasm and permit the collateral circulation to supply the distal area, but repair is better.

I know of no injury that requires more skill in management than the fractured elbow in a child. I make it an invariable rule in a child to x-ray both elbows and not try to remember or guess what the normal should be. By actually comparing one side with the other one can usually determine whether or not there is any displacement of fragments or disturbance of the normal relationships at the elbow.

Avulsion Fracture

In a previous section I discussed fracture of the epicondyle in relation to dislocation. This same fracture may occur as an avulsion fracture by muscle violence without dislocation of the elbow. Not infrequently the medial epicondyle will be pulled off by massive flexor pronator muscle contraction together with abduction stress on the forearm without dislocation of the elbow. This avulsion will be of the muscle and lateral ligament attachments at the elbow (Fig. 203). An identical force may completely avulse all or a portion of the flexor pronator muscle group at the elbow. I have seen this happen most often in football players who throw the ball with maximum exertion and terrific force in order to "throw the bomb." In this effort, the whole aponeurosis may be pulled off without any bone, or a single strip of it may be pulled off, such as the flexor carpi ulnaris and the flexors to the ring and little fingers. This acute injury is manifested by severe pain, early swelling, tenderness and particularly pain during the pronation flexion function. The symptoms are more severe with avulsion of the muscle and aponeurosis than with avulsion of the epicondyle itself. Avulsion of the epicondyle occurs in the young patient before the epiphysis is united, whereas a muscle avulsion occurs after the epiphysis is closed in an older person. Treatment for this condition is obviously replacement of the aponeurosis by direct suture. This should be done as early as possible since, as pointed out elsewhere, contracture of the muscle soon makes it difficult to get it back. However, if it comes off in a single mass, it may well be replaced with the

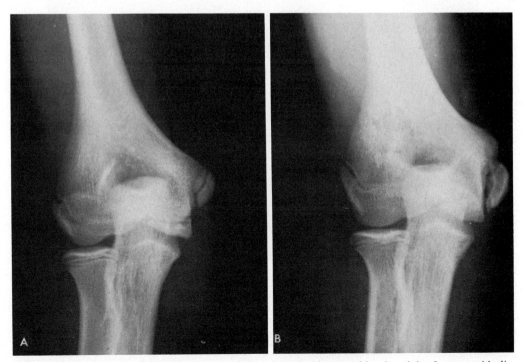

Figure 203. *A*, Normal elbow. *B*, Anteroposterior view showing an old epicondylar fracture with displacement of the fragment downward. At the time of operation it was impossible to replace this greatly enlarged epiphysis. It was removed and the aponeurosis sutured to the epicondylar ridge.

elbow flexed and the forearm supinated. The treatment for delayed avulsion is a reconstructive problem which may require some muscle substitutions.

Perhaps of even more concern, since it is so readily overlooked, is the circumstance of violent muscle contraction (as in throwing) which separates the apophysis from the major bone but does not grossly displace it. X-ray pictures will often appear to be negative unless they are carefully compared with the opposite side, when you will see slight widening of the epiphyseal line in relationship to normal (Fig. 204). In these instances the injury does not seem to be too severe but the recovery is very slow and often the symptoms increase rather than improve with the passage of time. The young athlete suffers distressing recurrence of his elbow pain and ineffectiveness in the use of his arm, usually with restriction of extension. This condition should be treated by immobiliza-

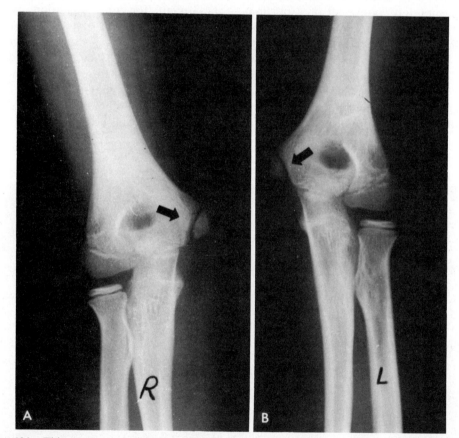

Figure 204. This 11 year old male was pitching four weeks ago, threw very forcibly off balance to first base and had right elbow pain. He tried to pitch further but had to quit. The elbow swelled. On examination everything appeared to be negative. He gradually improved until he tried to pitch again. Every time he tried to throw his condition worsened. On examination his complaint was all around the medial epicondyle. There was thickening but not gross swelling. There was pain particularly in gripping and pronating the forearm against resistance. *A,* X-ray shows the right elbow with what might be interpreted as being a normal epiphyseal plate until compared with the opposite elbow, *B,* where you will notice that the epiphyseal plate is narrower and smaller. Even in four weeks' time the epiphysis had enlarged in size and traversed downward a few millimeters. Ultimately this may well have regressed to the point of Figure 203. The patient was treated by immobilization for another four weeks with uneventful recovery except for some enlargement of the epicondyle.

tion for a relatively short time, 4 to 6 weeks, until this has reunited. The apophysis ordinarily will continue to grow without any further symptoms. Anytime a young pitcher or football thrower complains of pain on the inner side of the elbow and x-rays appear to be negative, your index of suspicion should be quite high. In some instances, as indicated in Figure 203, the incomplete displacement will become complete, at which time it is difficult to obtain a normal elbow.

It is possible for the olecranon to be avulsed by violent contraction of the triceps as the forearm is forcibly flexed, but this is unusual. If there is a complete fracture of the olecranon by such a force, the triceps attachment is, of course, disrupted. This should be repaired surgically regardless of the size of the fragment. If there is simply a "skin" of bone pulled off, it should be treated exactly as tendon avulsion; namely, removal of the fragment and suture of the tendon to bone. If the fragment is larger it should be attached to the olecranon by internal fixation. The olecranon process fits into the trochlea fossa of the ulna, and perfect positioning of the fragment is necessary to assure normal function. This cannot be obtained in the usual case by immobilization of the elbow in complete extension. Then, too, accurate and firm internal fixation permits rapid rehabilitation, whereas immobilization of the elbow in extension for a period long enough to permit the olecranon to unite will give rise to a great deal of difficulty in obtaining normal flexion later.

Direct contusion of the olecranon with the elbow flexed may result in fracture of the olecranon process. This may be comminuted and accompanied by anterior dislocation of the forearm on the humerus. This dislocation is usually spontaneously reduced before the patient is examined. Careful manipulation may determine whether or not there is instability of the ligaments in this direction. If this dislocation has been present, it greatly complicates the recovery. If the olecranon is broken it may be replaced and held by internal fixation. It may be necessary to remove some of the comminuted fragments in order to prevent overgrowth of callus. If the fragments are small and at the proximal tip, they may be removed and the triceps sutured to the remaining olecranon.

BURSITIS

The olecranon bursa lying between the tip of the olecranon and the skin is the bursa most commonly involved in bursitis at the elbow (Fig. 205).

Acute Bursitis

Acute contusion to the point of the elbow will usually result in hemorrhage into the olecranon bursa. The bursa distends with blood and there is synovial irritation. If this injury is seen early the blood may be aspirated, hyaluronidase injected and a pressure dressing applied. This will ordinarily relieve the condition, although it may be necessary to aspirate more than once. More frequently, the condition does not receive early care since the symptoms and disability may not seem severe. The

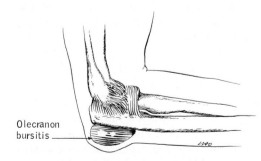

Olecranon bursitis

Figure 205. Olecranon bursitis.

synovial irritation continues and a chronic bursitis ensues.

Occasionally following an injury or indeed without injury, an infection occurs within the bursa and an acute suppurative bursitis ensues. The area is hot, inflamed and red and the patient presents the ordinary signs of infection with malaise, fever, pain, restriction of motion, tenderness and swelling. If upon examination the bursa is found to be full of fluid, this should be aspirated and a culture made. In the meantime the arm is immobilized in a sling and treated with continuous hot packs. An appropriate broad-spectrum antibiotic should be given in the hope that the acute inflammation will subside without the necessity for drainage. If the symptoms persist and aspiration does not relieve the effusion, the bursa should be drained surgically. Usually following acute inflammation and drainage the bursal walls become adherent and this automatically cures the bursitis. For the duration of the acute inflammation it is important that the arm be immobilized to avoid constant movement of the elbow. This is particularly true if an incision has been necessary. We advise an incision at either side of the bursa and the usc of a through-and-through tissue drain, which should be removed in a very few days as the inflammation subsides. Occasionally the infection will progress to spontaneous rupture of the bursa, since the skin over the back of the elbow is rather thin. The rupture usually occurs at the point of the olecranon and may leave a painful, adherent scar.

Much more frequently the bursitis is not suppurative. The bursa simply fills up with fluid under tension because of synovial irritation. This should be treated by aspiration followed by injection of a corticoid into the bursa and use of a pressure dressing. Repeated aspiration may be necessary, but with proper treatment the acute bursitis will usually subside without apparent residual.

Chronic Bursitis

Since acute bursitis is frequently overlooked, minimized or undertreated, a chronic bursitis of the olecranon bursa is quite common. In this case the sac gradually enlarges, at times becoming quite tense with fluid. At other times the bursa is simply boggy and thick. Through the course of many weeks and months some of these bursae attain amazing size. The author has seen some as large as 7 inches long and 4 inches wide — a veritable bag of water dangling from the point of the elbow. When seen in the early stages bursitis can often be relieved by aspiration, injection of a corticoid and pressure dressing, with the aspiration repeated at suitable intervals to prevent tension within the sac. Once the chronic bursitis is well established, surgical excision is usually the only means of obtaining permanent relief. Cartilaginous, or occasionally calcific, nodules may develop in the floor of the bursa which are readily palpable beneath the skin. They may become quite tender to pressure, giving rise to severe discomfort particularly when one rests his weight on the elbow. Surgical excision is simple since easy access can be obtained to this area. It is important to remove all of the bursa. Tacking the redundant skin to the underlying tissue may serve to prevent reaccumulation of fluid in the space and hence recurrence of the bursitis. Immobilization is imperative and must be continued until the wound is healed (3 weeks).

Radiohumeral Bursitis

Radiohumeral bursitis is frequently called "tennis elbow" and confused with epicondylitis. The radiohumeral bursa lies directly under the flexor pronator aponeurosis and it permits the aponeurosis to slide freely over the humeral condyle and the radial capsule. Gripping will cause pressure on this area and will cause pain simply by tensing the aponeurosis over the bursa, if the latter is inflamed. There usually is not sufficient bursal fluid to cause fluctuation. On examination the tenderness is localized over the radial head rather than over the epicondyle.

This condition responds well to local treatment with injection of a long-acting local anesthetic and a corticoid followed by elimination of the movements that cause pain. Indeed, it responds very well to the same therapy that relieves an epicondylitis.

OSTEOCHONDROSES

Osteochondritis dissecans is not common in the elbow except in certain activities. The baseball pitcher, for example, is very prone to injury of the articular cartilage with resulting "joint mice," pitting of the cartilage and chondromalacia. X-ray diagnosis of osteochondritis dissecans in articular cartilage at the elbow is difficult. Usually it is not seen until the fragment becomes detached. Indeed, it appears that the deposits may be largely in the nature of concretions formed within the joint as the result of chrondral tags and synovial irritation. While these occasionally will reach an amazing size (Figs. 206 and 207), they are usually very small and give trouble simply by being impinged between the olecranon and the back of the humerus (Fig. 208). Surgical removal is quite successful, although repetition of the same activity that caused them to form may cause recurrence. At the time of removal the joint should be carefully explored and any suspicious areas of loose cartilage carefully trimmed away. The joint should be thoroughly lavaged to wash out small rice bodies. If the foreign bodies appear to be the result of chronic synovitis, the elbow can be treated by the usual meas-

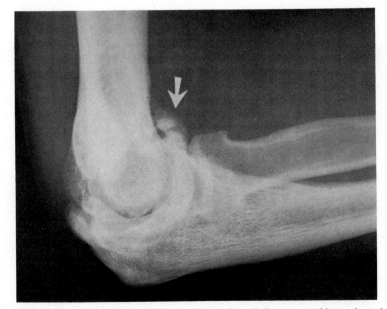

Figure 206. Excessive ossification following dislocation of elbow treated by early active use.

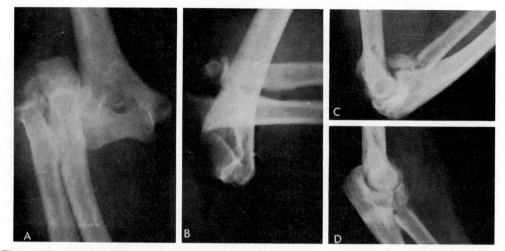

Figure 207. *A* and *B,* Anteroposterior and lateral views of severe fracture-dislocation of the elbow, fracture of radial head and ulnar coronoid. *C,* Radial head removed. Remaining coronoid caused extensive ossification in the capsule. This ossification may also be the result of damaged periosteum around the radial neck. *D,* Same as *C,* in extension, showing range of motion.

ures of injection, local heat and protection. In chronic synovitis extensive effusion in the elbow is not common. The capsule is not redundant and is not prone to distend as it does in other joints during acute inflammation. Complete avoidance of the forceful action that caused this condition may be necessary to prevent prompt recurrence.

OSTEOCHONDRAL FRACTURE OF THE CAPITELLUM

One type of osteochondral fracture or "osteochondritis dissecans" is frequently overlooked and misdiagnosed. The complaint is of pain in the lateral side of the joint, not in the radial head or on the epicondyle of the humerus but on

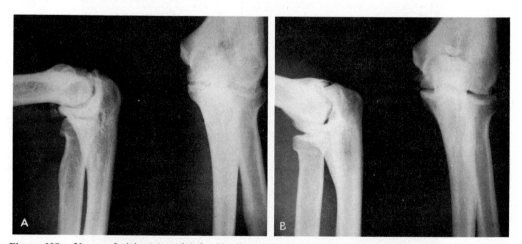

Figure 208. X-ray of right (*A*) and left (*B*) elbow of professional football player who had gradually increasing disability culminating in sharp restriction of motion of the right elbow after he fell on his elbow. This is a chronic traumatic bilateral arthritis which markedly improved by surgical removal of the foreign bodies and spurs. No other joints were involved.

the condyle itself right at the joint line down to the articular margin. A history of a previous fall on the outstretched hand or some similar trauma may be helpful, since this type of injury would force the radial head directly into the arc of the capitellar articular cartilage. It may not have been seriously symptomatic at the time, very similar to osteochondritis dissecans at the knee.

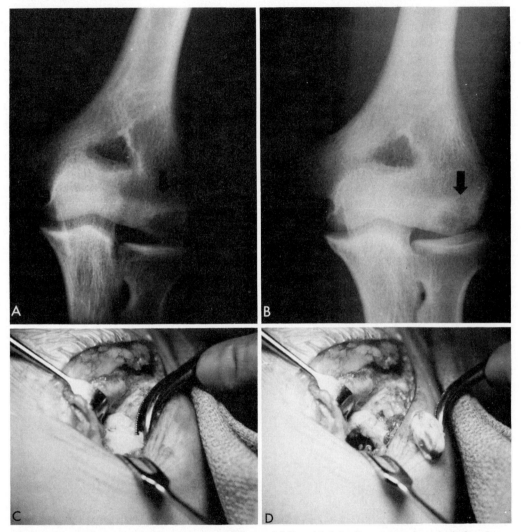

Figure 208A. This 14 year old male was wrestling and fell on his left elbow several weeks before I saw him. His complaints were gradually increasing pain on motion, hurting as he raised the arm, popping in the elbow when he rotated it and severe pain on snapping the elbow straight. He was comfortable in his sling. On examination there was tenderness on the lateral condyle at the joint line. Neither the radial head nor the epicondyle was tender. Surgical incision revealed a large foreign body consisting of a major portion of the lateral condyle lying completely free in the joint. This left a gross defect that had been tentatively diagnosed as a cyst. The bed was relatively fresh bleeding bone. Treatment was removal of the fragment and drilling of the bed. *A,* X-ray shows the radiolucent area adjacent to the subchondral bone on the lateral condyle that could be interpreted as being a cyst, chondroblastoma or chondral fracture. Arrow points to the defect. *B,* Subsequent film seven months postoperative shows satisfactory filling in. *C,* Surgical photograph of the lateral condyle with the fragment in situ held in Kelly forceps. *D,* The defect and the fragment removed from the joint. Note the relatively fresh bed indicating recent injury.

The complaint is of aching pain and especially of pain on forced snap extension of the elbow, as in throwing the baseball. X-ray examination may be negative but often the x-ray reveals a cystic appearing radiolucency within the capitellum extending down toward the articular cartilage. This may be diagnosed as a chondroblastoma. This is a typical location for this tumor insofar as the articular cartilage is concerned, although the elbow is not as common a location for this lesion as is the knee — or it may be called a bone cyst. Although it does not have the trabeculation one might expect to find in a multilocular cyst, it has the appearance of a unicameral bone cyst (Fig. 208A). At surgery the true pathologic condition is revealed, namely a large osteochondral fragment including the articular cartilage, the fragment leaving a gross defect in the articular portion of the capitellum. If the fragment is large and fairly fresh, it may be replaced and pinned in situ. Usually it has become chronic and the best treatment is to remove the fragment and curette the bed down to bleeding bone. If the bed is sclerotic it should be treated by curetting out the fibrous tissue and then drilling multiple small drill holes using a Kirschner wire into the bed. Since the elbow is non–weight bearing, the results are predictably good. Whether the defect fills with fibrocartilage or hyalincartilage, it seems to function well. Repeat operation is rare, fortunately, so we can only speculate on the anatomic result. Functionally it is very satisfactory especially in the young person (under 18 years of age) in whom it most frequently occurs.

CHAPTER 10

INJURIES OF THE FOREARM

ANATOMICAL CONSIDERATIONS

While to a large extent injuries to the forearm concern function of the wrist and hand, there are certain anatomical considerations in the forearm proper that merit review (Fig. 209). Whereas in the upper arm there is a single bone surrounded by a mass of muscle, the forearm contains two bones with the rather complex interrelated movements that were described in the chapter on the elbow. The ulna, being large at the elbow and small at the wrist,

serves to give good stability between the humerus and the forearm. This humero-ulnar articulation permits motion in only one plane, flexion and extension. The ulna is fixed to the humerus and does not rotate so that the position of the entire shaft of the ulna is constant in relationship to the upper arm. At the lower forearm the radius is the larger bone and it alone articulates with the carpus. The radiocarpal joint is of the ball and socket type, which permits motion in any direction. The range of motion permitted is due to ligamentous limitations rather than any bony

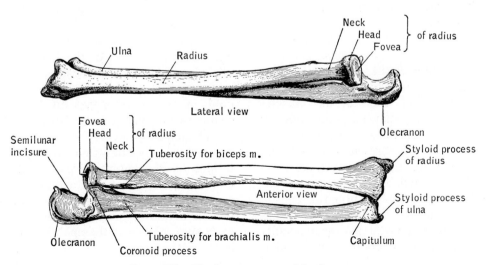

Figure 209. The bony anatomy of the forearm.

block. The axial relationship of the radius to the carpus and hand is constant in the sense that there is little rotary motion between the carpus and the radius. Pronation-supination of the hand occurs by the rolling of the radius and carpus as a unit around the axis of the fixed ulna.

While the two bones of the forearm are essentially parallel to each other, the radius arches enough to allow considerable space between it and the ulna in the middle third, whereas they are in contact at the proximal and the distal radioulnar joints. The integrity of these two joints is entirely ligamentous. Each joint consists of a small saucerlike bed for the radial head at the upper end of the ulna and a small fossa for the ulna on the lower radius. The two bones are firmly bound together by the interosseous membrane. The fibers of this membrane are so interdigitated and decussated as to permit rotation of the radius over the ulna while maintaining constant tension of some of their fibers. The upper end of the radius is firmly fastened to the ulna by the orbicular ligament. At the distal end the ulna is bound to the radius by a similar arrangement so that these ligaments give considerable inherent stability to the two joints. On either side of the interosseous membrane lie the blood vessels and nerves. An extremely intricate complex of muscles attaches along the shafts of the two bones. The synergistic action of these muscles carries out all the complicated motions of the wrist and hand, each of the muscles having a somewhat different function depending upon the relative position of the hand and the forearm and the arm.

This is not the place for a more detailed discussion of the anatomy of the forearm. The reader is urged to consult a good atlas of anatomy, and he is bound to be amazed by the ingenuity with which the function of the hand is assured. The entire dorsal surface of the ulna is subcutaneous so that from the tip of the olecranon to the ulnar styloid the bone can readily be palpated beneath the skin. The only subcutaneous areas on the radius are at its proximal and distal extremities.

CONTUSION

The forearm is very subject to contusion because of the substantial area of subcutaneous bone. This is doubly true since the forearm is toward the distal extremity of the most active member of the body and so often comes in violent contact with an opposing player or an obstacle. Hence, a contusion may result from a fall on the olecranon process with the elbow flexed or from a direct blow against the subcutaneous shaft of the ulna.

Contusion of the Skin

In either of the above instances the result is damage to the skin with typical excoriation, pain, local swelling and hematoma. The most frequent complications that may arise are olecranon bursitis at the elbow and a periostitis along the ulna. Ordinarily, contusion of the skin presents minimal disability and *treatment* should be largely of a local character: aspiration of the hematoma, injection of long-acting anesthetic, pressure dressing followed by application of cold in the early stages to be subsequently changed to heat. The area can be adequately protected by a pressure pad and usually contusion need not interfere with athletic participation. Chronic periostitis, if it results, may require more comprehensive treatment with injection of a corticoid and more extensive physical therapeutic measures.

Contusion Involving the Musculotendinous Structures

Of more consequence than contusion of the skin is contusion involving the musculotendinous structures. This is particularly pertinent in the lower forearm where the tendons become subcutaneous as they converge toward the carpal tunnel on the volar side and toward the extensor aponeurosis on the dorsum of the wrist. In these circumstances the catching of a tendon and its sheath between the striking object and the underlying bone may well result in a serious and disabling *traumatic tenosynovitis*. In this condition there is a history of a direct blow followed by discomfort of a moderate degree. After 12 to 36 hours the pain increases and is particularly aggravated by motion of the part involved. For example, if the extensor carpi ulnaris tendon is involved there will be pain on dorsiflexion of the wrist against resistance, pain on passive palmar flexion of the wrist and pain on gripping. All of these activities are well nigh essential to athletic competition. If the tendon happens to be the long supinator, the pain will be on function of this muscle, and so on. It behooves one to make a careful analysis of the symptoms involved in order to determine what tendon is involved. Usually the pain will be well localized over the area of the contusion.

Treatment of a traumatic tenosynovitis demands rest of the involved tendon. It is completely futile to try to "work it out," or to use extensive physical therapy and at the same time encourage use. The part must be put at functional rest and the best criterion of the adequacy of immobilization is relief of pain. *Painful motion should be eliminated.* This may mean restriction of motion of the wrist in either rotation or flexion and extension and also interdiction of gripping. If a little time is taken to explain to the athlete the purpose of asking him not to exercise the part to the extent of causing pain, he can usually be permitted to exercise just short of the pain-producing movement and so continue his rehabilitation to some extent. Local treatment is of value and injection of the involved tendon sheath with local anesthetic and one of the corticoid preparations is worthwhile. Care should be taken not to inject into the tendon, which not only is ineffective but may cause degenerative changes in the avascular tendon. It is, however, more successful in the chronic than in the acute stage. In the acute stage rest, local heat and protection will usually result in good recovery. Recovery is likely to be more complete following a tenosynovitis caused by contusion than one caused by strain. Very frequently a chronic tenosynovitis results. This will be discussed later under the proper heading.

Another complication of contusion is *fracture*. If the condition appears to be severe, the bone tenderness is acute, and function is painful, careful x-ray study should be made to rule out fracture.

Contusion higher in the forearm involving the belly of the muscle is similar in nature to muscular contusion anywhere and requires the same treatment, namely, aspiration, local injection of an anesthetic, compression, cold followed by heat and protection against motion. However, contusion of the muscles of the forearm presents an additional problem in that the motions of these muscles are extremely complex and so may cause considerably more disability for a given degree of contusion than elsewhere in the body. Very early rehabilitative use of the fingers can nevertheless be permitted, always short of pain. Protection may consist simply in prevention of competition and careful instruction. For certain sports it is possible to support the wrist and so wrap the forearm that the injured muscle can be protected. This extensive wrapping should be carefully removed once competition is over to permit resumption of pain-free function.

STRAIN

Strain is a common problem in the forearm, where many tendons glide together in the same sheath or separately. Any one of these musculotendinous units may be subject to strain from overexertion caused by a single active contraction of the muscle against too much resistance, from overstretching of the musculotendinous unit or from chronic overuse of the unit. The unit may be damaged by the actual disruption of some of its fibers by stretching, by a single violent contraction of the muscle beyond its capacity, or by repeated contractions of the muscle beyond its fatigue quotient.

Acute Strain

In acute strain the symptoms are pain along the area of strain, usually at the musculotendinous junction or at the attachment of the tendon to the bone. At this stage, overstretching or active contraction of the unit will cause pain at the area of strain. As the condition continues a tenosynovitis develops with irritation between the tendon and its sheath or mesotendon. This results in hyperemia, local swelling, inflammation and exudation of fluid. As the tendon continues to slide within the irritated sheath, sticky adhesions result and the so-called snowball crepitation is elicited; i.e., with the finger over the tendon, soft crepitation can be felt as the tendon slides up and down the sheath. This motion is painful and becomes increasingly so as use is continued. If the

condition progresses, the tenosynovitis may become adhesive, in which state the tendon fails to slide and dense adhesions form between the tendon and sheath. In other circumstances the tendon itself thickens and becomes constricted by its sheath.

If the strain is in the muscle belly the pain will be muscular and more diffuse. This results from either congestion within the muscle or rupture of some of the muscle fibers, or both. In extreme cases the strain may be so severe that continued use may cause a rupture somewhere in the unit. This may be of the fibers of the muscle itself or at the origin of the muscle or the attachment of the tendon. Very careful analysis of the condition will permit one to determine the exact location and nature of injury and so suggest the treatment. Only by careful examination can one properly regulate the treatment of the condition since the treatment will vary from no specific treatment to surgical repair of the lacerated unit.

Treatment of the acute strain depends upon the severity of the condition and the exact unit involved. The principles of treatment are rest, local heat and protection. In the very early stage an ice pack and compression bandage may be used, particularly if hemorrhage within the muscle is suspected. Within a few hours cold should give way to local heat. Until the severity of the condition is determined it is wise to immobilize the forearm in a position that will relax the involved unit. If the muscles to the fingers are involved, immobilization should include the hand. A word of caution should be sounded against prolonged immobilization of the fingers. In the first place, the fingers do not tolerate immobilization well and the joints tend to stiffen very rapidly. In the second place, active unresisted motion of the fingers will put very little strain on the injured area, the exception being a case of acute tenosynovitis involving the tendons to the fingers themselves.

The strain and, indeed, the resulting tenosynovitis much more commonly involve the muscles to the wrist so that immobilization is adequate if it terminates at the distal palmar crease with the wrist placed in the slight cock-up position. Careful inspection of the forearm should be carried out at frequent intervals in order to determine the progress of the condition. As soon as unresisted movement of the wrist is pain-free, complete immobilization may be discontinued and protection substituted. In a strain of moderate severity this will usually be a week or ten days. If the condition has gone on to tenosynovitis, the treatment must be more prolonged and more intensive with absolute immobilization of the affected tendon and some sort of inductive heat that can be given through the splint. Once crepitation is detected, meddlesome testing should not be carried out for at least a week, since repeated irritation only encourages adhesions and complete rest will permit resolution of the lesion. There is no place for local injection in the case of acute tenosynovitis. Only occasionally will there be sufficient fluid in the tendon sheath to justify aspiration.

Chronic Strain

Management of chronic strain can be extremely difficult for the doctor and disheartening to the athlete. In the usual case the strain is caused by the very activity that the athlete wants to carry out and resumption will cause its recurrence. The condition should be managed by rest and local heat. Careful analysis of the cause of the strain may reveal some unusual habit or posture that can be altered to place less strain on the involved muscle. As in so many conditions, it is important that use of the muscle be held within the limits of discomfort and pain and that overuse be carefully avoided. In the management of chronic tenosynovitis the same general dicta apply. In this circumstance, however, local treatment is of considerable value and injection of a corticoid into the involved tendon sheath may speed up the recovery markedly. There are no areas in the forearm proper in which constricting tenosynovitis is a problem. (See de Quervain's disease, page 295, and Carpal Tunnel syndrome, page 296.)

FRACTURE

The forearm is a common location for a fracture in the young individual, usually caused by a fall on the outstretched arm. Hence, in any instance following a fall in which there is pain with swelling and disability, fracture should be suspected. X-ray examination of the forearm is easy and should be carried out in case of any doubt. One common error in x-ray examination is to get anteroposterior and lateral views by simply rotating the hand on the film. This does not rotate the ulna, and while it results in anteroposterior and lateral views of the radius, the ulna is shown in the same plane. The forearm epitomizes very well the rule that the adjacent joints should be visualized. In making an x-ray of the forearm, the elbow and the wrist should be included. If there is any suspicion of epiphyseal separation or of some abnormality of the forearm, films of the opposite extremity should be taken for comparison.

A detailed discussion of the *treatment* of fractures of the forearm will not be given here since it is available in many good textbooks on fractures. A few points pertinent to the athlete should be mentioned, however.

Since the radius rotates around the ulna in pronation-supination of the forearm, one should be particularly careful to immobilize the elbow in case of fracture of the radius even at its distal end. An undisplaced fracture of the radius may become displaced by rotation of the forearm.

The so-called *greenstick fracture,* in which the forearm is bent and one cortex of the radius or ulna is broken and the other is intact, may trap the unwary. It is too easy to simply straighten the bone out and apply a splint or indeed a circular cast. Often as the fracture heals, however, the deformity recurs, and on removing the splint marked bowing of the forearm bones is found (Fig. 210). This is particularly likely to happen if a solid cast is used, since the cast becomes loose as the muscles atrophy and the swelling subsides. As a general rule, the greenstick fracture should be completely broken and this will usually require anesthesia. An exception is in the youngster in whom the dorsal cortex at the lower end of the forearm is buckled by a fracture

equivalent to a Colles' fracture in the adult. The angulation can sometimes be straightened by a quick snap without anesthesia. Following fracture of the forearm the young athlete should wear some protection on this arm for several weeks.

Typical *Colles' fracture* is quite unusual in the athlete, since ordinarily there will be a distal radial epiphyseal dislocation or fracture slightly higher in the forearm.

Subluxation of the distal radial epiphysis has considerable significance and requires careful handling in order to minimize the danger of growth disturbance. If the pain of the so-called strained wrist is actually at the lower end of the radius, x-ray examination is mandatory. If the x-ray shows any abnormality in the epiphyseal plate, films of the opposite wrist should be made for careful comparison. Many times the so-called sprained wrist will actually be a slipping of the epiphysis (Fig. 211). In this instance the subluxation either was

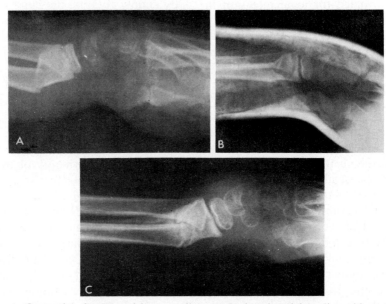

Figure 210. *A,* Greenstick fracture of lower radius. *B,* Reduced and in splint without breaking the dorsal cortex. *C,* Recurrence of deformity in splint. This deformity may correct spontaneously since the child was only 7 years old and modeling is already beginning. Surgery is not indicated.

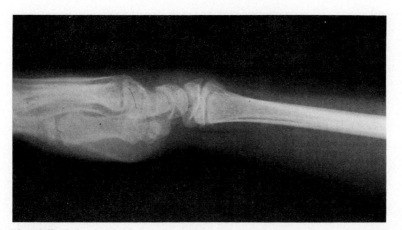

Figure 211. "Sprain" of the wrist. Note the buckling of the dorsal cortex which indicates that this is the same injury as shown in Figure 212, which either was spontaneously reduced or was incomplete to start with. No reduction necessary. Splints should be applied. Note that the displacement is actually through the distal radial epiphysis.

incomplete or was spontaneously reduced. In spite of normal appearing x-rays there will be persistent pain along the distal radial epiphyseal plate. Even if there is no displacement, the wrist should be immobilized until this tenderness disappears. If the epiphysis is displaced (Fig. 212) it should be reduced promptly and completely with as little trauma as possible. In any case of real or suspected damage to the epiphysis, the parents should be warned of the possibility of growth disturbance with consequent radial shortening (Fig. 213). This does not often occur but may be quite deforming when it does. This same type of injury may result in a dislocation extending partially through the plate with a fracture extending up the radial shaft (Fig. 214). This also requires very careful reduction. Growth disturbance here may lead not only to overall shortening but to angulation, which is even more distressing than shortening. This case should be very carefully followed and if angulation begins, the viable part of the epiphysis should be closed to prevent increasing deformity.

Complete fractures of both bones

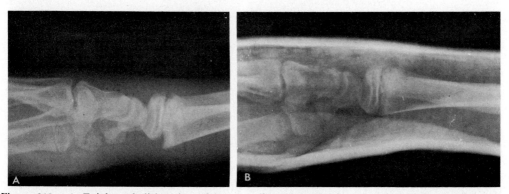

Figure 212. *A*, Epiphyseal dislocation of lower radius. Note the fragmentation of the dorsal cortex indicating that a part of the epiphysis is probably intact. Should premature closure occur in one portion of this epiphysis and not in another, deformity may occur. *B*, Atraumatic but complete reduction gives some insurance against premature closure.

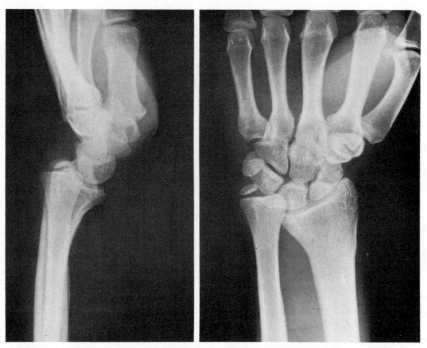

Figure 213. Radial shortening from epiphyseal disturbance some years following epiphyseal fracture of the lower radius. Note complete dislocation of the distal radio-ulnar joint, the ulna being distal to and behind the carpus. This was extremely disabling. Correction was carried out by shortening of the ulna and osteotomy of the radius.

of the forearm in the adolescent or adult are extremely difficult to reduce properly and hold in position by external means. One must bear in mind that in this category of patients one will wait in vain for correction of the deformity by growth modeling. The beneficent effects of further growth which are so notable

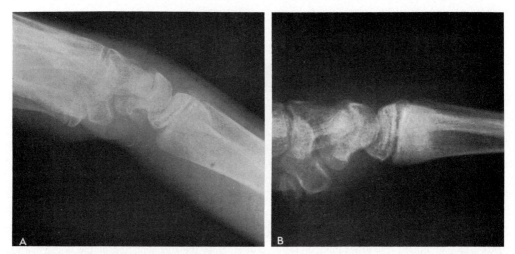

Figure 214. *A*, Fracture-dislocation of lower epiphysis of the radius. Note the epiphyseal dislocation on the palmar two-thirds of the plate with fracture of the shaft dorsally. *B*, Early accurate repositioning will minimize the chances of epiphyseal disturbance and growth deformity.

in the child will not be seen. Forearm fractures with displacement illustrate well the aphorism that fractures do not spontaneously improve in the splint. If the reduction looks bad before the splint is applied it is going to look worse when the splint is removed. There is no place for optimism in the management of a fracture in the athlete. Every effort must be made to restore the bones to their normal position. This is particularly true in the forearm where the interrelationships with the wrist and hand are extremely intricate.

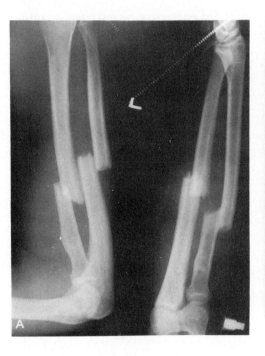

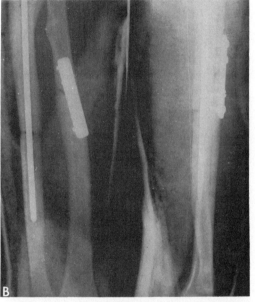

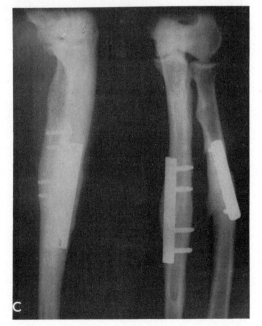

Figure 215. This 19 year old male was playing football and fell on the outstretched left hand when another player fell across his arm. He heard a cracking and had severe pain in the forearm with obvious instability. An air splint was applied and he was sent to the hospital. *A*, X-ray shows the fracture with the forearm in the air splint. Complete overriding of both bones. Closed reduction was impossible. *B*, Open reduction was readily carried out with a plate on the radius and intramedullary pin in the ulna. *C*, The ulna failed to unite. The pin was removed and bone graft applied, with excellent union. Note proper spacing between radius and ulna with slight bowing of the radius away from the ulna. This is extremely important in function of the forearm. This boy missed one season of football.

With two parallel bones in the forearm one must pay particular attention to their alignment (Fig. 215). In the child some correction of malalignment may be expected with growth, particularly in the axis of flexion of the adjacent joint. Hence, some posterior or anterior bowing may be acceptable in the adolescent. This is not so with lateral angulation noted with relative shortening or lengthening of one bone. This deformity does not correct with growth or with modeling. The bone itself may appear to be straight but the length will not increase. So an angulation at the wrist is inevitable. This deviation, usually radial, will not only be disfiguring but will be to some extent disabling. Therefore, in the adolescent or young adult accurate realignment and correction of shortening are imperative, even if this should require open reduction and internal fixation.

Fractures of both bones of the forearm in this age group are a major injury requiring excellent care and fraught with danger not only of disfigurement but also disability. Definitive treament initiated early will be extremely gratifying. One must not shrink from open reduction if this is required to obtain perfect function. The adolescent is not a "child" and must not be treated as one. In treatment of fractures of both bones of the forearm, we should use that method which has the best chance of restoring normal function of the extremity.

CHAPTER 11

INJURIES OF THE WRIST

ANATOMICAL CONSIDERATIONS

The wrist covers the area from the distal end of the radius and ulna to the proximal end of the metacarpals (Figs. 216 and 217). This includes the eight carpal bones, the proximal articular surfaces of the metacarpals, the distal articular surface of the radius and the fibrocartilage at the distal end of the ulna. There is no articulation between the ulna and the carpus, the two being separated by a fibrocartilaginous disc which also separates the wrist joint proper from the distal radio-ulnar joint (Fig. 218). The shallow concavity of the distal end of the radius is extended ulnarward by the articular disc, which thus serves to broaden the carpal articu-

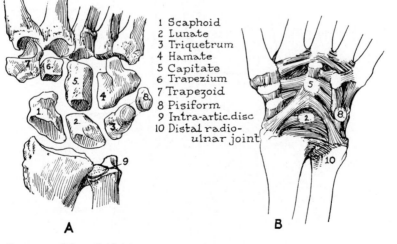

1 Scaphoid
2 Lunate
3 Triquetrum
4 Hamate
5 Capitate
6 Trapezium
7 Trapezoid
8 Pisiform
9 Intra-artic.disc
10 Distal radio-
   ulnar joint

A

B

Figure 216. Structure of the wrist joint.

A, The bones of the carpal mechanism, opened on their volar surfaces, are irregular in size and shape but fit perfectly like the pieces of a jigsaw puzzle (after Grant).

B, Many strong ligaments hold the carpal bones firmly in place, connecting their volar surfaces to the radius, the metacarpals and to each other.

The intra-articular disc separates the wrist joint from the distal radio-ulnar joint, and acts as a soft-part hinge upon which the radius swings around the ulnar head in supination and pronation. (From McLaughlin, Trauma.)

291

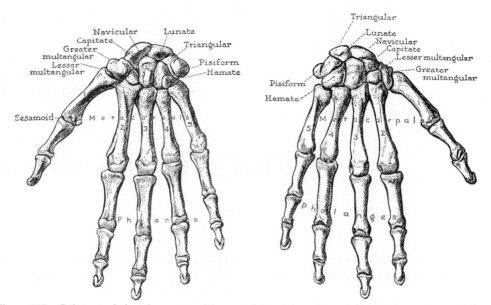

Figure 217. Palmar and dorsal aspects of bones of the right wrist and hand. (From Anson, Atlas of Human Anatomy.)

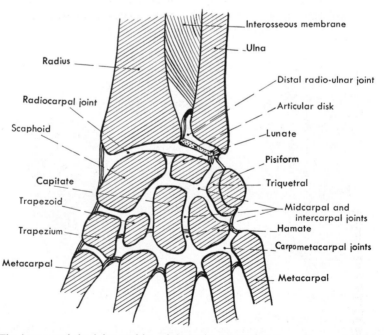

Figure 218. The bones and the joint cavities of the wrist. Note that the radiocarpal and inferior radio-ulnar joint cavities are separate and distinct; that the midcarpal joint is continuous with the intercarpal joints between both the proximal and distal rows of the carpals; and that the carpometacarpal joints, except for that of the thumb, are continuous with the intermetacarpal joints and with the distal parts of the intercarpal joints, but have no communication with the midcarpal joint. (From Hollinshead, Functional Anatomy.)

lation. At the radiocarpal joint the proximal row of carpal bones together form a smooth convex surface that articulates with the concavity at the lower end of the radius.

The amazing complexities of the articulations of the carpal bones will not be discussed in detail here. It is important to recognize the relationships of these bones to one another and to the forearm and hand. The greater part of the motion at the wrist takes place between the carpals as a unit and the radius. However, there is a definite amount of motion in each of the intercarpal joints. The navicular bone, the most radial of the proximal row, is long and boat-shaped and extends the furthest distally of this proximal row. In a transection through the wrist it will be noted that the capitate and to a lesser extent the hamate extend proximally into a concavity formed by the navicular, lunate and triquetrum. The two multangular bones are relatively short. Thus, the navicular extends across the two rows of the carpals, its distal portion actually extending more than halfway down the length of the capitate, a fact which makes it particularly vulnerable to injury on forceful motion through the midcarpal joint.

The entire lower end of the forearm, metacarpals and carpals are firmly bound together by the volar carpal ligaments, which make a dense impenetrable ligamentous mass on the palmar surface of the wrist. Dorsally, the ligaments are much weaker. These volar ligaments, and particularly the radial and the ulnar collateral ligaments, have various main components. The pisiform bone actually lies within the tendon of the flexor carpi ulnaris so that in effect the flexor carpi ulnaris attaches to the pisiform and in turn to the rest of the carpus through the strong ligaments extending from the pisiform to the metacarpals and to the hamate. Injury to the pisiform, therefore, is in a somewhat different category than injury to the other carpal bones.

In addition to the strong ligaments that bind these bones together there is a heavy band, the volar carpal ligament, which extends from the greater multangular bone across to the hook of the hamate. By virtue of this ligamentous strap the volar carpal tunnel is formed, three sides of which are made up by the carpal bones themselves and the roof by the ligament (Fig. 219). Through this tunnel pass the flexor tendons to the fingers together with the me-

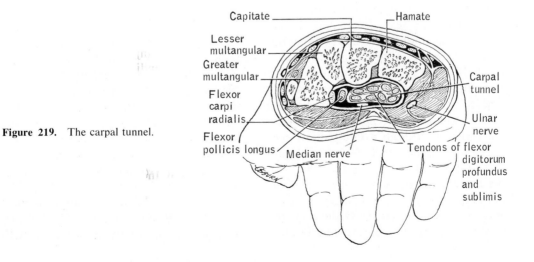

Figure 219. The carpal tunnel.

dian nerve. This sets the stage for the carpal tunnel syndrome. While the carpal bones are not in a true sense subcutaneous, they are covered only by ligaments, tendons, blood vessels and nerves, there being no muscular pad in the vicinity of the wrist.

CONTUSION

Contusion of the wrist is a frequent occurrence. It is not usually due to a fall but rather to a direct blow by the knee or headgear or foot when the outstretched hand is lying on the ground. Owing to the multiplicity of tendons in the wrist, the resulting injury is much more likely to involve them than the skin or bone. Hence, at the time of such an injury the wrist should be carefully examined for associated injury to the underlying structures. If the contusion seems severe, x-rays should be taken not only in the anteroposterior and lateral but in the right and left oblique planes. The carpal bones are not frequently fractured by a direct blow unless the crushing injury is especially severe. Tendon injury is quite common from contusion, which, if overlooked or minimized, may progress to a chronic tenosynovitis with all its attendant disability.

TREATMENT. Contusion of the wrist is treated by the usual measures according to its severity. If there is any doubt as to underlying injury to either tendon or bone, a splint should be applied. If there is no involvement of the radio-ulnar joint, the splint may be limited to the forearm. A good test for the adequacy of the splint is to rotate the forearm through a complete arc of pronation-supination. If this causes pain the splint should go above the elbow. In the early stage the splint may be incorporated into the compression bandage and an ice pack used. Ordinarily the contusion is not too severe and an elas-

tic bandage wrapped over a protective pad will be adequate, the more extensive treatment being reserved for the complications.

Laceration also will be found fairly commonly in the wrist although not as frequently as in the hand. This will be discussed in some detail in the section on the hand.

STRAIN

The general treatment of strain in this area was discussed in the section on the forearm. Since there are no muscles in the wrist proper, muscular strain does not occur here. However, this area is particularly vulnerable to tenosynovitis. The tenosynovitis may be the result of contusion of the tendon sheath, the tendon being caught between a blunt object and the hard bone, or it may be caused by a single violent muscular contraction against resistance or by violent passive motion. The most common cause for tenosynovitis in the wrist, however, is chronic overuse. With the multiplicity of tendons, tenosynovitis may become a highly complicated problem. It will require the usual type of treatment, namely, local injection, rest, heat and protection as indicated above.

Tendon Rupture

Each of the many tendon attachments in the region of the wrist is subject to strain, those particularly vulnerable being the flexors and extensors of the wrist. The same forces that cause tenosynovitis may rupture some of the tendon fibers at their attachment (second degree strain). Usually the force is a violent passive motion rather than an active contraction of the muscle. The history is of a fall with resultant pain at the site of the attachment of the tendon. The injury may easily be confused with contusion of the wrist or sprain or carpal fracture, the significant finding being pain on active contraction of the muscle involved. Thus, if the extensor carpi radialis is avulsed from its carpal attachment, active dorsiflexion of the wrist against resistance will cause pain. This is not ordinarily the case in a sprain or a fracture. If possible it is important to determine the degree of injury. The detachment is usually not complete.

TREATMENT. To relieve pain the wrist should be immobilized in the position in which the involved tendon is relaxed. If this tendon is an extensor the wrist is put in the cock-up position. If it is the flexor, the wrist is placed in flexion. This immobilization, which is most readily accomplished by plaster splints, must continue until the healing is complete, after which the wrist is carefully protected for the remainder of the playing season against the particular motion that caused the injury.

If the condition becomes chronic and there is persistent tenderness at the site of the tendon attachment and discomfort on active use of the muscle, local treatment is of some value. In these instances we advise injection of the area with a long-acting local anesthetic followed by a corticoid preparation. Steroid injections should not be made into the tendon but into the peritendinous area. Necrosis of the tendon may occur if the injection is into its substance. A test of the effectiveness of the injection is that the pain and tenderness must be completely relieved following the anesthetic injection. This will indicate that the condition has been correctly located. It should be remembered that many of these tendons have extensive insertions, particularly into the ligaments at the wrist and at the bases of the metacarpals. Following complete relief of pain and tenderness by anesthetic injection, a corticoid is injected into the same area. In the chronic condition it

may not be necessary to immobilize the wrist completely but the patient should be warned against any activity that causes discomfort. Some sort of wrist wrapping or strapping is advisable. Since the wrist flexors and extensors are tight whenever the fingers are made into a tight fist, forceful gripping should be discontinued during the treatment period, particularly if it causes discomfort. X-ray study should be carried out in any such condition involving the wrist. Occasionally a small flake of bone caused by avulsion of the tendon fibers if visualized in the x-ray will permit localization of the injury.

If the detachment is complete (third degree strain) it should be repaired surgically.

Certain peculiar characteristics of the wrist predispose to the pathological entities now to be described.

de Quervain's "Disease" (Constrictive Tenosynovitis)

As the tendons to the thumb cross over the lower end of the radius on its radial aspect, they pass through tunnels made up of grooves on the lower end of the radius and a fibrous retinaculum forming the roof. In particular, the long abductor and short extensor of the thumb pass directly over the styloid process of the radius and multiple tendons of the abductor may pass through the same sheath. This sheath is subcutaneous. Tenosynovitis in this area is quite common, usually as a result of overuse of the wrist and thumb. These tendons slide through the tunnel not only in movements of the thumb but on movements of the wrist with the thumb fixed. As the condition progresses, the tendon tends to swell and the sheath to thicken and a situation arises analogous to "trigger finger" so that, while one tendon slides through the groove, another one hangs and doubles up. In the early stages it may then slip through the

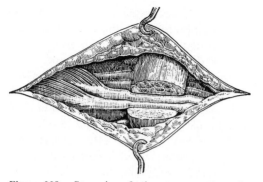

Figure 220. Stenosis of the two tendons in one osseofibrous canal. (K. L. Loomis, Journal of Bone and Joint Surgery, Vol. 33-A, 1951.)

constriction with a palpable click (Fig. 220).

During the early stage of this condition, use of the wrist is increasingly painful. An actual swelling appears over the styloid of the radius which on palpation is very firm and tender. At this stage the tendons will slide through the tunnel although with discomfort. A good test for this condition is to grasp the flexed thumb with the fingers, thus fixing the thumb in flexion. Then adduct the wrist. This will cause severe pain in the area of the constriction, since by this maneuver all the tendons are forced through the tunnel at the same time. The condition may progress until no motion of these tendons through the tunnel is possible.

If the condition is diagnosed in the early stage, *treatment* consists in immobilization of the wrist including the thumb if motion of the thumb is painful. Injection of the tender area with a long-acting local anesthetic and a corticoid may have some value. Care should be taken not to perforate the tendons themselves with the needle, since this may increase the swelling or cause later necrosis. Local heat is a useful adjunct and if treatment is carried out promptly the condition should subside. Once it establishes itself it is very prone to recur.

Fortunately, surgical treatment is extremely effective. Through a small transverse skin incision across the radial styloid, the thickened tunnel can be visualized and its roof carefully divided. Care must be taken to isolate and protect the cutaneous nerve that passes over the styloid process. It may be necessary to unroof more than one compartment in a well established case, since the adjacent compartments frequently become involved. Attention must be called to possible variations in the insertion of the abductor pollicis longus tendon (Fig. 221). The best procedure is to actually resect the entire roof of the tunnel rather than to split it, since the condition may recur as the separated edges heal. A few days of immobilization after the operation will suffice and recovery is usually prompt and complete.

Carpal Tunnel Syndrome

The carpal tunnel syndrome develops from unusual anatomical relationships on the volar aspect of the wrist. The eight flexor tendons of the fingers and the flexor pollicis longus pass through the constricted confines of the carpal tunnel (Fig. 219). The median nerve also passes through this canal. This vulnerable and compressible nerve lying in this confined space with the incompressible tendons is the innocent bystander that bears the brunt of early compression. The syndrome may be initiated by direct trauma, such as a fall on the outstretched hand, which causes swelling and thickening of the volar carpal ligament. It may be initiated by tenosynovitis of the flexor tendons. It is not an infrequent complication of an injury such as a Colles' fracture or indeed fracture of any of the carpal bones. An occasional case is caused by an actual mass intruding into the tunnel. This may be a ganglion, an exostosis, a solid

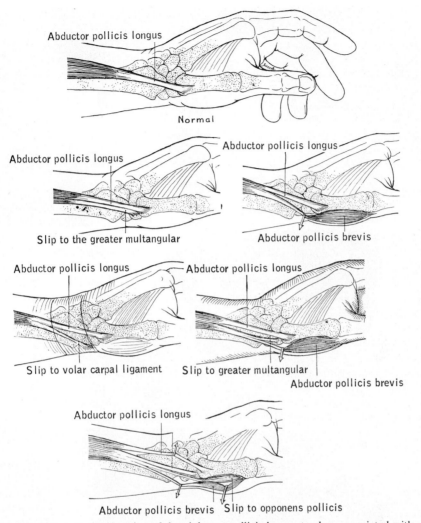

Figure 221. Variations in the insertion of the abductor pollicis longus tendon, associated with stenosing tenosynovitis. (T. Lacey II, H. L. Goldstein and C. E. Tobin, Journal of Bone and Joint Surgery, Vol. 33–A.)

tumor, a fragment of one of the carpal bones, a dislocation of the carpal bones, or an adventitious bursa. We recently had a case in which the typical findings were caused by a calcific mass, apparently a calcified bursa, within the tunnel itself (Fig. 222).

The essential ingredient of the carpal tunnel syndrome is either swelling of the structures within the tunnel or constriction of the tunnel, or both. Under these circumstances pressure on the median nerve is evidenced first by tingling in the distribution of the median nerve at the tips of the index and long fingers. The unwary physician may be deluded into believing that the involvement is in the fingers or in the nerve higher up in the arm. The characteristic distribution in the long and index fingers should lead one to suspect this condition. Careful examination then will elicit tenderness to deep pressure on the volar ligament which may increase the pain and paresthesia in the median distribution. Atrophy of the thenar muscles is a late

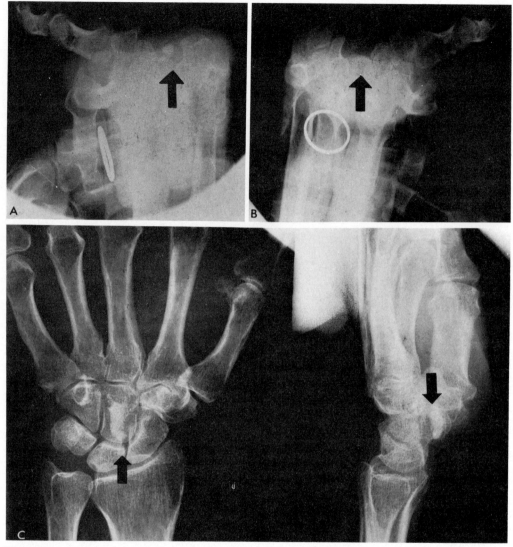

Figure 222. Patient is a 20 year old female. Spontaneous onset with typical gradual increase in pain and numbness of index and long fingers. X-rays show calcified mass in the carpal tunnel. *A*, Tunnel view showing mass. *B*, The opposite wrist for comparison (see Fig. 223 for x-ray positioning). *C*, Anteroposterior and lateral views of same patient.

manifestation. The condition should be diagnosed long before this occurs.

X-RAYS. A careful radiographic study may be very valuable and should always be done. Anteroposterior, lateral and right and left oblique views may reveal spurring, osteoarthritis or actual fracture. The carpal tunnel view is extremely important (Fig. 223). Comparative views of the opposite wrist must be

done in all projections. The carpal tunnel view may show unusual configuration or, as in this case, invasion of the foreign substance.

TREATMENT. If the syndrome is diagnosed early, immobilization of the wrist may give relief since it accomplishes two things. In the first place it puts the swollen parts at rest and thus permits subsidence of the inflammation.

In the second place it prevents the tendons from sliding up and down over the nerve. If the condition does not respond promptly to conservative treatment or if it shows signs of progression it should be treated surgically. Surgical treatment is highly successful but in this area it is not for the uninitiated.

SURGICAL TECHNIQUE. A proper tourniquet is essential. After preparation of the skin, the hand is placed supine on a suitable table. There are several landmarks for the incision, which begins above the wrist directly over and parallel to the palmaris longus tendon as it passes down to its insertion into the palmar fascia. The incision is just to the ulnar side of the flexor carpi radialis tendon. It begins about 2 inches above the distal carpal crease and extends down to this crease. At this point

the cut passes laterally along this crease until the most proximal end of the thenar crease is reached. It then extends distally into the palm along the thenar crease to a point where the thenar muscle mass terminates (Fig. 224). The skin flap is reflected, including the attachment of the palmaris longus which is left in the flap.

The palmar carpal ligament is readily defined as a broad transverse band extending from the thenar to the hypothenar eminence. Its proximal and distal margins are defined. An instrument is passed under the ligament and along the flexor tendons. The entire breadth of the ligament is carefully divided, the incision being protected by an underlying instrument (a grooved director or hemostat). The tunnel is now carefully explored by displacing the ten-

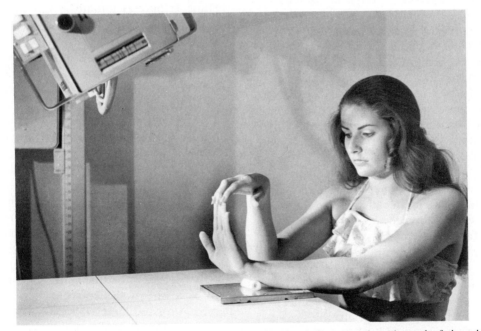

Figure 223. Radiographic position for carpal canal. With the patient seated at the end of the table, extend the forearm parallel with the long axis of the table. Center the radial styloid to the center of the cassette. Place a 2 centimeter thickness roll of gauze or plastic foam under the wrist. Hyperextend the wrist until the hand is in a vertical position slightly rotated radially to prevent superimposition of the hamate and pisiform bones. Let the patient hold this position with the opposite hand. With the tube angulated 25 to 30 degrees to the long axis of the hand, direct the central ray approximately 3 centimeters above the base of the fourth metacarpal.

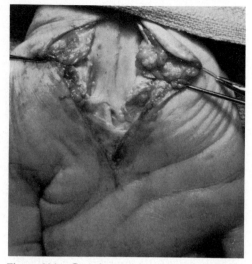

Figure 224. Carpal tunnel syndrome, classic. Constriction of the palmar carpal ligament. Note the palmar carpal ligament has been resected and reflected with the retractor.

dons out of the groove to permit careful inspection. The median nerve is readily visible together with the many tendons. If there is extensive synovial thickening, it should be removed very carefully to expose the underlying structures. If there is definite constriction of the median nerve, a saline neurolysis, accomplished by inserting a small needle into the nerve sheath above the constriction and forcing saline within the sheath to dilate it at the constricted area, is advisable. This is probably less traumatic than mechanical neurolysis, which entails splitting the sheath by sharp dissection. If irreversible changes of the nerve have not occurred recovery will be complete. Great care must be taken not to damage the recurrent thenar branches of the median nerve which usually come off the main trunk of the median nerve just proximal to the distal edge of the ligament. The cut edges of the ligament should be trimmed back to leave at least a ½ inch defect as an assurance against reunion of the palmar carpal ligament. A forearm splint is applied for protection for two or three weeks, depending on

how well the wound heals and on the extent of the pathologic condition found. The fingers should be left free after the first 48 hours.

Ulnar Nerve Entrapment

Very similar to the carpal tunnel syndrome is the entrapment of the ulnar nerve branches to the fourth and fifth fingers and to the intrinsic muscles of the hand. As the ulnar nerve winds around the hook of the hamate it may get caught between this bone and the overlying ligament. The etiology of this condition is more often chronic overuse of the wrist than acute injury. The symptoms pertain to the ulnar nerve and include pain along the hypothenar eminence and in the fourth and fifth fingers. The entrapment may cause aching through the palm and cramping of the intrinsic muscles. Paresthesias of the skin are frequent. This condition is long lasting. It may eventuate in atrophy of the intrinsic muscles of the hand, since this deep branch of the ulnar nerve does supply almost all of the intrinsic muscles of the hand. Because of the relatively less vulnerable superficial branch of the ulnar nerve, there may be no sensory involvement. This makes the condition even more puzzling. Surgical treatment is indicated if this condition does not respond promptly to immobilization. The nerve or ligament should not be injected with any local anesthetic, since this can only increase the pressure. Surgical release of the ligament will usually suffice, for surgical release of the ligament and fascial tissue overlying the nerve will usually permit complete recovery if the condition has not persisted for too long.

Strain or Fracture of the Pisiform Bone

Anatomically the pisiform does not actually make up a part of the carpal joints. Basically it lies within the tendon of the flexor carpi ulnaris but it has a small articulation with the hamate and this attachment, continuing down to the carpus through the ligament, connects the pisiform to the carpus. Forcible strain on the flexor carpi ulnaris tendon may cause injury here quite similar to that of injury around the patella. The tendon may avulse the pisiform (Fig. 225). The pisiform may be pulled loose from its attachments or the bone may actually break. The injury commonly occurs from a fall on the outstretched hand when the wrist is in dorsiflexion and the tendon is stretched tight. Tenderness along the palmar aspect of the hand often sharply localized over the pisiform bone should lead one to suspect pisiform damage. On careful examination the flexor carpi ulnaris tendon can be palpated to its attachment in the bone and determination made of the exact location of the lesion. Both dorsiflexion of the wrist with radial deviation and active contraction of the flexor carpi ulnaris will cause pain. X-ray ex-

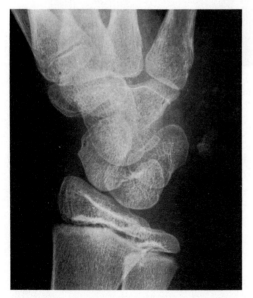

Figure 225. Avulsion of the pisiform by the flexor carpi ulnaris tendon. Bone removed and tendon repaired to the carpus.

amination may or may not reveal involvement of the bone.

TREATMENT. The condition is treated as a strain. Acute dislocation of the pisiform may occur and should be recognized by comparing x-rays of the two wrists (Fig. 226). A carpal tunnel view is unusually valuable here. It is not possible to reduce and hold this bone by closed methods due to the distracting effect of the tone of the flexor carpi ulnaris muscle. Early open reduction with threaded K-wire fixation of the bone to the carpus and repair of the ligaments may be effective. Much more often the bone should be removed and the tendinous attachment of the flexor carpi ulnaris secured to the adjacent carpal capsular ligaments (Fig. 227).

If rupture is complete and the pisiform is dislocated, it should be removed and the tendon repaired. If the condition is treated as a contusion the progress of recovery will be disappointing, since constant re-injury by use of the involved muscle may prolong and even prevent recovery. In a chronic injury in this region calcification within the tendon is quite prone to occur, the result of a chronic tendinitis with degenerative change or of calcific deposit within the hematoma.

Injury of the Triangular Cartilage

The fibrocartilaginous extension of the radiocarpal joint lying between the ulna and the carpus is subject to injury in sprains or fractures about the lower end of the forearm. The symptoms are of tenderness and pain not on the ulnar styloid but in the sulcus between the ulna and carpus. This is particularly elicited by lateral motion of the wrist, either by impingement as the wrist is pulled into adduction or by distraction as it is pulled into radial flexion. Rupture of the fibers of this ligamentous and

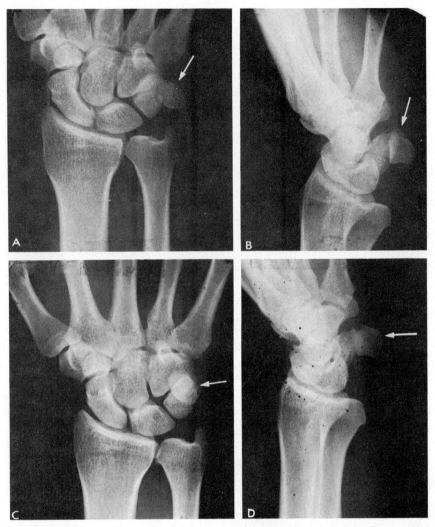

Figure 226. Acute injury to the wrist. Original x-ray interpreted as negative. Comparable multiple views of each wrist show the dislocated pisiform. *A* and *B*, Anteroposterior and oblique views showing dislocation. *C* and *D*, The normal wrist for comparison.

cartilaginous structure may result in hemorrhage and degeneration. Calcification is a late manifestation of this same condition.

TREATMENT. During the acute phase this condition will ordinarily respond well to immobilization although it is quite prone to recur. In the chronic stage local injection of an anesthetic plus a corticoid into the area may give considerable relief. If relief cannot be obtained the cartilage may be excised including the calcified area. Care should be taken not to damage the ulnar collateral ligament. If the ulnar collateral ligament is damaged it should be adequately repaired, since a large part of the stability of the wrist depends upon the integrity of this structure.

Dislocation of the Extensor Carpi Ulnaris Tendon

This tendon lies in a groove along the medial side of the distal ulna. Dislocation is manifested by a feeling of slipping as the wrist is rotated, and by pain in the area. Attempts to hold the extensor in the groove are not often successful. The condition will usually become symptom-free except for the slipping and requires no particular treatment.

GANGLION

Ganglion, which has been previously discussed (page 85), has a predilection for the dorsum of the wrist, where it often causes disability particularly on forceful use. There is lively controversy as to the exact cause of the mass, many believing it to be a degenerative change and others considering it a synovial herniation either from the carpal joints or from one of the tendon sheaths. It probably arises from a variety of causes. In the wrist it usually presents itself as a soft, fluctuant, nontender mass distal to the dorsal carpal

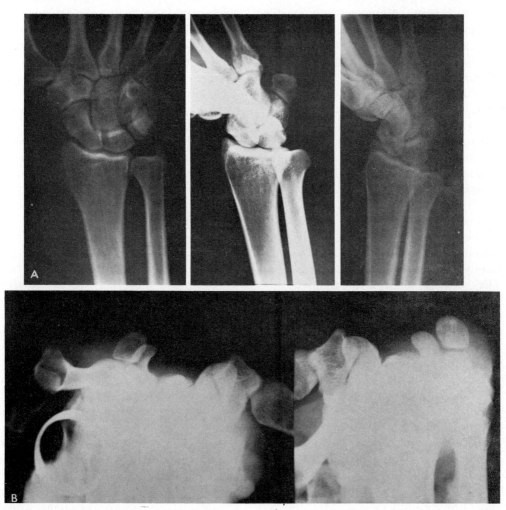

Figure 227. *A*, Patient "sprained his wrist" six months before and experienced constant pain with impairment of grip. Note subluxation of pisiform; symptoms relieved by excision of the pisiform and reattachment of the tendon to the carpal ligaments. *B*, Carpal tunnel view; note the narrowing of the joint between the pisiform and triquetrum, demonstrating some displacement as compared to the opposite side. (For x-ray positioning, see Fig. 223.)

ligament. It may protrude between any of the various tendons of the back of the hand but seems to be most common directly over the capitate. The condition seems to follow chronic strain or chronic sprain of the wrist but in many instances there is no history of trauma. It must be differentiated from an effusion within the tendon sheath and from other types of soft tissue tumor. Sometimes amazingly firm, it may feel like a cartilaginous or bony mass under the skin. The mass is usually movable but not freely so since it has a firm underlying attachment. Effusion in a tendon sheath is infrequent on the back of the wrist and it is ordinarily not as firm as a ganglion and is more linear. In the case of the firm tumor, x-ray examination should be made to rule out possible bone involvement.

TREATMENT. A ganglion may spontaneously regress and disappear altogether, or it may disappear and then reappear. The time-honored methods of breaking the sac and of aspiration will usually fail. I have not had satisfactory results from the injection of corticoid, as has been reported by others. If the mass is troublesome, causes pain or is too unsightly, it should be removed surgically. The success of surgical removal depends upon adequate repair of whatever defect is found. Sometimes the tumor can be dissected out intact. In still other instances it will be diffuse so that the presenting part is comparable to the top of an iceberg in that the mass covers a good deal of the posterior carpus beneath the tendons. If the ligaments are split or if there is a defect in the capsule of the wrist, careful suture is necessary after removal of the ganglion. If there is a pedicle communicating to the tendon or carpal joints, as is often the case, it should be carefully closed. After removal of a ganglion the hand is immobilized in a cock-up wrist splint for at least three weeks. True enough, this

may result in some restriction of motion of the wrist which may persist for several weeks, but in my experience recurrence is much less likely if the wrist is protected during the healing period.

Ganglion may occur on the palmar aspect of the wrist or on the flexor tendons to the fingers. Treatment is the same whatever the location.

SPRAIN-SUBLUXATION-FRACTURE-DISLOCATION

Since by our definition *sprain* is a ligament injury, it is relatively uncommon in the wrist. Most of the so-called sprains—and the diagnosis is a frequent one—are not sprains at all but are strains of the tendon attachments or injuries to the bone. The ligaments of the wrist permit a large amount of motion in the radiocarpal joint but very little motion in the intercarpal joints. The massive ligaments on the volar aspect of the wrist are so strong that in hyperextension the injury is more likely to be a fracture of the carpal bones which may be incomplete or a contusion of the articular surfaces or possibly chondral fracture, rather than a tearing of the ligaments. It is felt by some that in hyperextension there may be actual slipping of one row of carpals on the other which permits damage to the dorsal carpal ligaments although this is rather difficult to demonstrate. Suffice it to say that in the very common dorsiflexion injury of the wrist, the damage is usually on the dorsal aspect. One should therefore be very wary of the diagnosis of sprain of the wrist, i.e., ligament damage, in the common dorsiflexion injury. On dorsiflexion of the wrist pain is more frequent over the back of the wrist and forearm than over the front although the greatest stress on the ligament would appear to have been on the volar side. If there is tenderness over the carpus, careful x-ray study should be made and the carpal bones closely studied as to both their position and condition.

If the x-ray study is negative, as it usually is, and a diagnosis of "sprain" is made, the *treatment* is by immobilization with the wrist in slight dorsiflexion for two or three weeks, unless the symptoms completely subside before this time, and by physical therapy. If facilities permit, the splints may be removed for daily treatment always within the limits of pain-free motion. When athletic participation is permitted the wrist should be carefully strapped to prevent re-injury, since these conditions tend to be quite chronic. At the end of the period of immobilization further x-ray study should be carried out since linear fractures through the carpal bones may well be revealed in this second picture when they did not show in the first. The common carpal fracture is through the navicular at its midpoint since the navicular takes a good deal of stress of the wrist, whether it be in dorsiflexion or palmar flexion, because of its position bridging the two rows of carpals.

Subluxation and *dislocation* may accompany ligament injury and in the wrist they have some peculiar characteristics. Dislocation of the radiocarpal joint is extremely uncommon although it has happened as a result of violent action (Fig. 232). A complete carpal dislocation is also uncommon and is obviously a serious injury (Fig. 233). Both of these conditions present manifest deformity and disability, hence are readily diagnosed and ordinarily receive good treatment. The diagnosis of the exact dislocation through the carpus offers great difficulty, but careful x-ray study of the normal as well as the injured wrist in several positions will cut down the margin of error. It is particularly important that these conditions be diagnosed early since, as with most dislocations, the longer the dislocation remains unreduced the greater will be the likelihood of recurrence and of permanent residual disability. So in the presence of major swelling, pain and particularly deformity of the wrist, prompt definitive treatment must be sought if there is any question as to the extent of injury or the perfection of reduction.

Dislocation of the Lunate (Semilunar Bone)

The most common dislocation in the wrist is of the lunate (Fig. 228). The shape of this bone lying between the massive capitate and the lower end of the radius makes it particularly prone to volar dislocation since the bone is narrow in its dorsal portion and quite wide at its volar margin. Forceful compression of the lunate against the capitate by dorsiflexion of the wrist slips this bone forward much in the manner of an apple seed pinched between the fingers (Fig. 228, *B*). The dorsal carpal ligament, which is attached to the lunate, gives

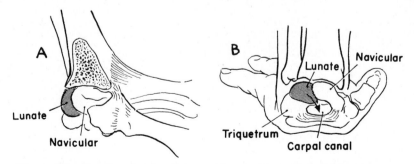

Figure 228. Drawing showing dislocated lunate. (From McLaughlin, Trauma.)

way and the lunate slips forward, its convex proximal surface lodging along the undersurface of the capitate. If the dislocation is more pronounced the bone may be completely extruded from the space and may locate almost anywhere on the volar surface of the carpus. If the disrupting force is relatively mild the subluxation or dislocation may reduce spontaneously, but the damage to the dorsal carpal ligament will remain. Indeed, this may be the mechanism of sprains of the wrist in which the force is dorsiflexion but the ligament injured is actually on the side that is not overstretched.

It is extremely easy to overlook a dislocation of the lunate (Figs. 229 and 230). Clinically, the wrist will be painful. It will be tender on the dorsum just distal to the lower end of the radius. Brawny swelling will usually prevent palpation of the space where the lunate should be. On the palmar aspect of the wrist, particularly if it is examined early, there is a palpable thickened area under the flexor tendons, quite unlike the corresponding area on the opposite wrist. Motion may not be acutely painful if the lunate is not locked under the volar ligaments; if the lunate is locked, motion may be completely prevented. In such a case careful x-ray study will reveal the deformity, particularly if the film is compared to a similar one of the opposite wrist.

Occasionally the displacement will be accompanied by neurological symptoms since the extruded lunate tends to compress the carpal tunnel. Frequently there will be paresthesia and pain in the median distribution of the hand, i.e., the first and second fingers, but in the acute injury these are easily overlooked be-

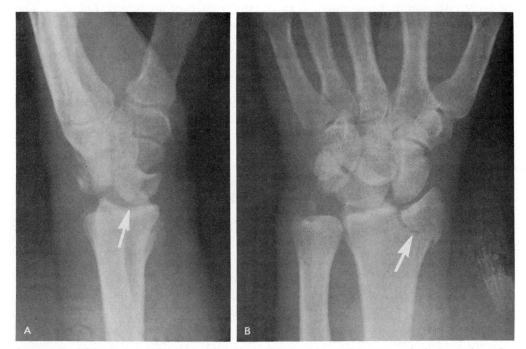

Figure 229. Dislocated carpal lunate. The patient fell forcibly on the outstretched arm and another player fell over him. Note *(A)* the complete forward displacement of the lunate in relation to the carpus. *B,* Anteroposterior view shows the fracture of the styloid of the radius and styloid of ulna. The carpal dislocation was overlooked in treating the radius and ulna. It was recognized later and the lunate was removed with consequent disability.

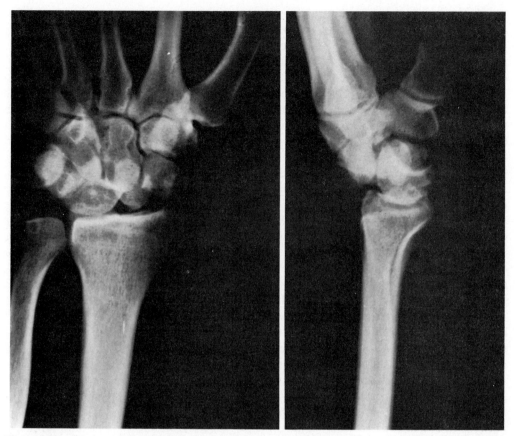

Figure 230. Fracture dislocation of the wrist. Note that in this case the navicular fractured and the lunate dislocated. Compare to Figure 229 in which the navicular remained intact and the radial styloid fractured as the lunate dislocated.

cause of the pain. It has been aptly said that the sprained wrist accompanied by symptoms of involvement of the median nerve in the hand is an indication of lunate dislocation (Fig. 228, *B*).

Treatment of these cases is often casual until late complications call attention to the diagnosis. By that time successful treatment will be virtually impossible. If the diagnosis can be made early, manipulative treatment is highly successful. Under complete anesthesia, straight traction combined with moderate dorsiflexion of the wrist opens up the space from which the lunate was displaced and direct pressure against the lunate on the volar surface of the wrist will slip it into position. Once the bone is reduced the wrist should be moderately flexed. This tends to close the space again and maintain the proper position. Following reduction the wrist is protected by splinting in semiflexion for three weeks. It should then be moved into a neutral position for the fourth week. After this it is protected against dorsiflexion for several more weeks, particularly if athletic competition is to be permitted. It should be emphasized that closed reduction should be prompt if it is to be successful. If the bone is going to reduce at all, it will reduce by gentle manipulation. Force is neither necessary nor advisable. If closed reduction fails, open reduction should be carried out.

In far too many cases the diagnosis is not made early and the patients present themselves several days or several weeks after the injury. Closed reduction should not be attempted after the lapse of more than a week since then it is virtually impossible to open the space and reduce the bone. Even if the dislocation is reduced it is with so much attendant trauma that necrosis is inevitable. Open operation is relatively successful if carried out within the first few weeks. After this period removal of the bone is probably more desirable than an attempt to force the lunate into its normal position. As is true in other dislocations, the longer the lunate remains dislocated, the greater is the likelihood of circulatory changes. For this reason many surgeons advise removal of the bone if it has remained dislocated more than two or three weeks. However, this does not give a normal wrist and I believe that in the athlete one should attempt reduction of the bone even if this means it later must be removed because of avascular necrosis. As might be expected, a dorsal incision is much to be preferred, and for two pertinent reasons. In the first place, considerable damage may be done to the remaining blood supply if the bone is dissected out from the front, since the only remaining attachment to the lunate is the volar ligament. Secondly, it is necessary to traverse very vital structures on the volar aspect of the wrist in order to reach the dislocated bone. Dorsal exposure, while it may present some difficulties in actually reaching the bone, will be much less traumatic from both standpoints. In the very late case in which a firm decision has been made to remove the bone, a volar incision should be made. I cannot emphasize too strongly that the principal peril in these wrist injuries is that the true diagnosis will be overlooked and hence the ideal opportunity for definitive treatment will be lost. Any of the other carpal bones may be dislocated although this is quite uncommon.

Perilunar Dislocation

In dislocation of the lunate this bone dislocates in relation to both the radius and the carpus so that there is a true dislocation of the lunate alone. In the so-called perilunar dislocation (Fig. 231) the lunate remains with the radius, and the carpus dislocates on the lunate and radius. This is almost never a pure dislocation. Usually either the navicular bone dislocates and the whole bone remains with the radius and the lunate or, more commonly, the navicular fractures at its vulnerable waist and its proximal fragment remains with the lunate and the radius. There are many possible combinations; for example, the entire proximal row of carpal bones may remain with the radius and the dislocation be intercarpal, or any combination of these bones may remain with the radius.

TREATMENT. This is an extremely serious type of fracture-dislocation and bodes ill for normal function of the wrist. For this reason this type of dislocation should be handled by the specialist. It is extremely important not only to get a perfect reduction but to maintain it. This dislocation is notably unstable because of the extensive damage to the carpal ligaments. Each of the carpal bones must fit exactly against the other if function is to be normal. Even if reduction of the displacement is obtained, one still must deal with the fracture so that the overall problem becomes very complicated. Time is of the very essence since the dislocation rapidly becomes irreducible because of massive fibrosis through the wrist. Should this occur, wrist fusion is practically the only procedure offering some salvage of function of the wrist.

Chronic arthritic changes are com-

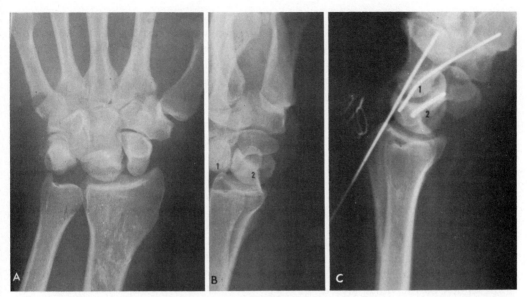

Figure 231. Perilunar dislocation. Note that the lunate has remained with the radius whereas the rest of the carpus is dislocated dorsally. This case is unusual in that the navicular is intact. Frequently the proximal half of the navicular remains with the lunate, the remainder of the bone dislocating with the rest of the carpus. The "1" on the dome of the greater multangular in *B* should appose "2" on the concavity of the lunate as in view *C*.

mon in these fracture-dislocations even under the most favorable circumstances. It behooves one to be precisely analytical in his studies of these obviously serious injuries to the wrist. X-ray diagnosis of a fracture-dislocation through the carpus is difficult and only by very careful study, with x-ray comparison of the injured wrist and the normal one, can one have a reasonable hope of success. One should be particularly suspicious in the sprain that is slow to recover or of the wrist that feels thick from front to back. For this reason no wrist injury should be treated for a long period of time without repeated careful observation since the deformity, which may be obscured by swelling, may become quite evident once the swelling has been reduced.

Dislocation of the Navicular

A rather unusual injury of the carpus is dislocation of the navicular.

This injury is much more readily determined by x-ray study since the radial-carpal relationship is more obviously disturbed than in the lunate dislocation. It is unusual for this dislocation to occur as an isolated injury; it is frequently the residual of an incompletely reduced perilunar or intercarpal dislocation.

TREATMENT. If the dislocation is seen and recognized early it may be reduced by manipulation. The wrist is placed in complete ulnar flexion to open up the space between the styloid of the radius and carpus, after which the navicular may be rotated in position by direct pressure of the fingers. It must be obvious that this can be much more readily accomplished early than late. As with most dislocations, the longer the navicular remains displaced, the more likelihood there is of an aseptic necrosis of the bone. If the dislocation is recognized after several weeks, an attempt at open reduction may be carried out. If to obtain open reduction the navicular will have to be forced into position or held in position by forcible radial flexion of the wrist, it may be advisable instead to remove it. However, if there seems to be some possibility of restoration of the circulation to the bone, reduction can be tried and fusion of the wrist or excision of the navicular done at a later operation if the first procedure fails.

Sprain-Fracture

Avulsion of the ligament from the bone results in a sprain-fracture. Careful x-ray study made in various positions may reveal the flake of bone lifted up from one of the carpals or from the lower radius or the ulnar styloid. As a general rule, sprain-fractures require longer for union than simple sprain. In some instances painful nonunion may develop between the flake of bone and the parent bone. In such a case it may be necessary to remove the fragment surgically and suture the tendon to its original bed.

Avulsion of the Ulnar Styloid

The styloid process of the ulna may be pulled off by the ulnar collateral ligament. This is in reality an injury to the ulnar collateral ligament and should be treated as such. It usually will heal with fibrous union without instability. If instability does occur, or if the area is painful on function, the styloid should be removed and the ligament sutured to the lower end of the ulna.

Avulsion of the Radial Styloid

The styloid process of the radius is not as vulnerable as is the styloid of the ulna, nor are its ligament attachments as strong. Usually a force that will break the styloid of the radius will either tear the radiocarpal ligament or break the lower end of the radius. A sharp ulnar flexion of the wrist with little or no dorsal component may cause avulsion of the radial styloid (Fig. 234). In such a case the symptoms will be those of sprain. There will be pain on ulnar deviation of the wrist but little pain on flexion and extension. The tenderness will be at the tip of the styloid just at the base of the thumb. Careful examination will distinguish between tenderness over the navicular or over the base of the metacarpal of the thumb and that over the radial styloid. These areas are all subcutaneous and can be readily palpated. In palpating the dorsal surface of the radius one may be misled into believing that the condition is a sprain, since the tenderness will be lateral rather than dorsal. Any injury of this severity merits x-ray films taken in anteroposterior, lateral and oblique planes. Careful study of the films will be necessary to reveal the precise nature of the lesion. A very small fragment, hardly recognizable in the x-ray, should be treated as a carpal sprain. On the other hand, a significant amount of the styloid may be pulled away (Fig. 234). Poorly planned x-ray films may fail to reveal the displacement.

TREATMENT. Since this fracture involves the articular surface of the radiocarpal joint, it is subject to the same prerequisites of treatment as are articular fractures elsewhere. The fragment must be perfectly reduced and firmly held until union is secure or it must be removed and the ligament sutured to the radius. If the fragment is as substantial as in Figure 234, where it involves roughly two-fifths of the articular surface, it should be replaced. The main problem is recognition of the nature of the injury. It will be futile to try to replace the fragment and maintain fixation by any bizarre position of the wrist. Internal fixation is an absolute necessity.

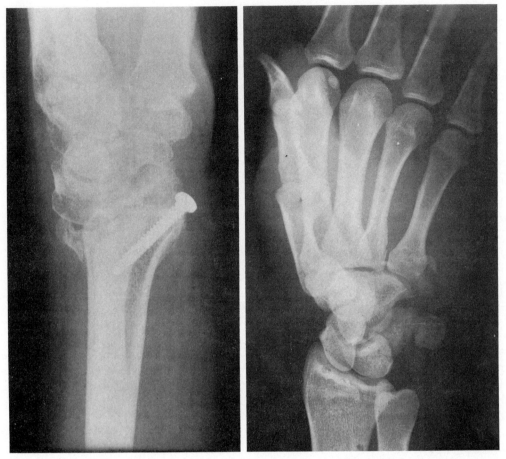

Figure 232   Figure 233

Figure 232. Radiocarpal dislocation. Result of a serious injury to the wrist. There was a fracture of the radial styloid which was reduced and held by a transfixion screw. The dislocation of the entire carpus on the lower end of the radius was not held reduced. Wrist fusion was the only solution to this painful wrist.

Figure 233. Fracture of hamate caused by forcible dorsiflexion and ulnar deviation of the wrist. At operation for removal of these fragments there was found to be very extensive ligament damage to the carpus indicating that the patient had had a carpometacarpal dislocation which had spontaneously reduced.

FRACTURE

Fracture of the Navicular

For reasons previously mentioned, the most common carpal fracture is of the navicular. The fact that the navicular bridges the intercarpal joint, that it is directly impinged upon by the lower radius on dorsiflexion and radial deviation of the wrist, and that it has a rather narrow waist all contribute to this injury (Figs. 235 and 236). The force is usually hyperextension as by falling on the outstretched hand—a force similar to that causing lunate dislocation or Colles' fracture. Following such an injury there will be pain through the wrist, not at the lower end of the radius but just distal to it. Careful x-ray study may well be negative. The diagnosis of sprain of the wrist is acceptable here if one is prepared to treat the sprain adequately, that is, by immobilization of the wrist for two or three weeks. At the end of

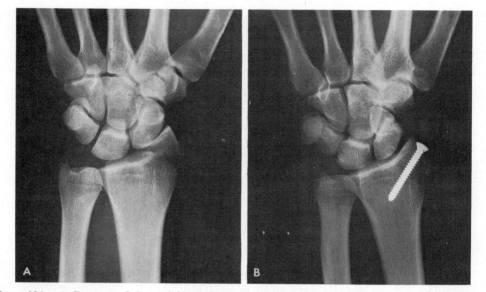

Figure 234. *A,* Fracture of the styloid of the radius; presumably the fragment was pulled off by the lateral ligament. *B,* Note perfect union one month following screw fixation.

two weeks the wrist should be re-x-rayed, care being taken to get oblique views (Fig. 237). Frequently a fracture line will be revealed in this second x-ray (Fig. 238). If the x-ray in two weeks is negative and symptoms still persist after four or five weeks, films should again be made with the wrist in various positions since the assumption must be that there is a fracture of the navicular until it can definitely be ruled out.

The *treatment of an undisplaced*

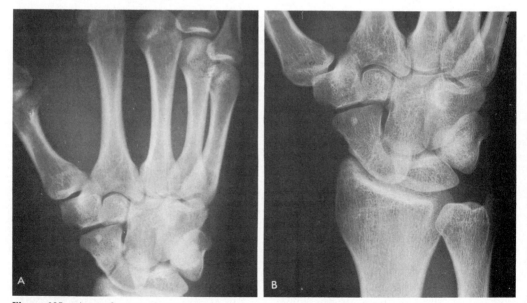

Figure 235. Acute fracture through the wrist of the carpal navicular (*A*). Treated by plaster cast with solid union four months later (*B*).

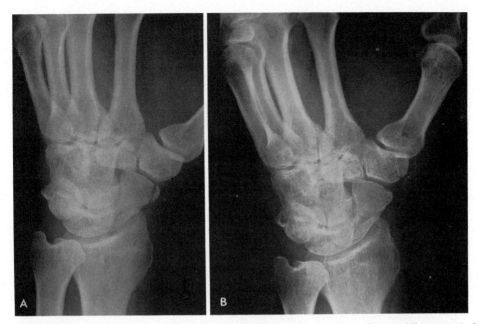

Figure 236. *A*, Avulsion fracture of the carpal navicular by traction on the radiocarpal ligament. *B*, Solid union four months later following cast immobilization.

fracture of the navicular is immobilization for a period long enough to permit the fracture to heal completely. This will be many weeks or months. The progress of union should be checked by x-ray. The original dressing should be anterior and posterior splints extending from the proximal interphalangeal joints to below the elbow with the wrist in slight dorsiflexion. The first phalanx of the thumb is included. This type of fixation is continued for a variable time depending upon the amount of swelling. If there is little reaction in the hand and no danger of constriction, a solid cast may be applied at the first visit. In the presence of considerable swelling, however, plaster splints with some compression are used instead, the cast being postponed until the size of the wrist has somewhat stabilized. In any event immobilization should be early and complete, with the hand in the grasping position. No bizarre position of the wrist is either necessary or desirable. Since complete immobilization is important

(Fig. 239) the gauntlet cast should be changed if it becomes loose, as it usually does. This may require a change of cast every two or three weeks, at which time the x-ray check of the progress of union should be made. When union appears to be secure across the fracture line, as revealed in a good oblique x-ray picture, the gauntlet may be supplanted by a leather wristlet or adhesive strapping. If athletic competition is to be permitted, dorsiflexion of the wrist must be prevented by an adequate support. In the fracture without displacement it may not be necessary to immobilize the thumb. My own practice is to include the base of the thumb to the metacarpophalangeal joint and thus permit phalangeal but not metacarpal motion.

In a complete fracture and particularly *in fracture with displacement or instability,* the type of immobilization described will not be adequate. The management of such a fracture requires the utmost in skill and judgment. If

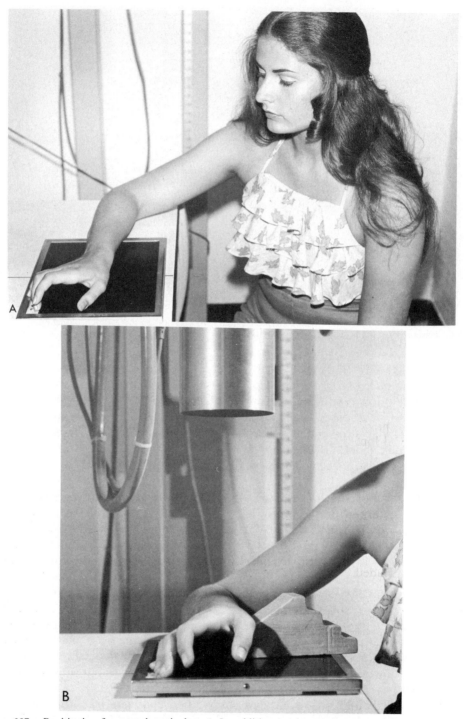

Figure 237. Positioning for carpal navicular. *A,* In addition to the routine views it is often helpful to position the patient's wrist in a routine anteroposterior view but with as much lateral deviation as possible. *B,* The oblique view is best obtained by supporting the palm of the hand on a non-opaque object such as a 35 degree angle balsa wood block. The wrist should be abducted as much as the patient can tolerate.

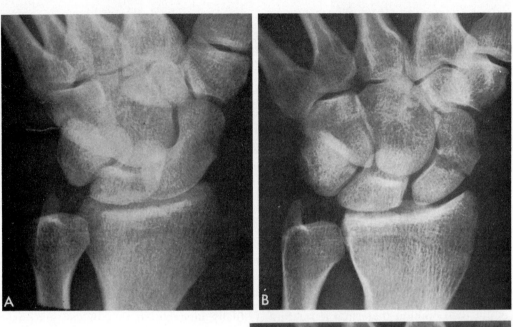

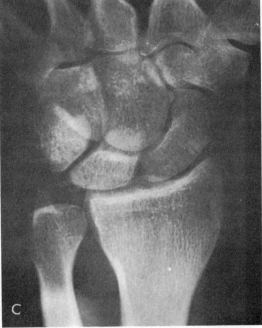

Figure 238. *A*, Acute sprain of the wrist. Note normal appearing navicular on the day of injury. *B*, Two weeks later showing some separation. *C*, Following several months of immobilization. Note the union.

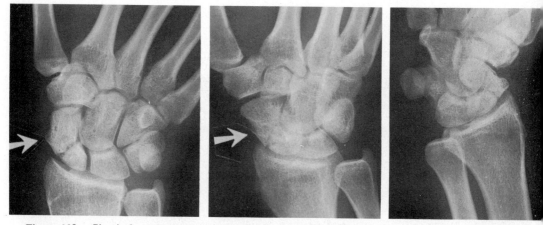

Figure 239. Classic fracture through the waist of the navicular showing fibrous healing with spur formation following inadequate immobilization.

there is displacement an attempt may be made by manipulation to reduce the fragments. The hand is checked in radial deviation or in ulnar deviation, flexion or extension, to determine what position makes the fragments the most stable. It is my own opinion that such a fracture should be treated by operation to obtain perfect reduction and held with transfixion screw or pins. By this method immobilization can be assured at the fracture site although at the expense of some further sacrifice of circulation to the fragments. If the fracture line is actually unstable so that in various positions the fragments can be shown to

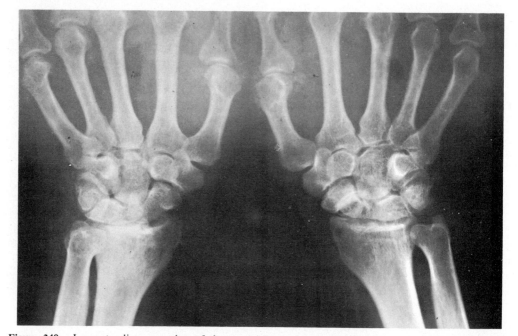

Figure 240. Long-standing nonunion of the carpal navicular fracture which occurred in football. Patient is now 60 with advanced degenerative arthritis of the radiocarpal joint and sclerosis of the adjacent margins of the fragments.

move on each other, it is extremely un-likely that simple immobilization of the wrist will prevent motion. Indeed, im-mobilization of the wrist does not pre-vent rotation of the forearm and in rota-tion of the forearm there is inevitably some torsion at the radiocarpal joint.

Following operation the same treat-ment should be carried out as for a frac-ture without displacement. The after-care of such a fracture requires sound judgment. There seems little justifica-tion for continuing immobilization for many months if union does not appear to be progressing or if the fragment has become sclerotic or cystic. True enough, prolonged immobilization has in some cases finally resulted in bony union, but in my experience these are few and far between. The displaced fracture that has been unrecognized and is discovered after several weeks is also probably doomed to nonunion. In the x-ray study as the union or nonunion de-velops, decision must be made in each case on whether to continue immobiliza-tion or to recommend some other type of treatment. If union is not at least pro-ceeding satisfactorily after three or four months, I would advise removal of the external fixation to allow function of the wrist.

Many of these ununited fractures are entirely pain-free and allow remark-ably good wrist function (Fig. 240). If this is the case surgery is not advisable, since any type of open reduction and grafting for delayed union or nonunion has a high percentage of failure. If symptoms persist and are disabling (Fig. 241) then one must consider the various possibilities for treatment of nonunion. I know of no treatment that can promise a normal wrist and the choice is a very difficult one. One must depend to a large extent upon the nature and condition of the navicular bone. If there is carpal ar-thritis and particularly arthritis of the radiocarpal joint, solid union of the na-

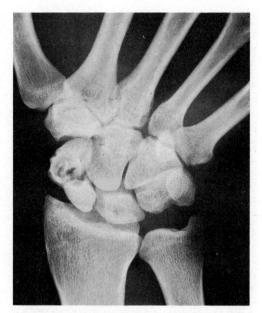

Figure 241. Untreated fractured navicular with resultant cystic changes and considerable dis-ability. This type of case is not amenable to bone grafting. The salvage procedure here would proba-bly be radial styloidectomy although this would not completely relieve the symptoms.

vicular will not relieve the symptoms (Figs. 242 and 243). If the fracture is central and the bone fragments are rela-tively viable, bone grafting should be at-tempted and is frequently successful. Since following this procedure there often will be chrondral damage around the fracture site, it is advisable to re-move the styloid of the radius (Figs. 242 and 243) so that the fracture line does not articulate across the lower end of the radius. Indeed, if the arthritis is local-ized to this area, a radial styloidectomy may be the treatment of choice either with or without grafting of the navicular. If, on the other hand, one fragment is small or there is comminution of one or the other fragment, these fragments should be removed (Fig. 244). Indeed, this probably should be done as a pri-mary procedure in such a case. Because of the very poor prognosis in nonunion, it is extremely important that these frac-tures be diagnosed early, since treatment

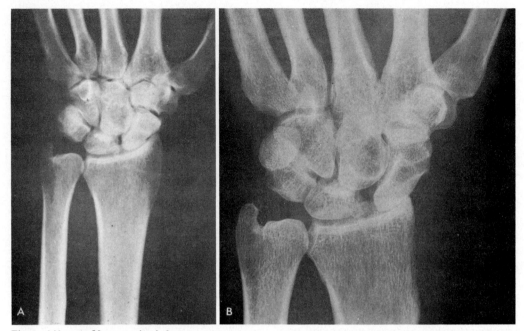

Figure 242. *A,* Unrecognized fracture through the waist of the carpal navicular which has gone on to union but with marked narrowing of the joint space and radiocarpal arthritis. This house painter was unable to work. *B,* His symptoms were ameliorated by radial styloidectomy.

of the acute fracture is highly successful while treatment of the nonunion is very unsatisfactory.

Should one be allowed to participate in sports following a fracture of the navicular? Most teams will not allow a member to wear a plaster cast; therefore, he should not be allowed to participate during the period in which union may still be expected. If injury has occured in spring practice and several months have elapsed and union is not expected, should the patient be allowed to participate? I have permitted this where it seemed that nonunion was inevitable and there was no justification for further immobilization. I recall one player who "sprained" his wrist in spring practice. The navicular fracture was revealed after several weeks and he was treated by immobilization throughout the summer without union and was permitted to play the following season wearing a suitable leather gauntlet. At

the end of the season, bone grafting was carried out (Fig. 245). Whether or not this is justifiable I think depends upon the drive of the particular patient and the importance to him of his participation.

Compression Fracture

Since the carpus is made up entirely of cancellous bone and since it is subject to compression forces such as a fall on the clenched fist or on the outstretched hand, it would seem that compression fractures of the carpal bones should be frequent. The fact that they are so rarely diagnosed does not necessarily mean they rarely occur. I am sure that many of the so-called sprains of the wrist which improve with that tardiness which is so aggravating to the athlete may well be compression fractures of the carpals. Diagnosis is virtually impossible by early x-ray. Later x-rays which might be expected to show some

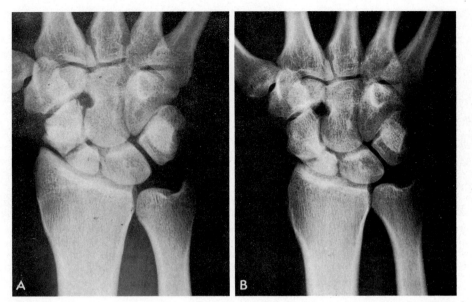

Figure 243. *A,* Fracture of middle third of navicular with nonunion and bone spurring on navicular and radial styloid. *B,* Treated by excision of the radial styloid and bone graft with navicular pegs. Solid union. Good clinical result.

atrophy or condensation of bone are extremely difficult to interpret because many of the bones are superimposed. Clinically the diagnosis of compression fracture is also difficult since the ordinary findings of this fracture are quite confusing at the wrist. Local tenderness is present whether the injury is a sprain

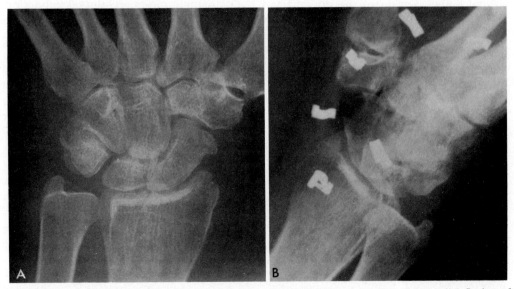

Figure 244. *A,* Compression fracture of the body of the navicular caused by sharp radial flexion of the wrist so that the bone is impinged between the radial styloid and triquetrum.

B, This painful injury was relieved by removal of the fragment. Athletics resumed. If recognized early, this condition should be treated by immobilization with the wrist in ulnar flexion so that the carpal capsule will tend to pull the fragment back into position.

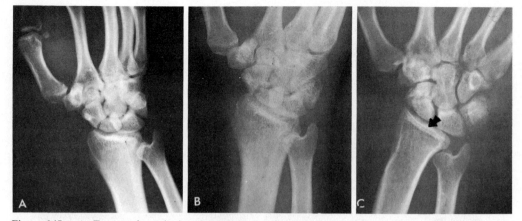

Figure 245. *A*, Fractured navicular through the wrist as an acute injury. This was immobilized in plaster for four months *(B)* with no bony union. The patient was allowed to play football with the arm carefully protected in a brace and at the end of the season radial styloidectomy with peg grafts of the navicular was carried out with solid union *(C)*. Arrow indicates well preserved radial navicular joint space.

or a fracture. Pain on forced motion is also likely in either. The unusual fact that many of the "sprains" of the dorsum of the wrist are caused by dorsiflexion forces may give a clue. It is possible that many of these dorsal flexion "sprains" may actually be compression or chondral fractures of one or the other carpal bones. Sprain of the dorsal ligaments of the wrist is caused by palmar flexion, which puts stress on these ligaments. Dorsal flexion is the usual force in the so-called sprain of the wrist but this puts no stress on the dorsal ligaments. On the contrary, dorsal flexion puts all the stress on the palmar side. Hence, pain on the dorsum of the wrist following falling on the outstretched hand is more likely from osteochondral damage to the dorsal part of the carpus than from sprain of the ligaments on the dorsal side. For this reason careful re-x-ray should be made after two or three weeks, particularly if pain persists on the dorsum. There may be fragmentation of the edges of the bones. Even though early x-rays are negative, a period of immobilization is imperative so that any chips of cartilage that may have been fissured or cracked will have a chance

to heal. This particular injury to the wrist should be treated with the wrist at neutral position or possibly with a little palmar flexion, whereas if the ligament is injured ("sprain"), the wrist should be treated in dorsal flexion. This is not difficult to determine if one has a high index of suspicion. The two conditions, i.e., palmar sprain and dorsal impaction, are easily distinguishable if one takes the trouble to make a definitive diagnosis.

No specific *treatment* is required for the acute condition other than rest and protection. Since this is also the treatment for a sprain, one does not err in applying protective support to any wrist injury provided he first assures himself that no condition is present that requires more definitive treatment. A compression fracture will heal much more slowly than the ordinary sprain. If the symptoms are persistent over a long period of time one may be unable to decide whether the lesion is a compression fracture, a synovitis or some type of chondral damage. Since all will require basically the same treatment, namely, protection against the motion that causes the pain, a definitive diagnosis may be academic except that the prognosis may be somewhat more grave in one condition than the others. The wrist should be protected against painful motion progressively by splint, by a leather wristlet, by adhesive strapping and finally by elastic wrapping. Only thus may we minimize the tendency for occurrence of chronic arthritis, which can be extremely serious in the carpus where there are so many interrelated joints. In the final analysis, the treatment for persistent chronic arthritis is fusion of the wrist. The intervening treatment should be physical therapy, local injection and other measures ordinarily employed for chronic traumatic arthritis elsewhere.

Kienböck's "Disease." The so-called Kienböck's disease (Fig. 246), which is a late involvement of the lunate, may well be the result of compression fracture of this bone. The condition is variously called osteitis, osteochondritis or malacia of the lunate and is most common in the adolescent. In this condition there is definite involvement of the lunate with bony changes, the bone going through various stages, i.e., atrophy followed by sclerosis and later decalcification, often with fragmentation resulting in marked change in shape of the bone. The deformity may be prevented by early recognition and protection. Should a youth with an osteochondritis of the lunate be permitted to participate in sports? Certainly he should not during the early stage. He should never play unless there is adequate protection applied in the nature of a gauntlet cast or a reinforced wrist and forearm splint. The period of resolution of this bone may require a couple of years. The same condition may involve the other carpal bones and requires the same treatment.

Chondral Fracture

Almost the same can be said about chondral or osteochondral fracture (see Chapter 4) as has been said above about compression fracture. It seems inevita-

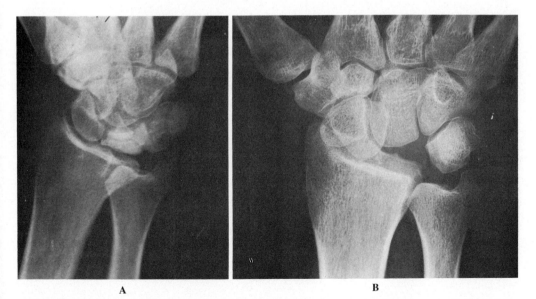

        A   B

Figure 246. *A*, Classic Kienböck's disease (osteochondritis of the lunate), old, in which the bone involuted incompletely leaving a sclerosed, deformed bone causing painful carpal function. *B*, The symptoms were relieved somewhat by removal of the carpal lunate. Early recognition of this osteochondritis and immobilization would have prevented this poor result.

ble that there will be serious damage to the cartilage of the carpus in many injuries of the wrist. These cannot be visualized by x-ray in the early stages. The late changes to be expected are those so often associated with chronic arthritis, namely, irregularity of the joint cartilage, narrowing of the joint space, painful motion and tenderness to pressure. If actual fragments of cartilage loose in the carpal joints could be recognized early, surgical excision would be the treatment of choice. They are, however, almost impossible to diagnose unless the fracture includes a small portion of bone. Many of the wrists that show small "flakes" of bone are very likely to have a rather large chondral fragment. I feel sure that if one would analyze the injury carefully and come to this conclusion, the final result would be markedly improved by early removal of this fragment. The mild chondral injury goes on to a good recovery. The moderate ones leave aching pain and pain on forced motion. The severe ones terminate in intercarpal arthritis.

SUMMARY

From the foregoing comment the conclusion is inevitable that successful treatment of the carpal injury can be expected only when one takes the pains to analyze the injury carefully. Diligent evaluation of the forces applied will be extremely rewarding. Precise clinical study with location of tender points by using the rubber end of a pencil may enable one to pinpoint the lesion. A painstaking study of the effect of the various directions of motion will give invaluable aid. In short, the treatment must depend upon a very careful and exact analysis of the condition one is treating. Only by such methods can one avoid the embarrassment and humiliation of realizing that he is dependent upon Father Time for his diagnosis. This is often to the extreme detriment of his patient. Once the lesion has been identified and a reasonable degree of recovery has occurred, rehabilitative exercises can be a major factor in preventing recurrence of the condition (see p. 804).

CHAPTER 12

INJURIES OF THE HAND

WITH GAEL FRANK, M.D.

ANATOMICAL CONSIDERATIONS

The hand is a highly complicated, intricate, mechanical device and sensory organ. Most functions of the upper extremity are directed at positioning the hand in the best manner to perform the intended task. Before undertaking any treatment of this complex organ, one should be thoroughly familiar with its functional as well as its gross anatomy and aware of the principles of treatment which have been developed over the past half century. Those not familiar with the treatment of hand injuries can do far more damage than that represented by the original injury by an oversight as simple as splinting the hand in a nonfunctional position.

Position of Function

The key to proper functioning of the hand is the overall configuration which the hand assumes in the resting position. This is known as the position of function, and it is the position which the hand assumes when the wrist is dorsiflexed approximately 45 degrees and the thumb is placed parallel with the forearm in a position of opposition to the fingers. The fingers are flexed 45

degrees at the metacarpophalangeal and interphalangeal joints. The importance of the position of function cannot be overemphasized. A hand which is stiff in a flat position is useful only as a paddle, whereas a hand which is stiff in the functional position is able to utilize even a small amount of motion to perform useful operations. In this position the intrinsic and extrinsic muscles are balanced and can perform with optimum efficiency (Fig. 247).

When the hand is in the functional position, its form assumes two arches. One is formed in a sagittal plane, with the metacarpals and phalanges forming the elements of the arch. The other arch is in the transverse plane and is seen best in the curve formed by the metacarpal heads. The transverse arch motif is carried proximally to the wrist, where the bony elements of the wrist form the carpal tunnel. The thumb represents a mobile post against which the fingers can function in pinch and grasp.

Joints and Ligaments

The bony elements of the hand are formed by the metacarpals and phalanges (Fig. 248). The metacarpal of the thumb articulates with the greater multangular in a saddle-type of joint.

323

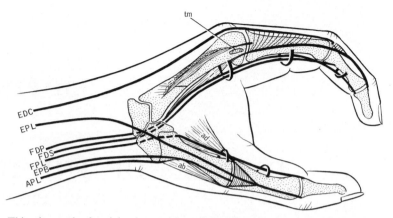

Figure 247. This shows the hand in the position of function. Notice in particular that a very small amount of motion in the thumb and fingers is useful motion in that it can be utilized in pinch and grasp. Notice the close relationship of the tendons to bone. The flexor tendons are held close to bone by a pulley-like thickening of the flexor sheath as represented schematically. With the hand in this position intrinsic and extrinsic musculature is in balance, and all muscles are acting within their physiological resting length. The key to abbreviations is as follows:

EDC, Extensor digitorum communis
EPL, Extensor pollicis longus
FDP, Flexor digitorum profundus
FDS, Flexor digitorum sublimis
FPL, Flexor pollicis longus
EPB, Extensor pollicis brevis
APL, Abductor pollicis longus

i, Interossei
tm, Transverse metacarpal ligament
l, Lumbrical
ad, Adductor pollicis brevis
ab, Abductor pollicis brevis

The capsule is thickened laterally and dorsally to form ligaments. This gives the joint a wide range of motion combined with good stability. The ulnar and radial lips of this metacarpal provide bony stability. This stability is lost when either lip, but most commonly the ulnar lip, becomes fractured. The four finger metacarpals articulate with the distal row of the carpal bones and with each other. These articulations form arthrodial, or gliding-type, joints. The metacarpals articulate with the proximal phalanges by means of a condyloid joint, a joint which allows motion in all planes except axial rotation. The interphalangeal articulations are of the ginglymus type, allowing motion in only one plane.

At the finger carpometacarpal joints very little motion is possible, and there are no specifically named ligaments. The capsule is thickened on the dorsal and the palmar sides to form ligaments. The capsules of the metacarpophalangeal and interphalangeal joints are thickened on the sides to form collateral ligaments and on the volar surface to form a volar plate. These joints articulate with a cam-like action. The heads of these bones are shaped like a cam, and the collateral ligaments are tightest in flexion and most relaxed in extension. Therefore, these joints should always be splinted in some degree of flexion when stiffness is anticipated, because from this position the fingers can eventually be straightened. This is possible because with straightening the ligaments become more relaxed. With the joint splinted in extension, flexion is extremely difficult, since it involves stretching the collateral ligaments, which are quite refractory to this type of stretching.

Binding the finger metacarpal heads and necks together are the very important transverse metacarpal ligaments. The lumbrical tendons pass anterior, and the interosseous tendons posterior, to these ligaments.

Skin and Fascia

The skin covering the hand not only provides cover but also contains the sensory end organs which give the hand its highly specialized sensory function and enable it to distinguish various sensations and to identify objects in a highly discriminatory manner. The skin covering the palmar surface of the hand and fingers is more firmly fixed to the underlying soft tissues than that on the dorsum of the hand. Beneath this skin there is a cushioning pad of fat separated into multiple compartments by fascial septa. This enables the hand to grasp objects with a tremendous amount of pressure with a surface which does not slip beneath the grasp. On the dorsum of the hand the skin is highly mobile. This is necessary because the wrist and fingers have a wide range of flexion and extension. In flexion the skin is stretched tightly across the convex surface, and its mobility is necessary to accommodate to the shape of the hand. The subcutaneous layer beneath this dorsal skin is primarily areolar tissue which makes possible gliding motion.

The fascia on the palmar side of the hand is primarily a deep layer, there being no superficial fascia in the palm. This deep fascia is divided into bands and septa termed *palmar fascia*, which separate the palmar structures and divide the subcutaneous tissue into compartments.

Blood Supply

The blood supply to the palmar surface of the hand is provided by two palmar arches formed by the terminal branches of the radial and ulnar arteries. The superficial palmar arch gives rise to the common volar digital arteries, excepting those to the thumb and the radial side of the index finger. These latter arise from the deep palmar arch. The deep arch gives origin to the metacarpal arteries, the first one forming a proper volar digital artery to the thumb and another to the radial side of the index finger. Through this complicated network of arches and anastomoses the hand is assured of a good collateral circulation and a very adequate blood supply. On the dorsum of the hand, the dorsocarpal arterial arch is formed by a branch of the radial artery and a branch of the dorsal branch of the ulnar artery. This arterial arch gives origin to the dorsal metacarpal arteries, which terminate in the dorsal digital arteries. This dorsal

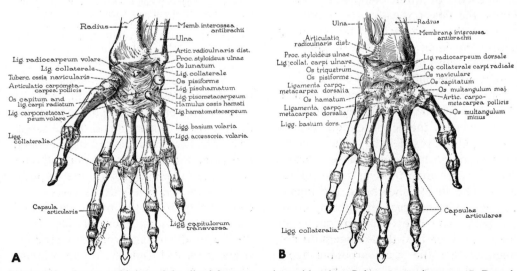

Figure 248.   Bones and joints of the distal forearm, wrist and hand. *A*, Palmar (ventral) aspect. *B*, Dorsal aspect. (From Anson, Atlas of Human Anatomy.)

anastomosis is not as important as the volar network in supplying the fingers and does not extend beyond the proximal interphalangeal joints of the fingers.

Nerves

The motor nerves to the intrinsic muscles of the hand arise from the ulnar and median nerves. The median nerve supplies most of the intrinsic muscles of the thumb and the two most radial lumbrical muscles. The ulnar nerve supplies the remaining intrinsic musculature of the hand and extends across the palm to supply the transverse head of the adductor brevis muscle of the thumb. Motor function of the hand results from a balanced action between intrinsic and extrinsic musculature.

Tendons and Associated Structures

An important consideration in regard to the flexor tendons of the fingers is that they are enclosed in a flexor sheath throughout most of their excursion through the palm and fingers. These flexor sheaths provide a gliding mechanism through which the tendons slide. Also, since the tendons must glide around two or three completely flexed joints, the flexor sheaths act as pulleys to keep the tendons from bowstringing across the interval. As one might suspect, the more joints crossed, the more important the pulley action of the flexor sheath becomes. In the fingers, where there are two flexor tendons and three joints to cross, the flexor tendon sheaths are quite restricted. The communications between these flexor sheaths are important in hand infections. The flexor sheaths to the index, center and ring fingers are interrupted in the palm, and infections originating in the flexor sheath of these fingers do not migrate past the metacarpophalangeal joints when carried along the flexor tendon sheath (Fig. 249).

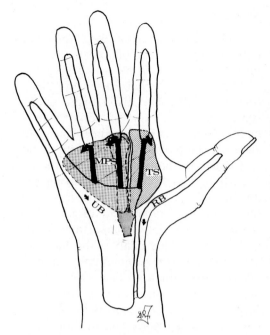

Figure 249. A schematic representation of the flexor tendon sheaths and the fascial spaces of the palm. To avoid confusion, it is important to remember that the tendon sheaths are termed bursae and the potential spaces deep to these bursae and their tendons are termed spaces. Notice that, whereas the flexor tendon sheaths of the little finger and thumb communicate proximally with their bursae, the index, center and ring bursae end at the metacarpophalangeal joints. Flexor tendon sheath infections starting in the thumb and little finger can therefore migrate proximally into the wrist, whereas infections in the index, center and ring fingers are limited proximally at the metacarpophalangeal joints. Should the infection from these three fingers point and drain at this proximal termination of the flexor sheath, they will drain into the potential spaces as indicated by the arrows. RB, Radial bursa. UB, Ulnar bursa. TS, Thenar space. MPS, Midpalmar space.

With the extensor tendons of the thumb and fingers there is no need for pulleys, so there is no extensor sheath for the thumb or fingers distal to the wrist. The intrinsic musculature of the hand is divided into the muscles of the thenar eminence, the muscles of the hypothenar eminence, the interosseous muscles arising from the metacarpals and the lumbrical muscles arising from the flexor digitorum profundus tendons (Figs. 250, 251 and 252). The primary function of the muscles of the thenar eminence is to bring the thumb into op-

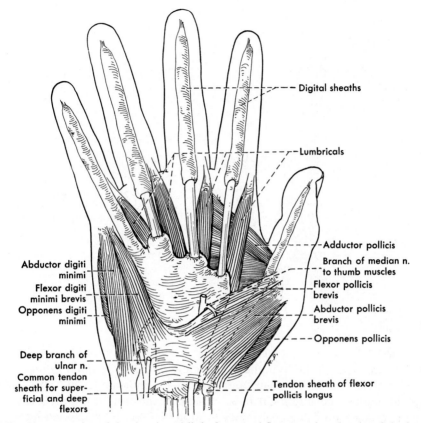

Figure 250. Short muscles of the thumb and little finger and flexor tendon sheaths of the hand. (From Hollinshead, Functional Anatomy.)

Labels in Figure 250:
Digital sheaths
Lumbricals
Adductor pollicis
Branch of median n. to thumb muscles
Flexor pollicis brevis
Abductor pollicis brevis
Opponens pollicis
Tendon sheath of flexor pollicis longus
Abductor digiti minimi
Flexor digiti minimi brevis
Opponens digiti minimi
Deep branch of ulnar n.
Common tendon sheath for superficial and deep flexors

Figure 251. The flexors of the interphalangeal and metacarpophalangeal joints. Note that each joint has its own special flexor or flexors. (From Hollinshead, Functional Anatomy.)

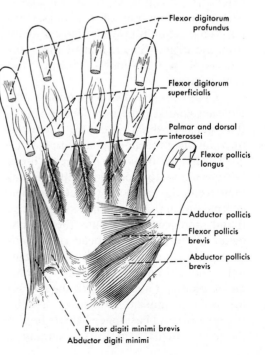

Labels in Figure 251:
Flexor digitorum profundus
Flexor digitorum superficialis
Palmar and dorsal interossei
Flexor pollicis longus
Adductor pollicis
Flexor pollicis brevis
Abductor pollicis brevis
Flexor digiti minimi brevis
Abductor digiti minimi

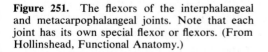

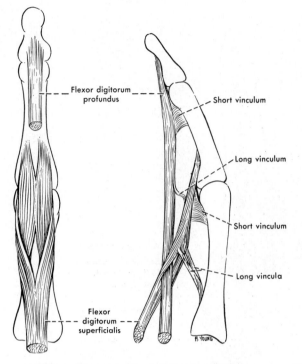

Figure 252. The flexor tendons on a finger, anterior and lateral views. (From Hollinshead. Functional Anatomy.)

position. The muscles of the hypothenar eminence control the little finger and help cup the hand. The lumbrical muscles flex the metacarpophalangeal joints of the fingers and, through their insertion into the dorsal hood mechanism, extend the distal interphalangeal joints. The prime function of the dorsal interossei is abduction of the fingers away from the center finger, that of the volar interossei is adduction toward the center finger.

Deep to the flexor tendons and their associated structures lie two potential spaces which become important only in the presence of infection (Fig. 249). The dividing line between these two spaces is formed by a septum running from the shaft of the center metacarpal along the palm toward the thumb and associated with the attachment of the transverse head of the adductor brevis of the thumb, The potential space lateral to the center metacarpal and superficial to the adductor pollicis muscle is known as the *thenar space*. That space which lies to the ulnar (medial) side of the septum is called the *midpalmar space*. As previously indicated, this space becomes important only in the presence of infection and will be discussed later.

CONTUSIONS AND ABRASIONS

The hand's location at the end of the extremity and its function expose it to a wide variety of traumatic episodes. Many of its functions automatically require an increased possibility of contusion. The athlete does not ordinarily receive severe crushing injuries such as those seen in industry. The most common contusions of the hand in the athlete come as a result of direct impact, such as from a foot on the outstretched hand with the fingers extended or from a blow of the fist against an opposing blunt object with the fingers closed. Very often these will result in a combination of an abrasion and a contusion or a contusion and a laceration.

Although the hand, and particularly the back of the hand, is prone to rapid swelling, hematomata are not common.

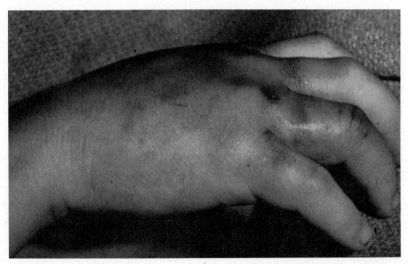

Figure 253. A large collection of blood on the dorsum of the hand should immediately alert the examiner to the possibility of a defect in the clotting mechanism. Before one injudiciously sets about to drain such a hematoma by aspiration or incision, a careful check should be made of any history of bleeding tendencies. This particular individual had hemophilia.

The blood on the back of the hand is much more likely to infiltrate up and down under the loose skin than it is to collect in a localized pool. On the palmar surface of the hand there is no room for excessive hematoma formation because of the very nature of the tightly closed spaces. The bleeding is usually in the form of extravasation through the tissues rather than collection into a pool. If an hematoma can be demonstrated, it should be treated by aspiration and a pressure bandage under strict surgical asepsis. When a large hematoma is seen on the dorsum of the hand, one should suspect a defect in the clotting mechanism such as is found in hemophilia (Fig. 253).

The Dorsum of the Hand

The skin over the back of the hand is so loose that it swells rapidly but is not subject to hematoma formation between the skin and underlying fascia. Certain complications do occur from contusion which should be thought of, particularly if the contusion appears to be of serious import. Nerve damage is not likely from direct contusion because the major nerves lie on the volar aspect

and are well protected. The tendons, however, lie subcutaneously and may be caught between the underlying bone and the contusing object. So, too, if the fist is clenched and the knuckle forcibly driven against a hard object, there may be chondral damage to the end of the metacarpal, damage to the extensor tendon as it passes over the metacarpal head, or a fracture or infraction of the head.

These areas, mainly subcutaneous, are readily available for careful physical examination. One can frequently determine whether there is a fracture of the underlying bone by simple palpation and careful manipulation. Active and passive motion of the fingers should be carefully checked to determine whether there is any loss of tendon function. Nerve function should also be noted. This can be done quickly and may save many headaches later. If the contusion seems severe with local tenderness, pain and swelling, an x-ray should be made and carefully studied.

TREATMENT. *Early treatment* of the contusion should be initiated by very careful cleansing of the skin with soap and water. The athlete is likely to be in an area where there is dirt, dust or various other contaminants and these may be ground into open cuts or abraded areas. The cleansing should be done at once. Copious amounts of running water and bland soap are much better than alcohol or various antiseptics. There is no necessity for painting the part with an antiseptic. Following such cleansing, the area can be protected by a water soluble unguent, a thin strip being appropriate. Some may prefer an antibiotic ointment, and I see no objection to this if inquiry is made as to any possible sensitivity. Once the skin has been carefully cleaned, attention must be given to the underlying condition. It is best treated by a compression dressing with a mechanic's waste or similar soft material placed over the contused area and snugly wrapped in place with an elastic bandage. An ice pack is then applied. Careful inspection of the hand is carried out after 12 hours, and if the swelling is under control the ice may be discontinued. It is inadvisable to use heat for the first 36 hours.

Subsequent treatment will depend upon the extent of the contusion. If the area remains swollen, edematous and painful, and particularly if there is pain on active extension of the fingers, one should protect the hand much longer because of the possibility of tenosynovitis, which may be quite crippling and last for many weeks. If function of the fingers remains pain-free, a rigid protective dressing may be applied over the back of the hand and snugly held in place by an elastic bandage. Participation in sports may be continued, always provided that function of the fingers is pain-free. Careful re-examination from time to time will detect any possible late complication such as involvement of the intrinsic muscles of the hand, localized phlebitis, lymphangitis, delayed tendon rupture and so forth.

The Palm

A particularly distressing injury to the hand is a contusion in the palm in which there is damage to the intrinsic muscles. This occurs most commonly at the base of the hand in the thenar and hypothenar eminences where the intrinsic muscles to the thumb and to the little finger are involved. This injury is of the "stone bruise" type and may require considerable time to subside. The palmar portion of the hand is a relatively closed space and any localized swelling here can be distressing. Contusion directly over the transverse ligament may give rise to the carpal tunnel syndrome (see p. 296). Contusion of the distal part of the palm may cause severe tenderness over the metacarpal heads so that gripping a hard object such as a golf club or a tennis racket may be painful. This condition may be very disabling; if it persists, later treatment may be necessary, consisting of local injection of a long-acting anesthetic and a corticoid preparation. Physical therapy, particularly with the heat modalities, is appropriate.

FINGERTIP INJURIES

Injuries to the athlete's fingertip usually involve the nail and the pulp, sometimes in combination with fractures of the distal tuft. These most commonly result from direct trauma to the fingertip.

Injuries to the Nail

The nail is very closely apposed to the bone, being separated only by the nail bed. Contusion here is likely to cause hemorrhage into the closed spaces under the fingernail or in the tip of the phalanx. As the hematoma develops, it causes pressure symptoms and throbbing pain that are very distressing. The immediate treatment is application of cold, the hand being held in direct contact with crushed ice or in ice water. If swelling subsides early enough, the severe symptoms may be prevented. Should blood accumulate under the nail at this early stage, it is advisable to drill the nail to relieve the pressure. This should be done under aseptic technique since infection in this space has extremely serious consequences. Everyone has his preferred method for drilling the nail. I prefer to drill carefully through with a convex type knife blade, such as a No. 10 Bard-Parker, which will drill through the nail without pressure. However, there are many other suitable ways to open this space, for example, burning through the nail with a red hot paper clip. After the bleeding stops, the cold may be discontinued, but heat should not be applied for 48 hours. A protective splint will usually give considerable relief.

Badly lacerated nails can be either repaired with suture or removed if damage is extensive. Various complications are seen in this condition, making careful examination of the area mandatory. In order to clean the area thoroughly, it is usually necessary to anesthetize the finger by injecting procaine into either side at its base. Once the finger is insensitive and the pain is gone, a more definitive examination can be carried out. The nail should be carefully studied. Frequently the root of the nail has slipped out from under the eponychial fold, and its proximal end is found lying on top of the skin (Fig. 254). In this case enough of the proximal end of the nail should be cut away to permit the nail to fall back into the nail bed. The finger is then dressed carefully with a petrolatum strip, and a splint is applied with moderate pressure. The nail must be carefully protected in the athlete. In many instances the root will not adhere to the nail bed, and protection will be needed until the new nail grows out from under the injured part. It is well to clip off the old nail just distal to the advancing edge of the new nail.

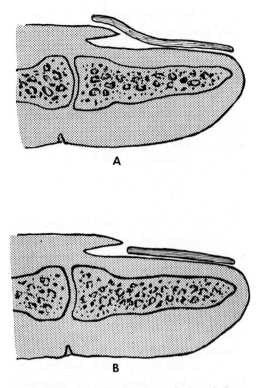

Figure 254. Lateral drawing of tip of finger showing *(A)* the nail avulsed from its root and lying on top of the skin on dorsum of the finger and *(B)* proximal end of nail cut off to permit the nail to fall back into the nailbed.

Avulsion-Lacerations of the Fingertip

If the injury is less than 1 cm. in diameter and if the bone is not exposed, treatment consists of simple cleaning of the wound and application of a sterile dressing. The wound epithelializes fairly rapidly and can be healed within two weeks. Wounds greater than 1 cm. in diameter without exposure of bone are treated by the application of a heavy split-thickness skin graft or a full-thickness skin graft taken from the volar surface of the forearm in the male or some less conspicuous spot in the female. If the patient has preserved the avulsed fingertip, it can be replaced after defatting as a full-thickness graft.

All the injuries just mentioned can be associated with fracture of the tuft or shaft of the distal phalanx. A fracture with significant displacement should be reduced insofar as possible to prevent the development of a deformed nail.

More severe injuries of the fingertip are not commonly seen in the athlete, but when they do occur they can be repaired by (1) excising enough bone to allow primary closure, (2) covering the defect with split- or full-thickness graft, (3) creating cross finger flaps, or (4) creating a palmar pedicle flap or an abdominal or axillary pedicle.

One must be extremely penurious in sacrificing the length of the finger simply to effect closure. It is far better to use a primary split graft and get the wounds to heal, deciding later on definitive treatment, including the possibility of amputation. It is not proper to rush a patient with such an injury to the emergency room and clip away the distal tip of the finger until one has analyzed the blood supply very thoroughly. In many instances what may appear to be a hopelessly unsalvageable fingertip may actually be viable when properly replaced (Fig. 255). We have witnessed

many instances in which a seemingly lost fingertip was saved by replacement of the avulsed portion as a full-thickness graft. Extreme conservatism must be practiced in sacrificing any tissue in the finger.

Before undertaking a complicated program of pedicle grafting, it is well to consider how important the added length may be to the patient, especially if this added length will be anesthetic. Injuries of the fingers are often lightly treated and all too often result in various deformities which may be quite painful in the very sensitive area at the end of the finger. We cannot overemphasize the importance of cleanliness in treating all these injuries.

LACERATIONS OF THE HAND

Lacerations of the hand may have extremely serious consequences and should never be minimized. The laceration penetrates the skin with the fingers in various degrees of flexion or exten-

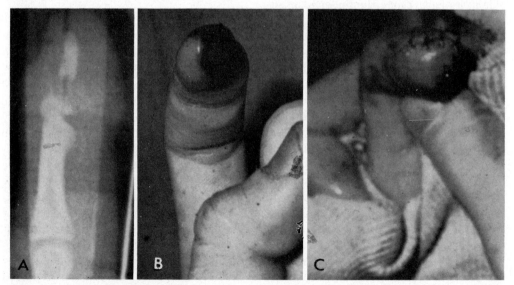

Figure 255.   This water skiing accident illustrates a principle of treatment of finger tip injuries. The patient sustained an extensive injury to the tip of the index finger which resulted in avulsion of a portion of the distal phalanx (A). This was repaired primarily, and the ischemic area allowed to demarcate, as indicated in (B). Once demarcation was complete it was possible to remove the gangrenous tissue and close the finger tip with the viable flap of skin on the radial side of the finger (C). Injudicious primary amputation would have resulted in a much shorter phalanx or anesthetic skin coverage on the finger tip.

sion. All too often when the cut is examined the finger may be in another position and superficial examination through the cut may reveal normal structures. It is dangerous to assume that the deep structures are not involved unless the cut is carefully examined with the finger in various positions.

TREATMENT. The first step in treatment of the lacerated hand is an assessment of the function of the part. This includes all motions of the involved area, both active and passive. One should then carefully check the nerve function, bearing in mind the distribution of the nerve which is likely to be injured. This check may be made without removing the dressing from the hand; in fact, there is no excuse for repeatedly removing the dressing to examine the hand if the laceration appears to be severe. As the player comes off the field, a sterile dressing should be applied immediately and a firm pressure bandage wrapped around the injured part. He should then be taken to the infirmary or hospital in which he is to receive definitive treatment. At that time, and at that time only, should the dressing be removed. After the dressing has been carefully removed and the wound has been thoroughly inspected, determination should be made of the type of anesthesia indicated. If there is disturbance of tendon function, if there is loss of nerve function or if there appears to be any joint involvement, it is advisable to use a general anesthetic, which makes easier the use of a tourniquet to control bleeding. Occasionally a tourniquet placed on the forearm is well tolerated and may be used with local or regional nerve block of the hand; in this case a general anesthetic will not be necessary. An x-ray study should be made to detect any abnormality of the bony structures of the hand.

After preliminary preparations, the patient is taken to the operating room and given the appropriate anesthetic, either nerve block or general. Any definitive treatment is best carried out under tourniquet control. The dressing is removed and the surgeon, wearing sterile gloves, should carefully inspect the hand. This is not the time for a detailed examination of the wound itself. The next step is a thorough cleansing of the hand. If necessary, a detergent is used to remove grease; otherwise, soap and water are employed to cleanse the entire hand with particular attention being paid to the site of the wound. The wound is thoroughly lavaged with running water.

The hand is now redraped with sterile drapes; the medical team puts on new gowns and gloves. Only then is the wound itself investigated. It is thoroughly lavaged again, all exposed areas being brushed with a sterile sponge. Examination should make it possible to determine the extent of involvement of nerve or tendon. It may be that a tendon has been partially cut. This can be determined only by moving the finger through a full range of motion while inspecting the tendon throughout the area which might have been exposed in this wound. Ordinarily it is not necessary to enlarge the wound simply for diagnostic purposes. If there is nerve damage, and if the wound is relatively clean, the wound should be enlarged enough to expose the nerve ends and permit nerve suture. If there is a combination of nerve and tendon damage, the tougher structures should be sutured first.

REPAIR OF LACERATED TENDONS AND NERVES. No attempt is made here to describe in full the repair of lacerated tendons and nerves, but a few principles should be emphasized. As a general rule, it is not advisable to suture lacerated nerves unless the wound is scrupulously clean. Lacerated nerves are best repaired at a later date after scarring in the perineurium renders them more easily sutured. The volar digital nerves can be repaired primarily in most instances. Lacerated extensor tendons can also be repaired primarily and delayed repairs are not necessary or advisable. With flexor tendons an entirely different situation exists, because they must glide in a very tight fibro-osseous compartment at the level of the fingers, and repair of the flexor tendons within the flexor tendon sheath of the fingers is not advisable. Certain rules have been established for repair of these particular tendons. The profundus tendon cut close to its insertion into the base of the distal phalanx can be advanced and sutured into the base of the phalanx, excising the distal segment of the tendon. Lacerations of both flexor tendons between the area just proximal to the insertion of the profundus tendon and the distal palmar crease are in "no man's land." If both sublimis and profundus tendons are lacerated in this location, it is best to obtain primary closure of the skin and do a flexor graft later.

If only the sublimis tendon is lacerated, repair is not indicated. If the profundus tendon is cut, and the sublimis remains intact, a tenodesis procedure fixing the distal interphalangeal joint in flexion or fusion of the distal interphalangeal joint in flexion will yield the most consistently satisfactory result.

If it is determined that the laceration is within the sheath and it nevertheless seems advisable to repair the tendon, the sheath should be partially excised. Never repair two tendons within the same sheath. If both the flexor digitorum profundus and sublimis have been severed within the same sheath, the sublimis should be sacrificed and the profundus alone repaired.

Tendon, as well as nerve, suture in the hand is a highly specialized procedure, and one should be thoroughly versed in the proper technique before attempting even a simple repair. Since becoming the team physician for the Meat Packers at the Marshall, Missouri, Wilson Plant, I have seen a large collection of "trigger fingers" as a result of traumatic tenosynovitis of the flexor tendon sheaths of the center, ring and little fingers. This results from a strong grip on a knife there, but probably occurs also in the athlete. Therefore, although these injuries are not common in the athlete, when they do occur they are extremely important. I know of one instance wherein the classic mistake of suturing a lacerated flexor tendon to the median nerve was accomplished once again. Needless to say, the function of neither the tendon nor the nerve was restored.

Following repair of the tendon or nerve, the extremity must be placed in the position that most relaxes the area of repair and held there for at least three weeks to permit the early stages of repair to take place. Following the three-week period, if the finger can be securely splinted with a dressing that is acceptable to the athletic authorities, participation in sports might be permitted.

Many of these injuries are locker room accidents, such as from thrusting the hand through a glass door, and may indeed involve multiple tendons. One of our patients was a young athlete who was in the hospital to have his knee cartilage removed. He attempted to close the transom window over his bed by driving the heel of his hand against the glass. The glass broke and the jagged edges sectioned all the flexor tendons and the median nerve at the level of the wrist. The only good thing about this accident was that he was in the proper locale to get early treatment. This could hardly be called an athletic injury, although it certainly was an injury to an athlete. In this instance we were able to repair the tendons and the nerve since the tendons at this level are not within a sheath.

PUNCTURE WOUNDS OF THE HAND

Puncture wounds of the hand are infrequent in athletes, although they are common enough in others. A wound in the hand by a sharp cleat is almost always a laceration, because the skin in the dorsum of the hand tears as the cleat hits it and skids. Puncture wounds may be caused by contaminants on the playing field or by sharp projecting points on the players' equipment. After a puncture wound, particularly on the palmar side, the hand should be carefully checked for disturbance of nerve or tendon function. If this function remains intact, the wound should be treated expectantly; that is, the surrounding area should be thoroughly cleansed, a sterile dressing applied and the wound regularly observed. If any sign of deep-seated infection appears, adequate drainage must be provided immediately, since infection within the closed spaces of the hand can be very severe and may lead to a crippling disability. The player should be instructed that if he experiences fever or malaise, or if he has aching or throbbing in the hand, he should report at once for a careful examination to determine the severity of the involvement. In the early stage there may be considerable deep soreness. This should not be confused with infection since infection is unlikely to develop for several days.

Here once more is illustrated the great value of careful primary examination. If the initial examination elicits no particular soreness anywhere in the hand, any soreness that develops after several days is much more significant. One must be particularly careful when treating the hand to prevent an iatrogenic lesion. An incautious scalpel or scissors may readily spread infection into the tendon sheath or palmar space or may actually sever a nerve or a vessel.

It is axiomatic that any puncture wound requires tetanus toxoid. A broad-spectrum antibiotic may be required.

In any penetrating wound one must always suspect the presence of foreign material, particularly glass. Clothing or similar material is not frequently carried into the tissues of the hand.

Human Bite

A wound in the athlete that has a particularly grave connotation is the "knuckle" wound caused by striking the human tooth. It is a contaminated wound and should be treated as such by meticulous cleansing of the part. Again, the extensor tendon, which is part of the capsule of the metacarpophalangeal joint, may be cut with the finger flexed. When it is examined with the finger in extension, the laceration of the tendon has now traveled considerably proximal to the cut in the skin and the defect may be completely overlooked.

TREATMENT. To treat such a wound as a casual "barked" knuckle is to court disaster. In the first place, infection from a human bite is one of the most difficult to treat. In the second place, there will remain not only a defect in the capsule but also irregularity of the metacarpophalangeal joint. In this instance the proper treatment is to retract the wound edges carefully; to lavage the wound thoroughly; to clip away any obviously necrotic tissue but to be very wary about sacrificing tissue. Then examine the tendon carefully by flexing the finger. If necessary the wound may be enlarged to permit careful suture of the tendon. When the skin is to be closed, the contused, devitalized edge may be trimmed away very sparingly. It is important to effect well-demarcated skin edges. The wound may be closed without drainage but must be watched very carefully. The patient should be observed for signs of any developing infection. One should give a prophylactic broad-spectrum antibiotic in any case. If infection is imminent or actually present, the skin edges should not be closed. They should be opened if the wound was closed primarily and infection supervenes.

INFECTIONS OF THE HAND

There is no place on a team for a player with an infected hand. His dressing should not be changed in the dressing room or training room since the spread of infection to other members of the team may be disastrous. This applies as well to any infection elsewhere. If a player has an abrasion that is contaminated and draining pus, he should be barred from the dressing room until the purulent stage has passed. The hand should be treated with warm saline dressings. After the suppuration has cleared, the abraded area should be carefully protected with unguent and a suitable dressing. Even at this stage the player should be warned not to peel his dressing off and throw it on the floor or in the shower or any other place where it can contaminate the room.

Infection about the Fingernail

Although not strictly in the category of an athletic injury, this subject should be considered here since it frequently involves the athlete. Indeed, it may often follow relatively minor injuries about the nail with impingement of the paronychial fold against the side of the nail.

Simple contusion of the nail or along the side of the nail may cause some abrasion or laceration of the skin. An inflammatory reaction about the nail produces the familiar picture of a red, inflamed, swollen nail fold. This may be

an extremely distressing condition and may materially handicap the athlete, particularly if it is on the thumb or first or second finger. In the early stage it is best treated by heat applied locally. It should be carefully explained to the player that adequate care in the early stage may well prevent considerable disability later. Soaking the area several times a day or continuous warm soaks and the use of a heat lamp may prevent suppuration.

If an abscess develops it should be drained. If the involvement is close to the nail, an instrument can be passed between the nail and the paronychial fold and the nail lifted gently, permitting the pus to exude through this defect. This route of drainage has the advantage of not requiring a cut on the skin. It has the disadvantage that the nail fold tends to close down readily over the nail and the abscess does not drain. If this occurs, or if the infection seems to be away from the nail, a straight linear incision parallel to the nail edge will usually suffice for drainage. The incision is carried down to the abscess. Ethyl chloride applied locally will suffice for anesthesia. This incision will tend to gape open rather than to seal and drainage will be adequate. Hot soaks should be continued, and the dressings applied should be sufficiently protective to prevent contamination of the finger from extrinsic infection and to prevent the finger from being the source of contamination to the patient or to others.

An infection of the base of the nail may have more serious consequences, because it tends to burrow under the proximal edge of the nail at the root and so to form a subungual abscess. Prompt, adequate drainage must be carried out or else the nail bed may be destroyed and permanent damage result. If the pus has actually elevated the proximal section of the nail, this portion should be removed to permit exposure of the nail bed at its root, thereby preventing further undermining. As much of the nail should be removed at the proximal end as is undermined by the infection; otherwise the detached nail lying over the nail bed will serve to form a pocket of infection. Following complete drainage by resection of the base of the nail, the area must be carefully protected to prevent external contamination of the wound and the spread of infection to other parts of the body. If the drainage has been carried out promptly, there is every reason to expect regrowth of the nail. If drainage is delayed, destruction of the nail root and bed will lead to gross and often painful deformities of the nail.

Felons

A felon is an abscess located within the fat pad of the fingertip. The important consideration here is that pus creates pressure in the closed septal spaces, which exist primarily to provide a cushioning effect from the fat on the palmar side of the finger. When these spaces become infected, abscess pressure builds up, because it is not easily decompressed by expansion of the skin. The abscess continues to invade tissue adjacent to it, gradually enlarging until the whole fingertip may become involved. This can lead to osteomyelitis of the phalanx if the abscess is not adequately drained (Fig. 256, B).

TREATMENT. Treatment consists of incision and drainage: by making an adequate incision along either the medial or lateral border of the phalanx. Combining both in a fish-mouth type of incision is usually not necessary or desirable. It is important to decompress all involved compartments (Fig. 256, A). The wound should be held open with petrolatum gauze or a through and through rubber drain. It should be allowed to close in two or three days

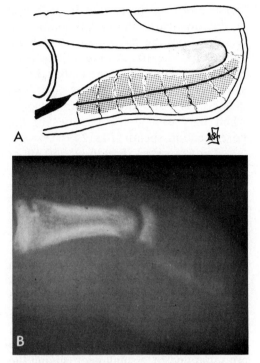

Figure 256. *A*, Illustration shows the importance of an adequate incision and drainage of a felon. The pus is contained in compartments, and all compartments must be decompressed to prevent erosion of bone and osteomyelitis. The line of incision is outlined extending through all compartments. *B*, An unfortunate result of an inadequately treated felon which led to osteomyelitis. Most of the bone of the distal phalanx was destroyed. Treatment of an abscess, even in this day of modern miracle drugs and antibiotics, is still drainage through an adequate incision.

when the inflammatory reaction has subsided. The tragic complication of osteomyelitis of the phalanx should never be permitted to develop.

Flexor Tendon Sheath Infections

Infections in the fingers which enter the flexor tendon sheaths will present symptoms of swelling and pain along the flexor sheath, limited painful extension and flexion contracture. Infections entering the little finger or thumb flexor sheath will travel proximally to the wrist and palm and may join to form a horseshoe abscess. Infections in the index, center and ring finger sheaths will stop at the metacarpophalangeal joints. Infections from the index finger which escape the sheath at the metacarpophalangeal joint will enter the thenar space; infections in the ring and long fingers will enter the midpalmar space when they escape the confines of the flexor tendon sheath (Fig. 249).

TREATMENT. Treatment of all of these infections requires proper drainage of the abscess from the space or bursa involved. This drainage should be preceded and followed by continuous hot sterile soaks until the infection subsides.

The collar button abscess is one in which the primary abscess cavity is located deep to the palmar fascia and only a small portion of the abscess is seen superficial to the palmar fascia. This gives two abscess cavities which are separated by a small neck, giving the appearance of a collar button. It is important to recognize that the most superficial portion of the abscess does not represent the entire abscess. A similar situation exists with a felon in which there can be a small collection of pus immediately beneath the dermis overlying the more important felon beneath.

Traumatic Inflammation of the Flexor Tendon Sheath

Repeated trauma to the flexor tendon sheath can result in an inflammatory reaction with swelling that restricts the normal gliding of the flexor tendons within their sheath. This is especially true of the already thickened portion of the sheath that forms the pulley at the level of the distal metacarpal. A small nodule already present in the flexor tendon can become impinged on either the proximal or distal side of the pulley, creating either a snapping sensation or complete locking of the finger in either the flexed or extended position.

This is the so-called *trigger finger*. It can be treated initially by rest and anti-inflammatory agents such as phenylbutazone systemically or cortisone injected into the sheath.

Frequently surgery is necessary to correct the problem. Surgical treatment is directed toward removing the thickened pulley at this level. It should be performed under general anesthesia or by adequate regional block. A tourniquet is a must, as is adequate visualization of the involved portion of the flexor tendon sheath. Adequate excision of the pulley and a portion of the adjacent sheath will prevent a distressing recurrence of the problem.

STRAIN (MUSCULOTENDINOUS INJURIES) IN THE HAND

With the vast complex of muscle-tendon units in the hand it is obvious that strain will occur frequently.

There are two basic categories of these muscle-tendon units: the long flexors and the long extensors, which are entirely tendinous in the hand; and the intrinsic muscles, in which the entire musculotendinous unit is contained within the hand itself.

Strain in the hand is due to two primary causes. One is excessive overuse against resistance and the second is overstretching of the unit beyond its normal extensile range. In the intrinsic muscles of the hand the former cause is by far the more common and usually results from repeated use beyond the total capacity of the unit rather than a single excessive contraction. This is not a common injury in athletic competition but may occur in sports such as gymnastics or those requiring constant gripping, such as rowing, tennis or golf. The initial symptoms are cramping and fatigue of the muscles involved with pain on function against resistance. If the activity is discontinued at this stage, recovery is prompt and without residual. Continuation of overuse may result in persistent muscle spasm or even contracture. Tenosynovitis is not common in the intrinsic muscles of the hand since the tendons do not have a synovial sheath.

Strain in the long musculotendinous units may be manifested in the forearm near the musculotendinous junction. This has been discussed previously (see Forearm). There may also be a tenosynovitis in the palm or more distally in the fingers. There may be irritation at the attachment of the tendon to the phalanx. Irritation or strain of the attachment of the wrist flexors and extensors as they reach the base of the metacarpals may cause symptoms in this area. Those conditions which result from overuse must be treated primarily by rest. Rest is the essential ingredient for recovery. Other modes of treatment that may accelerate recovery are the use of local heat, particularly the penetrating modalities, and the local injection of an anesthetic and a corticoid. These are of considerable value if the irritation is specifically within the sheath or tendinous attachment or even at the musculotendinous junction. Injection is much more successful if the condition is local. A local spot of discomfort over the dorsum of the base of the second metacarpal with tenderness on pressure and pain on dorsiflexion of the wrist against resistance may be interpreted as strain of the attachment of the extensor carpi radialis, and local injection of this area will give prompt and often permanent relief, provided that the etiological factor is eliminated. To relieve such a case the hand and wrist should be supported by a forearm splint with the wrist in dorsiflexion. When competition is resumed, the wrist should be taped. Keeping in mind that the cause is overuse rather than overstretch, one must be careful to avoid active use of the muscle. Hence, a serious involvement of the carpal flexors or extensors will prohibit participation in athletics.

Whereas strain of the short flexors is most often within the muscle and is due primarily to overuse, long flexor involvement may well be in the tendon and is frequently due to overstretch, particularly against resistance. For example, a wrist that is forcibly dorsiflexed with the wrist flexors contracted may suffer strain of the flexors. This strain may be anything from a slight separation of some of the fibers in the musculotendinous junction or at the attachment of the tendon in the hand (mild) to a complete avulsion (severe). Symptomatically, there will be pain at the site of involvement, pain on active contraction of the muscle and pain on passive stretching of the muscle. If the rupture is complete, there will be loss of function of the muscle. In this case there may be bunching up of the muscle as it contracts with the distal end of the tendon pulling free, so that the muscle may actually shorten while the wrist does not flex.

If the tendon is avulsed, surgical treatment is indicated and the tendon should be sutured to its attachment. Much more frequently the strain is partial (mild to moderate). The treatment in this instance will be protection, first against overstretch, second against overuse. This protection must be continued for a sufficient time to permit the strength of the tendon to be restored. With only slight involvement (mild) little or no immobilization will be needed, whereas if there is extensive tearing (moderate), protection must be provided for several weeks. One can usually assess the degree of involvement by the rate of subsidence of symptoms and so regulate the degree and extent of immobilization of these long flexors. If there is irritation within the tendon sheath the part must be immobilized. Injection of a steroid into the tendon sheath together with physical therapy is of considerable value. Corticoids must not be injected into the tendon itself. Rupture may result as a direct consequence of their adverse effect on collagen formation. Function should be resumed very slowly here or there will be prompt recurrence of symptoms. Although it is difficult to elicit in the hand, snowball crepitation can sometimes be felt along the tendon sheath. If present, it is diagnostic.

Avulsion of the Flexor Digitorum Profundus Tendon

This lesion is seen very infrequently but can occur. It is usually avulsed from the attachment to the base of the distal phalanx. The earlier the lesion is recognized, the better the chances of obtaining a satisfactory result from surgical repair. Inability to actively flex the distal interphalangeal joint and problems with the flexor tendon sheath strongly suggest an avulsed tendon. This, together with a high index of suspicion, will lead to the correct diagnosis in those rare instances of tendon avulsion without x-ray evidence of avulsed bone.

SPRAIN-SUBLUXATION-DISLOCATION

It should be emphasized again that injuries to the components of the hand are extremely serious from the functional point of view. One must always bear in mind that almost the whole function of the upper extremity rests in the capability of the fingers and thumb. Despite this fact, injuries to the hand proper are often considered minor injuries and all too frequently the treatment

they receive can be classified as minor, too. The treating physician does not recognize the magnitude of the maximum deformity occurring at the peak of injury unless an accurate history is taken or unless stress films can be obtained. Much damage to ligaments will have occurred before the joint is returned to normal. Since there is a considerable difference functionally and anatomically between the thumb and the remaining fingers, or more accurately between the first ray and the remaining rays of the hand, they will be discussed under separate headings.

THUMB RAY

Carpometacarpal Joint

Since the thumb is the opposing member of the group, it of necessity must have more mobility. The carpometacarpal joint is extremely mobile, its action in effect being that of a universal joint so that it moves in all directions—flexion and extension, adduction and abduction, circumduction and rotation. For this to occur the stability of the joint to extremes of motion must be maintained almost entirely by ligaments and other soft tissues, since there is no bony restriction to any particular motion. Forced motion in any direction beyond the strength of the ligamentous support will cause a sprain which may be mild (first degree), moderate (second degree) or severe (third degree). If the force is continued, a subluxation or dislocation will occur. For example, forceful wide abduction of the thumb produces hyperextension of the carpometacarpal joint, which throws a strain on the anterior portion of the capsule. If the force is arrested, the injury may be mild or moderate and a sprain results. If it continues, the injury will be severe, and the base may dislocate as it passes out through a rent in the capsule. The thumb in this case is actually bent backward over the wrist owing to complete disruption of the anterior structures of the joint. Similarly, the dorsal capsule may be injured by hyperflexion. The foolish habit of grasping the thumb within the fingers and then striking a blow with the clenched fist tends to rotate the base of the metacarpal dorsally and to rupture the dorsal ligaments. Subluxation is more likely to occur here than dislocation, although disruption of the capsule may be complete. There may be sprain of the lateral, and less frequently of the medial, components.

TREATMENT. Treatment will vary according to the severity of injury. Mild sprain of the carpometacarpal joint is extremely common and causes pain around the joint, tenderness to pressure over the area and pain on reproduction of the motion that caused the injury. Within a few hours the area of the base of the thumb will be swollen and edematous and almost any motion will cause pain. Treatment should be directed toward reduction of any residual subluxation and protection of the joint against stress until the healing is complete (Fig. 257). If the injury is mild, simple adhesive strapping will suffice to prevent overstretch (Fig. 260). If the injury is moderate to severe, the joint should be immobilized by plaster fixation in a position which would be assumed by grasping a 3 in. ball (Fig. 247). It is not necessary to immobilize the fingers but the splint should include the hand and wrist and the thumb as far as the middle of the proximal phalanx. The duration of the immobilization will vary with the severity of the injury. As a general rule, the cast should be left on about three weeks and the thumb should be protected against strain by adequate taping for the next three weeks. Later the thumb should be protected during con-

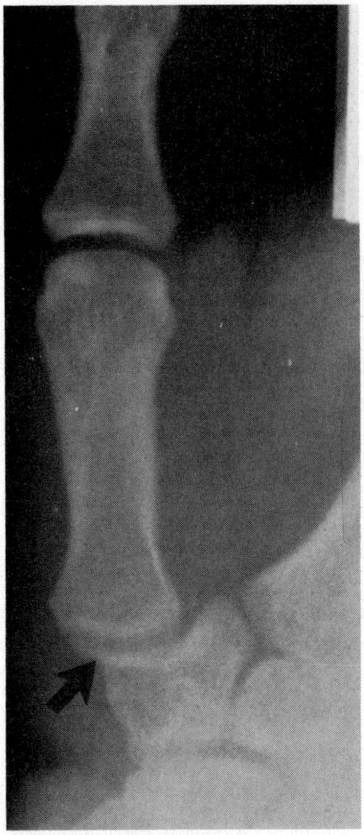

Figure 257. This patient sustained subluxation of a carpometacarpal joint in a bowling injury. Notice the lateral subluxation of the base of the first metacarpal (arrow). Although the injury appeared to be quite minimal on x-ray, the patient was in severe pain until the subluxation was reduced by traction and pressure at the base of the thumb.

tact sports if the ligament rupture was complete.

If there is subluxation or instability of this joint, great care must be taken to immobilize the joint in its normal relationship. If the subluxation cannot be reduced and held by simple plaster fixation, traction should be applied. In these cases immobilization will be considerably longer since at least six weeks is needed for the ligament and capsule to unite firmly, even under the most favorable circumstances.

Simple dislocation of this joint is not a frequent injury. If the force is sufficient to disrupt the joint, a fracture-dislocation will occur (Fig. 258, *A*). The so-called Bennett fracture leaves a small portion of the lip of the metacarpal fixed to the anterior capsular ligaments, whereas the remaining portion dislocates. This is discussed in the section on fractures.

It may be that when a frank dislocation does occur it is reduced spontaneously, and by the time it is seen by the physician there is no deformity. If dislocation persists it should be reduced by traction along the long axis of the thumb and by gradual abduction while local pressure is placed on the dorsal aspect of the proximal end of the phalanx to force the metacarpal back into its normal carpal relationship. If it is unstable in this position, some form of internal fixation such as percutaneous insertion of a K-wire is advisable, since it is extremely difficult to hold it by plaster alone. While the thumb is held manually, a transfixion pin may be drilled through the base of the metacarpal and

into the adjacent carpal or into the adjacent second metacarpal (Fig. 258, *B*). Ideally it probably would be better at this time to open the dorsal aspect of the joint and repair the ligaments. The fact that one so often sees a hypermobile, painful and even subluxating joint following this injury would suggest that some improvement in treatment is indicated. The usual error is that of inadequate immobilization rather than incomplete reduction. After dislocation of the thumb the athlete should wear supportive strapping for the rest of the season (Fig. 260).

Treatment of the chronic sprain is difficult since continued participation in sports causes frequent reinjury. The first requirement is an adequate support that is tolerable to the patient and yet protects the joint. Adhesive strapping is not dependable since someone is required to reapply it and frequently it is not done properly. An injury may occur while the strapping is off. A little slip-on protector that fits around the wrist can

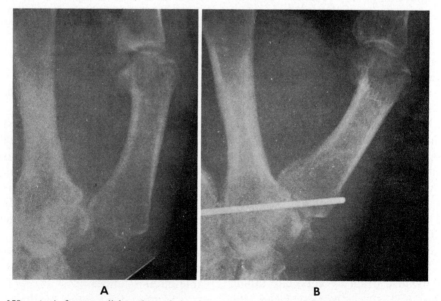

A   **B**

Figure 258. *A*, A fracture-dislocation of the first metacarpal on the trapezium by a force similar to that causing a Bennett fracture. *B*, Excellent postoperative fixation was obtained in the same case as *A* by transfixation through the metacarpal base into the base of the adjacent metacarpal. (For positioning for x-ray, see Fig. 259.)

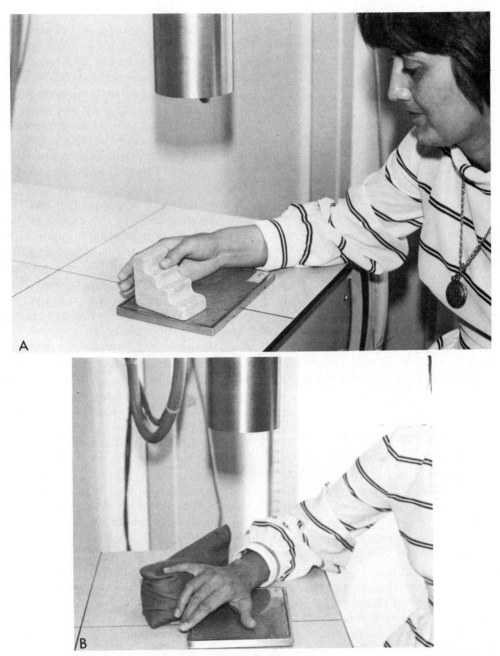

Figure 259. To visualize the carpometacarpal joint of the thumb, the most comfortable position for the injured patient to assume should be the choice. *A,* Posteroanterior view. Place the hand in a lateral position with the thumb abducted and supported on a nonopaque pad. Direct the central ray to the base of the thumb. *B,* Lateral view. Pronate the forearm. Support the slightly elevated palm enough to place the lateral aspect of the thumb, slightly abducted and flexed, on the cassette. Direct the central ray to the base of the thumb. These same views show the Bennett fracture.

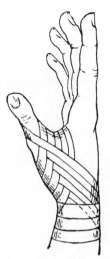

Figure 260. Basket weave strapping of thumb. (Courtesy of Rawlinson, Modern Athletic Training, © 1961 by Prentice Hall, Inc.)

be devised by the bracemaker and is quite effective. At the time of acute recurrence of chronic sprain local injection of a corticoid into the joint is effective, and the usual physical therapeutic measures also help.

Metacarpophalangeal Joint

The metacarpophalangeal joint of the thumb (Fig. 261, *A*) permits motion primarily in flexion and extension. However, there is an element of adduction and abduction permitted by the convex-concave lateral curvature of the head of the metacarpal and base of the phalanx. The collateral ligaments definitely restrict adduction and abduction. This joint is extremely vulnerable to sprain, because as the thumb is abducted the metacarpal becomes fixed, and the force applied to the end of the thumb is directed against the metacarpophalangeal joint. When the lateral stress is toward either adduction or abduction, the sprain is to the collateral ligaments. When the force is in straight extension, the strain is to the anterior capsule. If

the force is limited, the resultant injury is low-grade and no instability results. If the force continues, subluxation occurs as the result of tearing of the stressed ligament (Fig. 261, *B*). Thus, if the force is abduction, the medial collateral ligament will be avulsed (Fig. 262) or torn (Fig. 263), the phalanx and metacarpal will separate and the joint will open on the medial side. As soon as the force is released, the thumb falls back into its normal position and reveals no obvious abnormality. The pain will be along the medial side of the joint and, as with sprains elsewhere, in the final analysis the determination of the degree of lateral instability is of utmost importance. If the force involved is hyperextension, the metacarpal head thrusts forward through the anterior capsule (Fig. 264). Here again, if the force is relieved, the joint may slip back into position and be spontaneously reduced.

A sprain to the area of the metacarpophalangeal joint may cause chronic disability for months or years or even permanently. Inadequate treatment of an initial injury is mainly responsible, since it permitted the ligament and capsule to heal with redundancy. Thus recurrent subluxation is easily produced. Many baseball players, particularly catchers, have such an involvement, and the least hyperextension of the thumb or flexion of the thumb across the palm will cause recurrence of the painful, swollen joint. The thumb should be immobilized for at least three weeks if the injury seems severe. It should then be protected for several more weeks by very comprehensive strapping that permits only a minimum of motion in the metacarpophalangeal joint but leaves the distal phalanx relatively free. The degree of immobilization and duration of protection will depend upon the response to treatment. As long as the interphalangeal joints are given motion relatively early (within three weeks),

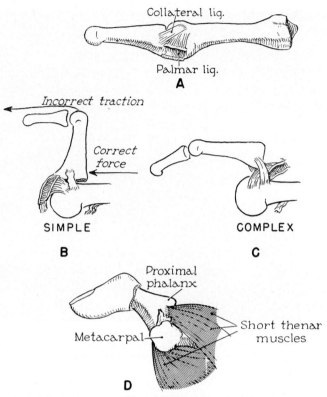

Figure 261. Simple and complex metacarpophalangeal dislocation. *A*, The volar aspect of a metacarpo-phalangeal joint capsule is reinforced with a palmar ligament, or fibrocartilage. *B*, In a simple dislocation the phalanx is hyperextended and the palmar ligament hangs like a curtain over the metacarpal head. Traction may pivot the phalanx on the intact collateral ligaments and interpose the palmar ligament between the bones. The phalanx should be pushed into place. *C*, The finger is hyperextended more nearly parallel to, but not on, the metacarpal in a complex dislocation. The volar joint capsule and palmar ligament are interposed and usually prevent reduction by manipulation. *D*, In the metacarpophalangeal joint of the thumb the short thenar muscles augment the pivot force, thereby predisposing to complex dislocation. (From McLaughlin, Trauma.)

one need not fear immobilization. I have yet to see an instance of restriction of motion in this metacarpophalangeal joint that could be attributed to overlong immobilization. Protection of the joint in the young is particularly important. One has only to experience a recurrent or chronic sprain of this joint to appreciate the seriousness of the resulting handicap to the budding athlete.

With a *complete dislocation* (Fig. 264), the very fact that the dislocation reaches the doctor unreduced is a warning signal. Under ordinary circumstances this dislocation will reduce spontaneously. If it does not do so at once, or if it does not do so spontaneously, the injured person himself almost certainly will have grabbed the thumb and pulled it into position, oftentimes with the eager help of one of his teammates. Hence, if the dislocation will reduce by simple traction and manual manipulation, it will already be reduced before the doctor sees it. If this dislocation is seen almost immediately, one is justified in attempting an atraumatic manipulation without anesthesia. The traction should be in the long axis of the deformed phalanx, whatever its position. Direct distal pressure of the operator's thumb against the base of the phalanx

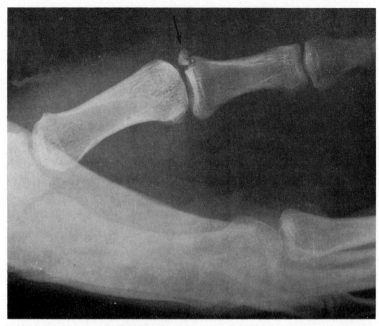

Figure 262. Lateral ligament injury of the metacarpophalangeal joint of the thumb avulsing the corner of the proximal end of the phalanx. This is really a ligament injury and requires repair by either pinning the fragment or removing the fragment and repairing the ligament.

will slide it into position as the phalanx is flexed. This dislocation cannot be reduced by traction along the long axis of the metacarpal since this simply locks the dislocation in position.

If a complete dislocation does not reduce readily by such methods, one should proceed to open reduction on the assumption that the metacarpal head is caught in the rent in the capsule or between the long flexor tendon and one of the intrinsic tendons. The hand should be prepared for surgery, the anesthetic given and a second attempt made to reduce the dislocation under anesthesia. If it does not reduce promptly with minimal stress, manipulation should not be pursued since it only damages the periarticular structures. Open operation should be carried out at once. It should be emphasized here, as in all dislocations, that time is of the essence and one must not wait days or even hours before final reduction is carried out.

Lateral stress injuries are treated using the same principles as for hyperextension injuries with the exception that surgery is performed to repair ligaments rather than to effect reduction. If complete instability is demonstrable following acute injury, repair of the involved ligament is indicated (Fig. 263). If x-ray shows an avulsion fracture with separation, the ligament should be opened and repaired (Fig. 262).

POSTOPERATIVE CARE. If the injury is moderate or if deformity is spontaneously reduced, or if open reduction has been done, the thumb should be treated by immobilization of the joint, plaster splints being my preference. The splints in this instance go out beyond the interphalangeal joint extending back to the wrist and down onto the thenar eminence. It is not absolutely essential to immobilize the wrist. After the splint is applied, motion of the thumb itself should not increase the discomfort. If it

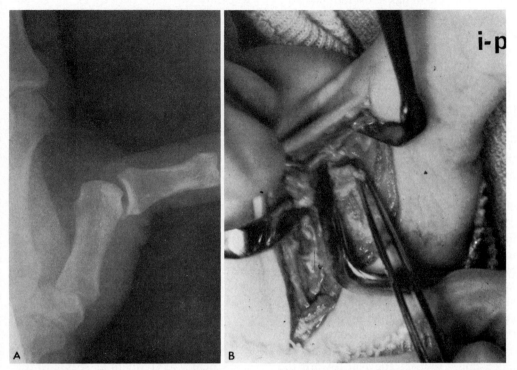

Figure 263. This demonstrates a lateral deviation injury at the metacarpophalangeal joint of the left thumb with a complete tear of the collateral ligament of the ulnar side. *A*, A stress film showing the extent of dislocation possible. *B*, An operative photograph of the torn ligament held in the forceps. Here the orientation is the same as on the x-ray, looking into the dorsomedial aspect of the metacarpophalangeal joint through the first web space. The dorsal creases of the interphalangeal joint are marked with i-p.

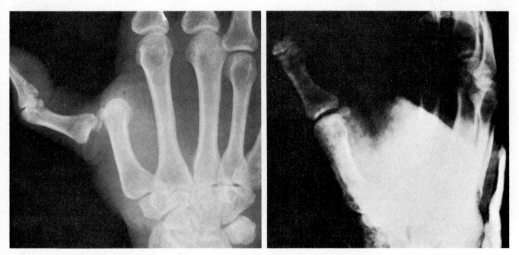

Figure 264. Complete dislocation of the metacarpophalangeal joint of the thumb. This could be reduced only by open reduction since the flexor tendons were looped around the metacarpal head.

does, the wrist should be included until the muscle spasm has subsided, possibly a week. After approximately a week in splints a thumb spica cast may be used to complete three weeks of immobilization. Since the ligaments are not securely healed at this stage, the thumb should be carefully taped to prevent the motion that puts stress on the involved ligament. This should continue for at least three additional weeks. After this the thumb must be taped during athletic participation until all tenderness is gone.

A sprain of the medial collateral ligament of the metacarpophalangeal joint of the thumb may be extremely distressing in the athlete, particularly if he has to handle the football. Actually the pinch of the thumb opposing the fingers in grabbing the ball to throw it or pass it back, such as by the center, depends upon the stability of this joint. Because this joint is unstable, when the pinch occurs it simply opens up. When the index finger presses the ball toward the thumb, it opens this inner side of the

joint up and results in serious disability. Recently we had two cases at essentially the same time. One was a center and one was a quarterback, on the same team (Fig. 265). Both obtained excellent results from reconstruction by advancement of the cuff of the capsule without any additional reinforcement. It requires considerable study of the anatomy of this portion of the hand in order to recognize the various components. It is a much more favorable injury if the ligament is actually torn off the metacarpal head, which was true in each of these cases, and reconstructive repair was carried out by simply detaching the ligament from the scar which had formed, advancing it down on the shaft and securely suturing it through with drill holes through the metacarpal shaft.

Interphalangeal Joint

Sprain of the interphalangeal joint is not nearly as frequent as sprain of the other two joints of the thumb. The lev-

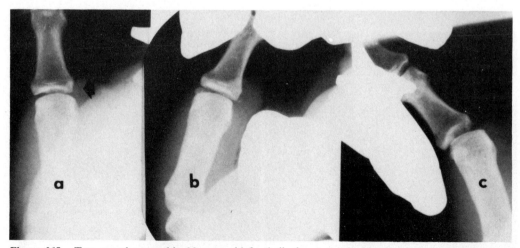

Figure 265. Two months ago this 22 year old football player caught his thumb in the equipment of another player when he was blocking and threw the thumb into wide abduction. He continued to play with a tape splint but now has complete instability of the ulnar side of the metacarpophalangeal joint of the thumb. He is unable to grasp the football in order to throw it. *A*, Shows neutral position. The small fragment is pulled off the ulnar side of the base of the proximal phalanx of the thumb. *B*, Stress, toward the radial side. *C*, Stress, toward the ulnar side. Note the phalanx actually subluxes off the metacarpal head.

erage factor is such that more strain is applied to the other joints than to the interphalangeal joint. Lateral motion of the distal phalanx may tear the opposing collateral ligament and the pain will be on the same side of the thumb as the applied force. Since the interphalangeal joint is a hinge joint, there is no appreciable lateral motion and the joint should be carefully checked for lateral instability. If instability is evident or if a small fragment of bone is revealed in the x-ray, one must assume that the collateral ligament has been avulsed or torn and the protection should be correspondingly protracted. If one can diagnose with certainty a complete tear of the collateral ligament, primary repair of the ligament is the treatment of choice. All too frequently the instability is not recognized until several weeks following the initial trauma when swelling, pain and disability persist and one notices the phalanx is deviating to the opposite side. At this time one may belatedly discover instability of the collateral ligament. Reconstruction is then necessary rather than repair and is correspondingly difficult and less successful. If injury to the interphalangeal joint is relatively severe, immobilization is indicated for at least three weeks followed by protective strapping for three more weeks.

Finger Rays

Metacarpal Area

Sprain may occur at the carpometacarpal, the metacarpophalangeal and the intermetacarpal head area.

Sprain at the *base of the metacarpal* is not common. This entire area is firmly bound together by the dorsal and palmar ligaments of the wrist and hand so that they are firmly adherent not only to each other but to the carpus. There is little lateral motion in these joints and lateral stresses are not readily applied.

The sprain is much more likely to involve the wrist than the carpometacarpal joint, since the same force puts stress on both areas and the wrist is much more vulnerable than the carpometacarpal joint.

At the *distal end of the metacarpals* the joints are in effect universal, permitting flexion and extension, adduction and abduction and circumduction, but not axial rotation. Extremes of these motions may cause a sprain of the capsular ligaments. The digits most likely to be injured in collateral sprains are the index and little fingers, since either one may be forcibly abducted away from the hand, whereas it is much more difficult to abduct the other two fingers to the extent required to damage the capsular ligaments.

The most common injury is damage to the transverse metacarpal ligaments. The same force that pulls the fingers apart may tear the ligament binding the metacarpal heads together and this may occur at any space. That is, the long and ring fingers may be forcibly separated and tear the ligament between the third and fourth metacarpals. This is much more likely than a tear of the capsular ligament of the metacarpophalangeal joint. This injury is readily overlooked. It is usually minimized but may cause weeks or months of disability of the hand and, indeed, may lead to chronic sprain with repeated reinjury and resultant disability. The injury is readily recognized if the hand is examined with the condition in mind, since simple separation of the two involved fingers will cause severe pain. The most common areas are between the fourth and fifth metacarpals and between the second and third. Treatment is relatively simple. If the hand is dressed in a manner so as to hold the fingers together, free motion can be permitted to the phalanges, and athletic competition can actually be continued if fixation is firm enough to prevent separation of the metacarpal heads. Protection should be continued for another three weeks. This injury is not particularly disabling, and essentially free function of the hand can be carried out so long as the patient wears the protective dressing.

The force most likely to cause a sprain of the metacarpophalangeal joint is hyperextension. In this instance the anterior capsule becomes tight. As the force continues the capsule may tear. The injury may be mild or moderate or it may be a complete avulsion (severe) leading to dislocation. It may involve a single finger or more than one.

Symptomatically, any sprain involving the metacarpals will present tenderness at the area of the tear, and pain will be caused by reproduction of the motion that caused the injury.

Sprain of the metacarpophalangeal joint may be severe enough to cause actual dislocation. This is infrequent and is readily recognized as a very serious injury which demands definitive care by an experienced physician. Dorsal dislocation of the base of the phalanx at the metacarpophalangeal joint occurs as a result of the same hyperextension that causes sprain of the anterior capsule. As the force continues, the proximal phalanx moves backward over the metacarpal. The anterior capsule tears and the soft tissues are pulled dorsally, being displaced posterior to the metacarpal head. The phalanx dislocates onto the back of the metacarpal where it stands at a 90 degree angle to the metacarpal. As mentioned previously, it is quite unlikely that this dislocation is seen in its original position; inevitably someone has attempted to straighten the finger. If an attempt has been made by simply flexing the phalanx, it will usually result in sliding the phalanx back along the dorsum of the metacarpal and impinging a flap of capsule between the phalanx and metacarpal head. Such manipulation

is to be condemned and should be avoided by the physician who attempts reduction (Fig. 266, A to D).

If the deformity is of the right angle variety, reduction can frequently be accomplished by applying pressure distally along the base of the phalanx in the direction of the long axis of the metacarpal while the finger is maintained in hyperextension. This permits the base of the phalanx to slide over the metacarpal head, and as it resumes its normal position in relation to the metacarpal head, flexion of the finger will reduce the dislocation. An attempt may be made to carry out this manipulation without anesthesia provided the dislocation is seen very early and also provided that there has been no traumatic attempt to carry out reduction earlier.

If the finger and metacarpal are parallel with the phalanx resting on the back of the metacarpal neck, it is unlikely that the dislocation can be reduced without anesthesia. In such an instance it is well to be prepared to perform a surgical procedure at the time the anesthetic is given since it may be impossible to reduce the dislocation even under anesthesia. Under anesthesia traction may be placed on the phalanx along the axis of the metacarpal. Many times this maneuver will successfully reduce the dislocation. If it does not, the phalanx may be very carefully hyperextended to an angulation of 90 degrees to the metacarpal placing it back in the position it occupied at the time of the dislocation. This may remove the interposed tissue and permit classic reduction. If such a reduction cannot be done without undue force, the attempt should not be continued, and one should proceed to an open reduction in order to disengage the interposed tissue and permit the metacarpal head to move backward under the phalanx (Fig. 267). Since the structures blocking reduction are located anteriorly, the inci-

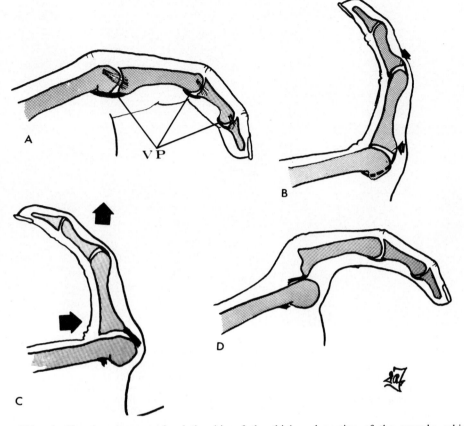

Figure 266. *A,* Showing the normal relationship of the thickened portion of the capsule, which is termed the volar plate. Notice that it attaches well proximal to the head of the proximal bone. *B,* Illustrates the first effect of hyperextension, which is either sprain of the ligament or avulsion of its attachment to the bone (arrows). *C,* The end point of complete hyperextension, with a torn capsule and dislocation of the involved phalanx. The arrows indicate the direction of the forces which should be used in reduction. If the phalanx is merely straightened, the situation in *D* will possibly prevail, with the head of the proximal bone protruding through a rent in the capsule.

sion must be in the palm. The head of the metacarpal becomes caught between the flexor tendons medially, the lumbrical laterally, the volar plate distally and the transverse elements of the palmar fascia proximally. A transverse incision over the metacarpophalangeal joint will give excellent access to these structures. A midlateral incision will result in a three-hour bungling attempt at the same thing. Following reduction, immobilization should be carried out for about two weeks, but it is not necessary to immobilize the interphalangeal joints. Thus, rehabilitation can start at once.

Finger Area

Sprain of the interphalangeal joints may be caused by hyperextension of the joint, which causes the anterior capsule to be torn (Fig. 266, *A* and *B*), or by excess lateral motion of this hinge joint (Figs. 268, 269). The interphalangeal joints have definite collateral ligaments which are tight in flexion and relatively loose in extension. Lateral angulation of the phalanx will cause damage to the collateral ligament. This usually occurs with the involved joint in extension. A torn collateral ligament may be a very painful injury and may result in disabil-

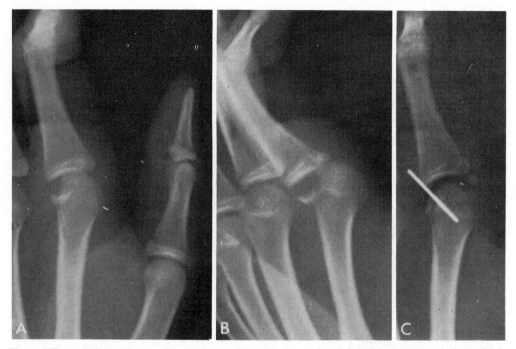

Figure 267. *A* and *B*, The anteroposterior and lateral views of a dislocated metacarpophalangeal joint of the index finger. Avulsion of the attachment of one of the collateral ligaments to the first metacarpal has taken a small piece of bone with it. Dislocation of this joint should be opened through an incision in the palm because the metacarpal head becomes caught between the lumbrical tendon laterally, the long flexor tendons medially, the capsule distally and transverse fibers of the palmar fascia proximally. In this instance the avulsed ligament was repaired through a separate dorsal incision *(C)*.

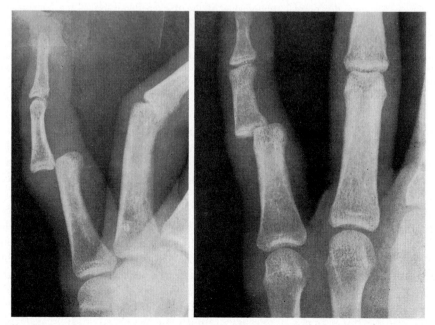

Figure 268. Dislocation of proximal interphalangeal joint of the little finger. This dislocation usually entails severe injury to the collateral ligaments and is likely to heal with swollen, stiff joint or instability, or both.

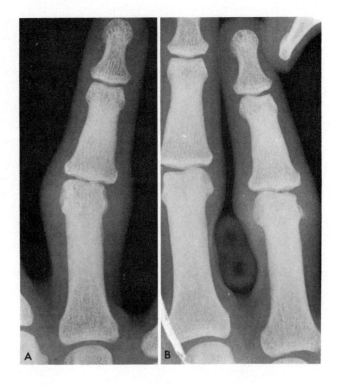

Figure 269. A neglected injury to a collateral ligament of the proximal interphalangeal joint results in a finger which is unstable in lateral deviation. *A,* The joint remains chronically swollen. *B,* A stress x-ray shows correction of the deformity.

ity if left untreated. On the other hand, if it is immobilized, disability may result from stiffness. Careful examination of the finger will permit one to determine whether or not there is instability. If there is instability the joint should be immobilized in extension with appropriate lateral deviation to close the joint on the involved side. This should be maintained for about two weeks. After that, some motion may be permitted, but flexion beyond 90 degrees should not be permitted for at least four weeks.

Sprain of the anterior capsule can be demonstrated by pain when an attempt is made to completely extend this joint. If the injury is severe, it may actually be possible to hyperextend the joint. In such an instance the joint should be immobilized in moderate flexion for two or three weeks. If there is no instability but only pain, it should suffice to protect the finger for a week or 10 days and then permit motion, warning the patient that he should not permit

complete extension. If athletic competition is permitted, either in game or practice, the finger splint should be replaced during actual play for at least four weeks since relatively minor repetition of the original injury may cause recurrence.

Dislocation of the interphalangeal joints is ordinarily caused by the same forces that cause sprain of the anterior capsule (Fig. 270). As the hyperextension continues, the anterior capsule tears, and the head of the more proximal phalanx thrusts through the palmar surface of the joint; it may, indeed, pierce the skin. Such an injury should be regarded as very serious (Fig. 271). It is frequently spontaneously reduced, particularly if incomplete. Even if the dislocation is complete, it will usually be reduced by the time one sees it if it is readily reducible.

In the dislocations that do not reduce, the head of the phalanx is usually caught either in the capsule or in the

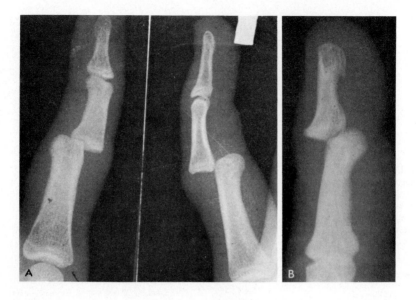

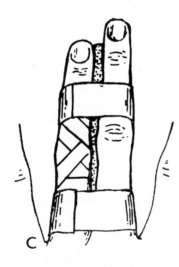

Figure 270. *A,* The anteroposterior and lateral views of a dislocated proximal interphalangeal joint. Usually this can readily be reduced by hyperextending the dislocated joint and applying distal pressure to the base of the middle phalanx. When the overriding has been corrected the joint is flexed. *B,* A similar situation in the distal interphalangeal joint which is reduced in much the same manner.

C, The taping for a sprained or dislocated finger. Flex the injured joints slightly. Using ½ inch adhesive tape, apply a basket weave over the injured joint. Place ⅛ inch thickness of soft sponge, felt or cotton between the fingers to prevent maceration. Using ½ inch tape, strap the finger to an adjoining finger which will act as a splint, leaving the index finger free if possible. (Courtesy of Rawlinson, Modern Athletic Training, © 1961 by Prentice Hall, Inc.)

flexor tendon. If this is seen immediately after the injury, it may be reduced by manipulation. The first step in the manipulation is to reproduce the hyperextension to unlock the base of the dislocated phalanx and then, by traction along the line of the dislocated phalanx, the base of the bone can be readily pushed down into contact with the head of the more proximal phalanx. If it does not reduce readily, procaine block may provide adequate anesthesia because muscle relaxation is not necessary. If the dislocation is open, the wound is given a very thorough cleansing using copious amounts of soap and water. The head is then reduced. If it is an early injury, the skin edges are sutured as a primary procedure.

Following any of these dislocations, the finger should be immobilized with the joint in some flexion. The finger should not be flexed to 90 degrees although this may seem to hold the dislocation more firmly. In this position the collateral ligaments are under undue tension, and healing occurs with the ligament too long.

The dislocation may occur without actually tearing either collateral ligament. After the finger is reduced, particularly if the procedure is performed under anesthesia, careful check should be made to determine whether or not there is instability. If instability is present, one should seriously consider repair of the collateral ligament. In many of these conditions there is redundancy of this ligament with migration of the more distal phalanx toward the opposite side, and a painful, unstable, nonfunctional joint may result.

The same components are present in dislocation of the interphalangeal joint as are present in dislocation of the knee. It is a serious injury and may well result in permanent disability, particularly if treatment is too casual. One should study the x-ray carefully, partic-

ularly after reduction, since it may provide evidence of an avulsion of the ligament or possibly a fracture of one of the margins of the phalangeal base. The belief is growing among many orthopaedists that severe and complete tears of the collateral interphalangeal ligaments should be treated by surgical repair. It is very difficult to obtain reliable figures relating to the rate of permanent instability in these cases. Many patients are treated quite casually and never see the doctor. The ones who do, have severe dislocations which will not reduce or old ones which have already healed but which have instability. Certainly it is very difficult to repair an old tear. Reconstruction is not very satisfactory. Hence, there is the tendency to recommend surgical repair early if there is gross instability in the involved joint. Remember that the most stable position in the interphalangeal joint is at 90 degrees of flexion rather than at complete extension. In complete extension most

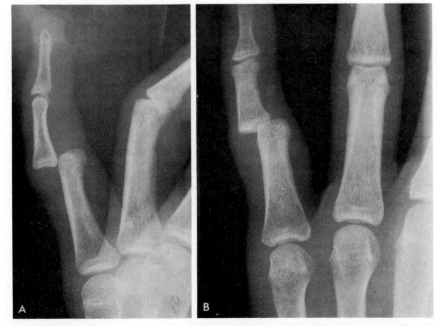

Figure 271. *A* and *B*, Dislocation of the proximal interphalangeal joint of the little finger. This dislocation usually entails severe injury to the collateral ligaments and is likely to heal with a swollen, stiff joint or instability, or both.

interphalangeal joints do have some lateral motion.

Chronic Sprain of the Interphalangeal Joints

A joint that has sustained repeated sprains or several inadequately treated sprains, or even the joint that has been treated properly, will occasionally become swollen and stiff, and defy all efforts at rehabilitation. Local steroids or systemic phenylbutazone are helpful, and avoiding repeated trauma provides the best complete cure of the painful swollen joint that is incompatible with satisfactory hand function.

FRACTURE-DISLOCATIONS

When the dislocation is associated with a fracture, the fracture will frequently appear to be the primary injury; however, attention should still be directed toward reducing the residual subluxation of the joint. Frequently when the subluxation is reduced, the fracture fragments will mold themselves into proper position. If the deformity of the phalanx is a volar subluxation, this should be corrected and held with a K-wire inserted percutaneously across the joint. Similarly if the subluxation is dorsal, it can be reduced and held in position with a K-wire. Molding of the fracture fragments will sometimes offer surprisingly good results (Fig. 272). If a medial or lateral subluxation fractures one of the condyles of the phalanx, it can be similarly returned to its normal position by reducing the subluxation and holding the condyle in place by a K-wire inserted percutaneously without opening the fracture site. Occasionally, however, it must be opened.

If a small fragment of bone attached to the capsule at the base of the phalanx is pushed distally at the time of the dislocation, it can be returned to its normal relationship by hyperextending the joint (Fig. 273). If the small chip is merely avulsed and returns to its normal position with flexion, the finger can be immobilized in moderate flexion for two to three weeks (Fig. 274).

FRACTURES OF THE HAND

In dealing with fractures of the individual bones of the hand, it is important to remember that each presents unique problems, but none of the problems associated with the healing of the fracture should overshadow the importance of obtaining satisfactory hand function. The necessity of obtaining a good x-ray reduction should be weighed against the possibility of producing joint stiffness and tendon adherence. On the other hand, malposition of a fracture cannot be tolerated if it interferes with the balance between intrinsic and extrinsic function, which is achieved with the hand in the position of function. Frequently immobilization of the hand in this position will help with the reduction of the fracture. It is important to remember that the tendons glide in close proximity to the bones in the hand, and careless treatment of fractures will result in adhesions of tendon to bone.

Fractures are caused by indirect violence or by direct violence with a direct blow to the bone involved. Indirect violence with hyperextension or medial or lateral angulation produces damage to any one of three elements. The first element is composed of the ligaments and their bony attachments, the second element is the epiphyseal plate and the third is bone. Treatment of the ligamentous injuries, including their bony attachments, has been discussed previously and will be found in the section on sprains. Epiphyseal fractures and fractures through bone present es-

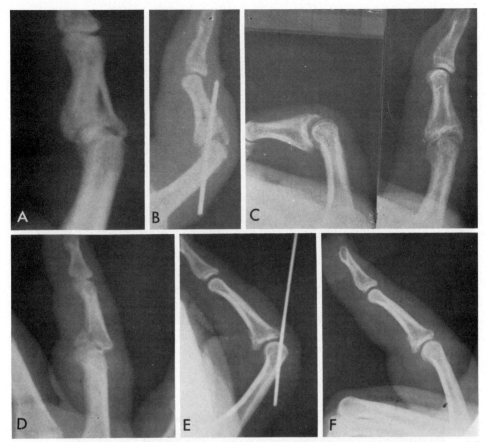

Figure 272. *A,* A volar fracture-subluxation of the proximal interphalangeal joint. *D,* A dorsal fracture-subluxation. *B* and *E,* Each injury was treated by reducing the subluxation and holding the joint in the reduced position using a K-wire strategically positioned so as not to cause separation of the fracture fragments. *C,* Although a perfect x-ray result was not obtained, notice the complete range of motion obtained. There was no swelling about the joint. *F,* A much better reduction with an equally good functional result. This same situation exists at the base of the proximal phalanx at the metacarpophalangeal joint.

sentially the same problems of treatment and will be discussed together. In fractures of the epiphyses and in fractures close to the joints the reduction should be as nearly anatomic as possible. Again, since the thumb and fingers present unique problems, they will be discussed separately.

THUMB RAY

Metacarpal Area

The same forces that produce dislocation of the thumb may also cause fracture. A fracture peculiar to the thumb is the *Bennett fracture,* which is in reality a fracture-dislocation of the carpometacarpal joint with fracture of some portion of the medial proximal margin of the base of the metacarpal (Fig. 275, *A*). The same force that will cause dislocation by direct force down the shaft of the metacarpal, such as a blow with the fist, drives the base of the metacarpal proximally and dorsally. Instead of the anterior capsule tearing, the bone breaks. The injury causes not only fracture-dislocation of the metacarpal but

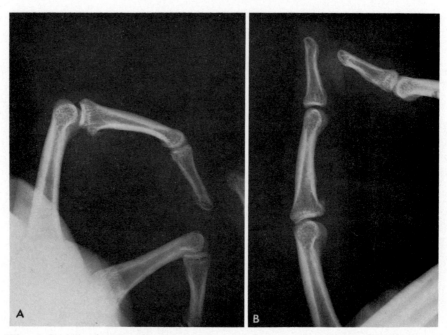

Figure 273. *A*, Snubbing fracture of the anterior flange of the proximal end of the middle phalanx. *B*, Note reduction of the fragment by extension of the finger.

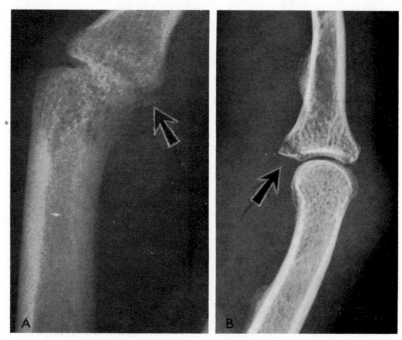

Figure 274. Avulsion injuries of the volar plate pulling small fragments of bone from the base of the phalanx. *A*, A very small flake of bone. *B*, A larger chip of bone. Frequently, careful questioning regarding the mechanism of the injury and oblique x-rays in several planes will elicit the presence of these fragments when they might otherwise be overlooked.

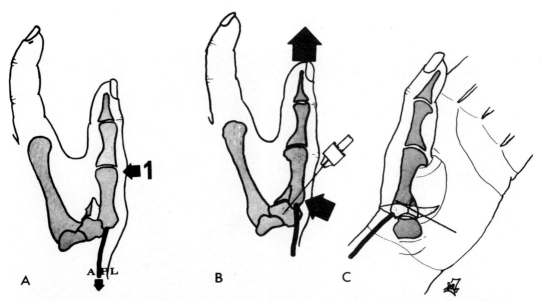

Figure 275. *A*, The mechanism of production of a Bennett fracture with a force as indicated (arrow 1). This force drives the thumb into the palm and results in a fracture of the ulnar lip of the base of the metacarpal, which holds the base on its saddle-like articulation. The abductor pollicis longus (APL) contributes a deforming force by pulling the base of the thumb from its saddle. *B*, The principle of reduction with closed percutaneous pinning. Longitudinal traction is placed on the thumb, and pressure is applied at the base of the thumb, in order to reposition the metacarpal on the greater multangular so the fracture is reduced in the same manner that fracture-dislocations of the fingers are reduced (see Fig. 272). Notice how an intact periosteum helps mold the fracture. The K-wire must not enter the fracture site, since this will merely cause distraction of the fracture fragments. *C*, The principle of open reduction of this fracture. The fracture is visualized through an incision at the base of the thumb and held in the reduced position with one or two small threaded K-wires inserted across the fracture site. These are best inserted with a motor drill.

also tearing of the dorsal ligaments and capsule of the metacarpophalangeal joint. On examination the thumb appears foreshortened. It is thick at its base with prominence of the base of the shaft of the metacarpal. Traction-abduction readily reduces the dislocation and one may not suspect the fracture unless x-rays are made (Fig. 259). On relaxing the traction, the deformity promptly recurs (Figs. 276 and 277).

Theoretically traction and abduction with pressure against the base of the phalanx should adequately hold this fracture. This method is unnecessarily cumbersome and ineffective. If traction is elected, skeletal traction should be used through either the distal end of the metacarpal or the shaft of the proximal phalanx. The wrist must be flexed to the

ulnar side, the thumb widely abducted with traction along its long axis. The cast is applied in this position, care being taken to place a felt pad at the pressure area on the base of the metacarpal. Elastic traction is then applied by an outrigger (Figs. 278 and 279). The pull is along the long axis of the metacarpal. This position must be maintained for several weeks until union is fairly firm. The traction can then be removed, but the cast must be replaced holding the thumb in abduction. It is notably difficult to hold this position and recurrence of deformity is frequent (Fig. 280). An alternative method of holding the reduction involves insertion of a K-wire to hold the base of the metacarpal on its saddle (Figs. 275, 276 and 277).

Since an inadequate reduction will

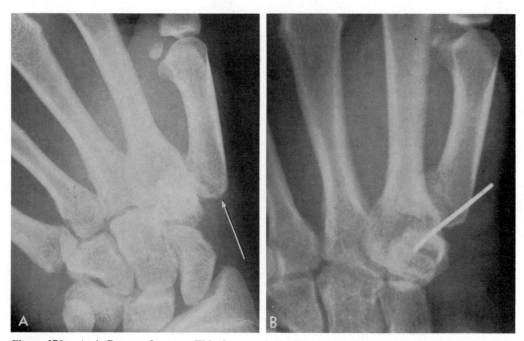

Figure 276. *A,* A Bennett fracture. This fracture is completely unstable, *B,* Reduction is best maintained by internal fixation. The wire shown is not well placed but did hold. (For x-ray positioning, see Fig. 259.)

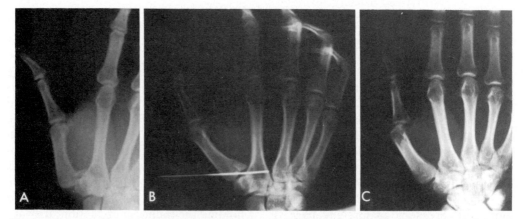

Figure 277.   This 19 year old male received pain and disability of the thumb during a football injury. *A,* X-ray shows the dislocation of the base of the metacarpal with the triangular fragment of bone remaining adherent to the ligaments. *B,* This was treated by closed reduction and transfixion pin across the base of the metacarpal of the thumb and into the base of the metacarpal of the index finger rather than into the carpus. This gave very adequate fixation. *C,* Shows complete healing. (For x-ray positioning, see Fig. 259.)

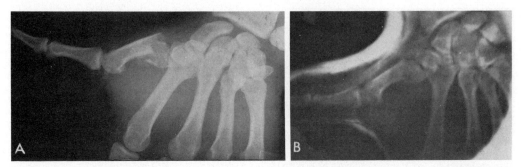

Figure 278. *A,* Transverse fracture of the base of the thumb with displacement. *B,* Fixation in wide abduction maintained by plaster cast.

lead to osteoarthritis later, the best result is obtained by a nearly perfect reduction. Our preference is to try to reduce the fracture under anesthesia by manipulation and traction. If reduction is good, percutaneous threaded K-wire fixation across the base of the metacarpal through the fragment and into the carpus is attempted. If this is successful and if it holds firmly, a gauntlet thumb spica is applied. If it fails to reduce or if the fixation fails to hold, primary open reduction should be carried out and completed by properly placed internal fixation of the shaft to the fragment without involving the carpus if possible. This will permit motion of the thumb before the fixation is removed, which may be a quite important factor.

With *fractures of the shaft* and of the neck of the metacarpal of the thumb it is important to obtain and maintain good position. The fracture of the middle of the shaft of the metacarpal will

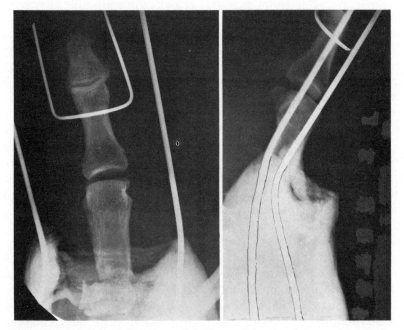

Figure 279. Transverse comminuted fracture of the base of the thumb, treated by traction. Note distraction of the carpophalangeal joint.

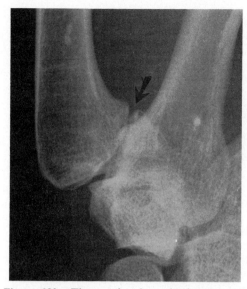

Figure 280. The result of an inadequate reduction of a Bennett fracture. There is nonunion of the fracture (arrow) and osteoarthritic spurring about the carpometacarpal joint.

cross toward the base of the fifth metacarpal head, not toward the second. This permits opposition of the thumb to the various fingers. The so-called mallet finger, or baseball finger, is unusual in the thumb and treatment is the same as in the fingers. The same is true in fractures involving the interphalangeal joint and in crushing injuries of the tip of the distal phalanx.

FINGER RAYS

The subject of fracture of the metacarpals and phalanges is a voluminous one. The reader is referred to standard works on fractures or treatment of injuries to the hand for adequate detail. Some of the details particularly pertinent to the athlete will be reviewed.

Metacarpals

Fracture of the *base of the metacarpal* (Fig. 282) occurs from a direct blow against the end of the metacarpal, which transmits the force down the shaft as exemplified by the blow with the clenched fist. It may also be caused by a direct crushing force over the back of the hand as it rests on a solid surface. The metacarpal bases are so closely bound together that the fracture is not displaced. Diagnosis may be made by history of the character of the injury and by the local findings. Tenderness will be extreme at the site of the break (Fig. 283). Direct pressure over the injured area is painful. Pain is elicited by tapping the end of the bone, the force being transmitted down the shaft of the metacarpal to the fracture site.

Careful x-ray study is important since in many instances the fragments are impacted. This combined with the fact that the bones normally overlap may make x-ray interpretation difficult. One may be amazed to see, after several

usually angulate dorsally and may be reduced by abduction of the thumb and pressure over the fracture site. It may be held in this position by an appropriate plaster cast. If the position is not secure or does not hold, open reduction with internal fixation or percutaneous insertion of K-wires is the treatment of choice.

Fractures of the proximal phalanx of the thumb are not nearly as common as those of the fingers (Fig. 281). If a fracture is complete, it is much more difficult to hold because of the extreme mobility of the normal thumb. Fixation should be with the thumb in flexion, at both the metacarpophalangeal and the interphalangeal joints. This may be maintained by a suitable plaster splint until swelling is stabilized. Then a plaster cast is applied. It is imperative to secure good position in order to preserve the function of the thumb. One must be particularly careful that there is no rotation of this phalanx. When the thumb is flexed into the palm, it should

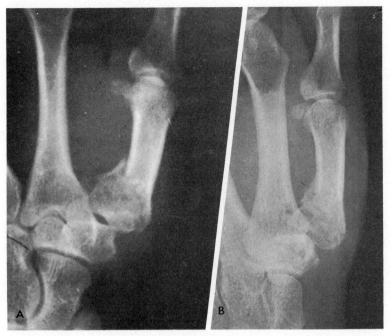

Figure 281. *A*, An example of a fracture at the base of the thumb metacarpal produced by essentially the same force as that causing a Bennett fracture. However, this is an impacted fracture of the base and is corrected by simply abducting the thumb, thus straightening the angulation (*B*).

weeks, fractures that did not appear at all on the original x-ray. A particular effort should be made to assess any possible dislocation. Since the palmar ligament is so much stronger than the dorsal, the force may drive the shaft backward, break off the anterior margin of the metacarpal and permit the shaft of the metacarpal and dorsal part of the proximal end to displace dorsally (Fig. 282). This can be readily palpated immediately after the injury but is later concealed by swelling, edema and infiltration of blood. Very careful lateral x-ray views in several planes may be necessary to actually demonstrate this dislocation.

One may be chagrined after treating

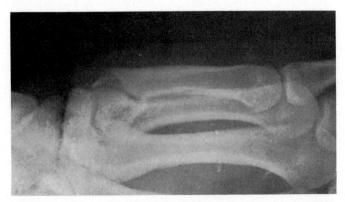

Figure 282. An oblique fracture at the base of the metacarpal; notice the shortening. This can be corrected by traction with a Z-wire of fishhook type inserted into the neck of the metacarpal.

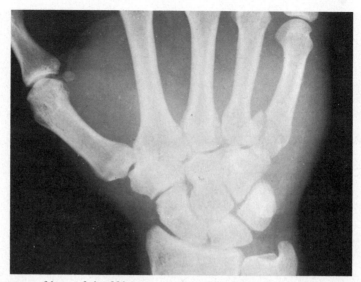

Figure 283.   Fracture of base of the fifth metacarpal resulting from a blow with the clenched fist against the opponent's head. This comminuted type of fracture requires traction – in this instance straight traction – for reduction and fixation.

what appears to be contusion or sprain of the hand to find gross deformity of one of the bases, particularly of the second and third metacarpal. On the other hand, if the injury is recognized early it may be reduced by traction. It may be difficult to maintain reduction by cast fixation only. Internal fixation is relatively simple since the bone may be transfixed by percutaneous insertion of K-wire after reduction without actually opening the fracture site. After reduction, transfixion wires may be placed through the metacarpal into the undisplaced proximal fragment. A little ingenuity will be well rewarded provided the diagnostic acuity has been sufficient to reveal this lesion. If the fracture is incomplete or without displacement, simple immobilization of the wrist and hand is adequate. It is not necessary to immobilize either the metacarpophalangeal or the interphalangeal joints. Protection should continue as long as the symptoms persist. The inherent stability here is such that in many circumstances immobilization may be discontinued within two weeks.

As the location of the injury moves distally to involve the *metacarpal shaft,* management becomes more complicated. Many fractures of the third or fourth metacarpal, being surrounded on two sides by intact bone, may be without displacement and so require little treatment. Angulation of the shaft of the third or fourth metacarpal is not common. If it occurs, it should be reduced by traction on the fingers, direct pressure over the metacarpal adjacent to the fracture site and then transfixion of the shafts by Kirschner wire drilled across and through the two adjacent and intact metacarpals above and below the fracture site (Fig. 284). These can be cut off beneath the skin and virtually no external immobilization is required after the first few days. This internal fixation is more likely to be necessary in the oblique than in the transverse fracture (Fig. 285). The long spiral fracture ordinarily will maintain adequate position and a few millimeters shortening of the bone will be of little consequence. When the fracture involves more than one metacarpal, or when it involves the second

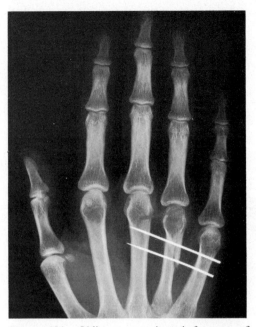

Figure 284. Oblique, comminuted fracture of the shaft of the fourth metacarpal, treated by manual traction and K-wire transfixing two intact metacarpals. This is an excellent method.

or fifth, stability is much less secure. It has been our experience in the athlete with a fracture and displacement in the shaft of either of these metacarpals that some sort of internal fixation is advisable. This is particularly true because fixation by plaster is cumbersome and very often fails.

If plaster fixation is elected, the wrist should be dorsiflexed. Direct pressure is applied over the metacarpal adjacent to the angulated fracture site while traction is placed on the involved finger. If the fracture is unstable, skeletal traction may be necessary using any of the various methods, such as a Z-hook K-wire through the dorsal cortex of the distal fragment or transfixation traction through the proximal phalanx laterally. After traction is applied and the fracture is reduced, a palmar splint should be applied with the wrist dorsiflexed, the metacarpophalangeal joint

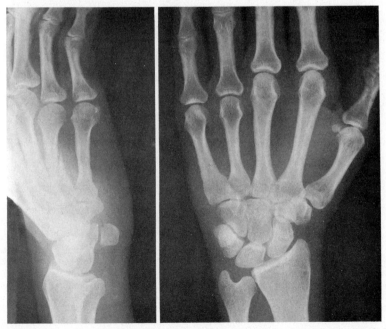

Figure 285. Spiral oblique fracture of the middle of the shaft of the fourth metacarpal. Note that in the anteroposterior view the fracture line is not visible, although the bone does look somewhat shorter. Because of the shortening, traction is indicated even though the fracture should heal well without treatment.

semiflexed and the proximal interphalangeal joint rather sharply flexed (90 degrees). This should be supported by a posterior splint plus a felt pressure pad adjacent to the fracture site which permits direct downward pressure against the angulated fracture fragment.

This pressure must never be exerted directly over the fracture site since it may force the extensor tendon into the fracture site and lead to adhesions (Fig. 286). This position is maintained by manual traction until the splint is hardened. Sometimes additional felt pads

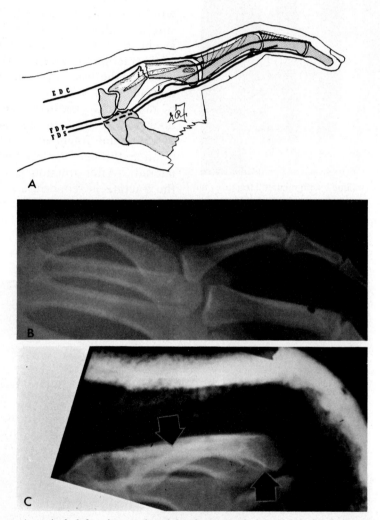

Figure 286. *A,* A typical deformity produced by fracture of the mid-shaft of the metacarpal. Note that once the intrinsic-extrinsic balance of the finger is upset, a series of deformities is produced, each one contributing to another deformity. In this example the angulation of the metacarpal produces tension on the extensor digitorum communis (EDC) which in turn hyperextends the metacarpophalangeal joint. This places tension on the lumbrical (1), which helps produce more bowing at the fracture site, and also places tension on the flexor digitorum sublimis tendon (FDS). The first principle to observe in treating fractures of this type is to place the hand in a position of function which will correct the deforming forces. *B,* An x-ray of this type of fracture. *C,* A very satisfactory reduction obtained by splinting the hand in the position of function. If additional pressure padding is needed to help maintain the reduction, felt is used. It is never placed over the fracture site but adjacent to it; this avoids pushing the tendons into the fracture site (arrows).

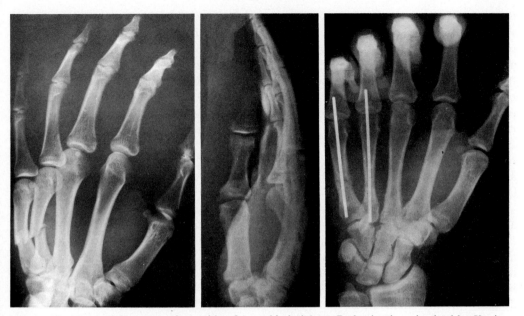

Figure 287. Fractured metacarpals resulting from athletic injury. Reduction is maintained by K-wires. These wires transfix the metacarpal head and should be removed as soon as the union is solid enough. The fingers should be immobilized until the wires are removed.

can be inserted after the splints harden. After the plaster sets, some sort of outrigger must be applied to maintain traction on the involved finger. Bear in mind that this cannot be done with the fingers in extension but must be done with the fingers flexed.

It is much more difficult to treat a metacarpal fracture by skeletal traction than it is by some form of internal fixation. Consequently, if the fracture is not adequately supported by the cast alone without traction, I would abandon further efforts to hold it and would use internal fixation. Internal fixation is carried out with wire loops or a small plate or by K-wire transfixion of the fractured metacarpals to the intact ones. Another method is to use an intramedullary pin inserted into the distal end of the bone with the metacarpophalangeal joint in complete flexion (Fig. 287). It should not be left in place for more than three or four weeks.

It must be emphasized again that fractures of the metacarpals are serious injuries. If one intends to treat them, he should properly prepare himself by adequate study of the various factors involved not only in causing the deformity but in preventing its recurrence.

Fractures of the *neck of the metacarpal* are very common, the most frequent being of the fifth. They are often caused by the impact of the knuckle of the clenched fist against someone's skull as he ducks a blow to the face. The result is almost always a flexion deformity with the head rotated over the neck, so that the head presents itself in the palm. Examination of the metacarpal bone will show why forward rotation of the head causes such prominence in the palm of the hand. The head normally hooks forward to be much more prominent on the palmar than on the dorsal surface. Forward angulation causes this normal prominence to be exaggerated. On examination this abnormality is readily palpable. This fracture is usually impacted but should not be left unreduced. It should be noted that there is usually more trouble with the third and fourth heads than with the others since they are less mobile, and any gross displacement of the head into the palm will cause disability not only by the impingement of the head but by pressure on the nerve and restriction of motion of the joint.

These fractures are usually readily reduced. Anesthesia is required. Under anesthesia it may be possible to manipulate the head by pressure of the surgeon's fingers over the shaft dorsally and pressure backward with his thumb against the head. It may be impacted so much that this simple manipulation is ineffective. In such a case the proximal phalanx can be utilized to push the head dorsally on the metacarpal shaft after flexing the metacarpophalangeal joint to 90 degrees. One should not be deluded into believing he can flex the proximal phalanx into the palm, apply a pressure dressing and so reduce the fracture. The fracture must be disimpacted and re-duced before any dressing is applied. Very frequently, it may be held in a simple splint, maintaining the fingers in semiflexion (Fig. 286).

If the fracture seems unstable, it has been advocated that greater stability can be obtained by flexing the proximal phalanx to 90 degrees and splinting the finger in this position on the theory that pressure upward on the phalanx and downward on the back of the hand will hold the position. My experience with this method is not favorable. It is my belief that if the fracture will hold in this position, it will probably also be held securely by a splint in the functional position. It is impossible to keep constant pressure on the back of the hand and on the distal end of the proximal phalanx in an active individual.

If the fracture is unstable my preference is to transfix it with a K-wire (Figs. 287 and 288). With the uncomplicated case one can go through the end of the knuckle and down the shaft of the

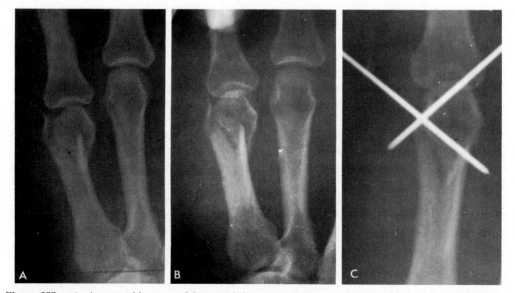

Figure 288. *A,* An unstable type of impacted fracture of the neck of the metacarpal. Once the impaction was corrected, the metacarpal would not maintain its normal length because the head kept slipping into maximum deformity *(B)*. *C,* K-wires were inserted to maintain the reduction. Each K-wire obtained purchase on the head and also into the neck. These wires were inserted percutaneously without opening the fracture site.

metacarpal. This wire can be removed at the end of three weeks since the fracture stabilizes itself rapidly. The more serious injuries of the hand involving multiple metacarpals with fractures and dislocations will require a high degree of skill and no effort should be spared to restore the function of the hand to normal.

Phalanges

Proximal Phalanx. The *proximal phalanx* is more commonly fractured than the other two phalanges. This is primarily due to the fact that the entire leverage of the fingers is brought to bear on the proximal phalanx, whereas in the middle one there is a much shorter lever arm. Any of the phalanges may be fractured by a direct blow. This may be caused by a football cleat as the hand is stretched out on the hard ground or by catching the finger between two hard opposing objects such as the football helmet and the ground or the fiber pad on the pants against a helmet or a shoe. This type of fracture from crushing injury is ordinarily stellate and without displacement. Whichever phalanx is involved, it may be treated by simple immobilization of the bone, including the joint above and the one below, provided there is no rotational deformity.

The finger is not often broken by direct impact, as in boxing, since the flexed position tends to protect it from this force. The more serious fractures usually result from leverage action. In the proximal phalanx this action is usually hyperextension of the fingers, the same force that causes dislocation of the proximal interphalangeal joint or the metacarpophalangeal joint.

At the *base of the proximal phalanx* the injury may actually be a fracture-dislocation. As the phalanx slides backward over the metacarpal head the dorsal margin is broken off by direct impingement

against the metacarpal or the palmar margin is pulled off by traction of the capsule. The dislocation in this instance is usually spontaneously reduced, since the head does not tend to lock out of position. The result is the player's presenting himself with a painful, swollen, very tender metacarpophalangeal joint without obvious displacement. However, if the fractured fragment is large enough, instability results and the joint will subluxate (Fig. 272). The tenderness will be at the base of the phalanx rather than over the metacarpal head. Careful x-ray examination will reveal the triangular-shaped shadow of the fragmented bone. If the fragment is the posterior cortex, the metacarpophalangeal joint must be placed in extension in order to get apposition. If it is the palmar border, the finger should be placed in flexion (Figs. 274 and 292, *C*). Following the repositioning of the finger, careful x-ray study should be made to determine the exact alignment of this fragment (Fig. 292, *B*). If it is not correctly positioned and held, the fracture should be treated by open reduction and pinning with a small threaded K-wire. Since the joint surface is involved, the aphorism "the nearer the joint, the more perfect the reduction must be" is pertinent.

This same type of fracture may occur on the lateral margins of the index or little fingers as a result of forced abduction of the finger away from the midline (Fig. 262). These injuries are in effect capsule or ligament injuries and should be treated as such (Fig. 290).

The *shaft of the proximal phalanx* may be fractured at any level by the same hyperextension force; the break occurs most commonly through the middle third (Fig. 291). The fracture is transverse or oblique and the distal fragment will angulate dorsally (Fig. 292, *A* and *C*). It may or may not be completely displaced. If the fracture is a sta-

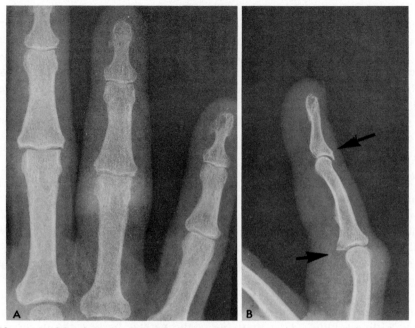

Figure 289. *A*, Avulsion fracture of the palmar lip of the proximal end of the middle phalanx as a result of hyperextension of the finger. This mild displacement requires no treatment other than fixation of the finger in a splint. *B*, Note the old baseball finger deformity in the distal phalanx (arrow) and the healed fracture of the middle phalanx.

ble fracture or can be made one, it may be supported in complete flexion of the finger by simple splint fixation. This applies particularly to the transverse fracture and more so to the transverse fracture in which the fragment is angu-

lated but not displaced. Careful manipulation will reduce the angulation, and the fracture will be quite stable as the finger is held with all the interphalangeal joints and the metacarpophalangeal joint in complete flexion (Fig. 292, *A*, *B* and

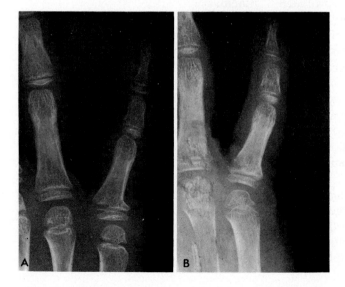

Figure 290. *A*, Transverse fracture and epiphyseal dislocation of the proximal phalanx of the fifth finger, treated by manipulation and splint. *B*, Solid union. No growth interference.

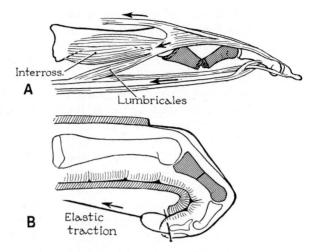

Figure 291. Fractures of the proximal phalanx. *A*, All the muscle forces acting upon a fracture of the proximal phalanx collaborate to produce an angular deformity, apex forward. *B*, Proximal phalanx fractures must be immobilized by well fitting splints with the finger flexed. Unstable fractures may require supplemental traction. (From McLaughlin, Trauma.)

C). It can be held in this position for about three weeks by a well-padded dorsal splint and then gently mobilized. In the young individual the resulting stiffness is not permanent.

We have not found it necessary in these cases of transverse fractures to use traction in the flexed position, preferring the following dressing (Fig. 292, *C*). The involved finger is joined to its immediate neighbor; i.e., if the ring finger is the one involved, include the little finger; with the index finger, the long finger; with the long finger, the ring finger. This serves two purposes. It permits the fingers to be held in this posi-

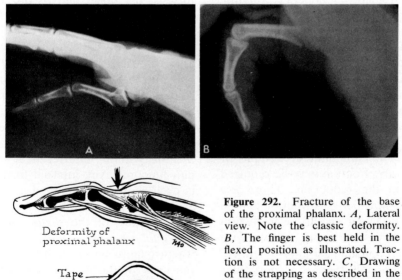

Figure 292. Fracture of the base of the proximal phalanx. *A*, Lateral view. Note the classic deformity. *B*, The finger is best held in the flexed position as illustrated. Traction is not necessary. *C*, Drawing of the strapping as described in the text. (Modified from Ochsner and DeBakey, Christopher's Minor Surgery.)

tion without strain and provides some stability from the adjacent finger for not only angular but also rotary position. After the finger is flexed, a piece of adhesive tape is started over the metacarpal head, passed over the finger, down into the palm and up along the palmar surface of the hand and wrist. It is advisable to place a strip of sheet wadding between the two fingers and through the flexor creases of the fingers. This position, when held by these two strips of tape, will be quite secure. A strip of one inch tape is then passed from the back of the hand, through the palm just proximal to the tip of the flexed fingers and back onto the dorsum of the hand. This serves to anchor the palmar strips. The whole is then included in a firm wrapping of gauze bandage. The fingers need not be flexed beyond the point of comfort, and if the hand is uncomfortable after the dressing is applied, it should be loosened sufficiently so that there is no feeling that the joints are overflexed. If the hand swells or the fingers feel numb, the tips should be carefully checked for circulation. This dressing may be buttressed if desirable by a plaster or plastic-type splint about two inches wide, beginning at the tips of the fingers and extending over the dorsum of the hand. This will protect the hand against a direct blow on the injured area.

If the fracture is unstable, as will be the case in a comminuted, oblique or spiral fracture, traction may be required to maintain the reduction. There are many ways in which this traction can be applied. The finger should be in flexion since it is unwise to apply traction with the metacarpophalangeal joint extended. On the other hand, there is no particular objection to extension of the proximal interphalangeal joint. We prefer a plaster cast which includes the wrist and hand and goes down to the proximal interphalangeal joint on the palmar sur-

face and to the metacarpal heads on the dorsal surface. The plaster should be molded so that the proximal joint can be flexed at least 45 degrees. An outrigger, such as a bent piece of coat-hanger wire, can be incorporated into the back of the cast behind the fingers and flexed to the same angle as the proximal phalanges. Traction can then be applied to the fractured finger distal to the proximal interphalangeal joint. This can be done by a small K-wire passed through the base of the distal phalanx or a fish-hook type wire drilled into the dorsum of the middle phalanx. Traction can be exerted by rubber bands. It is undesirable to include more than one finger in the traction, but the splint should include an adjacent finger.

Open reduction of the fracture of the proximal phalanx is usually not necessary. It is neither desirable nor easy since internal fixation is very difficult to apply to this phalanx. It is not for the uninitiated. Intramedullary fixation can be carried out by passing the wire through the distal end of the proximal phalanx with the middle phalanx flexed at 90 degrees (Fig. 293). The finger must be supported with the joint flexed until the wire is removed since the wire will interfere with, and cause irritation from, motion. The wire may damage the proximal articular surface of the middle phalanx unless movement is prevented. There is not room in the finger for plate fixation without interference with tendon function. Any internal fixation that is used should be removed as promptly as stability will permit.

Fracture of the *distal end of the proximal phalanx* usually is a flexion fracture quite similar to fracture through the neck of the metacarpal. The distal end of the phalanx is snubbed downward toward the palm with palmar angulation of the distal fragment. This is usually a *transverse type* of fracture, often impacted. It can be readily re-

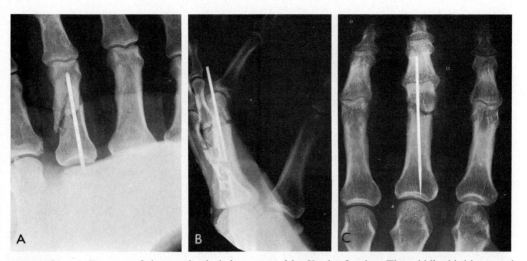

Figure 293. *A*, Fracture of the proximal phalanx treated by K-wire fixation. The middle third is treated by a wire through the proximal end of the phalanx. *B* and *C*, Similar type of fracture with the wire through the distal end. This is the more acceptable of the two procedures.

duced by hyperextension of the middle phalanx with pressure against the shaft of the proximal phalanx. The fragments will frequently move into position and be quite stable. In this instance the finger must be immobilized in complete extension in order to prevent recurrence of deformity. The pull on the anterior capsule of the joint by the extended middle phalanx will hold the head of the proximal phalanx in the proper position. The finger should not be maintained in this position more than two weeks since undue stiffness will result. At the end of two weeks the finger should be slightly flexed and the splint continued.

Our preference for a splint for the transverse type of fracture is carefully molded plaster applied as follows: A small splint about 1 in. wide and six layers thick is begun at the base of the finger on the palmar surface, passed over the end of the finger and back to the metacarpophalangeal joint. This is placed over the single layer of compacted sheet wadding. The splint should actually be applied with the finger in the position in which it is to be held, so that the splint will not cause undue pressure

such as might occur if it is applied before the finger is positioned. After the splint has set, a few circular turns of 1 in. gauze bandage may safely be applied from the base of the finger to the distal interphalangeal joint, leaving a gap at the tip of the finger covered only by gauze. This will permit the finger to be inspected for circulation. If this dressing is uncomfortable, it must be changed. Pressure necrosis can almost always be avoided by careful follow-up care, because the finger should not be painful once the fragments are reduced.

"T" fracture of the distal end of the proximal phalanx poses a more severe problem since it is quite unstable. Frequently the "T" fracture can be stabilized by careful reduction and transfixation across the condyles with a threaded K-wire. It may then be treated as a stable fracture. The interphalangeal joint will not tolerate gross irregularity of the articular surface and open reduction should be resorted to if it is needed to secure good apposition.

Rotation of the distal fragment is of extreme importance in fractures of the proximal phalanx (Fig. 294). Rotation

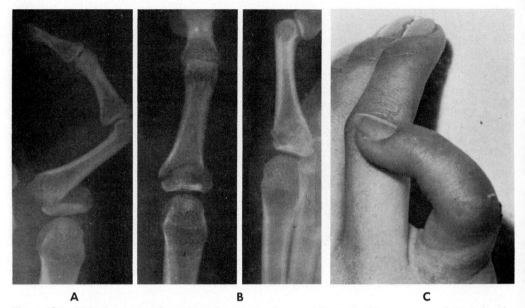

A   B   C

Figure 294. This shows the effect of rotation upon a fractured finger. In this case most of the deformity is due to rotation. The injury was produced when the finger was caught and the hand rotated. *A,* The fracture. *B,* Anteroposterior and lateral views show the reduction is obtained by simply correcting the rotation. This type of fracture should be splinted with the adjacent one or two fingers in flexion to be sure that proper rotation is maintained, or the final result may resemble *C,* which shows marked rotation. Note flexed finger rests on its neighbor, a non-functional position.

causes a concealed deformity which results in the finger flexing in the direction of the long axis of the forearm rather than toward the tubercle of the navicular. Normally as the fingers are flexed together into the palm, only the long finger flexes directly downward toward the tubercle of the navicular. However, if flexed individually, all fingers converge toward the base of the thumb, so if a line is drawn down the axis of each flexed middle phalanx, these lines will converge to the navicular tubercle at the wrist. Hence, any fixation of the finger should be in this axis rather than along the axis of its metacarpal, This is particularly true in the unstable fractures. The traction must be directed along this line. It is distressing to have a healed fracture in which the fingers overlap as they flex because the physician failed to recognize the converging long axis of the flexed fingers.

Middle Phalanx. Fractures of the middle phalanx present many of the same problems as those of the proximal phalanx. The fractures of the base of the phalanx should be treated in the same way. In any fracture without displacement a simple finger splint, preferably of aluminum, will be adequate to maintain all the joints of the finger in a semiflexed position (Fig. 289). It should be emphasized that the phalanges do not require long immobilization. To do so invites adhesions of the closely overlying tendons.

In complete fractures of the middle phalanx that are unstable, the deformity will vary considerably according to the location of the fracture because of the tendon attachments to this finger (Fig. 295). The extensor tendon has an attachment to the base of the phalanx, whereas the flexor sublimis attaches to the middle of the palmar surface of the phalanx. If the fracture lies between these two tendon attachments, the distal fragment will move forward with the sublimis tendon; the proximal fragment will be pulled backward by the extensor retinaculum. If the fracture is transverse it may be stable after reduction. The finger may be splinted in extension (not hyperextension) by simple plaster or aluminum splint. It should be noted that the splint must be rigid and so applied and maintained that it will hold a constant position without direct pressure over the fracture site.

In a fracture distal to the sublimis attachment (Fig. 295), the angulation of the proximal fragment is forward in the same manner as in the proximal phalanx and the same treatment will be necessary; that is, the maintenance of flexion of the fingers in all joints. This may be accomplished by the same apparatus as indicated for the proximal phalanx. If the fracture is comminuted or spiral and unstable, it should be treated by traction, in this instance with the splint extended slightly beyond the proximal interphalangeal joint and traction applied to the distal phalanx along the long axis of the middle phalanx, which will ordinarily be at about 45 degrees of flexion from the extended position. This traction may be by K-wire through the base

of the distal phalanx or by pulp traction at the tip of the phalanx. Our preference is K-wire through the distal phalanx. Once the fracture is fixed, careful x-ray study should be done to determine that the alignment is correct. The importance of rotation in fractures of either the proximal or distal phalanx should be emphasized. Rotation in the long axis of the finger will change the relationship of the interphalangeal joints with each other and present an obvious deformity after healing occurs.

AVULSION OF THE CENTRAL EXTENSOR TENDON SLIP AT THE PROXIMAL INTERPHALANGEAL JOINT (BOUTONNIÈRE DEFORMITY). A tendon avulsion problem which gives a classic deformity is usually less well recognized than the baseball finger deformity discussed in the following section. The lesion is avulsion of the central slip of the extensor mechanism at the proximal interphalangeal joint. Unfortunately, the resulting boutonnière deformity with inability to actively extend the proximal interphalangeal joint does not always lead to the correct diagnosis and the injury is then seen after a flexion contracture of the joint takes place. The correct

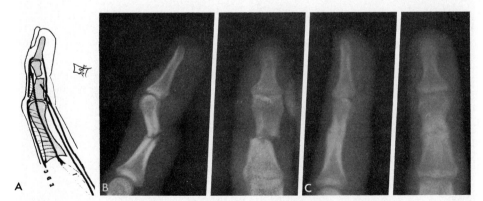

Figure 295. The type of deformity seen in fractures of the shaft of the middle phalanx. Here the lumbrical is relaxed and the deformity is maintained by the pull of the flexor digitorum sublimis attaching to the distal end of the proximal fragment, very close to the fracture site (*A* and *B*). *C*, The final result is obtained by splinting the finger in the position of function with a little extra padding placed over the distal interphalangeal joint. There should be no padding placed on the volar side of the fracture to push the flexor tendon into the fracture site. If something is placed in the palm, it should be a soft roll of felt, never a hard roll of gauze.

diagnosis might be made earlier if it shows on x-ray. When seen late the flexion contracture must be corrected before surgical repair will be successful. This contracture can be corrected with the application of a dynamic splint. A simple splint is the so-called clothespin splint or a reverse finger knuckle bender, available in prefabricated forms from several of the surgical supply houses. This same splint can also be used to prevent deformity while healing takes place in the incompletely avulsed tendon for which surgical repair is not elected. As noted earlier, the diagnosis is the key to correct treatment and would be made in more cases if x-ray evidence of avulsion with a bone fragment were present, but it is not.

An untreated boutonnière deformity will require reconstructive surgery.

Distal Phalanx. Fractures of the distal phalanx are almost always *crushing injuries* except for the avulsion fracture of the flexor or extensor tendons. This crushing injury may involve the tuft at the tip of the finger, in which case the fracture itself is of much less significance than the crushing injury (Fig. 296). It may involve the shaft or indeed extend back to involve the base and articular surface. Usually these fractures require no treatment other than the treatment of the soft tissue injury. However, the two more distal phalanges of the finger should be immobilized by a metal splint in order to protect against a direct blow and to prevent later deformity. In the occasional case in which there is a transverse fracture through the shaft with displacement and instability, the fracture may be reduced and readily stabilized by an intramedullary K-wire drilled through the distal end of the finger and down to the distal inter-

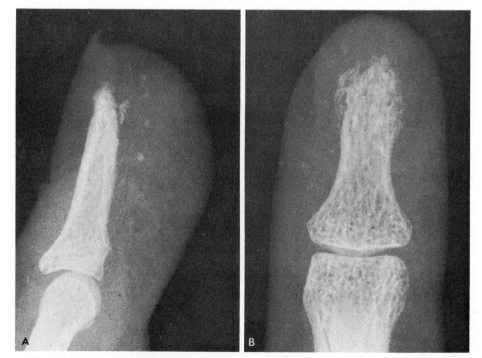

Figure 296. Tuft fracture, lateral *(A)* and anteroposterior *(B)* views. Note swelling of the tip of the finger.

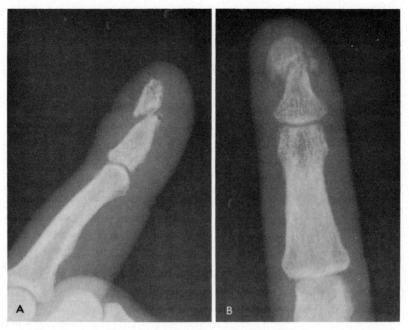

Figure 297. *A*, Compound crushing injury of the distal phalanx. This was treated by simple dressing. The wound healed but the finger remained so painful that the patient was unable to work for four months. *B*, X-ray revealed malposition and nonunion. Treated by resection of the fragment with good recovery.

phalangeal joint. Angular deformity of the distal phalanx should not be ignored since it may cause distressing disability (Fig. 297).

If the fracture is directly across the base of the finger and seems unstable, the wire may be passed across the joint and down into the middle phalanx. In this instance the finger should be immobilized in the position in which the fracture is most stable, preferably in a few degrees of flexion. The threaded wire should be removed as soon as healing has accomplished stabilization, which will occur at two or at the most three weeks. If the fracture involves the articular surface in the nature of a "T" fracture or a fracture across one angle of the base, it may be transfixed by drilling the wire laterally across the finger after reduction of the fracture. If reduction cannot be obtained otherwise, open reduction should be done using a transverse incision distal to the fracture.

Great care should be taken not to involve the nail root lest deformity of the nail result.

TENDON AVULSION INJURIES WITH OR WITHOUT A BONE FRAGMENT. Fractures of the base of the phalanx involving the dorsal or palmar surface are almost always *avulsion fractures,* in which the flexor or extensor tendon pulls off a segment of bone as the distal phalanx is hyperflexed or extended. Unfortunately, a fragment of bone is not always avulsed with the tendon and the physician looking for the "classic" case overlooks the injury. This is doubly unfortunate because pure tendon injuries require surgical repair more often and earlier than those involving avulsion of a chip of bone. In injuries of the dorsal surface involving the tendon, which give rise to the so-called *baseball finger* (Figs. 298, 299 and 300), it may be possible to immobilize the finger by flexion of the proximal and extension of the dis-

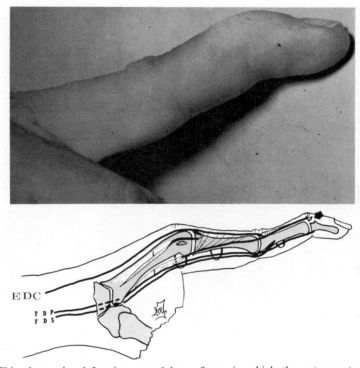

EDC

F D P
F D S

Figure 298. This shows the deformity caused by a finger in which the extensor tendon is avulsed from the base of the distal phalanx. Any attempt to extend the distal phalanx results in an imbalance between the intrinsic lumbrical tendon and the extrinsic long extensor tendon. The metacarpophalangeal joint is slightly flexed. The proximal interphalangeal joint is hyperextended and the distal interphalangeal joint is flexed. Tension on the fracture fragment can be alleviated by flexing the proximal interphalangeal joint and hyperextending the distal interphalangeal joint. The finger can be maintained in this position by casts or a K-wire, but maintaining it with a splint is very difficult. In an old nonunion the intrinsic-extrinsic imbalance can be relieved by sectioning the attachment of the long extensor to the base of the middle phalanx.

tal interphalangeal joints. The plaster can be applied dry to the finger over a tube gauze covering. The finger is then dipped into water and the finger held until the plaster hardens. This method of applying the cast avoids much fumbling and loss of position during setting of the plaster.

We have been unable to hold this fracture satisfactorily by simple splint fixation and have not been particularly pleased with the method of passing an intramedullary K-wire down the distal phalanx and across the extended distal interphalangeal joint, then out through the palmar cortex of the middle phalanx to transfix the proximal phalanx. We have had better success in passing the K-wire across the extended distal joint and down into the middle phalanx, stopping short of the proximal joint. One must supplement this by splinting, holding the middle phalanx flexed.

Most of these fractures should be treated by open reduction and internal fixation. If the fragment is large enough, it may be reduced and held by a transfixion pin through the fragment and into the distal phalanx. If the fragment is too small for this, it may be held by wire suture passed through the fragment from the fracture line back through the tendon and looped back to emerge into the fracture line again. It then passes through holes drilled in the distal phalanx to emerge on the palmar surface of

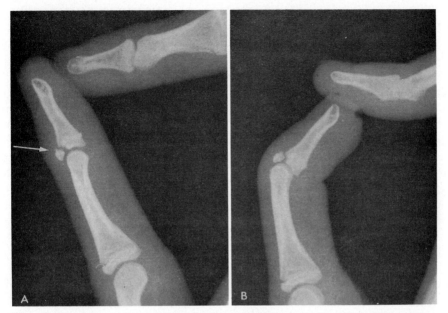

Figure 299. Baseball finger. *A,* Note fragment is not reduced by extension of the phalanx, *(B)* nor does it widely separate by flexion. However, the patient lacked complete extension. Treated by open fixation.

the finger. It is then tied over a button. A pull-out wire will permit its easy removal after healing. Great care must be taken not to cause pressure necrosis on the skin of the palmar surface of the finger by the button or the splint.

Avulsion fracture of the flexor tendon attachment may be fixed in similar

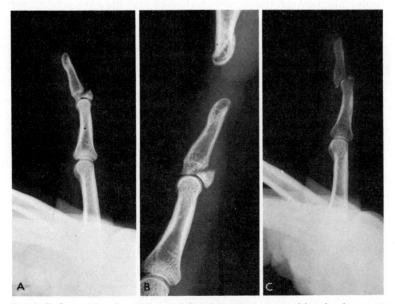

Figure 300. Baseball finger showing *(A)* the deformity, *(B)* poor position by hyperextension of the finger and *(C)* poor result, with dislocation of the phalanx, because of improper immobilization. It should be noted that this fracture involves over one half of the articular surface.

manner with the finger in flexion. Again, the preference is open reduction, obtaining fixation either with a small pin through the fragment and distal phalanx or by wire fixation utilizing a pull-out wire. In this instance the wire may be passed directly through the nail bed over a button on the fingernail. In either instance surgical repair should be supplemented by appropriate splinting, in the dorsal fracture with the distal phalanx extended and in the palmar fracture with the distal phalanx flexed.

OPEN FRACTURES

Open fractures are quite common in the finger due to the fact that the bone is so close to the skin, particularly on the dorsal surface. They should be treated as open fractures are elsewhere. If the injury is seen early enough, very careful and thorough lavage of the tissue may permit primary closure. If seen later, the wound should be left open and appropriate drainage used. It must be closed as soon as possible since long-standing chronic infection of the finger will result in stiffness of the inter-phalangeal joints. It is impossible to clean a finger adequately without anes-thesia, either local block or general. Great care should be taken not to sacri-fice any skin. Even if there is some question as to the vitality of the skin, it should be saved, and a decision made later as the line of demarcation is formed.

ARTERIAL INJURIES

Following direct trauma to the palm of the hand, an occasional case of thrombosis of the palmar arterial arch and its tributaries occurs. It is most prevalent in older people but happens occasionally in young athletes following direct trauma to the ulnar border of the hand. The symptoms are point ten-derness and swelling over the hand, most commonly located on the ulnar border of the hand. The fingers may be pale and cool compared with the oppo-site hand. The symptoms are most pro-nounced in cold weather.

Physical examination discloses ten-derness, swelling and evidence of de-creased circulation. Allen's test should be performed in cases in which throm-bosis of the palmar arterial arch is sus-pected. The test is performed by oblit-erating both the radial and ulnar arteries at the wrist with pressure from the examiner's fingers. The patient is then asked to open and close his hand repeatedly until blanching occurs. Pres-sure over the ulnar artery is then re-leased and the pressure on the radial ar-tery is maintained. If the ulnar artery is patent, an almost immediate erythema develops throughout the palm and fingers. If the ulnar arch is obliterated in the palm, this erythema will not occur.

In the presence of the findings just mentioned an arteriogram and surgery consisting of thrombectomy performed through multiple arteriotomies, or other appropriate surgery, is indicated.

CHAPTER 13

INJURIES OF THE CHEST

RIBS

ANATOMICAL CONSIDERATIONS

In discussing functional anatomy it is very difficult to separate the trunk from the extremities and the various parts of the trunk from each other since, by the very nature of their function, the extremities depend to a large extent upon the trunk not only for stability but also for mobility (Figs. 301 and 302). So, in the chapters on the upper extremities we have perforce included a good deal about the chest. The discussion in this section will be largely confined to injuries of the chest proper, excluding the spine but including the sternum.

The thorax is the most rigid part of the human trunk. Not only are the vertebrae much more firmly integrated in the dorsal spine than in other areas but the formation of a rough oval by the spine, ribs and sternum serves to stabilize the whole structure. Each rib articulates with its appropriate vertebra and is firmly attached by strong ligaments not only to this vertebra but to the one above and to its fellow ribs above and below. The end of the rib abuts directly against the articular process on the body of the dorsal vertebra on the lateral surface of the pedicle, and the articular

tubercle of the rib articulates on the anterolateral tip of the transverse process of the same vertebra. The capsular ligaments hold the rib firmly against the body of the vertebra and against the transverse process. There also are dense ligaments extending vertically from the transverse process above to the upper surface of the rib below so that the ribs are not only held firmly against the vertebrae but are bound to each other and to the adjacent transverse processes. These attachments are so firm that they are rarely damaged.

The oval of the chest is much smaller at the top. The first ribs together with the first thoracic vertebra and first piece of the sternum form a much smaller and more circular ring than those below. The ribs down to the 7th are progressively longer. The upper seven ribs are attached directly to the sternum by the costicartilage. The costicartilage is short in the upper three or four ribs, becoming progressively longer in the lower ribs. Whereas the costicartilage on the first rib may be no more than a fingerbreadth in length, the lower ones extend for several inches. The ribs are relatively horizontal at the top, running more and more obliquely downward until the 12th ribs may actually be more vertical than horizontal. The 8th,

381

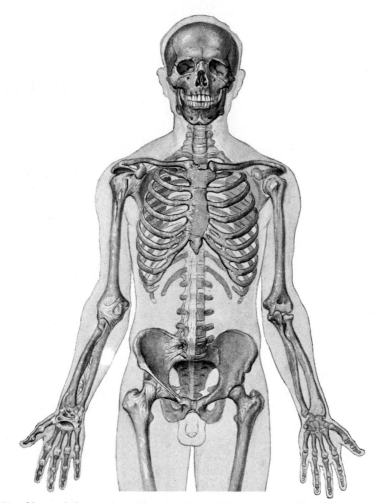

Figure 301.   Upper skeleton, viewed from the front. (From Anson, Atlas of Human Anatomy.)

9th and 10th ribs do not attach to the sternum but each of their costicartilages attaches to the costicartilage of the rib above. The distal tips of the 11th and 12th ribs are ordinarily free of any bony or cartilaginous attachment to the thoracic cage. The general alignment of the ribs is oblique from above, downward and forward.

The muscles which elevate the ribs, consisting of the intercostals and many other accessory muscles, serve to pull the ribs upward and forward so that the anteroposterior diameter of the lower chest is increased by elevation of the ribs. Correspondingly, the anteropos-

terior diameter of the chest is diminished by depressing or compressing the rib cage. The ribs are quite elastic in a child and become increasingly brittle as age advances. In the young athlete there still remains an amazing degree of elasticity. Some of this results from the shape of the chest itself. Some of it is in the costicartilages but there is a good deal of "spring" in the structure of the rib proper.

The ribs are largely subcutaneous in the anterior half of the chest, but in the posterior half the lumbar muscle mass covers the thorax. The intercostal muscles have a shingling effect, since each intercostal arises from the anterior margin of the inferior surface of the rib above to course downward and forward to attach to the posterior margin of the superior surface of the rib below. The intercostal vessels and nerves pass forward from the spine, nestling in a groove on the undersurface of the rib. The intercostal muscle protects this bundle from an external blow, but the nerves and vessels are readily damaged by an injury to the rib above. The constant position of the neurovascular bundle makes it readily available for local injection. The abdominal muscles attach to the lower ribs in front to give fixation from the bony thorax to the pelvis below.

The ribs are further secured each to the other by the intercostal membrane. The anterior intercostal membrane is an extension of fascia over the external intercostal muscle. This muscle extends from the articular process of the vertebra around to cover about four-fifths of the rib; the remaining one-fifth is covered by the intercostal membrane which extends forward to attach to the sternum. Similarly, they are held together posteriorly by the posterior extension of this membrane, the posterior intercostal membrane. The internal intercostal

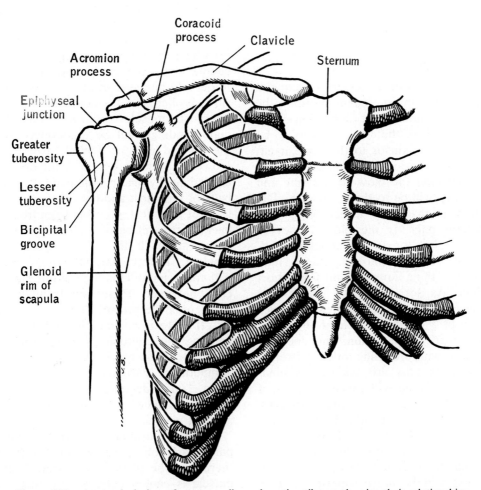

Figure 302. Anatomical view of sternum, ribs and costicartilages, showing their relationships.

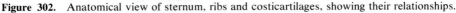

muscle is in two layers, the more superficial layer extending from the sternum two-thirds of the way backward to be continued in the spine as the posterior intercostal membrane, so that the ribs are held together by this membrane both posteriorly and anteriorly.

The sternum is in three pieces (Fig. 302), the manubrium, the body and the xiphoid. The first rib articulates on the manubrium, the second on the junction of the manubrium and body, the third, fourth, fifth and sixth on the body, and the seventh on the junction of the xiphoid and body. These costicartilages are firmly adherent to the sternum and to each other by interdigitating ligaments, the so-called sternal intercostal ligaments.

CONTUSION

Contusion of the chest is frequent, the resultant injury depending upon the location of the trauma. Contusion of the anterior half of the chest is likely to be either to the skin or to the bone itself, whereas posteriorly the muscles of the back cushion the blow to the ribs and the injury will be to these muscles. The history is that of a direct blow with resultant pain. If the blow is severe enough, the "breath is knocked out" and subsequent muscle spasm may make breathing quite difficult for a short period. As soon as these preliminary symptoms are over, the patient becomes aware of a localized area of the chest that is tender to palpation. This does not interfere with breathing unless extremely deep breaths are taken. Examination at this time will reveal an area of localized tenderness, either directly over a rib or in the skin. If the periosteum is involved there will be considerable tenderness on the rib itself, whereas if the skin is involved the tenderness will be more superficial. This

distinction can be made by sliding the skin upward or downward over the rib. If the tenderness remains constant in the skin, one can assume that the contusion is of the skin and subcutaneous tissues. If the tenderness remains on the bone, regardless of what area of skin is over the bone, one can assume the damage is to the bone.

Contusion of the chest wall does not often require extensive *treatment*. If there is a complicating hematoma, it may be aspirated. There is much more likely to be infiltration of blood and this may be injected with hyaluronidase early and a corticoid preparation several days later if symptoms persist.

Another complication is fracture of the ribs. If several ribs have been fractured, the diagnosis can be made quite readily on the basis of severe pain on breathing, crepitation, ecchymosis and edema along the chest wall. If, as so frequently happens in athletes, a single rib is broken, the adjacent ribs with the intercostal muscles splint it well and the major findings will be tenderness over the rib and pain on forced inspiration. However, if compression of the chest is carried out by placing one hand over the back of the chest and the other over the front of the chest, pressing from front to back, there will be pain along the point of contusion if the rib is broken or cracked. Rarely, lateral compression will cause pain. This sign is not significant, however, if pressure is made directly over the bruised area.

If there is no complication accompanying the contusion, no splinting is required. If the player is to continue in competition, particularly in a contact sport, an adequate protective pad should be placed over the contusion to prevent re-injury.

In the muscular areas of the chest, particularly on the posterior one-third, there may be painful contusion as the muscle is caught between the ribs and the striking force. This is treated as a muscular contusion anywhere, including the complication of hematoma. Myositis ossificans is not common in the muscles in the back of the chest. In the front of the chest, the lower portion is almost entirely subcutaneous. The superior anterolateral portion of the upper chest is covered with the pectoral muscle which fans out over all of the upper ribs as it extends out to its attachment on the humerus. This muscle is subject to all the injuries inherent in the muscular system and may receive a painful contusion with hematoma formation. Some of the fibers may be avulsed from the attachments to the ribs. This becomes essentially an injury to the shoulder rather than the chest, however, since the disability is primarily in use of the arm.

Overlying the pectoral muscle is the breast. The breast of most males is a recessive structure but it may receive a painful contusion. This may result in inflammation locally centered around the nipple and areola with redness, tenderness and local heat. The breast which has been quite inconspicuous may become quite prominent. On examination there is a palpable hard ring surrounding the nipple which is tender to touch. Serous fluid may exude from the nipple. This is really an inflammatory condition resulting from contusion and should be treated as such with local heat and protection. The acute symptoms may subside leaving a firm, palpable area around the nipple which may be moderately tender and should be protected by contact pads. Occasionally a painful fibrous nodule remains which may require excision.

With more participation in athletics by girls, something should be said about the female breast. The adolescent with immature breasts needs no particular protection but any injury to the breast should be treated promptly and adequately and athletic competition eliminated until inflammation has subsided. Early application of cold followed by heat and protection and support by a binder or brassiere should be maintained as long as there is swelling or inflammation. The more mature breast should be protected by an adequate brassiere during strenuous athletic competition. This not only will tend to protect the breast from direct blows but will prevent overexuberant motion of the breast during strenuous activity. Any contusion of the breast that does not respond promptly to local treatment will require consultation with a physician experienced in the management of breast conditions. The adolescent girl will tend to avoid any mention of a breast injury. The coaches and advisors should advise the girls to report promptly any discomfort in this area.

Be very wary of any persistent localized nodule in the female breast. Of equal importance are the symptoms of generalized chronic mastitis with aching pain, deep tenderness, and a tendency for "caking" of the gland.

STRAIN

Since a multitude of muscles attach to the chest, almost any manifestation of strain may occur. Strain may be caused by violent exertion or by overstretching of the muscles. The symptoms will depend entirely upon the area involved. In the long muscles of the back of the thorax, this condition may be indistinguishable from, or may be part of, a lumbar strain. In the front of the chest the strain may involve the muscles of the abdominal wall where they attach to the lower ribs. Strain may also involve the intercostal muscles although this is not frequent since they are well protected by other muscle structures and these muscles do not often act forcibly enough to rupture their fibers. A strain is much more likely to involve an area connecting to the chest than the chest itself. This is particularly true of the scapular muscles, i.e., strain of the rhomboids will occur either at the scapular attachment or along the spine much more frequently than at the costal attachment. Similarly, the serrati may more likely be injured in their substance or at their attachments to the shoulder than in their costal origins. Careful analysis of the active motion that causes the pain will usually determine the proper muscle group although it may be quite difficult to relate it to a specific muscle.

Strain of a muscle at its attachment to the rib is likely to be more painful than it is disabling. There may, however, be considerable attendant muscle spasm which will tend to splint the chest and interfere with deep breathing. It actually may prevent certain types of activity. A strain of the abdominal recti attached to the lower ribs may interdict a sport such as rowing or wrestling where forcible use of the abdominal muscles is required. Similarly, spasm of the shoulder muscles may interdict throwing.

TREATMENT. Since most of the attachments to the chest are diffuse muscular ones, they do not lend themselves well to local injection. After one has determined what muscular activity causes pain, this activity should be restricted, either by appropriate splinting or simply by reducing the activity of the individual. If the muscles attaching to the scapula are involved, the arm should be put in a sling. If there is serious involvement of the abdominal muscle attachments, the patient should be put to bed with the head rest and knee support elevated in order to flex his spine and relax the abdomen.

Treatment will depend entirely on the muscles involved. Local treatment may be of some value. In the early stages application of ice will minimize the inflammation and blood infiltration. Later, local heat will give considerable comfort and promote improved circulation. Many of these injuries will be relieved by wearing a snugly fitting binder on the lower ribs. Any webbing band such as a rib belt (Fig. 303) or Elastoplast strapping or, indeed, simply wrapping the lower chest with an elastic bandage may relieve the symptoms considerably. As with many muscular strains, complete recovery may be very tedious. Just about the time the player begins to get rid of his muscle spasm and have some expectation of recovery, he is likely to step up his activities to the point where he reactivates the process. The classic measures of rest, heat and gradual rehabilitation are quite pertinent here.

If after the first week or ten days there remains an area of persistent tenderness, local injection of this area with a long-acting local anesthetic plus one of the corticoid preparations may dramatically relieve the symptoms. Infiltration of several levels along the origin of the muscles to the ribs may be necessary. Our method usually has been to outline the areas of tenderness to palpation and check against active contraction and

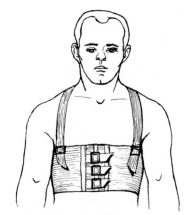

Figure 303. Drawing of rib belt on a patient.

passive stretching of the involved muscle. If these measures cause pain in the area where there is palpable tenderness, one may assume there is local inflammation at this spot. These areas are carefully infiltrated with a local anesthetic. Proof of the effectiveness of the procedure will be complete elimination of pain on palpation, active contraction and passive stretching. If the pain is not relieved, at least while the anesthetic is effective, the involved area has not been adequately infiltrated. If the pain is relieved, this same area should be infiltrated with a corticoid and the patient should be encouraged to continue his activities but to avoid excess of either active or passive motion.

An example of the condition just described is found in the serratus posterior which rises from the lower ribs and passes over to the lumbar aponeurosis in the midline. There may be an area of tenderness extending from the inferior angle of the scapula directly down over the ribs which corresponds to the attachment of this muscle. Complete expansion of the chest or leaning toward the opposite side will cause discomfort here. Actively pulling toward the involved side will also cause discomfort in the same area. If these feelings of discomfort can be eliminated by injection of a local anesthetic, one may assume he has reached the area of the trouble. This local treatment should be supplemented by inductive heat. In many cases, support by appropriate strapping will be of value.

Muscle ruptures are unusual about the thorax. They are very difficult to diagnose unless they involve the small attachment of a single large muscle such as that of the latissimus dorsi to the upper extremity. This does not directly involve the chest since the chest component of this muscle is an extremely extensive attachment to many ribs and is not susceptible to strain.

FLOATING RIBS

Some mention should be made of the characteristics of the 11th and 12th ribs — the so-called floating ribs. The tip of the 12th and many times the 11th rib does not reach the sternal attachment and has no costicartilage as such. These ribs articulate with the spine with a single articular facet having no tubercle and no head so that there is much less stability and comparatively free motion at the spine. They are invested in the abdominal musculature and completely surrounded by muscle attachments. These ribs do not actually participate in respiration to any major extent and are more likely to be involved in injury of the spine than of the chest. They will be discussed in relationship to injury of the spine.

SPRAIN-SUBLUXATION-DISLOCATION

The areas subject to ligament injury in the chest are primarily at the vertebral and the sternal attachments of the ribs.

Vertebral Attachment

As has been mentioned above, the ribs are bound firmly at their vertebral attachments. The degree of motion in this area is necessarily quite restricted and the forces which cause tension against these ligaments are primarily compression forces against the chest or rotation forces. The excursion of movement is relatively small so that there is no forcible lateral bending at a costal vertebral joint, such as might occur at the knee. A direct blow on the rib itself is more likely to break the rib than to knock it loose at either end. A compression force applied to the whole thorax in the athlete is usually from front to back and the major strain of this force is applied at the angle of the ribs owing to flattening of the oval of the chest by the compressing force. The greatest strain is correspondingly felt at the widest extremes of the oval. There are instances of damage to the vertebral joint. In this case the symptoms will depend upon the degree of involvement. If the sprain is mild, there will be point tenderness over the injured ligament and but little discomfort on movement of the chest. In the athlete, this area is well covered by the lumbar muscles, making the diagnosis of a mild sprain virtually impossible.

If the sprain is more severe, there may be some pain on deep inspiration or on forced rotation motions of the chest. Here, also, the isolation of the injury is extremely difficult since other conditions may cause essentially the same symptoms. It is difficult to separate forceful motion against the ligament of the joint from overstretching of a neighboring muscle. Active contraction of a muscle may cause pain in the injured joint in the same manner as it would if the muscle itself were injured.

I have never seen a complete dislocation of the proximal end of a rib in an athlete. It is possible that subluxation or spontaneously reduced dislocation may occur and be unrecognized. *Treatment* in any event will be symptomatic: early application of cold followed later by heat and protection against that motion which causes pain. If a localized spot of tenderness can be palpated or if there is constant localized pain by pressure on the involved rib, local injection with a long-acting local anesthetic may give prompt relief. And if it does, this is diagnostic.

If deep inspiration causes discomfort, a rib belt (Fig. 303) may be used to restrict inspiration. If rotation or flexion motions of the chest cause pain, these may be eliminated by adequate strap-

ping of the back. Strapping in this instance should consist of strips extending from the shoulders to the pelvis and parallel to the spine. It is my practice to use 3 inch tape with three or four strips to each side, each overlapping about 50 per cent. These strips can be anchored by circumferential tape extending from the pelvis to include the lower rib cage. Cross-stretch adhesive gives much firmer fixation (Fig. 304).

The strapping will to a considerable degree restrict forward or lateral bending and is equally applicable for ligament sprains and muscle sprains of the back. Physical therapy, particularly with inductive heat, will expedite the recovery. Active participation in sports may be impossible for several days while the condition is acute, but after a lapse of a week or ten days, particularly with adequate strapping, participation may be resumed in the ordinary case.

Recent studies have indicated that occasionally a subluxation remains

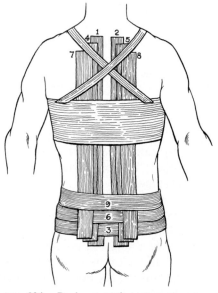

Figure 304. Back strapping to prevent rotation and flexion motions of the chest. Included also is a rib belt. The two are not usually used together. The rib belt does not add to the back support.

unreduced or there may be an actual dislocation of the rib, in which case the symptoms are that of a second degree sprain but more severe; that is, local tenderness, local muscle spasm and painful motion. In addition, there may be the symptoms of irritation of the neurovascular bundle which passes very close to this articulation. There may be symptoms of intercostal nerve involvement, either hyperesthesia indicating some neuritis or hypesthesia indicating pressure. Manipulation has been proposed for this condition. Hyperextension of the spine in this local area allowing the shoulders and arms to fall backward with backward pressure against the anterior portion of the chest may be effective. Successful manipulation results in complete relief with only residual soreness remaining. If a dislocation goes unreduced, chronic symptoms develop such as spurring or degenerative arthritis of the costovertebral joints. It has been suggested that open operation with resection of the proximal end of the rib including its articulations will give substantial relief. I have never had occasion to carry out this procedure.

Anterior Attachment

Ligament injuries at the anterior end of the rib are considerably more frequent than those of the posterior end. Possibly it should be said they are more often recognized. Although the ribs are firmly bound to the sternum, these ligaments are more subject to sprain than the posterior ones by virtue of the forward thrust which occurs with lateral compression of the chest or by direct force applied to the sternum, which drives the sternum backward while the ribs swing forward (Fig. 302). A sprain of the chondrosternal joint should be distinguished from injury to the costochondral junction, which will be discussed under fractures.

The player will complain of tenderness in the chest localized over the area of injury. This area is readily palpable since it is subcutaneous. Often, the symptoms may be confined to a single chondrosternal articulation. Pressure directly over the joint or pressure over the adjacent sternum will usually cause discomfort. The symptoms will vary with the degree of injury. If the sprain is a mild one, there will be local tenderness and possibly a little local swelling—and that is all. If the injury is severe but still short of avulsion of the ligament, the local symptoms will be more intense. There will be no displacement. The tenderness will be more diffuse and will be accompanied by local swelling. There may be infiltration of blood or even hematoma formation directly over the joint. Deep inspiration will cause pain definitely localized at the involved joint. If there has been an actual subluxation or spontaneously reduced dislocation of the joint, the symptoms will be even more severe. The subluxation may recur on deep inspiration or on lateral compression of the chest. Some degree of subluxation may persist, apparently caused by dehiscence of the anterior ligament while the posterior ligament remains intact so that the rib will slide forward in relationship to the sternum. There may be a palpable prominence. In the early stage this may be reduced by direct pressure. This movement may cause an audible snap and will certainly cause pain.

Treatment of these injuries is quite unsatisfactory if they are severe. The mild (first degree) injury may be handled without support but with local injection of an anesthetic plus hyaluronidase and application of heat locally. In the more severe injury where there is pain on motion of the chest, the chest should be strapped with adhesive or a suitable rib binder to prevent further stress on the ligament. The binder should not be put on tightly enough to increase the pain but should be used primarily to prevent wide expansion of the chest. If there is a chronic subluxation, it will be virtually impossible to hold the involved rib down in its normal position.

An acute subluxation, as with dislocation, may require open exposure for fixation. A threaded fixation pin passing through the rib and into the sternum will hold the rib in place. If the separation is at the costochondral junction, the pin can be threaded through the rib and into the cartilage, preferably far enough to reach the sternum. This gives temporary fixation; ultimate recovery must be by plication and repairing of the capsular ligaments, reinforcing them with periosteum and with the soft tissue at hand. This procedure is not successful unless it is done within the first two weeks, since scar formation is not compatible with successful reconstruction. Since the subluxation is usually diagnosed after it is a chronic condition, surgery for this situation is rarely indicated (see Chronic Subluxation, p. 395). One must be satisfied to immobilize the chest to eliminate pain and accept the minimal deformity caused by undue prominence at the tip of the rib. The injury may be extremely tedious to the player because of its chronicity and there will be many disheartening episodes of recurrence of pain following forceful activity.

The technique of injection of the chondrosternal area is quite simple. Repeated infiltrations should be used until all pain and tenderness is eliminated. Because of the interdigitation of the ligaments, the injury may be more widespread than first suspected. It may be advisable to infiltrate into more than one area. I do not find it necessary to infiltrate the joint itself as frequently as I do the surrounding ligament. Once the pain and tenderness are eliminated, these same general areas should be carefully infiltrated in the early case with hya-luronidase and in the more chronic case with a corticoid.

In the chronic case, as has been mentioned above, player participation in sports is often not permissible. If the rib binder is applied snugly enough to prevent deep breathing, it may seriously interfere with the player's ability since it will be necessary for him to breathe deeply in the course of his participation. One must carefully evaluate the source of the discomfort. If it is from direct pressure or direct contact, the discomfort may be prevented by a suitably placed protective pad. If the pain is actually caused by compression of the chest, I know of no appliance that will completely eliminate it. However, a snugly fitted rib belt or corset will tend to hold the chest in a more circular position and so may well eliminate the stress at this particular point. If on the other hand the pain is caused by deep inspiration, it can be checked by a suitable binder. In most conditions I do not approve of local injection to permit participation but in this particular condition, and especially if it is restricted to one or two ribs, it is difficult to believe that injection to eliminate the pain would increase the hazard of further injury. One may give the player substantial relief by local infiltration. The question of surgical treatment of these conditions does not often arise. If the pain seems to be from a chronic traumatic arthritis of the joint or from calcification in the anterior fissure of the joint, one may be persuaded to resect a portion of the costicartilage adjacent to the sternum. I have never had occasion to do this as a result of athletic injury or in order to permit participation.

A frank dislocation of the rib that persists should be reduced at the earliest possible moment. Dislocation of an isolated rib is rarely seen but it may be more frequent than is apparent because so often the dislocation reduces spontaneously. If seen, the deformity should be promptly reduced. For reduction, either local or general anesthesia is usually required since, if the dislocation would readily reduce, it probably would have been reduced before it reached the doctor. After injection of a local anesthetic, the rib may be snapped back into position by pressure over the chest and direct pressure with the thumb over the rib end. If it cannot be reduced by manipulation it may be reduced by making a small incision across the chondrosternal joint paralleling the rib. The rib can be gently levered into place with an elevator. Following open reduction an attempt should be made to repair the ligaments. If the rib tends to slip back out of joint it may be fixed by a suitable transfixion pin through the end of the rib and into the body of the sternum. Such treatment is rarely necessary. Following open reduction, a rib belt should be applied with a felt pad directly over the dislocated rib.

FRACTURE

Fractures of the ribs are relatively common in athletes. They usually are caused either by a direct blow from a blunt object, in which instance there is likely to be a fracture of a single or at the most two ribs, or by forceful compression of the chest in one of its diameters, in which case there may be single or multiple fractures. In the first instance, the player will give a history of a blow on the chest which may be forceful enough to "knock out his wind" and cause severe localized pain. As he gets his breath and tries to breathe deeply there is severe pain. Muscle spasm tends to splint the chest and to prevent deep breathing. The result is rapid, shallow respiration due to the combination of air hunger plus pain on inspiration. In the second instance the player may give

a history of being crushed in a pile-up or of falling forcibly on his side with the ball or a helmet between him and the ground. Here again he will have difficult breathing accompanied by severe pain. Careful examination at the time of injury will elicit tenderness localized directly over the rib or ribs. There is pain in this same area on deep breathing. Compression of the chest, even though direct pressure on the involved rib is avoided, will cause pain. For example, if the 6th rib is broken at the anterior axillary line, pressure made directly backward on the sternum will cause pain in the area of the fracture and deep inspiration is painful. Any attempt at coughing or sneezing is disastrous. The player grabs his chest and attempts to restrict its motion manually. There may be a palpable defect in the rib if the fracture is complete, and it may be possible to elicit crepitation. Manipulation to elicit such is not justifiable.

Fracture can be differentiated from a simple contusion by the fact that a contusion does not usually cause pain on motion of the rib. X-ray examination must be made but is often unsatisfactory in the early stages. A negative x-ray does not rule out fractured ribs. The obliquity of the rib, the depth of the thorax, the intervening soft tissues, together with the oblique nature of the fracture line and the frequent lack of displacement, make the fracture very difficult to recognize. An exception is the unusual complete fracture in which the ends are separated.

TREATMENT. *Complicated Fracture.* The vast majority of fractured ribs are uncomplicated by any more serious condition. In the occasional case, however, the complications may be more critical than the injury itself. Fortunately, the bones of the young athlete are elastic enough that they do not usually splinter and present sharp-pointed fragments. When splintering does occur in the fractured rib, the sharp fragment may damage the internal mammary artery, or penetrate the lung and cause pneumothorax, or even penetrate the pericardium. A more frequent injury is damage to the intercostal vessels and nerves which will result in rather marked local swelling and formation of a hematoma.

Following an injury to the chest, if the patient does not promptly recover from the initial period of difficult breathing one should carefully investigate the possibility of internal injury. The patient may remain short of breath, may become somewhat cyanotic or may complain of increased difficulty in getting enough air. All of these things suggest decreased lung capacity. If these conditions come on rapidly, a critical situation may arise in which immediate decompression of the chest is necessary. In such a case the patient should obviously be taken at once to the hospital where, after careful x-ray study to determine the degree of collapse of the

lung or shift of the mediastinum, a decision is made on aspirating the air or blood (Fig. 305). If the hemothorax is small, it is probably better left alone. If the hemopneumothorax only partially collapses the lung, closed drainage of the pleural cavity will be the likely course. The vast majority of these cases fortunately are not emergent in character and ample time may be taken to complete the diagnosis. In cases of doubt, consultation should be obtained from one versed in the treatment of such conditions in the chest.

There will occasionally be subcutaneous emphysema from fracture of the ribs, with leakage of air into the soft tissues causing diffuse swelling which extends along under the skin and causes characteristic crepitation. This condition may reach alarming proportions, even to the extent of a swelling of the neck that extends to the level of the angle of the jaw. It rarely requires any very radical or specific treatment. If there is any likelihood of internal injury,

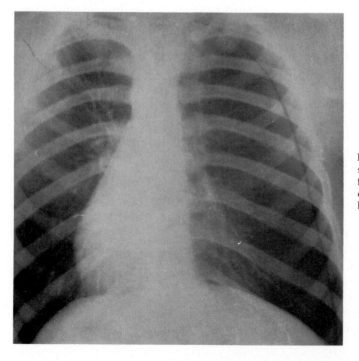

Figure 305. X-ray (retouched) showing collapse of right lung following trauma. Note absence of lung markings in periphery of lung.

the patient should be hospitalized until all doubt concerning the presence of a serious complication has been resolved. Needless to say, x-ray study should be repeated since there may be quite rapid changes in the chest which may change the indications for treatment.

Uncomplicated Fracture. In the absence of any complication, local treatment may afford the player considerable relief. If there is a marked pain and muscle spasm, local anesthetic may be infiltrated into the intercostal nerve, at least a hand's breadth proximal to the fracture (that is, toward the spine). The needle is inserted directly under the margin of the rib, the plunger carefully withdrawn to be sure there is no blood, and 4 to 5 cc. of the agent is injected. The injection of a single rib may be quite effective, but it is usually necessary to inject two or three or even four ribs before relief is complete. If a long-acting anesthetic is used the relief may be quasi permanent since a good deal of the pain was caused by the muscle spasm pulling at the fracture site. While the spasm will be relieved by injection, the recurrence of pain can be prevented only by support of the chest.

Once the pain is relieved, the chest should be properly immobilized to prevent motion of the rib. In any injury below the upper two or three ribs, the support should be circumferential and to the lower chest. It is not necessary to strap directly over the fractured 5th rib, for example. The purpose of the dressing is to splint the chest and prevent expansion of the thorax and elevation of the ribs. This can be done by pressure around the lower ribs and never needs to be any higher than the top of the xiphoid. There is little to be gained by strapping half of the chest since this certainly does not restrict expansion to any marked degree. I do not like adhesive tape because of the inevitable irritation of the skin due to the constant sliding of

the skin on respiration. A commercial or homemade rib belt, which need not be more than 4 to 6 inches wide, can be pulled snugly around the chest and may be adjusted by the patient himself. His discomfort index is a very good criterion for the tightness of the dressing. He may loosen it at night when he is breathing easily and may want to tighten it during the day when his activities are more extensive.

Another advantage of the rib belt is its usefulness in strapping the female chest. Nothing is more futile than trying to strap adhesive over the breast. In the first place it cannot be placed tight enough to give any real restriction and in the second place there is such insecure foundation that it has little effect on the underlying structures. In addition, it is extremely uncomfortable. If the lower chest only is constricted, the problem of the pressure on the breasts is eliminated.

The support should be continued as long as the discomfort in the ribs is greater than that from wearing the restraint. This will vary considerably in different individuals. For at least six weeks a binder should be worn during any contact sport. Into the binder should be incorporated a local rigid pad to prevent a direct blow on the area. The rib may remain quite tender for many weeks. I do not believe one is justified in injecting the intercostal nerves in order to permit participation of the player with *recently* fractured ribs.

In the case of injury to the upper two or three ribs, the pain may be more closely related to motion of the shoulder and neck than it is to expansion of the chest. This can be readily checked by appropriate test movements. If chest expansion does not hurt, there is no advantage in using a rib binder. There may be some value in strapping directly over the shoulder, the straps beginning in the back and crossing across the base of the neck, over the clavicle and down over the front of the chest. This strap tends to minimize elevation of the shoulder girdle when the arm is thrown up in the air. Considerable comfort may be obtained by carrying the arm in a sling. The support of the sling is not so important as the fact that the sling limits the use of the arm to routine movements with the arm at the side and, hence, forcible activity of the shoulder girdle is restricted.

Nonunion is not a common complication of fractured ribs. Malunion is of little importance. If there is troublesome pain and discomfort from a malformed rib that rubs against its fellow, this segment of the rib may be removed without noticeable disability. Before this is undertaken, diagnostic check should be made by intercostal nerve block to make sure that the pain can be relieved.

Fracture of the Ribs Below the Diaphragm

As has been mentioned previously, the lower ribs, particularly the 11th and 12th, have no firm fixation anteriorly and participate more in the abdominal muscle mechanism than in the chest. It should be emphasized here, however, that blows over the lower chest involving injury to the ribs below the diaphragm are potentially abdominal injuries and should be treated as such. The danger of complication is much more real than is the danger of the injury to the rib itself since the underlying structures of the spleen on the left and the liver on the right might well be injured. This will be discussed in detail under injuries of the abdomen.

COSTOCHONDRAL INJURY

The rather unusual anatomical situation in which the anterior end of the rib attaches directly to the corresponding end of the costicartilage sets the stage for an annoying and sometimes quite disabling injury to the chest.

Acute Injury

Following trauma, instead of rib fracture there may be an actual dislocation at the junction of the cartilage and the rib. Occasionally the same general circumstances will arise in fracture through the costicartilage itself. The symptoms vary depending upon the level of involvement. If the injury occurs in any of the upper seven ribs where there is direct attachment to the sternum, it can usually be diagnosed quite readily (Fig. 302). The dislocation may be incomplete and without displacement and will be manifested only by tenderness at the costochondral junction with pain on forceful expansion of the chest or on direct pressure. Such a condition will usually subside without the necessity of treatment.

If the dislocation is complete there may be an actual offset and overriding so that the tip of the rib rests in front of the costicartilage. In many cases I am sure that the dislocation is originally complete and is spontaneously reduced. The patient will present himself for examination complaining of pain in the anterior chest, which is particularly notable on coughing or sneezing. Since the area is readily palpable, he will have determined that he has a spot of localized tenderness and swelling one or two fingerbreadths lateral to the sternum. Careful examination will reveal the localized character of the lesion with pain on direct pressure, pain on pressure against the corresponding rib in the axillary line, and pain on pressure downward on the sternum. There may or may not be a palpable deformity and it may be possible to elicit a click as alternating pressure is applied on the sternum and on the involved rib or costicartilage. The subluxation may be minimal and be very difficult to determine, or the rib may completely dislocate. X-ray is of little value in this condition. The costicartilages are not visualized by x-ray. The rib deformity is not sufficient to be revealed by even the stereoscopic film.

TREATMENT. If there has been no demonstrable displacement or if there is no palpable click, one may assume that at least a major portion of the ligamentous investiture is intact and treatment can be directed toward preventing further injury and relieving the discomfort. The latter is accomplished by local injection of a long-acting anesthetic agent. The chest should then be firmly bound in the lower one half with either a rib belt, Elastoplast or similar strapping. The purpose of strapping is to prevent wide excursion of the ribs. If there is any possibility of recurrence of the subluxation, a direct pressure pad may be incorporated in the strapping with a piece of felt 1½ by 2¾ inches placed over the inner end of the rib but not overlapping onto the cartilage. In the male this can be strapped firmly in place with adhesive strips. This part of the dressing may be quite uncomfortable. Straps over the shoulder should be used if the lesion is high and insecurity is apparent at this level, otherwise not. Adequately protected, this lesion may heal within six to eight weeks. Costicartilage union is very slow, as is separation between the rib end and the costicartilage.

Chronic Subluxation

Far too often the player does not present himself until the condition already has become chronic and one is then faced with a different problem. Here again, *treatment* will vary according to the amount of instability in the area. If there is no instability so that the major complaint is pain, the condition may respond well to injection of a local anesthetic and a steroid in the usual fashion; that is, the anesthetic agent is injected until the area is symptom-free, after which the same area is infiltrated with a corticoid preparation. The patient should be warned that he may have increased pain beginning after several hours and continuing for several hours. He may then expect improvement. If none is seen after three days the chances are that this treatment will fail. If there is improvement but after a week or ten days the symptoms recur the area should be reinjected. It may be necessary to repeat the injection three to four times, and one expects to obtain longer and longer periods of remission of symptoms after succeeding injections until finally but little residual remains. In the occasional case a single injection may be effective permanently. There is no necessity for repeating the injection if the symptoms do not recur or if the first injection does not give relief.

In the case with or without displacement in which the symptoms persist and are severe enough to be disabling, one has to consider surgical intervention. The symptoms in such a circumstance are due to a pseudoarthrosis with, in effect, a chronic traumatic arthritis in a false joint. This may be remedied by means similar to those used at the acromioclavicular joint, namely, resection of enough of the opposing surfaces so that they do not actually rub together. One must be careful, however, that in so separating the bone and cartilage he does not end up with instability and a snapping joint. After ½ to ¾ inch of the cartilage is resected the chest should be put in various positions and subjected to various pressures to make sure that the ribs and the cartilage do not interfere on chest movement. Fusion of the rib to the cartilage surgically is extremely difficult, and I can think of no justification for internal fixation in an effort to obtain union in an old case.

If the chronic case includes subluxation or dislocation, instability is already present and treatment must be based on different principles. Whereas in the case without subluxation the symptoms are presumably due to chronic irritation with minimal amount of motion, the case with subluxation contains a built-in aggravator since every time the rib slips over the cartilage the irritation is increased. It should be emphasized that the mere fact that it is slipping is not sufficient justification for surgical treatment. In the occasional case the slipping makes the patient so nervous that there may be sufficient justification but the justification is then the nervous tension and not the slipping itself. If the slipping is symptomatic and it causes pain or spasm or local swelling, there is little hope of a cure short of surgical intervention. Local measures such as injection and heat may be palliative but the chances are they will fail. There is no justification for strapping in the chronic case. The relief given will be purely temporary and indeed the strapping may be more of an aggravation than a relief. If the symptoms justify it, treatment is surgical removal of a section of the costicartilage or of the end of the rib so that the two do not impinge. The fact that the end of the rib remains somewhat unstable will usually not be a problem. This rib is firmly bound to the one above and below and does not have wide excursion. In fact, it may actually slip less after resection since there is no lever action to slide it up over the costal cartilage and catch it in this position.

Costicartilage injury is usually not severe enough to require elimination of athletics. In the acute case, however, the dislocation should be reduced and held by strapping. Following the reduction, contact sports should not be permitted during the eight weeks required

for union to become secure. Fortunately, this condition is not a common athletic injury.

STERNUM

ANATOMICAL CONSIDERATIONS

The most anterior portion of the chest is the sternum which in the newborn is in many segments corresponding to the ribs. These segments later fuse to form three separate bones. The upper one, the manubrium, carries the attachment of the first rib and the upper portion of the second; the middle segment, the body, contains the attachment of the lower one-half of the 2nd rib and the whole attachment of the 3rd, 4th, 5th, 6th and sometimes the 7th ribs; and the lower segment, the xiphoid, hangs from the distal end of the body, its upper portion sometimes giving attachment of the 7th costicartilage. The 7th costicartilage usually attaches along the junction of the body and the xiphoid. The bone is subcutaneous throughout anteriorly and is readily palpable. Posteriorly, it protects the vital structures of the upper mediastinum.

Since in athletic injury we are usually dealing with young individuals it is of some importance to recognize the considerable variations in the time of fusion of the segments which make up the body. In the child under 6, the sternum will usually present six different segments much as the sacrum does (Fig. 313). As growth progresses, the third and fourth segments are fused around the seventh year to form the body. Hence, an x-ray of a 10 or 12 year old youngster will show definite segmental lines between the first, second and third pieces of the body. The second and third will fuse around the fourteenth year and the first and second are not fused until age 21. Any one of these segments may delay in fusion, particularly the first and second. Contrariwise, there may ultimately be a fusion between the body and manubrium and indeed between the body and xiphoid so that in an elderly person the sternum may appear as a single, solid bone. Hence developmental facts are important from the standpoint of injuries since one must be wary not to interpret a persistent fusion line as a fracture.

The superolateral angles of the manubrium carry the articular facets for the clavicles. Just below this is the facet for the first costicartilage. The second costicartilage, on the other hand, fits into the notch formed by the manubrium and the body. The manubrium is a heavy, thick bone. It is prominent and bulges forward at the lower end so that the most prominent portion of the sternum is the junction of the manubrium and the body. The body is somewhat thinner and elongated, roughly rectangular in shape and tends to slope slightly forward so that the lower ribs are more prominent at the costochondral junction than are the upper ones. The xiphoid process may actually be recessed behind the body and its proximal end may be somewhat posterior to the distal end of the body. The tip of the xiphoid hangs free in the infrasternal notch and carries the attachments for the lineae albae and abdominal muscle aponeurosis, particularly those of the recti. There is usually free motion at the xiphisternal junction. There is normally no demonstrable motion between the manubrium and the body.

There are many aberrations in rib attachments which are not particularly significant clinically as long as one keeps in mind that the ribs do not necessarily attach in a consistent pattern. For example, the 2nd rib may be horizontally attached to the manubrium and the 3rd may attach at the manubrial-body junction. Whereas usually the 7th rib is the last rib to attach directly to the ster-num, it may carry attachments also to the 6th rib and the 6th rib may attach directly to the 5th.

CONTUSION

Since the sternum is directly subcutaneous it is readily subject to contusion. The periosteum or skin is damaged by a blow from a hard object. If the blow is a severe one, there may be considerable shock reaction so that the player breathes with difficulty and will believe he has had a serious injury. However, the shock is well cushioned by the bony thorax and the intrinsic organs are well protected so that the effect is transient. After this transient period the patient will note tenderness along the sternum, usually localized in a particular area. There may be local swelling, infiltration of blood and symptoms similar to those of contusion of any subcutaneous bone. If the condition is uncomplicated, deep breathing or compression of the chest will not increase the tenderness.

Treatment is usually not necessary. Local treatment, if used, is by local injection and cold followed by heat. There is no need to strap the chest but a protective pad should be worn unless the athletic equipment carries such protection. In football the shoulder pads protect the sternum very well, the injury frequently occurring when the players are without pads. One may expect uncomplicated and complete recovery.

SPRAIN-SUBLUXATION-DISLOCATION

The same forces causing contusion of the sternum may cause sprain. We have discussed elsewhere sprain of the costochondral junction (page 389). Sprain of the ligaments connecting the manubrium and body is possible but quite unusual since there is seldom enough motion at this joint to permit ligament damage. Sprain will frequently occur by actual subluxation; that is, the body will be displaced rather than angulated backward on the sternum. The same force that would break the bone may separate the connection between the two causing a ligament injury, hence the lesion is really subluxation. The general contour of the chest causes the subluxation to be spontaneously reduced.

The patient presents himself with pain directly at the manubrium-body junction. Examination at this time will reveal tenderness here. Rarely, pain may be elicited by alternate pressure on the manubrium and body. Ordinary breathing does not cause discomfort but there is sharp recurrence of the pain on ballottement with the heel of the hand against either the body or the manubrium.

TREATMENT. If the condition is acute, contact sports should be eliminated for the first week or ten days. Subsequently a tailored plastic pad, hollowed out to protect the sternal angle and diffuse the force over the entire anterior thorax, may be placed over the sternum, particularly out over the adjacent ribs. This will usually be adequate to prevent recurrence of the trauma. If the condition is more chronic, injection of a local anesthetic plus a corticoid with the usual physical therapeutic measures may be effective.

If the dislocation is complete and persistent (Fig. 306), with the one bone caught over the other, it can readily be reduced under anesthesia by appropriate measures, first to separate the bone and then to slip one over the other (Fig. 307). Usually the bones will maintain themselves in a stable normal position unless the injury has been a major one — and this is not likely in athletes. It

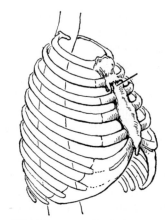

Figure 306. Fracture through upper portion of body of sternum with distal fragment overriding proximal one. Similarly the body and manubrium may overlap. (Redrawn from DePalma, The Management of Fractures and Dislocations.)

may be possible to reduce the dislocation without use of an anesthetic. The supine patient is positioned with a sandbag transversely under his shoulders slightly below the spine of the scapula. The arms are raised above the head and allowed to drop backward, thus overextending the dorsal spine (Fig. 307). As the head drops backward the dislocation will frequently reduce. The dislocation is almost always of the manubrium over the body so that, if it does not go into position, manual pressure placed against the dislocated edge of the bone and directed toward the head will usually effect reduction. Frequently closed reduction will be accomplished but the dislocation promptly recurs. In this case internal fixation is required. It should be done under direct observation by surgical exposure.

If the dislocation cannot reduce by manipulation even under anesthesia, open reduction is required. A transverse incision is made directly across the sternal angle. This will permit one to lever the fragment gently back into position. Following open reduction the junction, if it seems unstable, should be fixed by three or four wire loops which extend only through the anterior cortex of the sternum.

Since only a major force will dislocate the sternum one should be alert to the possibility of a visceral injury. Even if the immediate shock reaction with difficulty in respiration and a tendency toward collapse is only brief, the patient should be placed in bed for careful observation. X-rays of the chest should be made to determine the possibility of an injury to the structures beneath the sternum, and a careful check for hemoptysis is indicated. One may expect difficulty in respiration from the dislocation itself if it is acute.

Sprain at the xiphisternal junction is not common since the anterior posterior motion at this junction is quite free in the young individual. A blow in the substernal notch may seem quite severe but usually the resultant disability is small. There is little likelihood of any dislocation at this joint.

FRACTURE

The same forces that cause dislocation of various segments of the sternum

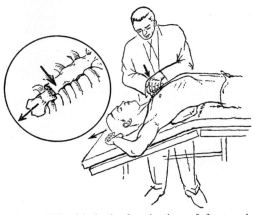

Figure 307. Method of reduction of fractured sternum. If necessary an assistant may apply traction by grasping patient's arm at the axilla and pulling cephalad. Insert shows detail of the forces applied in reduction. (Redrawn from DePalma, The Management of Fractures and Dislocations.)

may also cause fracture. The manubrium, a large bone almost cuboid in shape, will successfully resist almost any force tending to break it transversely. The fracture is usually through the upper portion of the body of the sternum and is caused by the identical forces applying in manubrial-body dislocation. The body is driven forcibly backward while the manubrium is held forward by the rigid first and second ribs so that the upper portion of the body tends to override the lower. This fracture may be complete or incomplete, with or without displacement (Figs. 308, 309 and 310). The complete fracture has undoubtedly had displacement at one time. Since there is a strong tendency for the chest to resume its normal contour, the displacement corrects itself.

The history will be of a severe blow with immediate loss of breath. There is a relatively prompt recovery from the general symptoms but pain persists in the sternum. If the fracture is complete there will be pain on even ordinary respiration so that respiration will be shallow. If the fracture is incomplete, normal respiration will not cause pain but deep inspiration will. Examination will reveal tenderness in the immediate area of the fracture site, with local swelling. Any deformity, if present, will be readily palpable in the early stages. Such a patient should be promptly x-rayed. Adequate x-ray visualization of the sternum is difficult but by positioning the patient in a few degrees of rotation with the sternum toward the cassette one can shift the sternum to the side of the spine and get a satisfactory anteroposterior view (Fig. 311). The lateral view may be instructive if there is displacement (Fig. 312). X-rays may be quite deceptive, however, since the various symphyses of the body of the sternum may be interpreted as fracture lines (Fig. 313). A spontaneously reduced fracture

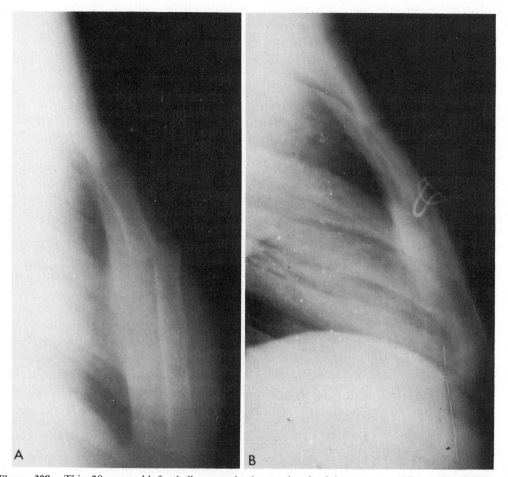

Figure 308. This 20 year old football quarterback was involved in an automobile accident. When seen 1 week post-injury, examination revealed extreme tenderness over the body of the sternum with definite, palpable offset between the first and second segments. *A,* X-ray confirms this position with the proximal end of the body overriding the distal end of the manubrium. Note there is complete fusion between the manubrium and xiphoid which indicates this is actually a fracture rather than a dislocation. Under anesthetic this could be readily reduced by manipulation but there was no position in which the reduction could be maintained. *B,* Open reduction and internal fixation with wire loops passing through the anterior one-half of the bone secured good fixation. Six months later he returned to playing football as a quarterback, asymptomatic.

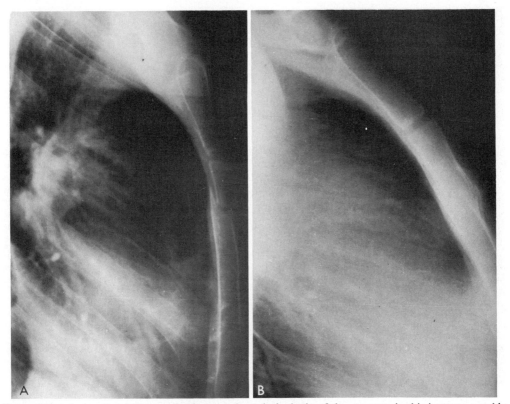

Figure 309. *A*, Another instance of a fracture through the body of the sternum, in this instance a stable fracture which went on to uneventful union *(B)*.

is usually not unstable but alternate pressure above and below will often cause pain at the fracture site.

Treatment is local with application of cold, followed by heat and compression of the chest by a rib binder or by circumferential adhesive. The test of effectiveness of the dressing is relief of the discomfort on normal breathing or ordinary activity.

A displaced fracture in which the fragments are caught or locked on one another should be reduced (Fig. 308). If the fracture line is oblique the displacement will tend to be minimal and is not important. The degree of disability will depend almost entirely on the stability with or without strapping. Contact sports should not be permitted the first few weeks unless the patient is completely pain-free on deep breathing and

on direct compression of the chest. The sternum can be protected from direct blow with padding, as indicated above, the heavy plastic pad resting on the anterior ribs and protecting the sternum from direct contact. However, this dressing will not eliminate chest expansion so it must be supplemented by adequate strapping.

COMPLICATIONS. One must be constantly aware that acute fracture is a major injury and may be accompanied by damage to the underlying structures with hemorrhage into the pleura, pneumothorax or subcutaneous emphysema. These conditions may develop insidiously over several hours. For this reason the patient with a sternal fracture should be kept recumbent in a hospital and carefully observed for signs of intrathoracic injury such as increasing dif-

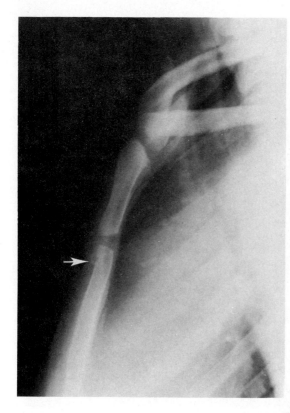

Figure 310. During an automobile accident this 16 year old girl struck her chest on the steering wheel. Her immediate symptoms were inability to breathe freely followed by persistent pain in her chest and severe pain on sneezing or hiccupping. X-ray reveals the snubbing fracture of the proximal end of the body of the sternum on the ventral aspect. This was treated symptomatically by a rib belt.

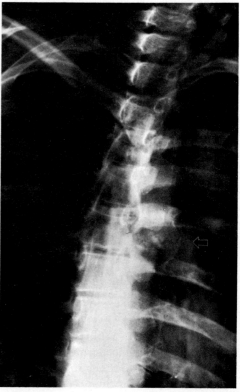

Figure 311. Fracture across body of the sternum. Note fracture line across the body, not through the line of fusion.

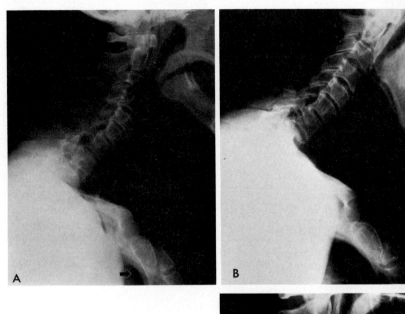

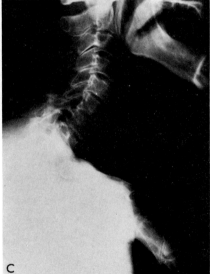

Figure 312. Patient fell directly on top of his head, receiving injuries to his neck and chest. An x-ray at the hospital revealed fractures of the spinous processes of C-5 and C-6 with displacement. Ambulatory treatment was instituted. Patient developed emphysema accompanied by difficulty in breathing and was re-examined six days later. A recheck x-ray of the cervical spine showed the fractured spinous processes and also revealed a fracture of the manubrium of the sternum with gross forward and upward displacement. Management by cervical traction cleared up the chest symptoms and materially reduced the deformity. *A* and *B*, The recheck films six days after injury. *C*, Six weeks later. Solid union, asymptomatic.

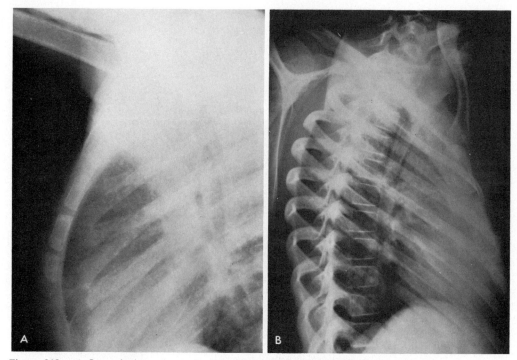

Figure 313. *A*, Lateral view of sternum in a child showing unfused separate segments. *B*, Note the closing spaces between the segments of 2-3-4 which will fuse to become the body and the much wider space between 1 and 2 which will persist. *B* is of a child older than *A*.

ficulty in breathing, impending shock or acceleration of the pulse, so that definitive treatment may be carried out if needed.

PENETRATING WOUNDS OF THE CHEST

A penetrating wound of the chest is not an athletic injury but may occur in the athlete. Any suspicion of penetration of the chest by a sharp instrument demands immediate hospitalization for careful clinical and x-ray study and prompt attention by a surgeon competent to handle conditions of the heart and lungs. There is no time for vacillation in penetrating chest injuries. One should assume that the worst has happened until he can prove that it has not.

CHAPTER 14

INJURIES IN THE AREA
OF THE ABDOMEN

ANATOMICAL
CONSIDERATIONS

The area under discussion is that from the diaphragm above to the pelvis below (Figs. 314 and 315). The abdominal area has two functions. One is as a cavity to support and protect the contents. The other is as a continuation of the trunk to support the body weight

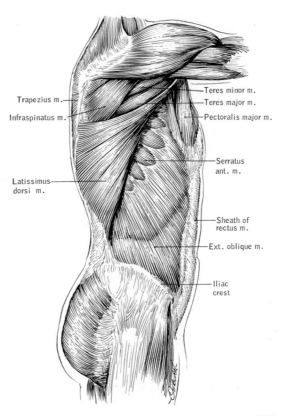

Figure 314. Lateral view of abdominal area showing the interdigitation of the abdominal muscles with the muscles of the back, shoulder and chest at the top and attachment to the iliac crest below. Note the external oblique attachments along the many ribs. The anterior attachment is to the fascia extending in front of the recti to converge at the linea alba in the midline in front.

Trapezius m.

Infraspinatus m.

Latissimus dorsi m.

Teres minor m.

Teres major m.

Pectoralis major m.

Serratus ant. m.

Sheath of rectus m.

Ext. oblique m.

Iliac crest

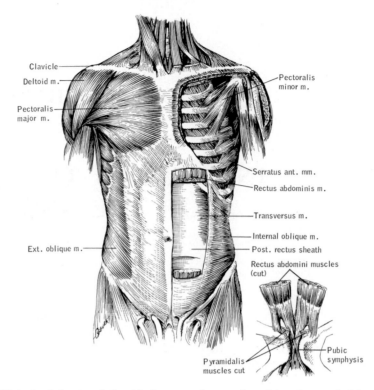

Figure 315. Note the intimate relationship between the muscles of the chest and abdomen. Also, the ingenious attachment at the pubis in the insert. Note the tendinae contained within the recti which may be subject to strain. Note the layers attaching to the iliac crest with the transversalis coming well forward on the crest while the obliques come only part way forward.

and to transmit musculoskeletal forces from the lower extremities to the body. Posteriorly, the lumbar spine gives the necessary skeletal support. In this area the massive bones completely surrounded by heavy muscle form a solid buttress which has some degree of mobility but provides a sturdy trunk with which to support the chest, upper extremities and head. It also serves to protect the abdominal contents from damage. Before the erect position was assumed, the great majority of insults to the abdominal area were posterior ones which the back is well constructed to withstand.

Extending from behind-forward are the abdominal muscles which traverse in several crisscrossing layers to converge into the fascia in front which in turn splits to include the vertical recti muscles and then converges at the linea alba in the midline. Superiorly, the lower ribs protect the upper part of the abdominal cavity and overlie the major portion of the liver, pancreas and spleen. Inferiorly, the abdominal cavity terminates in the pelvic cavity which has a strong, bony structure for protection of the urogenital tract. Anteriorly, the two recti muscles passing from the lower ribs to the pubis serve to help support the trunk by acting as a dynamic support helping to maintain the erect position. They also serve to assist the anterior spinal muscles in forward flexion of the spine. Thus, we have a massive group of muscles posteriorly, a relatively thin layer of muscle anteriorly and several overlapping layers extending peripherally from posterior to anterior. The whole makes an extremely synergistic muscle mass that permits motion in any direction—forward, backward, lateral, rotatory, or any combination of these—on the relatively flexible trunk of the lumbar spine.

Hence, it can be seen that injuries to athletes will fall into two very distinct categories although they may occur together: first, injury to the abdominal wall; second, injury to the abdominal contents.

INJURY TO THE ABDOMINAL WALL

The abdominal walls are subject to those injuries peculiar to the musculoskeletal structure. We will later discuss injuries to the posterior portion of the abdomen, namely, the lumbar spine (page 453). We have also elaborated upon thoracic injuries (page 445) but some further word is warranted on the subject of injuries to the lower ribs.

Contusion

Contusion of the abdominal wall is frequent but with the exception of certain specific areas the damage to the wall itself is not usually a serious condition. The muscles of the anterior and lateral abdomen are resilient. They overlie the soft abdominal content and, hence, are not severely injured by a direct blow. Occasionally a contusion against the tightly contracted rectus, as when a pitcher is struck by a batted ball, may cause a painful injury that may

even cause some bleeding into the recti muscles. Under these circumstances the treatment must be directed toward the muscular injury, namely, cold followed by heat and protection of the muscles until such time as the tenderness has disappeared. The physical condition of the athlete is such that he is not likely to have a severe contusion of the abdominal wall.

Contusion over the iliac crest at the attachment of abdominal muscles may be extremely distressing. This will be discussed elsewhere (Iliac Crest, page 472).

Contusion of the upper abdomen may cause injury to the ribs. The twelfth, the eleventh and to a lesser extent the tenth ribs are much more mobile than the ribs above. Since the proximal end is relatively free and the distal end does not have a bony attachment, an isolated fracture of these ribs is not common. The rib simply moves away from the blow. The contusion may cause periosteal reaction with a subperiosteal hematoma which may require local injection and some protection. It is extremely unusual to see any displacement of the fragments of a fractured rib in this area since in this instance the rib is well enclosed by the muscle mass and the stresses are such that there is no overpull on one fragment as compared to the other such as may be found in the clavicle.

The one fact of overriding importance in contusion of the abdomen is not injury to the wall but to the abdominal contents.

Strain

Since under our definition strain involves the musculotendinous unit and since the abdominal wall is essentially muscular, strain is a frequent occurrence. The symptoms will vary according to the location of injury. Thus, a strain may involve the recti with pain at or near the upper attachments or at the pubic attachments below or at the horizontal fibrous bands within the muscle itself. The strain may be from a sudden, violent effort which may actually cause rupture of the muscle fibers or some of the tendon attachments or it may be from continued overuse. In the first instance the onset will be acute with pain, muscle spasm, some rigidity and dysfunction. This may be readily distinguished from injury to the abdominal contents since the rigidity is localized to the muscle involved or at least to the group involved. Pain is aggravated by active contraction or passive stretching of the muscle. There occasionally may be some concern as to whether the painful muscle is due to acute inflammation of an underlying organ (appendix, for example) but with diagnostic acumen there should be no real confusion between them. Painful muscle spasm on the right side suggests appendicitis. However, the clinical symptoms are quite different since the patient with a diseased appendix will have signs of inflammation, some degree of peritonitis, positive laboratory findings and fever, none of which will be present in the acute strain.

In the great majority of cases, strain does not actually tear the muscle fibers and recovery is relatively rapid. In those instances of musculotendinous injury at the ribs, pubis, or iliac crest, the symptoms may be quite prolonged and cause a distressing degree of disability since resumption of athletics inevitably causes recurrence of the symptoms. The pole vaulter or high jumper who has strained his abdominal wall by excessive stress may require many weeks before he can return to active competition. In fact, he may never be able to return as long as he keeps trying to compete. The best treatment for this condition is to rest the muscle until the symptoms have subsided. This is not incompatible with rehabilitation since activity may be allowed so long as it is kept within the limits of pain. The primary problem, then, in abdominal strain is that of diagnosis, and careful attention to the actual physical findings will usually rule out any intra-abdominal complication.

It is difficult to use any appliance to protect the abdominal wall against strain and still permit competition. A well-fitted corset (see Fig. 353, page 457) will serve to give abdominal support and will restrict motion enough that passive tension on the injured area can be eliminated. The corset does little, however, in preventing the vigorous muscle contractions responsible for the symptoms.

Actual muscle or tendon rupture in the abdominal wall is an unusual injury, the exception being avulsion of the muscle from the iliac crest. I have never had to repair any other avulsion or ruptured muscle in the abdominal wall except avulsion from the iliac crest. However, any complete rupture should be repaired.

Hernia.   There is no necessity here to discuss in detail the various hernias involving the abdominal wall. It seems quite unlikely that any of them are caused by athletic injuries. However, it is inescapable that many hernias will become symptomatic by increased abdominal tension such as the straining of weight lifting or the violent exercise of the oarsmen. I believe that if a player has a symptomatic hernia and that if the symptoms are made more severe by athletics, either the hernia should be repaired or athletics discontinued. This is not to say that because the patient has a suspected hernia he should lead a sedentary life. I would recommend that this patient see a capable surgeon and be guided by his judgment as to whether or not the hernia should be repaired.

Following successful repair I see no reason for interdiction of sports.

INJURY TO THE ABDOMINAL CONTENT

In the abdominal area by far the most significant injury is the visceral one. When, following a blow or occasionally from violent exercise, abdominal symptoms arise, it is imperative to determine at the earliest possible moment the exact nature of the injury. *An intra-abdominal injury is an acute surgical emergency.* The team physician who is not a capable abdominal surgeon and who is not prepared to handle the extremely complicated situations which may arise from intra-abdominal injury will be unwise to carry out a policy of "watchful waiting" over any prolonged period. If there is *any* doubt in his mind as to whether or not there is injury to a viscus the patient should be transferred immediately to the care of the physician who will provide the definitive treatment should the need arise. These injuries are extremely infrequent in athletics but when they occur they may be disastrous, even fatal. This is another instance when timely diagnosis makes a simple problem out of what may otherwise develop into an extremely complicated one.

The injury may involve a solid viscus, such as the spleen, liver, kidney or pancreas. It may involve any portion of the gut. It may involve the peritoneum or mesentery, the bladder, or in the female, the genitalia. While in the final analysis it is extremely important to determine just what the nature of the injury is, by far the most important consideration is to determine whether or not *any* intra-abdominal injury is present. It is the problem of the abdominal surgeon to determine the diagnosis and the definitive treatment and he

must be given this opportunity at the earliest possible time.

Diagnosis

HISTORY. History is of vital importance, not only as a guide to what injury to expect but also to ascertain the progress of events up to the time of the examination. A detailed description of the accident is important. Was this a direct blow by a blunt object and if so what was the object? Was it the helmet, was it the knee, was it the heel? What was the position of the body at the time of the blow? What was the location of the injury? Was it over the back, which is well equipped to protect against trauma, or was it in the flank or anterior abdomen? Were the muscles tense and the player alert or was he relaxed and unguarded? The period of time from the blow to the examination and what happened during that time is of vital importance. Did the patient think he had a serious injury? Was he brought immediately to the doctor or did he report late manifestations, having minimized the original injury? Information should be obtained as to whether or not he has recently eaten. Was his bladder full or empty? Has he had a recent stool?

OBSERVATION. Observation of this patient is important. It may be that you were fortunate enough to be present at the time of injury and so were able to observe the actual development of the symptoms. The rapidity of their development is significant. The patient who has received a blow on the stomach or the so-called "solar plexus" may immediately present agonizing symptoms with air hunger, severe pain and cramping, which may lead to involuntary defecation and urination. If seen at once he may show symptoms of early shock. However, these symptoms subside rapidly, usually before medical attention can be obtained. Such a patient may be essentially well when he is examined by the doctor and is usually not cause for worry. However, the fact that he has survived the acute injury does not rule out the possibility of late manifestations from injury to a solid organ. The left lobe of the liver lying directly under the xiphoid is particularly vulnerable (Fig. 316). The right lobe of the liver extending down to the lower ribs is suspect in contusion of the right flank. While such a patient ordinarily presents no real problem he should be warned to report any recurrence of his symptoms.

If the patient is in immediate collapse and does not respond rapidly with or without treatment, he has an extremely severe injury that demands emergency care and immediate transportation to a hospital. In the less emergent situation the patient should be observed for pallor and cold, clammy skin; his respiration should be noted; he should be watched particularly for signs of impending shock which together with other symptoms will suggest hemorrhage.

PALPATION. Careful palpation will be extremely informative in abdominal injury. Rupture of a hollow viscus or indeed bleeding into the abdomen will almost always cause peritoneal irritation and muscle rigidity. This ordinarily will be diffuse. Localized rigidity in a certain area of the abdomen suggests a walled-off lesion with local bleeding or leaking from a viscus. If the abdomen is not tense and not rigid, one may proceed with a more detailed examination, palpating for tenderness around the spleen, liver and kidneys. Loss of peristaltic sounds may be quite significant since this is a frequent sign of early hemorrhage or other intra-abdominal injury.

LABORATORY. The laboratory may be of considerable value. In case of doubt, one should not wait for laboratory reports. Bloody emesis, bloody urine, bloody stool, all have significance. Change in the blood count usually will be only confirmatory since by the time hemorrhage is manifested by reduced hematocrit or hemoglobin, the decision should long since have been made that there was injury within the abdominal cavity.

X-RAY. X-ray examination is important but only in a positive way. A negative x-ray by no means rules out abdominal injury. Fracture of the lower ribs on the left may suggest damage to the spleen; on the right to the liver (Fig. 316). Fractured lateral processes may suggest kidney damage. Free air in the abdomen demands immediate attention (Fig. 317). Other findings such as obliteration or enlargement of the splenic shadow (Fig. 318), blurring of the psoas margin, change in the level of the diaphragm, generalized dilatation of the

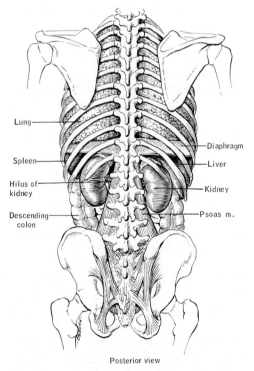

Lung

Spleen

Hilus of kidney

Descending colon

Diaphragm

Liver

Kidney

Psoas m.

Posterior view

Figure 316. Indicating the position of the spleen on the left side to demonstrate why a blow on the lower rib on the right might damage the liver and on the left the spleen. Note the liver on the right side.

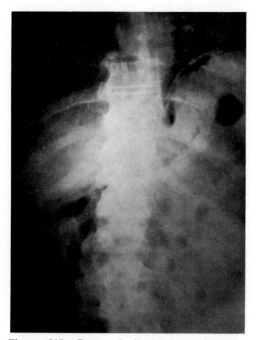

Figure 317. Ruptured diaphragm. Anteroposterior view shows air under left diaphragm and scattered throughout abdomen. Severe crushing injury to the chest.

shifting dullness in the abdomen due to free fluid. Abdominal tap may reveal free blood. It should be recalled that nausea and vomiting frequently accompany any type of abdominal injury and do not necessarily mean injury to the gastrointestinal tract.

Splenic injuries are particularly likely to be insidious since the symptoms here are due entirely to bleeding. This bleeding may be walled off and may actually stop only to be re-initiated by some other activity at a later time. The physician may be faced with the situation in which his patient is doing very well and then goes into a relatively sudden collapse. Splenic injury should have an extremely low mortality since the spleen can be removed without apparent handicap to the individual if done before dangerous collapse has occurred.

Liver injuries on the other hand are much more likely to be rapidly dangerous and carry a high mortality. As might be expected, the patients who die do so

bowel (Fig. 319) and dilatation of isolated loops of the bowel all have significance.

Specific Diagnosis

Although we are not at this stage primarily concerned with an exact diagnosis, a few words might be said about this problem. As a rule, injury to a solid viscus will be suggested by the history of the blow which makes one suspect the injury, by the location of the abdominal pain over liver, kidney or spleen, or by localization of tenderness and rigidity. The other significant findings are usually due to bleeding and as such are not particularly diagnostic as to the organ involved. They consist of the signs of blood loss, such as rapid pulse with low pulse pressure, dizziness, fainting, finally syncope, and the signs of impending shock. Examination may reveal

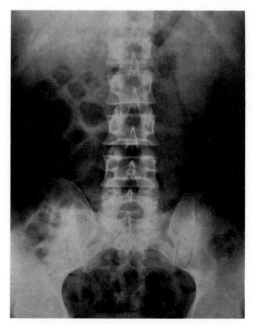

Figure 318. Flat plate of abdomen. Note the enlarged spleen in the upper left quadrant. Following injury this would suggest intracapsular hemorrhage.

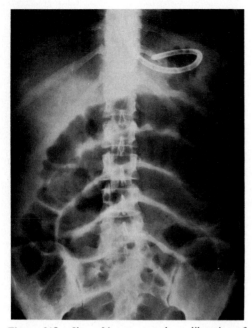

Figure 319. Ileus. Note tremendous dilatation of bowel.

quickly before they have had a chance to receive supportive treatment. There may be secondary abdominal symptoms from bile leakage as a late sequela to a relatively minor liver injury from which the patient has apparently recovered.

Pancreatic injuries are very uncommon in athletes.

Intestinal tract injuries are extremely uncommon in athletes or at least they are not commonly diagnosed. Contusion of the abdominal wall may well cause some contusion to the underlying stomach or intestines but these organs are pliable and usually "give" with the blow enough that they are not caught between the abdominal wall and the spine. This also is made much less likely since the player's stomach and intestine are usually empty.

The stomach is the organ of the gastrointestinal tract most frequently injured. Following such an injury there may be tarry stools or possibly coffee-ground vomitus which would make one suspect intrinsic damage to the stomach

or bowel. Either of these should put one on the alert but neither is necessarily serious. The injury of sufficient caliber to rupture the bowel will give immediate, serious symptoms with abdominal pain, tenderness and spasm, nausea, vomiting, ileus and other signs of peritonitis. Since such symptoms could occur without actual viscus rupture, some confusion may arise as to whether or not these symptoms are from the immediate shock of the blow or from the resultant complications. Here the rapidity of development of the symptoms is extremely important. If the vomiting is simply a process of emptying the stomach and if the symptoms of shock rapidly diminish, one may be permitted more latitude. Persistence of such symptoms and, more particularly, accentuation of these symptoms constitute an emergency which demands immediate hospitalization with appropriate examination and treatment.

Treatment of Injuries to the Abdominal Contents

It is not our intention here to give the detailed care of the patient with intra-abdominal injury. As indicated above, there is a diagnostic problem in determining whether or not the patient should be placed under the care of a competent surgeon. Some generalities about treatment are pertinent, however, since they serve to emphasize the necessity for diagnosis.

Treatment of any intra-abdominal injury is basically surgical. That is not to say that every patient must be operated upon but in the presence of a real or suspected intra-abdominal injury, surgery must be immediately available. It follows that the responsible surgeon must be in close touch with this patient and ready to carry out whatever procedure is indicated or may become indicated.

In the period prior to a definitive diagnosis, the cardinal points for treatment are bed rest under constant observation and repeated examinations by the physician who notes the local condition of the abdomen and the general condition of the patient. The patient should be covered but heat should not be applied to either abdomen or extremities. The patient's head should be lower than his feet. If he has abdominal distention, a gastric suction tube should be passed. If he is unable to void, an indwelling catheter should be used. His apprehension should be quieted but he should not be heavily sedated. Morphine or any of its modifications or derivatives should be avoided since they serve to lower the blood pressure still further. Of even greater importance is that opiates may screen vital symptoms. Barbiturates may be used. If the patient is obviously seriously injured and awaiting transportation to the hospital or arrival of the surgeon, certain other measures should be taken. An intravenous infusion should be started which not only gives the patient some support but also has the advantage of a patent vein which may be hard to obtain if the patient should go into collapse. Blood should be matched for transfusion if possible. Oxygen and suction should be available.

None of these measures is ordinarily necessary in abdominal injury received by direct blow in the athlete. If they are necessary, a very serious injury is indicated.

INJURY TO THE KIDNEY

It is probable that a mild degree of kidney injury is relatively common in any contact sport. In fact, it has been shown that red blood cells are frequently present in the urine from violent exertion alone. This has nothing to do with trauma to the kidney proper so that the mere finding of red blood cells in the urine does not necessarily indicate a kidney injury. Certainly not everyone who has pain in the flank has an injury to the kidney. On the other hand, anyone who has this type of injury does deserve examination to rule out the possibility of kidney damage.

Contusion

The most common injury to the kidney is contusion. This may be the result of a blow from a knee or helmet with the shock penetrating the muscles and transmitted to the kidney. The result of a minor contusion is slight kidney damage (Fig. 320) with local extravasation of blood under the capsule. This causes only mild pain persisting a few days. Red blood cells may be recovered from the urine. Such an injury is of no serious consequence and need not make the athlete overcautious once complete recovery has occurred.

Late manifestations are possible, principally localized infection in the hematoma area. This will be indicated by the general symptoms of infection plus local signs of urinary tract infection. In any kidney injury it is advisable to examine the patient and make a urinalysis some two weeks after the injury to determine whether any complication is developing.

A more violent blow may cause serious damage to the kidney (Fig. 320).

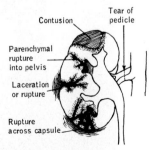

Figure 320. Anatomical view of kidney showing various types of injury.

The capsule may rupture with development of perirenal hematoma. There may be subcapsular hemorrhage which goes on to kidney necrosis. The rupture of the kidney may actually extend into its substance even to the extent of penetrating the kidney pelvis. The symptoms and signs will be related to the type of injury. In extrinsic hemorrhage, unless this is quite severe, the signs will remain quite localized with pain and muscle spasm in the flank and lumbar muscles together with painful function of these muscles. It may be difficult to distinguish this from muscular hematoma or contusion and the two may well co-exist. It may be impossible to determine the underlying kidney injury unless there are renal symptoms, particularly blood in the urine.

If the kidney substance itself is damaged, urine extravasation may occur. This must be extremely unusual in an athletic injury. In case of doubt, careful study by a competent urologist is in order. There may occasionally be serious hemorrhage from an injured kidney. It is important to determine not only the severity of injury but also the location since a major vessel may be damaged. The most outstanding signs here are those of hemorrhage. First these are local: signs of hematoma formation, extravasation of blood along the flank with tenderness, swelling, possibly positive x-ray findings. If these are accompanied by systemic signs of bleeding one is dealing with a surgical emergency. An intravenous pyelogram may give useful information. This can readily be taken during the course of examination.

INJURY TO THE BLADDER

Bladder injuries are extremely uncommon in athletics. The nervous tension of the athlete prior to competition is axiomatic. It is almost always manifested in repeated trips to empty the bladder. Since the collapsed bladder is

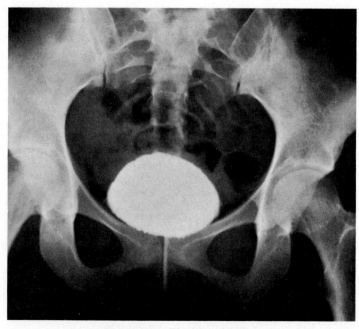

Figure 321.   The intact bladder.

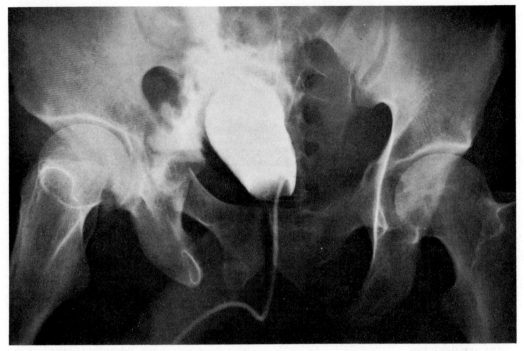

Figure 322. Severe fracture of pelvis with extravasation of urine from ruptured bladder.

practically never injured, the scene is not set for bladder rupture.

Contusion of the bladder may cause blood cells in the urine but otherwise no symptoms except some indefinite tenderness above the pubis.

Rupture of the bladder (see Figs. 321 and 322) is an extremely serious but quite unlikely complication. The patient should be asked to void. If he is unable to void, a catheter should be inserted and left in place. An intravenous cystogram is easily made but may be quite unsatisfactory. The injection of a measured amount of fluid into the blad-

der, followed by an attempt to recover the same amount, may be informative if radiopaque fluid is used. However, great care must be taken that the bladder is filled only by gravity flow. Pressure with a syringe may force extravasation from the ruptured bladder. The intravenous method is far better. Signs of shock with lower abdominal pelvic pain are also danger signals. An accurate visualization of the distended bladder may help. The presence of the dye outside the bladder indicates urine extravasation and urological consultation must be sought at once.

CHAPTER 15

INJURIES OF THE SPINE

The spine is readily subdivided into the cervical, dorsal (thoracic) and lumbar sections (Fig. 323). We shall consider these areas separately since the management of their injuries varies in many particulars.

CERVICAL SPINE

ANATOMICAL CONSIDERATIONS

From the standpoint of the athlete, the cervical spine is by far the most important part of the spinal column. It has two major functions. The first is the musculoskeletal function that provides support to the head in such a fashion as to permit the person to utilize the various sense organs, such as the eyes, ears and nose, to the best advantage. This requires enough stability to support the weight of the head, yet sufficient flexibility to permit the extreme ranges of motion which are necessary. From the evolutionary standpoint the neck has been one of the most adaptive areas. In various mammals there are wide differences, from the extreme length and flexibility of the neck of the giraffe whose small head perches an amazing distance from the trunk, to the apparent absence of neck in the pig

whose snout seems to extend right back into his body.

The other major function of the neck is to transmit the major nerves from the head to the rest of the body and to give them adequate protection. The requirements for these two functions are to a great extent contradictory. The best protection would be a rigid tube with the spinal roots and cord inside. The musculoskeletal function, which demands extreme flexibility, is ill designed to protect the nerves. The amazing ingenuity by which this is accomplished merits comprehensive study which cannot be given here.

Free flexibility of the head demands much more cervical motion than is available anywhere else in the spine. The degree of rotation that can be obtained from the oval vertebrae rotating each on the other is strictly limited. While this is very much greater in the cervical spine than in other areas by virtue of the relatively flat articular processes, still any major degree of rotation will simply subluxate or dislocate one facet on the other. Similarly, a much more localized range of flexion and extension is necessary to nod the head than can be obtained in any one ordinary vertebral joint or series of joints. Hence, the two top cervical vertebrae

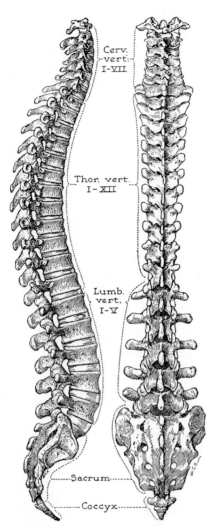

Cerv.
vert.
I–VII

Thor. vert.
I–XII

Lumb.
vert.
I–V

Sacrum

Coccyx

Figure 323. The vertebral column as seen in lateral and posterior view. (From Jones and Shepard, Manual of Surgical Anatomy.)

are entirely different in structure and function from the remaining ones. The first cervical vertebra (atlas) is a large ring bearing on its anterolateral sides the articular facets, those above articulating with the skull, those below with C-2. The neurocanal in C-1 extends forward to occupy the space which in other vertebrae contains the body. This forward extension is separated from the main neurocanal by a strong fibrous band, thus creating an open ring of three-fourths bone with the other one-fourth

a dense membrane. This space forms a socket to receive the odontoid process of C-2. Developmentally the odontoid is the body of the first cervical vertebra which has detached itself from the first vertebra to become a portion of the second. The superior articular facets of C-1 are long and shallow and on these facets the head can nod with a hinge motion. There is no rotatory or lateral motion between the cranium and the first cervical vertebra. This wafer of vertebra would readily dislocate were it not for its firm fixation to the odontoid of C-2.

So much for the flexion and extension of the head. The rotatory motion of the head which in the human is equally, if not more, important is provided at the atlanto-axial junction. The head and first cervical vertebra rotate as a unit around the pivot of the odontoid process of the second. The comparatively elongated articular processes permit this sliding motion between the atlas and axis.

The remaining cervical vertebrae are very similar to the dorsal vertebrae in general structure. There are certain variations characteristic of the function required. The massive cervical spinal cord with its extreme vulnerability to injury requires a large ring so that the cord can be suspended in the middle of the ring without direct contact with the surrounding walls. The other and opposing requirement, namely mobility, is obtained by the articular processes which in the cervical spine are relatively horizontal. The rather flat convex upper surface fits into the shallow concavity of the inferior articular surface of the vertebra above in a much more horizontal plane than in the dorsal area. The angle of these facets is about 45 degrees from the horizontal. This is much less secure than the hooks on any of the vertebrae below the cervical spine since in the dorsal and lumbar spine these articular facets are vertical. The bodies are relatively light since the weight to be carried is only that of the head. The spinous processes are long and extend horizontally backward in the upper portion of the neck but obliquely downward in the lower portion. They are bifid to add further to the area available for the attachment of the multitude of ligaments and muscles that provide good stability and yet free mobility. The seventh cervical spinous process is longer and more prominent and, hence, the most vulnerable to injury. The transverse processes of all are short and light because the massive muscles that attach lower in the spine are not present in the neck. Mobility is more important than strength. The foramina through which the rather large cervical nerve roots pass are relatively shallow. The nerves pass almost horizontally through the nerve root canals and so are quite subject to traction injury. The discs between the vertebrae are relatively shallow and much less strong than those below since there is less weight involved.

The vertebrae are bound together by the annular ligament with its dorsal and ventral thickenings that hold the bodies snugly but not rigidly together. The ligamentum nuchae extends from the external occipital protuberance to attach along the tips of the cervical vertebrae as far as C-7 and then extends downward as the supraspinous ligament. This ligament is a thin septum, wide from behind-forward, which serves to separate the muscles of the posterior portion of the neck at the midline. The interspinous ligaments lie between the spinous processes. The ligamentum flavum secures the laminae. The capsular ligaments bind the vertebrae at the articulations. Together, these ligaments stabilize the vertebrae in their relative position, each to the one above and the one below. In the neck they are much less stable than anywhere else in the column. This combination of extreme mobility plus the necessity for protection requires an amazingly intricate interdigitation of muscles as well as the support of many ligaments.

The muscles of the vertebral column are extremely massive in the lower back, becoming less massive but with wider excursion as the cervical spine is reached. Since the neck is an isolated column it requires support in the nature of dynamic guy wires in each direction. The fact that these musculotendinous guy wires can be varied in length permits the neck and head to be moved in any direction while maintaining a constant degree of support. Nowhere is the synergistic use of muscles better demonstrated than in the neck where the function of each muscle depends altogether upon the position of the head at the time the contraction takes place. It is not advisable here to discuss in detail the individual muscles of the neck since their number is legion. It suffices to say that the muscles are so arranged as to permit traction to be applied in any position of the head or the spine so that with appropriate contraction of one group and relaxation of others, synchronous motions occur. As might be expected, the heaviest groups of muscles are posterior. Many of the muscles of the neck pass distally to attach to the muscles in the shoulder girdle as well as to the trunk itself.

In front of the neck lie many vital structures that are poorly protected in the upright position. The veins and arteries on either side, the esophagus behind, the larynx and trachea in front are all quite vulnerable unless the head is held down to permit the chin and thorax to protect the front of the neck.

EMERGENCY MANAGEMENT

Injury to the neck has extremely serious connotations for major disability. If there is any question at all as to the severity of a cervical injury, it should be assumed that the most severe injury is present. Under no circumstances should the patient be asked to sit or stand. If he is lying on the ground with a possible serious injury to his neck he should not be moved until an evaluation of the situation has been made. This may require some time but delay of the game is of no consequence under such circumstances and the physician must not be hurried in his evaluation and so permit what may be fatal movement. If the player is conscious, a few words will determine his own feelings in regard to his neck. One should determine whether he has normal function of his hands and feet. This does not require a detailed physical examination but does entail sensible evaluation. The patient should then be moved to a stretcher and for this adequate help must be present so that it can be done without any motion between his head and trunk. Under ordinary circumstances the athlete will be conscious and he is better placed on his back with his head carefully supported. On occasion this may serve to dramatize and over-emphasize what turns out to be a relatively minor injury. On the other hand, it may save a life or prevent lifetime paralysis.

Once the player has been moved to a place for better examination, detailed study should be made at the end of which the physician should have a definite impression as to the severity of the injury. He should observe such deformity as may be indicative of unilateral or bilateral dislocation. He should attempt to localize the pain. Even if it is decided that the injury is only relatively severe and the patient can be moved to the hospital for evaluation, great care must be taken in his handling. The head may be stabilized by a sandbag on either side or by someone sitting at his side hold-ing his head. It may be stabilized quite well by a simple head halter which may be made by a muslin strip under the occiput and another under the chin with a weight hanging over the end of the carrier or bed. If it is decided that x-rays should be made, they must be made under the same precautions. Under no circumstances should the x-ray be made with the patient sitting up until one can be sure there is no instability of the neck. Once a diagnosis is made of a serious injury to the neck, consultation should be sought immediately with whatever person is going to carry out the definitive care. This may be the orthopaedic surgeon or neurosurgeon, or both. I cannot emphasize too strongly that the patient must not be asked to sit up. He must not have forceful manipulation of the head to see how well it will move. He must not be allowed to walk from the field. If he already is sitting or standing, this position may be maintained, again with greatest precautions.

In spite of utmost care, symptoms may develop insidiously. The patient receives his injury but may seem quite well, only to succumb to some inadvertent motion later. Any complaint of the neck by a player demands that he be removed from the contest and a definitive examination made. This will tend to minimize the tragedies that occur in the locker room or at home following the initial injury.

CONTUSION

Contusion in the vicinity of the neck has many serious connotations, not in relation to the integument, since the skin is rarely damaged, but because of the vital underlying structures. In the back of the neck, the blow may be received on the spinous processes, particularly in the lower cervical area, and since these are long the leverage exerted at their bases may be quite powerful. If the blow is received with the neck in forward flexion, the combination of tension on the ligament and muscle plus the striking force may break off a spinous process anywhere from its tip to its junction to the body. Such an injury will be painful. There will be local tenderness, particularly on dropping the head forward. Palpation will usually be unrewarding in fracture but careful x-ray study will reveal the lesion. A word of warning: X-ray of the lower cervical area is difficult and one must be sure he is visualizing the area of involvement. It is worthwhile to insert a hypodermic needle into the tender area at the time the picture is made in order to localize the tender spot in the x-ray.

If a fracture is found it should be treated appropriately as indicated below. Contusion of the bone without fracture is treated according to its severity. Ordinarily no treatment is necessary. Painful bruising of the cervical muscles may cause the usual complications of muscle contusion with hematoma formation (Fig. 324), muscle spasm, stiffness, pain, etc. In such an instance local treatment is of value with application of heat, pain-free massage and local analgesic balm. Some degree of protection with a cotton collar may speed up the recovery. Muscle spasm can be relieved by antispasmodics and participation in athletics should be minimized.

Occasionally a blow on the back of the neck will have a direct effect on the spinal cord and the resultant *shock* may cause transitory paralysis. Much more often there simply is a generalized feeling of numbness which is extremely transitory and of little significance. In case of persistent neurologic symptoms, such as numbness and paresthesia, a more thorough search for interspinal injury should be carried out. Certainly the

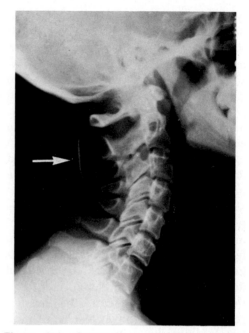

Figure 324. Calcification superficial to ligamentum nuchae following neck injury with hematoma. This mass does not move with the spinous process.

patient should be protected by observation and no contact permitted so long as there is any doubt. *Concussion* of the cord may be quite alarming but complete recovery is the rule.

At the side of the neck contusion is less frequent but may cause distressing symptoms by a direct effect on the brachial plexus with the feeling of shock to the neck and numbness in the arm. This is usually quite transitory and the player is able to shake it off. Occasionally there may be permanent damage to some of the components of the brachial plexus. Frequently the contusion may occur with the neck flexed in the opposite direction so that there may be strain as well as contusion.

In the front of the neck contusion may be quite severe. The athlete usually learns to protect the neck by carrying his chin low and forward so that the interval between the chin and sternum is relatively narrow. Given an opportunity, he will protect himself further by dropping his head forward when the blow is impending. The structures most likely to be damaged by a direct blow are the *larynx* and *trachea.* A blow to the throat may cause extreme distress, even to the extent of systemic shock. The player is speechless with severe dyspnea. He struggles for breath, is completely unable to phonate and for a period has the feeling of impending doom. Under ordinary circumstances he recovers quickly, the spasm of the vocal cords subsides and he is able to breathe more easily although the hoarseness may persist. Immediate treatment should be complete bed rest with a cold pack on the neck. Body activity should be discouraged in order to cut down on the oxygen requirement. Reassurance is vital but sedation should be given cautiously, particularly if there are signs of systemic shock. Recovery may be complete within a very few minutes with no damage done and the patient may be able to resume play. In the more severe case, there may be a hematoma, either intrinsic in the larynx or extrinsic from the muscles in the neck. If severe, this can be a dangerous complication. It usually is not. There may actually be *fracture of the thyroid cartilage,* of the *hyoid* or of the *trachea,* but this is not common in young athletes since these structures are quite resilient. If there is persistence of symptoms beyond the day of injury, careful laryngeal examination should be carried out, particularly if dyspnea persists. In case of doubt the patient should be hospitalized where oxygen, suction and intravenous therapy are available. Laryngoscopy is indicated if there is any question as to intrinsic injury. If signs of increasing intrinsic bleeding appear, the patient should be carefully observed since the neck will not tolerate much pressure either from the bleeding or from the attempt to arrest this by a pressure pack. It is axiomatic that if there is any persistence of these symptoms, the patient should be kept at rest and under careful observation.

It probably is not advisable to attempt to aspirate a hematoma in the neck unless all the facilities of the hospital are available together with a trained laryngologist. If the bleeding appears to be increasing and pressure more severe and ice packs do not control the situation, consultation is mandatory.

STRAIN

Muscular strain in the cervical area may be extremely complex. The large number of small muscles with multiple attachments are capable of different functions in different positions of the head. It is an area quite subject to strain. It may be very difficult to distinguish between strain and sprain or between sprain and muscle spasm caused by secondary nerve root involvement. While the athlete is quite subject to strain of the cervical muscles by violent movement of the head, he is also the subject of sprain of the joints with its attendant complications. Indeed, the strain and sprain may well coexist.

Diagnostically, there is some value in the history although it may be quite misleading. While strain may follow overuse of the muscles of the neck, it is even more likely to be the product of an avulsion force against a muscle resisting a violent motion. Since this same violent motion may cause sprain, subluxation, dislocation or fracture, a muscular strain may well be a secondary consideration. When strain occurs as a separate entity, active function as well as passive stretching of the involved muscle will be painful. The exact diagnosis becomes somewhat academic if the injury is a serious one. In the more minor injuries, diagnosis is not so difficult. The muscle spasm that follows this injury is a universal accompaniment of any injury to the neck and is of little diagnostic significance. Tenderness within the muscle itself or at its attachment may give a clue.

If the strain seems to be relatively mild, the *treatment* may also be mild. Local heat, rest and reduction of activity are important. All too often, what begins as a minor strain ends up as a rather severe spastic type wryneck which may be completely disabling while it lasts. The actual injury seems at the time to be minimal. It is not until 24 to 48 hours later that the constant irritation of the injured muscle causes spasm of all its fellows. This case requires more definitive treatment. Bed rest with light cervical traction, 4 to 6 pounds, is preferable to massive traction in the upright position (Fig. 325). It also has the undoubted value of being good treatment for any injury to the neck so that if one's diagnostic acumen has been somewhat at fault, at least the treatment is suited to whatever lesion may be present. Bed rest, cervical traction, local heat, muscle relaxants and mild sedation will result in prompt relief of symptoms. The danger is recurrence. If the strain is indeed quite mild and recovery is complete within 24 to 36 hours, no protection need be applied to the neck. The patient should be advised against forceful activities, told to move his neck as freely as he can but strictly within the limits of pain and not against resistance. If the case seems to be more severe and traction has been needed for several days, a cervical support such as a cotton collar (Fig. 326) may be necessary for two to three weeks. As in any strain, careful rehabilitation is needed to prevent prompt recurrence of symptoms. The protective factor here is not against motion of the neck as in sprain but against overuse of the muscle involved. This requires a cooperative patient who understands his problem. The posterior spinal muscles are the ones most commonly strained—the result of forcible extension of the spine against resistance as in the wrestler. However, any of the muscles may be involved in strain.

SPRAIN-SUBLUXATION-FRACTURE-DISLOCATION

Injuries to the spine are difficult to subdivide into specific categories of

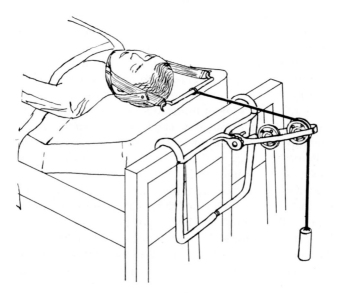

Figure 325. Patient in cervical traction. The traction apparatus is placed at the foot of the bed instead of at the head, with the type of halter as shown. Note that the traction is positioned so that the neck is held in extension.

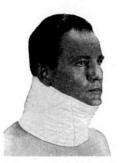

Figure 326. Cotton collar. The collar illustrated is a single strip of tapered quilted outing flannel, small end 3 inches enlarging to 6 inches and 6 feet long. Same can be made of alternating wraps of sheet wadding and gauze. This should extend far enough to support the occiput and chin.

sprain, subluxation, dislocation and fracture since one extends indistinguishably into the other and there is often a combination of all four. A much more serviceable classification can be made on the basis of the mechanism causing the injury. While there is a great deal of overlap and the motion may be much more complex than simple motion in one direction, nevertheless there is a predominant motion in one direction which is almost always the major cause of the damage. I suppose it is virtually impossible to have pure flexion of the neck without some degree of rotation or vice versa. Nevertheless, the injury characterizes itself by the prime mover.

Whereas the strain discussed above is caused by overuse of the muscle, sprain is caused by forcing a joint through an abnormal range of motion and the ligament designed to prevent this motion is damaged. Sprain of the neck is a very common injury and may be mild (first degree), moderate (second degree) or severe (third degree). The mild injury is of little significance and will require but little treatment. The moderate injury in which there has been some loss of ligament strength will require protection primarily from the forces that caused the injury. Much more complicated is the severe injury in which there is complete loss of integrity of the ligament. As this ligament loses its function, the motion that it is designed to prevent is unrestricted. The forces that ordinarily are controlled by this ligament are then transferred to other areas of the lever. This ligament injury may progress into subluxation in which the joint partially dislocates; or indeed the capsular ligament may tear completely and the joint completely dislocate. Other ligaments in the spine that are not related directly to the articulations may be involved. The interspinous ligament posteriorly restricts flexion of the neck. The anterior longitudinal ligament anteriorly prevents anterior separation of the bodies of the vertebrae and so hyperextension. There is usually some combination of ligament damage so that when the one ligament tears, the force is shifted to another ligament and damages this one also. This may continue until there is complete disruption of all the supporting ligaments and complete dislocation of one vertebra on another. So also a fracture may supervene. That is, as the ligament gives way one place, a fracture may occur elsewhere or, as the ligament holds, the edge of the bone comprising the fulcrum or counter-lever may give way. Some attempt will be made to describe these injuries under the categories of the forces applied.

Flexion Injury

Interspinous-Supraspinous Ligament Injury (Sprain). The supraspinous and interspinous ligaments which attach along the spinous processes from the occiput to the dorsal spine serve as a checkrein to prevent overflexion of the head. Although they are somewhat elastic, their fibers are not tight when the neck is in extension. They become increasingly tight as the neck flexes forward. The mechanism causing sprain is a forcible hyperflexion of the neck. As this force is applied, the cervical bodies are forced together. The vertebrae rotating on the sagittal axis of the articulations force the spinous processes to separate (Fig. 327). This force is arrested by the combination of the pressing of the intact bodies together and the checking action of the dorsal muscles and the ligamentum nuchae. If the force continues and the bodies maintain their integrity, the ligaments may tear (Fig. 327, A). This sprain may be mild (first degree), moderate (second degree) or severe (third degree).

The mild (first degree) sprain is of little consequence. There will be no particular weakness in the ligament. All the symptoms will be local with tenderness and pain at the site of injury. Ordinary cervical flexion within normal range will be pain-free. Forcing the neck beyond this range may cause some distress. This injury is not likely to arouse muscle spasm since the symptoms are mild.

In a moderate (second degree) sprain which involves some loss of function of the ligament, a portion of the ligament has actually been torn away. This may be within the ligament itself or may be at its attachment to one of the cervical processes. In this instance the symptoms will be more severe. The pa-

tient holds his head in extension and resists any attempt to flex it forward because of pain at the site of injury. There is localized tenderness. After the passage of several hours, there is likely to be muscle spasm of the posterior spinal muscles (Fig. 328); and the neck, instead of being pulled to one side or the other, is held in extension. The direction of force applied may indicate the expected location of injury. If the patient can rotate his atlanto-occipital joint, that is, nod his head without pain, one may assume the injury is below C-2. A further guide is the location of tenderness.

If there is sharply localized tenderness in the spinous processes or ligament, injection of this area by a long-acting local anesthetic if the patient is seen early or a corticoid preparation if he is seen later may give substantial relief. This injection may need to be repeated several times. In this case, traction is ordinarily not indicated since holding the head up will relieve the tension. However, this becomes quite tiresome and tension headache is common with spasm of the posterior cervical muscles. This patient will be relieved by a cervical collar that holds the chin up (Fig. 329). He may be more comfortable at night in light cervical traction although usually this is not necessary. Physical

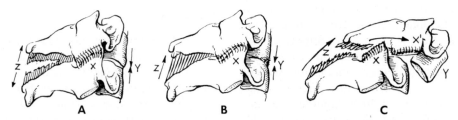

Figure 327. Flexion force. *A,* Forcible hyperflexion. The cervical vertebra rotates on the axis of the apophyseal joints (x). The cervical bodies (y) maintain their integrity. The interspinous ligament (z) ruptures.

B, Same force. The ligament (z) holds. The rotation is around (x) and the adjacent edges of the bodies of the cervical vertebrae buckle.

C, Same force. The interspinous ligament (z) gives way. The bodies (y) maintain their integrity. The center of rotation (x) advances (to x′) as the interarticular ligaments rupture to slide the inferior articular process of the upper vertebra in front of that of the lower with subluxation or dislocation.

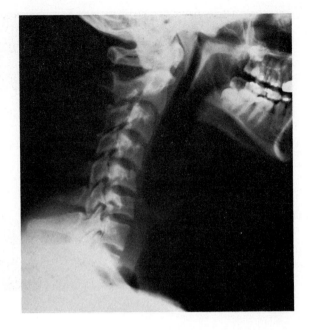

Figure 328. X-ray, lateral view, made with the neck in forward flexion. Note reversal of the curve, caused by muscle spasm of the lower cervical segment so that this is held in extension while the upper part of the neck flexes forward. This is indicative of muscle spasm such as accompanies strain or sprain.

therapy is of value here. Great care should be taken that any manipulative treatment is pain-free. This injury may be quite disabling to the athlete since six to eight weeks will be needed for the ligament to heal, which is enough to seriously disrupt his season. Rehabilitation exercises are extremely important since final stability depends upon strong cervical muscles (see p. 798). A well fitted cotton collar may permit him to

participate much sooner. The collar must be carefully fitted so that the ligament will not be reinjured by forward flexion of the neck.

If the ligament injury is a severe (third degree) one, there is complete separation of the ligament. The ligament may be torn off a single spinous process and the main body of the ligament may remain intact. This is a much less serious injury than that occurring when the ligament itself is pulled in two. If the ligament is ruptured either in its substance or off one of the processes, the symptoms will be quite severe with sharply localized pain. If palpated early, a defect may be felt in the ligament, particularly if the head is forced into some degree of flexion. Further flexion will be bitterly resisted. The patient will feel that his head is insecure and will tend to hold his neck quite rigid. Painful spasm soon supervenes and the head is pulled into hyperextension. At this time it may be quite difficult to determine the exact nature of the injury. Careful x-ray study may reveal an avulsion of a portion of the bone with the ligament (Fig. 330).

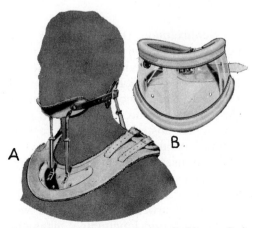

Figure 329. *A*, An adjustable cervical brace. *B*, A plastic cervical collar.

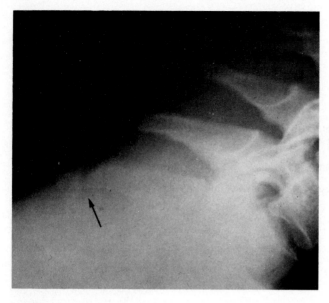

Figure 330. Avulsion fracture of the tip of the spinous process of C-7 following acute flexion injury. The articular facets and the bodies are spared.

X-ray made with the head and neck in flexion may reveal unusually wide separation of the spinous processes at some level. This is quite suggestive of ligament injury, particularly if this coincides with the level of local symptoms. There is normally a wide variation in the amount of separation of the spinous processes in the normal neck at different levels.

Treatment for avulsion of the tip of one of the spinous processes is surgical removal of the fragment and repair of the ligament. This treatment seems to be well accepted, especially since the diagnosis can be confirmed by x-ray. The same treatment would be ideal for complete ligament avulsion. Usually, however, this condition is not diagnosed in the early stage and is treated nonsurgically as a moderate sprain. Indeed, if the head is kept in hyperextension, thereby bringing into contact the tips of the spinous processes and with them the ligament ends, the ligament may grow together at near normal length. If this same force breaks the spinous process at the lamina or if it fractures the spinous process without displacement,

uneventful healing will occur by simple immobilization of the neck in extension. Avulsion of the tip is very prone to nonunion since the separation is usually wide. The treatment of a painful nonunion is excision of the fragment. Athletic competition should not be permitted until union is complete—either union of ligament to bone if the fragment is removed or bony union of the fragment to the vertebra.

Other Flexion Injury

Subluxation Dislocation. In the more severe flexion injuries of the neck, the damage is usually not confined to the interspinous ligament. As the neck is flexed, the cervical discs compress. The bodies are forced together in front and apart posteriorly and excess of motion occurs at the apophyseal articulations. If the interspinous ligament gives way while the body remains intact, the force is received on the laminal and articular ligaments as well as the posterior longitudinal ligament, which is relatively weak. As long as the front of the body remains intact, the dislocating force will separate the articulations and rupture the capsular ligaments, and a subluxation of the cervical vertebrae will occur (Fig. 327, *C*). Indeed, this may happen without actual rupture of the posterior longitudinal ligament. As the flexion is continued there is a shearing force of the head forward on the trunk that causes the superior articulations to displace forward over the ones below. If some of the ligaments are left intact—either the interspinous or the laminal or possibly the articular ligaments plus the anterior and posterior longitudinal ligaments—a great deal of stability is still present in the spine and the articular process of the vertebra above slips in front of the superior articular process of the vertebra below. This dislocation locks in the unreduced position. Subluxation followed by spontaneous reduction probably occurs quite frequently in flexion injuries of the neck. This is one of the reasons, already mentioned, why the neck should be carefully protected against a repetition of the flexion shearing force in order that complete dislocation does not occur with a subsequent injury.

In bilateral dislocation (Fig. 331) the head is characteristically held thrust forward but with hyperextension. The spinous process of the vertebra below is prominent with a corresponding defect above, while the proximal portion of the neck will appear to be flexed. The patient is usually extremely apprehensive and will resist any attempt to move his head in any direction. Indeed, he will often hold his head with his hands. I well recall being called to the hospital one Saturday afternoon to see a man who had ridden in his car to the hospital holding his head in his hands following an episode with a bull. He absolutely refused to take his hands away from his head, making the statement that if he did his head would fall off, nor would he re-

linquish his grasp to permit examination until he was supine in bed and even then only reluctantly.

This injury has serious potential for cord and root damage and a careful examination should be made for the presence of a neurological deficit. This absolutely must be done before any attempt at reduction is made. The injury is obviously a serious one but fortunately it is extremely infrequent in the athlete. It demands the prompt care of the orthopaedist. In the interim, the patient should be placed supine and the head should be protected by sandbags on either side. Since the exact nature of the injury will not be evident until x-ray study has been made, precautionary traction of a few pounds with head halter is imperative as soon as it can be applied. Needless to say, transportation must be made with extreme caution. Definitive care demands reduction at the earliest possible moment, hence the necessity for early diagnosis (Fig. 332).

The same flexion, forward shearing force that causes the dislocation mentioned above may continue with the destruction of the remaining ligamentous support at this level so that one body may slide forward on the other until the back of the neurocanal of one vertebra is at the level of the front of the neurocanal of the one below (Fig. 333). This applies a shearing trauma to the cord and may cause complete quadriplegia. With this injury there is such instability that the neck will frequently fall back into correct apposition and local physical and x-ray examination may be entirely negative. One must not be misled as to the severity of the injury by the negative x-ray. The same dislocation may have been complete and reduced and without cord damage only to have cord damage occur because the injury was not recognized and subsequent activity caused a dislocation.

As this dislocation occurs, the pos-

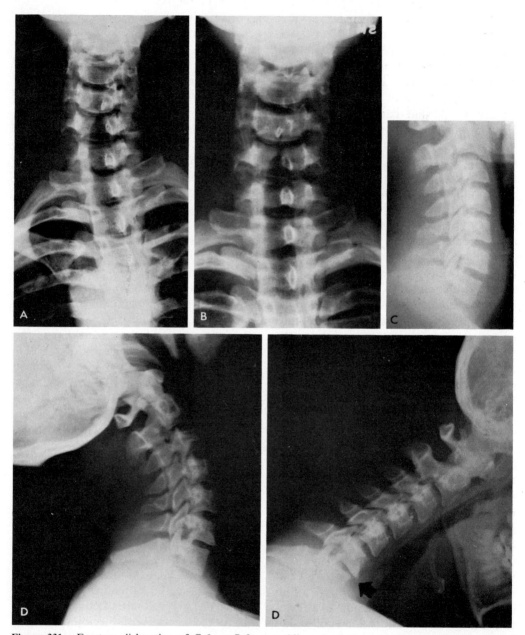

Figure 331. Fracture dislocation of C-6 on 7 from tackling. *A*, Anteroposterior view. Notice lateral displacement of mass of C-7 with rotation of C-6 forward. *B*, 24 hours in traction reduced the dislocation. *C*, Lateral view in traction shows no displacement, no obvious fracture. *D*, Recent lateral films in flexion and extension showing subluxation, with persistent collapse of disc between C-6 and C-7. This boy developed latent neurological deficit in the long thoracic nerve which has persisted.

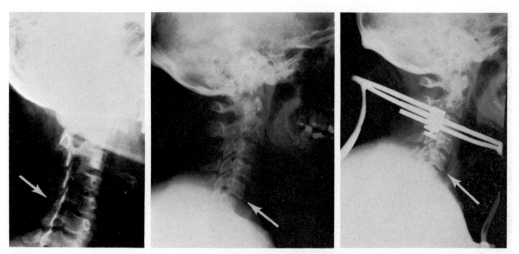

Figure 332. Fracture-subluxation of C-5 on 6 with fracture of the articular process of C-5. The deformity was corrected under traction, recurred in the brace and has persisted. Neurological deficit was persistent with hypesthesia in the right thumb.

terior portion of the neural arch may break and remain posterior (Fig. 334). This break may take place at the pars interarticularis or further back on the lamina. In any event, this protects the cord to a considerable degree since the shearing action of the posterior portion of the ring is prevented as the ring itself

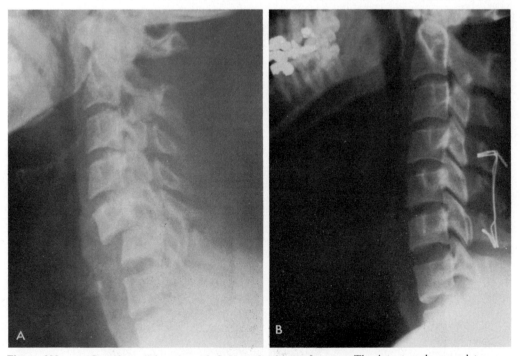

Figure 333. *A,* Complete dislocation of C-5 on 6 without fracture. The intact arch caused transection of the cord and complete quadriplegia. *B,* Postoperative picture showing complete reduction with internal fixation from C-4 to 6 plus bone graft. Partial laminectomy at C-5.

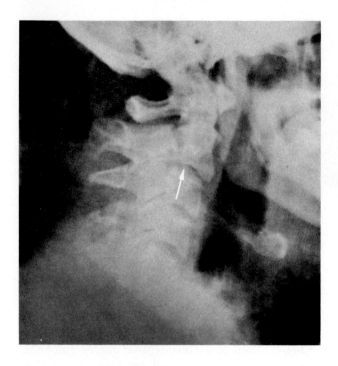

Figure 334. Fracture-dislocation of C-2 on C-3. Note that the fracture separated the arch and lamina from the body which relieved the tension on the cord and there was no neurological deficit. This picture shows the reduction and plaster fixation. Complete healing. Asymptomatic. Arrow indicates fracture.

expands. This accounts for the case of complete dislocation of the vertebra forward with no neurological symptoms. Careful x-ray examination will often reveal that the arch has remained posterior. Such cases serve to emphasize the importance of intelligent handling of the cervical injury. The same force that causes bilateral dislocation with forward flexion and shearing may well cause fracture of the articular processes which may complicate the recovery and result in painful joints.

A unique type of injury that may occur from forward stress is dislocation between the first and second cervical vertebrae (Fig. 335). It will be recalled that the odontoid is held firmly to the

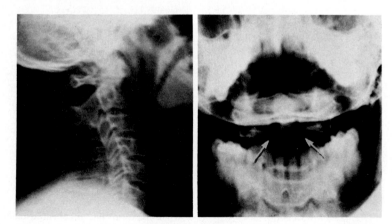

Figure 335. Fractured odontoid with forward subluxation of C-1 on 2. Only transient neurological deficit. Treated in traction, cast, brace with complete clinical recovery but some persistent subluxation.

anterior portion of the body of C-1 by the transverse ligament, which keeps the body of C-1 from displacing forward. On a sharp forward thrust of the head, particularly combined with some forward shearing, the odontoid is forced sharply against this ligament. If the ligament tears, the articular ligaments also give way and dislocation occurs leaving the odontoid within the neurocanal of the first cervical. The large vulnerable cord of this area is very likely to be damaged, with ensuing death. Occasionally there is a congenital shortness of the odontoid so that it can slip forward under the transverse ligament without actually tearing it. This is the so-called somersault dislocation caused by sharp hyperflexion of the neck. Many of these cases will not have serious nerve involvement. They may actually be in the nature of recurrent dislocation and slip forward and spontaneously reduce. If they do not reduce spontaneously, they can usually be reduced. Owing to the very large brain stem at this level, reduction is better done by mechanical traction with weights than by manipulation. The traction should first be with the neck well flexed, then gradually moved toward extension. This dislocation may be very difficult to distinguish from fracture of the odontoid since the latter, when it accompanies dislocation of the first cervical vertebra, is not readily seen in the anteroposterior x-ray. Careful study after the deformity is reduced will reveal the character of the lesion (Fig. 336).

A much more frequent injury appears to be the fracture of the odontoid from the body of C-2. In this instance there is much more leeway for the cord and it is much less likely to be impinged. This fracture may be complete or incomplete. The patient usually realizes that he is seriously hurt. The usual careful management should be carried out. Definitive diagnosis is made by x-ray.

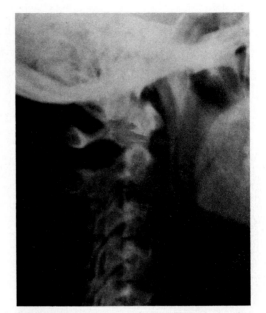

Figure 336. Fracture of the ring of the first cervical vertebra without displacement. No neurological deficit. Treated by plaster immobilization.

The severity of this major injury demands early, adequate treatment, which may well be surgical. Of some consequence is the incomplete tear with damage to the transverse ligament. The initial relatively minor injury may be followed by a fatal accident at a later time.

Fracture. Aside from the laminal fractures mentioned above, which are essentially a component of dislocation, there may be fractures of other portions of the vertebrae. It has been mentioned that the spinous process may break rather than the ligamentum nuchae tear. As the flexion force is applied and the spinous processes separate, the bodies are forced together and a fracture of the body may occur (Fig. 337, A). In fact, a fracture of the cervical body is more frequent than a complete tear of the posterior longitudinal ligament. If the fracture is not accompanied by a dislocation, the body may compress as much as 75 per cent. The front part of the body will be down to 25 per cent of its

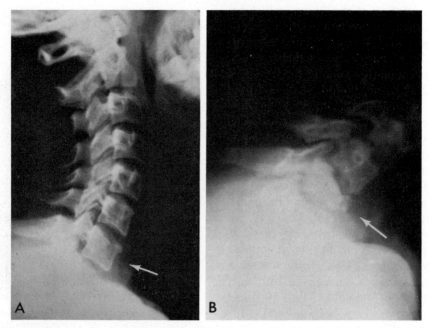

Figure 337. *A*, Compression fracture of C-7. This does not require reduction but requires protection so that the body does not collapse. A period of traction until the spasm subsides and then a Minerva cast would be adequate treatment.

B, Inadequately treated cervical fracture-dislocation. This is a flexion film made some months after the injury, showing anterior dislocation of C-6 and compression of C-7. A film made in extension determines gross instability because in extension the dislocation is reduced, indicating non-union.

normal height and the posterior part will maintain its normal height. Since the axis of rotation is at the articulations which are adjacent to the posterior portion of the body, the force is primarily applied at the extreme front. These cases are not often accompanied by cord damage since the neural canal is not impinged upon. The patient will have extreme forward flexion of the neck, and severe pain, with the feeling of insecurity that accompanies severe ligament injury or dislocation. The same careful study described above will reveal the fracture.

The fracture will require definitive treatment by traction to restore the bony contours and prolonged immobilization to permit union.

Roentgenographic study of the neck presents many difficulties and the team physician would be wise to consult a competent radiologist or orthopaedist before concluding that the x-ray of the neck is negative. The potentialities of permanent disability are so great that one can ill afford to "wait and see" in these injuries (Fig. 337, *B*).

Extension Injury (Dorsiflexion)

Anterior Longitudinal Ligament Injury (Sprain). The anterior longitudinal ligament extends throughout the cervical spine and serves to prevent separation of the anterior margins of the cervical vertebrae by hyperextension of the neck. As the neck moves into extension, the spinous process tends to impinge and, as the force continues, the lever changes from the first degree with the fulcrum at the cervical articulations to the second degree with the fulcrum at the tip of the spinous processes. Distraction force is applied to the anterior longitudinal ligament and to a lesser extent to the articular ligaments. This results in some degree of damage to the anterior longitudinal ligament. The anterior ligament may tear or avulse a fragment of the body (Fig. 338). If the ligament maintains its integrity there may be a fracture of the spinous processes. If the spinous processes hold, the ligament may tear. The tear may be of any degree and if it is severe enough may permit actual dislocation of the cervical spine. If the force is arrested the neck returns to its normal position and there are relatively few symptoms since the normal position of the neck puts no strain on the anterior longitudinal ligament. Usually the player knows that he has had a neck injury and examination will reveal that the pain and tenderness are anterior and that his symptoms are aggravated by extension of the neck.

If the injury is a mild (first degree) one, no particular treatment is indicated except that as a hedge a cotton collar should be applied. If the injury is moderate (second degree), the same treatment may be used as for the posterior sprain except that the neck should be placed in some degree of flexion rather than extension, whether it be in traction or a collar. The motion to be prevented by the brace is extension rather than flexion.

If the injury is severe (third degree) and there has been actual tearing of the anterior longitudinal ligament (Fig. 339), the symptoms will be more extreme and protection must be prolonged. This is the reason for mentioning that in the mild injury it is well to protect the neck until it is pain-free. The ever present danger is repetition of the force that caused the original injury. Riding in a car, participation in scrimmage, etc., should be ruled out without protection of the neck to prevent this motion. If muscle spasm supervenes, the head will be pulled forward by the bilaterally tight sternomastoid muscles. This may be extremely painful and to a considerable extent disabling since the patient has difficulty in raising his head to the erect position. It must be determined by examination that the difficulty is not actually from weakness of the dorsiflexors but from tightness of the forward flexors.

The severe case will require the same careful handling as any potentially serious injury of the neck. The patient should be put at bed rest with the neck in a position of slight flexion and light

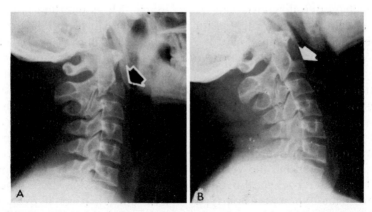

Figure 338. *A*, Fracture of anterior quadrant of C-2 with anterior rotation of the fragment. No neurological symptoms. *B*, Five months later solid union. All manipulative efforts to replace the fragment failed. This was undoubtedly an extension injury.

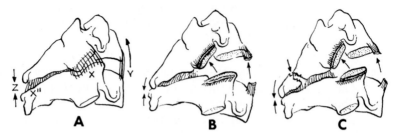

Figure 339.   Extension injury of the cervical spine.

A, Hyperextension forces the spinous processes together at (z), dislocates the front of the vertebra at (y). The center of rotation changes from (x) to (x″) as the spinous processes impinge and the vertebrae are torn apart.

B, Continuation of the same force dislocates the articulations, rupturing the discs and anterior and posterior longitudinal ligaments, and a frank dislocation may occur.

C, With application of the same forces, the spinous processes break which relieves the tension and the vertebrae fall back together without major damage to the cord.

traction (4 lbs.) applied. Muscle relaxants, sedation and local heat are all important. Attention should be called to the fact that the symptoms are very similar to those resulting from bilateral dislocation of the articular facets and careful x-ray study is needed to rule out possible bone or joint damage. Physical examination will help since in this instance forward flexion very carefully, even gingerly, applied will be pain-free whereas an attempt to extend the neck will cause increased spasm in the sternomastoids. On the other hand, with a dislocation of the neck the patient is quite willing to dorsiflex his head. A few hours of traction with local heat and sedation will serve to relax the spasm and a more definitive diagnosis can be made. The patient must be protected for several weeks against dorsiflexion of the neck. This is incompatible with active athletics.

Subluxation-Dislocation. If this same extension force continues, the anterior edges of the bodies are separated, the disc is disrupted (Fig. 339, *B*), the posterior longitudinal ligament tears, the articular ligaments tear and the vertebra may actually displace backward over its fellow below. This hyperextension type of injury is extremely serious and accounts for many of the cases accompanied by complete paralysis below this level, yet with entirely negative x-rays. The cord will tolerate posterior displacement even more poorly than it will anterior. This injury is not a frequent one in athletics. There is a limiting factor in that the lever of the spinous process is potentially a weak one and it may well give way (Fig. 339, *C*) at any time during the application of this posterior flexion. This buckling of the process may save the cord since it permits the vertebrae to rotate near the spinal canal rather than to open up on an axis of the posterior tip of the spinous process. The patient with paralysis will present no great problem to the examining physician since it is obvious he has a major injury. More puzzling is the injury that does not cause primary paralysis. Examination may be relatively negative. X-ray findings are negative. An incautious or unrestricted motion may lead to disaster. One should try to determine whether or not the direction of the force that caused the injury was extension or flexion. The initial traction in bed followed by a cervical brace should be designed to prevent extension of the neck. Permission to resume active athletic participation, if ever, will depend upon the individual case.

A present concern in the causation

of extension injuries is the modern headgear. There can be no reasonable doubt that today's headgear is a great improvement over the types previously used, particularly in the area of preventing blows to the head and face. However, there has been an unwelcome result from this improvement that is particularly related to cervical injuries. The plastic headgear is extremely solid and unyielding. Its posterior edge is no exception. In many types of headgear, the posterior edge strikes the upper cervical area so that, with the head in complete extension, the edge of the headgear drives toward the spinous processes. A major improvement in the headgear has been utilization of the face bar which has markedly diminished facial injuries. However, the long bar projecting well forward, as preferred by many, presents a convenient handle that the opponent may consciously or inadvertently grasp in his contact with the player. Indeed, he does not need to grasp it. The blocker coming up with the shoulder or elbow may catch the bar and forcibly extend his opponent's neck. The hazard is greatly increased if the bar extends well forward. A severe force is applied to the back of the neck by the combination of the leverage action on the front of the helmet and impingement of the unyielding back of the helmet against the spinous process. This may actually break off a spinous process, which is not of transcending importance. Much more vital is the fact that the back of the helmet may tend to support the tip of the spinous process so that it maintains its fulcrum as the front of the bodies of the vertebrae are separated. The force is concentrated at a single point, further encouraging extension injury.

There has been a great deal of study in regard to this problem of spinal injury from headgear in the last few years. Better design of the helmet with addition of a posterior roll or flap has been an improvement. The face bars have been better fashioned and do not protrude so far forward. Strict officiating with immediate, automatic penalty has sharply discouraged the temptation to use the face bar as a hand hold or as a lever.

Until lately the designers of helmets have concentrated on protecting the head of the wearer. Less thought has been given to the effect of the helmet on other portions of the player's or his opponent's anatomy. A recent modification of the helmet is designed to improve these conditions. A comparison of the helmet previously used by the University of Oklahoma and the one used now is seen in Figure 340. In Figure 340, A, the headgear is of solid, unyielding plastic with a small leather roll over the back edge of the helmet and no padding over the top of it. The new helmet (Fig. 340, B) has had the plastic back of the neck cut away and replaced with an apron so that it is impossible for the edge of the plastic to impinge against the neck proper. Formerly this same helmet had a strip of plastic foam beginning at the forehead and extending up over the crown of the helmet, about 6 inches wide, to serve as protection for the opposing player, but its use has been discontinued because of the additional weight and heat. The helmet also has plastic pads inside. While the players complain of it being somewhat hotter, it certainly seems to be more protective. The addition of the external and internal padding accounts for an increase of but 1 ounce in weight. Incidentally, the single face bar for protection has been supplanted in many places by double ones. These do not need to extend as far forward since they cover more of the facial area and so reduce the leverage somewhat. They are harder to grasp because of the spread between the bars. The blocker is also less likely

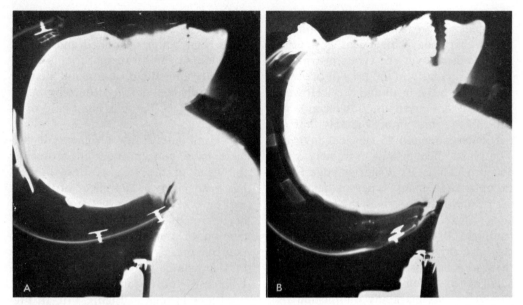

Figure 340. *A,* The older style helmet. Note the hard posterior edge of the helmet is directed at about C-6 and 7. However, it is at least 2 inches away from the spinous process with the head forcibly extended by pressure on the face bar.

B, The new style helmet. Note the soft leather roll against the skin with the hard plastic edge 1½ inches away so that the hard plastic edge is 4 inches from the bone. This is the same player.

to get his elbow, shoulder or knee under the bars since the lower one is considerably further toward the chest. The second bar adds about 10 ounces to the weight of the helmet but this probably can be reduced in newer models by using lighter weight material. These efforts to improve the protective helmet and face bar are certainly much more valid than condemning them and recommending their abandonment.

Rotatory Injury

Sprain. This sprain is usually the result of rotation of the neck so that the head is forcibly turned beyond the tolerance of the vertebra involved. The chin is pulled toward the opposite shoulder and excess strain is placed upon the ligaments as the neck is not only flexed to the side but rotated the same direction. These capsular ligaments tear to some degree. The force is released. The result is some damage to the ligament fibers with hemorrhage into the capsule and,

indeed, into the joint. In the vast majority of cases, no actual subluxation occurs. As soon as the head resumes its normal position, the spasm subsides but soreness will persist. In many cases, if the examination is made early, the level of involvement can be determined by palpation directly over the joint. Active function of the cervical muscles will not cause pain, even against resistance. If the sprain is on the left side of the neck, forcibly pulling the head to the left against resistance will not be painful. On the other hand, passive flexion and rotation to the opposite side to reproduce the force that caused the injury will cause pain.

If the sprain is a mild (first degree) one the symptoms will be few. The player will shrug it off. On the following day he will have soreness and stiffness in the neck but will usually recover completely without either treatment or protection.

If the sprain is moderate (second

degree) and some portion of the ligament is actually torn, the symptoms will be much more pronounced. Although the injury may not have appeared to be serious at the time of its occurrence, on the following day muscle spasm will intervene. Spasm of the muscles will have pulled the head toward the involved side and will resist any effort toward reproducing the motion that caused the sprain. The pain may become quite severe, not primarily from the ligament injury but from the resulting muscle spasm. The patient may present himself several days later with the ear pulled toward the shoulder on the same side and the chin rotated toward the same side with pain and spasm along the same side (Fig. 341, *A*). The treatment of this condition at whatever stage seen will depend upon the severity. If there is painful spasm, the best way to relax the spasm is by bed rest and light cervical traction, accompanied by local heat. Muscle relaxants will give relief. Indeed, the treatment is the same as that indicated for strain above. Here, too, the extent of the treatment will depend upon the symptoms. It may be that the spasm will subside in a few hours or a day or so but be assured that this spasm will return if the patient is allowed unprotected activity. This patient must wear a cotton collar or metal or plastic brace to protect the ligament against reproduction of the motion that caused the injury. Athletic competition cannot be permitted for several weeks if the injury was serious. If it appears to be less severe, the player should be protected with a cotton collar during the time of his participation.

Subluxation. If this force continues, subluxation or unilateral dislocation may occur. The spontaneously reduced subluxation gives the symptoms of the sprain mentioned above. In the cervical spine, the articular process may slide partially off and become locked in this position rather than dislocate entirely forward. This patient will have the same history of injury and the same complaints of pain as one with sprain, but the pain is usually more severe. He will have sharply restricted motion of the neck immediately so that he is unable to rotate his neck at all to the affected side. The chin will have turned toward the opposite side and the head will be tilted to the opposite side. The sternomastoid muscle on the involved side will be tight. The essential problem here will be muscle spasm due to tightness of the muscles that prevents

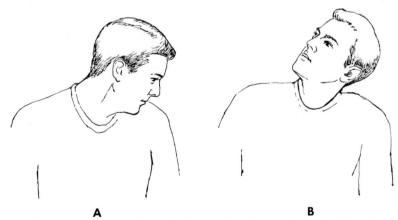

A   **B**

Figure 341. *A*, In sprain the head will be tilted and rotated in the same direction. *B*, In wryneck the chin will be rotated toward the opposite side and the head tilted toward the affected side. The left side condition is shown.

replacement of the dislocation. Subluxation may occur without actual ligament damage if the ligaments of the neck are somewhat relaxed. In the athlete it ordinarily occurs as an acute injury and with some damage to the ligaments. The reason for separating the two is that in the subluxation without actual ligament damage the joint is not affected and once the subluxation is reduced the patient is essentially asymptomatic, usually with no residual. This may be compared to the recurrent dislocation of the shoulder which has become so loose that it slips out without further damage to the ligament and, once the dislocation is reduced, it is pain-free. These recurrent subluxations may well be the result of an untreated sprain in which the ligament was allowed to heal with redundancy.

The case that is seen as an acute injury without previous history of subluxation should be treated as a severe sprain. It is important first to reduce the subluxation. This is accomplished not by massive overhead traction but by bed rest with 4-pound cervical traction, accompanied by local heat, muscle relaxants and sedation. I have yet to see one of these cases of subluxation persist overnight if the patient slept. This is not a complete dislocation and the articular processes are not locked. Reduction of a subluxation does not heal the ligament injury. As soon as the reduction is accomplished, the condition should be treated as a sprain and the neck protected against recurrence of the injury until the ligament healing is complete. This will take six or eight weeks.

Dislocation-Fracture. If this same force continues, a complete dislocation of the articular process occurs on one side. In this instance the articular process slips forward and lodges in front of the superior articulation of the vertebra below, where it is held securely in position. The patient will have had severe pain located at the side of the neck. Muscle spasm will be immediate. At examination the chin is turned away and the head is tilted away from the dislocation. The patient obviously has a serious injury and should be handled as such. True enough, if the injury was due to a rotatory force and the major ligaments are intact, the patient is in little danger. One cannot be sure, however, that the injury is not major and the same care should be assumed in management as in the case of complete bilateral dislocation.

Ill-advised attempts at manipulation should be discouraged. In the first place, manipulation is often unsuccessful and in the second place it may cause irreparable damage. Definitive treatment should be carried out by the surgeon skilled in this type of injury. If manual manipulation is to be attempted under anesthesia or without, the earlier it is done the more successful it will be. For manipulation without anesthesia the patient is sedated heavily and the head is tilted forward and rotated in the direction to increase the deformity until the vertebra is unlocked. The cervical spine is slightly flexed, traction is increased and the head is carefully turned and tilted back toward the injured side and into hyperextension. Repeated efforts to do this without anesthesia are unjustified. Under anesthesia the same manipulation may be carried out but must be done with utmost precautions, bearing in mind that the safety factor of the patient's muscles has been eliminated.

Many of these dislocations may be reduced by cervical traction although one is inclined to fear that, if reduction is too easy, one or both of the articular processes may be fractured. Following reduction of the deformity, light traction may be continued with the neck in extension or the patient may be promptly put in a Minerva type jacket (Fig. 342). The head should be placed in some hyperextension. The chin should be supported and the cast should extend over the forehead and rest on the iliac crest. Anything short of this cannot immobilize the neck. It should be borne in mind that the dislocation entails a ligament injury that will require the usual period for healing.

Many of the rotatory injuries are accompanied by lateral stress so that, as the head is twisted to the opposite side, the articular process slides forward on the involved side. A great deal of force is applied to the lateral mass of the vertebra on the opposite side from the inflicting force—that is, on the side toward which the head is turned and flexed. This may cause a fracture of the articular processes on the opposite side (Fig. 332) or any portion of the lateral mass. If this patient is treated as indicated above, the

fracture will not particularly complicate the picture since it will have healed by the time the ligament injury has. Casual treatment of the ligament injury combined with overlooking of the fracture may court disaster.

Unilateral subluxation and dislocation are extremely difficult to visualize by x-ray, particularly if they occur around C-6 and 7 where the intervening shoulders, particularly in a muscular individual, interfere with good visualization. In order to determine the nature of the damage it may be necessary to obtain repeated anteroposterior, lateral, oblique and stereoscopic views or even laminograms.

Many of these rotatory injuries are relieved by simple repositioning of the spine. It may be extremely difficult to persuade the eager athlete that he has an injury that demands prolonged treatment. One must exert every effort to prevent him from injudicious exercise in his effort to hasten his rehabilitation since this only results in prolongation of his recovery and even may result in permanent disability.

Torsion Injuries to Nerve Elements

Brachial Plexus and Nerve Root Injuries. While flexion and extension of the neck account for the major dislocations, in twisting injuries there may be serious involvement of the nerve roots. As the neck is forcibly rotated in one direction and flexed the same way, undue tension is placed upon the cords of the brachial plexus, particularly if traction is applied at the same time to the outstretched arm. For example, when the player is being tackled by his right arm and someone else is pulling his head to the left, considerable tension is placed upon the nerve structures. This may result in transitory paralysis of the arm with the familiar numbing or shocklike feeling which within a few seconds or

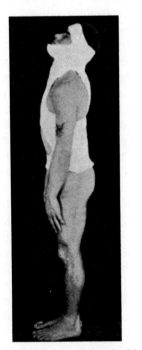

Figure 342. The Minerva jacket for high cervical fracture-dislocation. The forehead and parietal regions are included to limit rotation and nodding of the head which take place chiefly in the occipitoatloid and atlantoaxial articulations. In cases of lower cervical injuries the chin piece may be cut out if the forehead piece is firm.

minutes completely disappears. It may, however, result in more serious neurological pathology, even to the extent of tearing the nerve roots from the cord. This is an irreparable injury. Damage to the cords of the brachial plexus also may occur. This latter may well be remediable.

Following such an injury, any evidence of nerve involvement of the extremities that persists more than a few hours demands very careful study with an attempt to delineate the exact root or trunk involved. Frequently there will be a generalized involvement of the arm with diffuse numbness and a feeling of heaviness of the arm which gradually recovers. Certain specific neurological defects may be persistent, however, and may easily be overlooked. Damage to the posterior cord affecting the use of the triceps, for example, may be easily overlooked since the arm will readily fall into extension by the effect of gravity and several days may pass before the physician realizes that a loss of function of this muscle is actually present. It behooves him to make a careful neurological examination of the extremity after such an injury. The earlier this is done the better, since it provides a base for measuring the progress of the condition by successive examinations. In case of increasing involvement, surgical neurolysis may be indicated. The neurosurgeon should have the opportunity to determine the necessity and decide on the best time for the procedure.

Major tears of the roots are extremely rare. When they occur they are manifested by complete loss of function of the components involved. Unfortunately, they are not amenable to surgical repair. Fortunately, one is usually able to distinguish between damage to the more peripheral portions of the brachial plexus and damage to the nerve root. This is of vital importance since the plexus injury may be reparable.

ASSOCIATED CERVICAL INJURIES

Nerve Root Injury

Any of the above described forces may cause damage to the nerve roots ranging from brief irritation with a transient numbing, shocklike feeling in the arm, to complete severance of the root. As a rule, the important consideration is to determine if possible the exact nature of injury, so as to know what should be done with the patient. Once he gets well developed nerve root symptoms he is a problem for the neurosurgeon or the orthopaedist. There is nothing specifically diagnostic about nerve root pain. It may be caused with equal facility by the pressure of a cervical disc, by fracture of a portion of the nerve root foramen, or by pressure on the nerve root from hematoma or hemorrhage within the nerve. Certainly a diagnosis of nerve root syndrome is no more specific than one of bellyache or headache.

The nerve root symptoms caused by a sudden twist of the head that are transient and disappear rapidly are usually of little significance. Exceptionally they indicate a subluxation, particularly if the symptoms were the first of their kind to occur in this patient. Some players have repeated episodes of pain in the neck with nerve root symptoms into the arm which seem to be accompanied by no particular pathology in the neck. These must be interpreted as resulting from an impingement of the nerve, either due to hypermobility of a joint or to narrowing of the nerve root canal so that the nerve is pinched by a motion that ordinarily would leave it amply free. So also may adhesions about the nerve root cause traction on the nerve on an unguarded motion which ordinarily is prevented by protective muscle tension. While careful study may be rewarding in eliminating some remediable lesion, one is often in a quandary as to whether or not athletic participation should be permitted. The decision will depend partly on the patient's desire, mostly on the physician's own judgment of the situation.

Scalenus Anticus Syndrome

The scalenus anticus syndrome, like many other syndromes, has become much less frequently diagnosed as more specific diagnoses such as cervical rib, cervical disc and various vascular conditions are made. The symptomatology arises because of occlusion of the artery or vein and/or pressure of the brachial plexus caused by spasm of the anterior scalene muscle. Certain anatomic characteristics make this more frequent, particularly the presence of a cervical rib. The symptoms are usually of the lower roots of the plexus, with pain along the ulnar distribution, particularly whenever the arm is over the head. This is combined with a tendency toward vascular occlusion so that one is unable to work with his arms higher than his shoulders because of pain and the feeling that the arm "goes to sleep." This is not an athletic injury. It is mentioned here since it may at times be confused with cervical injury. A little attention to the history will help. A classic test is obliteration of the radial pulse as the arm is pulled over the head and the neck is pulled to the opposite side. A well established syndrome will require surgical treatment.

Cervical Rib Syndrome

This is mentioned along with the scalenus anticus syndrome since the two are quite similar. The presence of a cervical rib makes injury to this area of the plexus at the base of the neck somewhat more likely. A blow at the base of the neck over a cervical rib may well cause a sharp accentuation or may, indeed, initiate the neurological and vascular symptoms of cervical rib. Recognition of the possibility of a cervical rib will usually permit adequate diagnosis and treatment (Fig. 343).

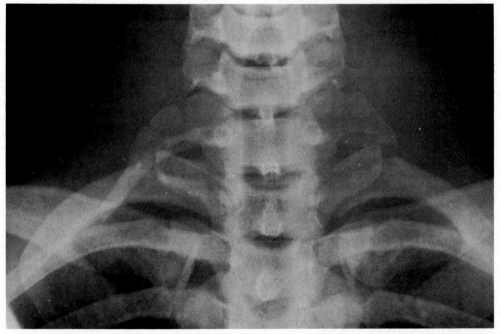

Figure 343. Bilateral cervical rib C-7. This is congenital and not necessarily disabling.

Injury to the Long Thoracic Nerve

Frequently occurring in conjunction with sprain or other injury at the base of the neck is injury to the long thoracic nerve. This nerve comes directly off the nerve roots and does not participate in the brachial plexus. It passes down and supplies the various serrations of the serratus anterior. Bruising or damage to this nerve may occur and pass unrecognized until distressing winging of the scapula is noted (Fig. 344). The cause may be a sharp blow at the base of the neck laterally that impinges the nerve against the lower cervical vertebrae. Since this is primarily a motor nerve, there is usually little pain or discomfort to guide the physician. There may be weakness or complete paralysis of the nerve, resulting in loss of fixation of the scapula to the chest wall so that, as the arm is pulled forward, the vertebral border of the scapula swings outward.

The ideal treatment for this condition has not been found. If it is recognized early, recovery would probably be expedited by immobilization of the arm in abduction and external rotation in order to hold the scapula against the chest wall and protect the muscles from undue strain. Since it is usually recognized quite late, there is some question of the value of immobilization. Surgical treatment is not acceptable since recovery will usually take place without it. The injury is usually a contusion rather than separation. Since the involved area is extremely inaccessible, making any sort of repair virtually impossible, neurolysis should probably not be attempted, even in late involvement. After a period of a few weeks there is no reason to forbid active use; in fact, athletic competition within the patient's capacity should be encouraged.

Injury to the Spinal Accessory Nerve

The spinal accessory nerve, located as it is somewhat superficially near the surface in the trapezius muscle, may be injured by a direct blow across the trapezius muscle. This injury may be confused with contusion of the muscle. The player may have difficulty elevating the shoulder toward the ear and will have severe aching pain. The injury requires no specific treatment other than physical therapy. Heat and superficial massage will usually relieve the symptoms, and restoration of the motor function of the trapezius muscle is rapid. For a few days there may seem to be serious paralysis.

Snapping Neck

Another and more common condition in the cervical area may give the

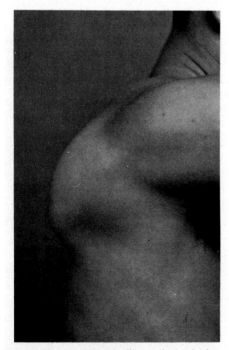

Figure 344. Photograph illustrating winging of scapula.

player and the physician a good deal of uneasiness. This is the presence of an audible and palpable click or snap of the neck on certain rotations. The cause of this popping or snapping is varied. It may be due to irregularity at the articulations. Much more commonly it is due to forcible snapping of a tendon over a bony prominence. As with most conditions of the neck, there is a very considerable apprehension factor which does not seem to be present in joints more distal from the head. The player who can pop his neck on certain rotatory movements is quite certain that he has gross pathology. He usually holds the neck stiff. He may become amazingly adept at this snapping since, if he learns to hold certain muscles tight, the audibility of the snapping becomes much more notable. There is undoubtedly a functional component in this condition and the player has a well nigh uncontrollable impulse to pop his neck whereupon he proclaims that he gets great relief.

The treatment for this condition is to prevent the snapping and with an understanding patient it can usually be stopped simply by having him stop demonstrating it. A word of warning should be sounded, however. One must make sure that no underlying pathological condition is present that needs to be treated, such as irregularity of the articular facet, tenosynovitis of a tendon, or muscle spasm that tends to bow the tendon across the bony prominence. For this reason, a fairly extensive regimen of physical therapy should be instituted. In the true "snapping neck," pain is not an important symptom while apprehension is. A very careful physical examination together with x-ray study may be followed by a frank conference with the player in which the situation is thoroughly explained. He is assured that he has no serious condition and that many joints are prone to snap. He should then be urged to avoid, if possi-

ble, getting in the position where the phenomenon occurs. Frequently after a suitable period either the snapping disappears or the player learns to ignore it.

Rehabilitation

Almost any involvement of the neck which is long-standing will require an extensive rehabilitative effort to prevent recurrence. See page 798 where exercises are detailed.

DORSAL SPINE

ANATOMICAL CONSIDERATIONS

The dorsal (thoracic spine (Fig. 323) is the most stable section of the vertebral column. No detailed description of the anatomy need be given here other than to mention a few pertinent points. The 12 dorsal vertebrae together with the ribs and sternum combine to form the bony thorax. The whole structure of the thorax is such that it tends to limit motion of the spine. The general contour of the spine is one of dorsal convexity, and extension from this position is resisted by the thoracic cage. The spine itself has a good deal of intrinsic stability, the vertebrae being very firmly bound together by the various ligaments. The articular processes are vertical and face in such a manner that the inferior processes of the vertebrae above lock behind the superior processes of the vertebrae below to completely prevent any forward displacement of the upper vertebrae on the lower unless there is a fracture of the arch. Sufficient displacement to permit the articular processes to displace upward the full length of the articulation is necessary before the joint becomes dislocated. The angle of these processes is such that the inferior processes on the superior vertebrae above fit within the arc of the superior processes of the lower vertebrae, the articular face of the lower vertebrae facing inward almost 45 degrees. The bodies themselves are slightly higher behind than in front, which causes the convexity and again adds to stability. The ribs, articulating as they do between two vertebrae, tend to reinforce the column at the level of the back of the bodies. The column is also supported by the very immobile articular processes.

The disc spaces are narrow and the discs have much less elasticity than either the cervical or lumbar discs. The spinous processes, rather than extending backward as in the cervical and lumbar spine, extend downward, overlapping each other as shingles on a roof. In many instances one actually rests upon its fellow below so that the leverage of the interspinous ligaments is greatly increased because these spinous processes actually have to separate as the

spine flexes forward. These processes immediately impinge as the spine is flexed backward. They are subcutaneous at their tips.

The stable dorsal spine serves for attachment of many of the muscles (Fig. 345) of the trunk, shoulder and arm. The trapezius muscle attaches to the spinous processes from the upper cervical well down to lower dorsal. In the lower part of the dorsal spine, it overlaps the long attachment of the latissimus dorsi, which attaches to the spinous process beginning mid-dorsal and extending to the pelvis. These are the most superficial layers of the muscles in the back and serve to enclose the deeper layers. These latter are broad, flat muscles and are not frequently subject to injury. The scapular muscles including the levator scapulae and rhomboideus major and minor underlie the trapezius in the upper portion of the dorsal spine and extend down toward

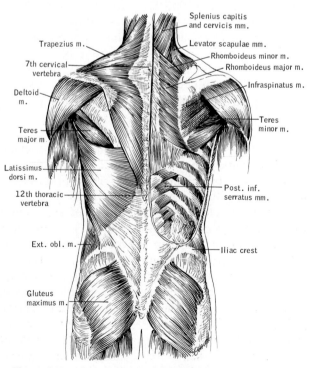

Figure 345. Anatomical drawing of muscles of back.

the level of the upper limit of the latissimus dorsi. Still deeper are the muscles running from the spine to the ribs — until we reach the sacrospinalis group which is a combination of many muscles whose course essentially parallels the spinal column. The sacrospinalis group fills the sulcus between the spinous processes and the bodies of the vertebrae and arc of the ribs. They interdigitate in such a manner that each tends to support the other. These muscles make up the so-called lumbar mass of muscle that extends from the occiput to the sacrum just lateral to the spinous processes. They all have multiple actions depending upon the inter-relationship between them. In one instance they may serve to stabilize the spine in a certain position while another portion moves; in another they may serve to move the spine; in yet another they may serve to anchor the spine while other muscles move some other portion of the body. The nerve supply is direct from the spinal roots and so is well protected and seldom damaged.

CONTUSION

Contusion of the spine is relatively common but is not often severe. The subcutaneous spinous process may receive a blow that crushes the skin against the protruding bone beneath or may damage the underlying bone. However, the most common contusion of the spine is of the muscles lateral to the spinous processes. These muscular contusions are similar to contusions elsewhere. One should make an effort to determine whether or not there is some underlying pathological condition. The contusion may cause a hematoma within the muscle that will require the usual treatment with cold pack, local injection and pressure, followed by heat.

The most common complication of

contusion of the muscle is residual stiffness, which causes aching pain and restriction of motion for a few days subsequent to the injury. This should be treated by heat, pain-free massage and careful exercise. If the contusion is over the spinous process there may be some periosteal reaction or reaction in the supraspinous ligament which will leave a painful, tender area very sharply localized to the involved area. It may be painful enough to suggest the possibility of a fracture. Indeed, there may be an infraction or crack in the spinous process which cannot be demonstrated by x-ray but which may be diagnosed clinically. The resultant painful area can usually be relieved by physical therapy. Local injection of a long-acting anesthetic is of considerable value here and should give rather prompt relief, although more than one injection may be necessary. If athletic participation is to be continued following contusion, a localized protective pad should be placed over the area.

STRAIN

The spine is particularly susceptible to muscular strain because of the multiplicity of muscles involved in holding the body erect. Strain of these muscles may be extremely distressing. In the early stages it may be rather difficult to distinguish strain from contusion since the contusion may cause some hemorrhage within the muscle and may well cause pain on function of the muscle. However, the early history may be a valuable guide in diagnosis. The patient may mention some unusual occurrence. In athletics it is usually a major effort while he is somewhat off balance, such as the shot putter throwing a 16 lb. shot from an imperfect stance. Strain in the athlete does not as a rule result from simple repetition of a motion, as it does in the industrial worker, since the athlete is usually in good enough shape that his muscles will tolerate the degree of strain he puts upon them in athletic use. Basically, the strain is caused by violent contraction beyond the strength of a muscle against a fixed resistance or by overstretching as the muscle attempts to resist this stretch.

On examining the patient with such an injury it is quite difficult to identify the exact muscle involved. In the shoulder girdle, where one may be able to check a certain specific function, as for example the rhomboid or levator scapulae, and find painful function limited to one motion, such identification may be quite simple, but in the spine one will consider himself fortunate if he can determine which group of muscles is involved and in some instances even which side of the back is involved since there is a great deal of generalized muscle spasm. There will be tenderness over the involved muscle and pain caused by passive stretching or active contraction. If, for example, the spinalis group is involved on the *right side,* one will find tenderness just to the right of the spinous process. Pain is elicited by passive forward flexion, whereas active forward flexion within limits even against forceful resistance is pain-free. Passive backward bending will be pain-free since the involved muscle relaxes in this motion, whereas active backward bending against resistance (as for example with the patient lying prone and raising his chest from the table) will cause pain. Passive flexion to the right is pain-free. Active flexion to the right against resistance will cause pain. To the left side passive flexion is painful and limited active motion even against resistance is not. If the condition is fairly severe and well established there will be tenderness and spasm in the whole group of spinal muscles as they endeavor to restrict the motion of the

spine and to reduce the pain. In this instance the spastic muscles themselves may become painful, even though not originally involved. Diffuse pain in the back is the result. The patient presents himself with a poker spine that will resist motion in any direction.

Treatment is general and local. If there is muscle spasm, muscle relaxants are of considerable value. Preparations are available today that have minimal sedative effect (carisoprodol) and these may suffice. The tranquilizers such as meprobamate may be used if there is an element of apprehension or nervous tension in the individual. Local treatment is directed at the local lesion and to relieve muscular tension. If there is an isolated tender area, a so-called trigger point, local injection of an anesthetic agent into this area will tend to break the reflex arc and relax the tension. Similarly, if there is evidence of rupture of the muscle fibers with hematoma formation, local injection of hyaluronidase may be of value. Physical therapeutic measures are important and should consist of local heat, massage and careful active motion limited to that which is pain-free. The patient may be placed in the prone position and hot packs used in a manner similar to the blanket packs in acute anterior poliomyelitis. Body whirlpool, if available, may be used although I think that heat is more effective when the patient is lying down. For this reason I prefer diathermy, infra-red, electric pad, or electric baker.

As soon as the muscle spasm is subsiding, rehabilitative measures may be commenced but should be carried out strictly within the limits of pain. Far too often in the athlete, the urgency of his participation persuades the doctor or trainer to rehabilitate him too rapidly, with recurrence a discouraging aftermath. It is difficult to protect the upper dorsal spine by a corset. The lower dorsal spine may be fairly well protected by a full length corset which the participant should wear whenever he is in active competition. Adhesive strapping of the back to limit the motion involved is quite valuable. Since the strain is usually of the posterior muscles, the strapping should be applied so as to prevent forward flexion and lateral flexion. I believe that parallel strips are very much more effective for this than criss-cross strips on the back. The back should be carefully prepared and shaved and the skin cleansed with ether before the strips are applied. One may use tincture of benzoin on the skin if he so desires. The most effective way of the strapping is shown in Figure 346. Strapping so applied is much more effective in limiting motion of the back than is a corset and is of course much less expensive if it is to be worn a relatively short time. Elastic adhesive cross-stretch may be substituted for regular tape and is considerably stronger. Elastic adhesive with long-way stretch is not adequate in this instance since its longitudinal stretch does not give enough support. Heat can be given right through adhesive tape. The tape is changed only when it becomes ineffective. Any adhesive that is dependent upon adherence to the skin for fixation will become ineffective if the patient perspires unduly. As the condition improves and less support is needed, one may shift to long stretch or to a corset, but some protection of the muscles should be continued for several weeks to prevent re-injury.

The *chronic back strain* represents a major problem. It is frequently the result of an acute strain that was not adequately treated. Every recurrence of the condition makes the final cure more difficult. It is frequently cured only after the season's athletic competition is over. The best treatment is physical therapy and protection. One is quite prone to accuse a player of being "chicken" or "dogging it" since in these

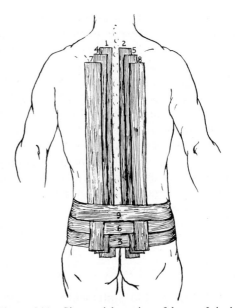

Figure 346. Six to eight strips of heavy 3 inch tape are cut long enough to extend from the base of the neck to the pelvis. The first strip is placed parallel with the spinous processes and just adjacent to them. A strip is placed on either side of the spine. This is anchored below by a circular strip placed just at the level of the trochanters and extending entirely around the trunk. The pubic hair is protected by a cotton pad. Transverse strips should be overlapped. It is important to get the first strip low enough to protect the inguinal canal. The second pair of vertical strips is then applied overlapping the first by one-half. The second horizontal strip is applied overlapping about one-third. This is continued until the strapping extends 4 to 6 inches on either side of the spine. This will require three or four pairs of vertical strips. It is not necessary to use cross lap strips above. Cross-stretch elastic tape is good here. Long stretch is useless!

back strains there are few, if any, positive findings. Little is to be gained, however, by insisting on strenuous activity in the presence of a painful back unless this seems desirable to establish the diagnosis. In the chronic condition there is usually not enough localization of pain to justify local injection. Frequently, the so-called fibrositis, which can be described as irritation of the fascial planes of the back, may be relieved by general therapy. We frequently use a combination of a muscle relaxant, salicylates and a cortisone derivative. Cortisone is well tolerated by the young athlete if the dose is small and is not continued too long. One should avoid long-continued use of any cortisone preparation. In the final analysis, since strain is basically overuse of the musculature, the ultimate relief must come from rehabilitation of the muscles. Dedication to long-continued rehabilitative exercises should pay dividends in diminishing and in finally eliminating the strain. (See p. 797.)

SPRAIN

Many of the statements we have made about strain may also be applied to sprain. It may be difficult in the spine to distinguish between the two. The same force that causes muscular strain may tear some of the many ligaments of the spine. Many of these ligaments are deeply placed, such as those around the articular processes and between the lateral processes and those extending between the lamina and vertebrae. About the only ligament that can be palpated easily in the dorsal spine is the supraspinous, which extends along the tips of the spinous processes. Injury to this ligament can be determined by localized palpable tenderness either along the course of the ligament itself or at its attachment to the bone. Extension of the spine should be pain-free but forward flexion will cause pain at the involved area if the supra- or interspinous or interlaminal ligaments are involved.

The direction of the motion that causes pain is the key for diagnosis of spinal ligament injuries. Given *right side* involvement with damage to the capsular ligament, one would expect the local tenderness and spasm to be on the right side in an effort to prevent stretching of this involved ligament. Forward flexion, either active or passive, is painful.

Backward flexion, either active or passive, is not. Homolateral flexion should relieve the symptoms and, indeed, the patient will stand pulled toward the right side. Contralateral flexion will increase the pain unless it is prevented by the spastic muscle. X-ray is of little importance in the diagnosis of sprain although x-ray should be made in a serious injury, if possible, in order to rule out bone damage. The one condition in which x-ray may be valuable is rupture of the supra- and interspinous ligaments. In this instance, as noted above, the tenderness will be right on the ligament. Sometimes a palpable defect may be felt. If the tear is complete, forward flexion may reveal greater separation of the spinous process than at the one above and below. This is an extremely unusual injury in the dorsal spine.

Treatment of a ligament injury of the dorsal spine is the same as that of ligament injury elsewhere, that is, protection of the ligament against stretch until it is healed. A period of bed rest may be necessary if the injury is severe. The back should then be strapped in a way to prevent the motion that causes the pain (Fig. 346). This is a good test of the effectiveness of the strapping. One should be extremely careful not to discard the protection too soon since recurrence is as likely in the spine as at the ankle or knee when the injury occurs in the latter.

DISLOCATION

The ultimate of sprain is dislocation (Fig. 347). This is extremely unusual in the dorsal spine. Even in the mayhem caused by the modern automobile, the dorsal spine is infrequently dislocated. As mentioned in the discussion of the anatomy, the vertebrae are very securely bound together and have a good deal of bony as well as ligamentous sta-

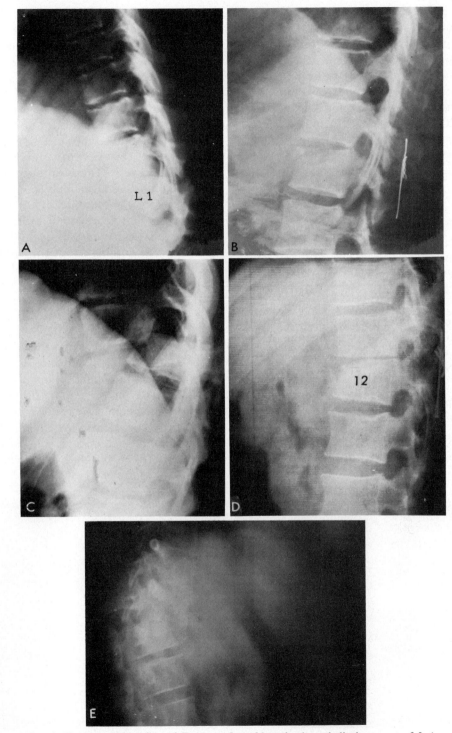

Figure 347. *A*, Fracture-dislocation of D-12 on L-1. Note backward displacement of L-1 and complete dislocation of the articular facet. *B*, Reduced and held with wire around spinous processes and spinal fusion. Neurological symptoms in lower extremities completely disappeared. *C*, Fracture-dislocation of D-11 on D-12. Paraplegia. *D*, Postoperative film showing internal fixation and graft. *E*, Complete dislocation of D-11 on D-12 without apparent fracture which resulted in complete paraplegia.

bility. If there is dislocation, the injury will obviously be a major one. I do not comprehend the so-called "dislocation" of the "manipulators," who will make an x-ray film and glibly describe a dislocation in a normal appearing spine. Following manipulation, this "dislocation" is reduced. Anatomically and physiologically such a thing is virtually impossible in the dorsal spine.

FRACTURE

Fracture of the dorsal spine is more common than dislocation but is extremely unusual in ordinary athletic competition such as football, basketball, baseball and track. Some of the more violent sports such as automobile racing, polo playing and the like do cause spinal fractures. The fracture may be of the body or of the arches or of the spinous or lateral processes.

Compression Fracture of the Body

Fracture of the body is usually caused by sharp forward flexion, the so-

called compression fracture (Fig. 348). The patient will give a history of sharp forward flexion such as falling violently on the buttocks or of having his head forcibly pushed between his knees. This tends to flex the very rigid dorsal spine, the posterior ligaments hold, and the force is taken by the anterior portion of the body of the vertebra. This cancellous bone gives way to a greater or lesser degree. The anterosuperior corner of the vertebra may be broken off or more commonly there is compression of the vertebra so that the cancellous bone is impacted into itself.

There is nothing about the ordinary compression fracture of the dorsal spine that will prevent ambulation so that the patient may actually be up and around in spite of his back complaint. On examination, although it may be difficult to determine the exact degree of injury, forward flexion will ordinarily cause considerable complaint. This may be elicited by having the patient lie supine. When the examiner flexes his neck to force the chin against the chest, there will usually be localized pain at the fracture area. This test will also be positive

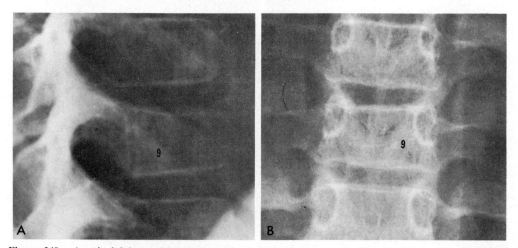

Figure 348. A spinal injury with compression of D-9. The patient suffered persistent localized pain. B, Careful study of D-9 reveals unilateral compression on the right. This can also be seen in the lateral view (A). Note that the superior surface of D-9 presents two cortical shadows, whereas the inferior surface shows a single shadow.

for ligament injury. Motion in any direction will probably cause pain, even in an impacted fracture.

Careful x-ray study will usually reveal this lesion although it may be easily overlooked if the deformity is mild and the x-ray film inadequate or inadequately studied. In the x-ray the vertebrae should be carefully measured anteriorly to determine whether a single vertebrae is narrower than its fellows. This may be extremely misleading, however, since frequently one or more dorsal vertebrae will be of smaller size than the others. Of more importance is the appearance of the bone itself. A fracture line may be visible. The bone may be compacted so that this particular vertebra not only appears smaller but seems more dense than its neighbor.

TREATMENT. In the young athlete if the compression is definite and amounts to as much as 25 per cent of the height of the body, I think an attempt should be made to reduce it. In the older person this amount of compression may be accepted in order to speed up healing but I do not believe this is acceptable in the youngster. The exact area involved is determined and an effort is made to correct the vertebra by manipulation. This will not correct by a simple convex bed if the bone is impacted. The usual methods of hyperextension in which the entire back is extended are needlessly handicapping to the patient since to be effective the extension must proceed to the point where all of the anterior ligaments are taut before there is any effect at all upon the broken vertebra. Local hyperextension is much more effective.

For local hyperextension I think the various modifications of the "jack method" are by far the best. In this method, with the patient supine on a suitable fracture table, the jack with suitable protective cap is placed directly under the spinous process of the vertebra involved. By elevating the jack the corrective pressure is applied to this vertebra alone and the back is locally extended (Fig. 349). This causes some local hyperextension of the adjacent vertebrae but it is not necessary to hyperextend the entire spine. Once the vertebra has come up to its normal height, a suitable plaster jacket can be applied, again without generalized hyperextension but with local extension, the pressure points being the pubis and sternum in front, the fracture site behind.

Although bed rest probably offers the best chance of maintaining the degree of correction obtained by manipulation, it is very difficult to keep athletic patients at bed rest. If the cast is applied with great care and if the spine is extended enough to place the entire weight on the articular processes, little is to be gained by enforced recumbency.

In any event there may be some loss of correction—a fact that prompts some surgeons to believe that no attempt should be made to correct a compression fracture. The cast should be worn for six to eight weeks to be followed by an adequate brace. In unusual circumstances a brace of the three point hyperextension type with pressure on the pubis and sternum and over the involved vertebra posteriorly may be substituted for the cast. X-ray examination will determine when union is complete but athletic competition should not be permitted for at least four months and probably six would be better. There is some danger of late aseptic necrosis of this vertebra if weight bearing is permitted too soon.

In minimal compression fractures of the vertebral body, rehabilitation can be much more rapidly carried out if the compression deformity is accepted. In these cases a protective brace need be worn only a few weeks until the fracture is well consolidated. In fracture of the

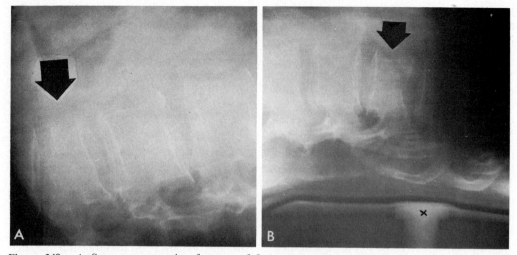

Figure 349. *A,* Severe compression fracture of L-1, preoperative view. *B,* Correction by the jack method. The "X" marks the head of the jack which actually is one vertebra above L-1. These x-rays were made with a surgical portable machine without a Bucky diaphragm, which accounts for their fogginess.

anterosuperior corner of the vertebra a differentiation should, if possible, be made between a snubbing fracture caused by flexion and an avulsion fracture caused by hyperextension, since in the latter protection should be in flexion rather than in extension. Often the history of the injury will provide a valuable guide. The increased pain on backward bending as compared to forward will also be significant. Sometimes the picture made on backward bending will show actual separation of this fragment.

Arch Fracture

Fracture of the lateral processes of the dorsal spine is extremely infrequent since they are well protected by the ribs. If it does occur, a corset, brace or body jacket may be worn until union has taken place. Fractures of the laminae or interarticular portions of the bone or of the articular processes themselves require very careful examination by x-ray for diagnosis. Adequate support by brace or cast should be worn for six to eight weeks to prevent painful excessive formation of callus or nonunion.

In fracture of the spinous process, protection should be against forward flexion. If there is separation of the fragment, a good deal of time will be saved by its early removal (Fig. 350) as a primary measure rather than to wait for nonunion and then remove the fragment if there is resultant pain. Separation is much more frequent in the upper dorsal spine and may be the result of avulsion of the tip by sharp forward flexion of the neck and upper spine or by a direct blow. It is occasionally caused by muscle jerk as described under the so-called "clay shoveler's fracture" in the cervical spine.

LUMBAR SPINE

ANATOMICAL CONSIDERATIONS

Whereas the dorsal vertebrae have a good deal of inherent stability as indicated above, the lumbar spine (Fig. 351) lying between the rigid pelvis and thorax is so designed as to permit greater mobility and yet provide inherent stability. The vertebrae in this area are massive. The convexity of the spine forward of this area is caused by bodies which are taller and slightly wider in front than behind. The entire arch is massive with heavy lateral processes extending well away from the midline to add additional leverage for muscle attachments. The laminae are heavy. The articular processes, which in the dorsal spine angulate to form a diagonal line with the body, in the lumbar spine are much more in the sagittal plane. While the processes on the vertebrae above do lock behind the one below they are at a good deal flatter angle. Hence, the mobility in the spine is largely in flexion and in extension in which the intervertebral joints serve more or less as an axis with motion permitted by compression and expansion of the disc and by separation and apposition of the spinous processes. There is little rotatory motion in the lumbar spine.

The muscles of this area of the back (Fig. 352) are very massive. The sacrospinalis group interdigitating up into the dorsal spine consists of heavy muscles arising from the pelvis to attach to the spinous processes and to the vertebral bodies and act as firm stabilizers of the trunk over the pelvis. The muscles of the abdomen complete the stabilizing effect in front. These muscles extending from the pubis to the ribs serve as anterior guy wires to provide active forward flexion and to prevent overextension. The heavy mass of spinal muscle also serves to protect the posterior portion of the abdominal cavity and prevent injury to the kidneys, spleen and liver.

CONTUSION

This area of the spine is frequently contused but fortunately the injury is usually not particularly severe. The only subcutaneous bones in this region are the tips of the spinous processes. These lie in a sulcus between the two erector spinae muscles so that the muscle ordinarily will absorb the blow unless it is by a relatively small object. Contusion of the muscle suffers the same complications as contusion of muscle anywhere. The history is of a blow with localized tenderness at the area of the blow and

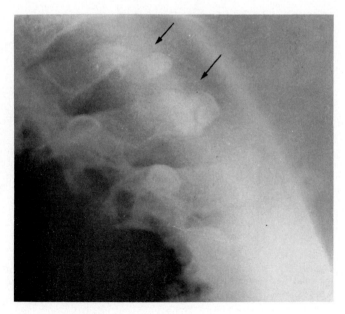

Figure 350. "Sprain" of the upper dorsal spine with persistent complaint. Early x-ray studies had not adequately visualized this area. More careful x-ray technique revealed the ununited fragments of the D-1 and 2 spinous processes. Uneventful recovery followed removal of the fragments but months of disability might have been prevented by more careful early treatment.

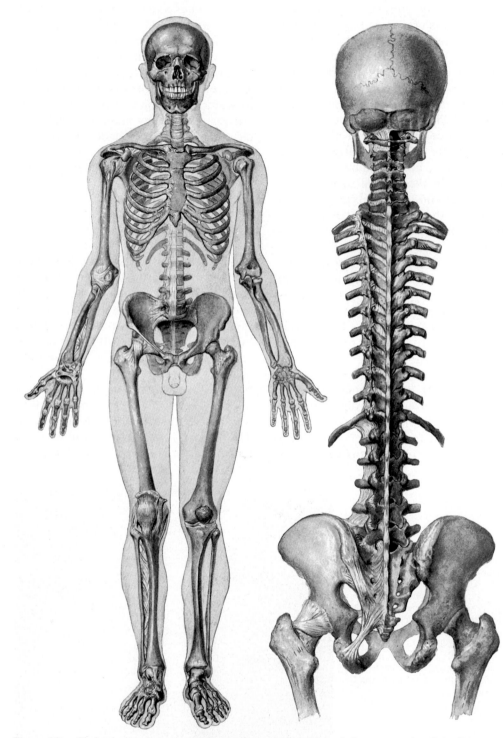

Figure 351. Skeletal view from the front and from behind. In both figures certain of the ligaments of the trunk and extremities are shown. (From Anson, Atlas of Human Anatomy.)

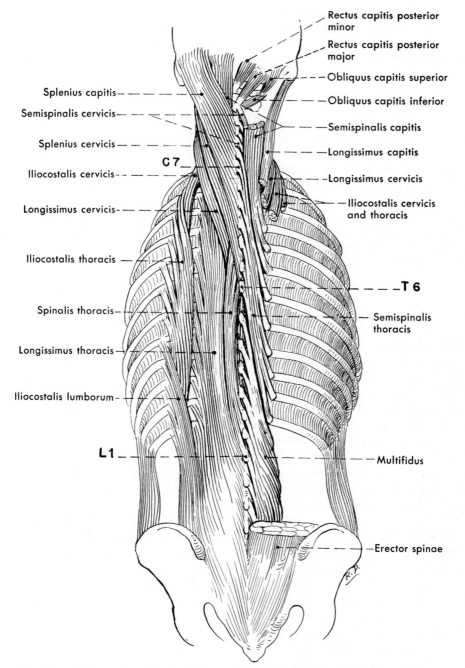

Figure 352. The chief muscles of the back (From Hollinshead, Functional Anatomy of the Limbs and Back.)

moderate pain on function. After a few hours muscle spasm supervenes which tightens up the whole group of muscles on that side, apparently in an attempt to prevent painful motion. At this time differentiation from strain may be very difficult. In a simple contusion, active muscle contraction is not especially painful.

If any *treatment* is necessary, application of ice followed by heat is indicated. If a massive hematoma appears to be present, an attempt can be made to aspirate it, although the location is difficult to determine in these heavy muscles. If the contusion seems to be severe, attention should be paid to the underlying structures to determine the possibility of a fracture of the lateral or spinous processes.

STRAIN

Muscular strain results either from overstretching or from overuse of the muscle. It may be difficult to distinguish from sprain. Fundamentally, any active motion of the involved muscle against resistance will cause pain. For example, if you have the patient stand erect and ask him to bend sideways and you resist this motion so that he does not actually bend, he should have a complaint of pain if the involvement is in the muscle but no complaint if the involvement is in the ligament. The muscle involved is palpably tender and passive stretching of the muscle will cause pain. If the strain is on the right side of the spine, active flexion to the right against resistance will be painful whereas in ligament injury it should not be. Passive flexion to the opposite side will be painful as soon as the injured muscle is put under stretch. Backward bending against resistance will be painful and forward flexion will become painful only when the excursion is sufficient to stretch the muscle.

The *treatment* of the acute strain is quite similar to that of sprain; that is, rest, protection and local heat. Protection is necessary, against active use of the muscle rather than against excessive motion. This is a good deal more difficult to accomplish. The patient should be instructed not to make any movement causing pain. If the area can be treated promptly and adequately, recovery will be prompt.

Unfortunately this condition is often inadequately treated and chronic strain supervenes with all of its implications. The only cure for chronic strain is prolonged rest until recovery is complete, after which gradual rehabilitation of the muscle can be carried out. If rehabilitation is too rapid the pain will recur. If athletic participation is begun during the recovery period a single overmovement may start the whole cycle over again. Localized trigger areas in the muscle may be present and, if so, injection of a long-acting anesthetic along with injection of a corticoid preparation into this area will be of benefit. This treatment is of little value in the case of diffuse muscle involvement, however. Muscle relaxants are useful, particularly in conjunction with physical therapy. Rehabilitation must be gradual, persistent, and kept within the limits of pain.

The actual protection of the back can be accomplished first by bed rest, later by a cast or brace, and finally by taping (Fig. 346). It is important to bear in mind, however, that taping is not as effective in strain as it is in sprain because, while the taping protects against overstretching of the muscle, it will not protect against muscle contraction.

A chronic strain tends to recur and can be extremely troublesome to the athlete. In many cases we advise a lumbosacral corset to help support the back and protect against overstretching—the same measure that is used in a case of chronic sprain. This is more effective than adhesive since repeated applications tend to irritate the skin. The corset should go well up over the lower ribs, particularly posteriorly, and well down on the sacrum if it is to provide much protection (Fig. 353).

Rehabilitation

As indicated in the dorsal spine, rehabilitation is extremely important, not only in complete recovery of strain but in avoiding recurrence. Proper exercises faithfully continued for many months may well prevent the recurrence of the strain since strain is, indeed, the result of using a muscle beyond its capacity. Hence, the greater its capacity, the less likely it is that it will be strained. (See p. 797.)

SPRAIN

Sprain is frequent in the mobile lumbar spine which has many ligaments giving support to the various joints. The supraspinous ligament, which extends along the tips of the spinous processes, is particularly susceptible. This sprain can be diagnosed by tenderness over the ligament or over the tip of the spinous process where the ligament attaches. Active contraction of the muscles to pull the spine into hyperextension is

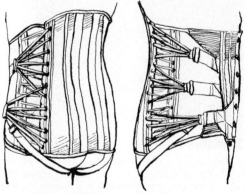

Figure 353. The lumbosacral corset.

pain-free, as is passive extension. Active flexion of the back, as in attempting to sit up from the supine position, is pain-free until tension is put on the process by forcing the head toward the knees. Passive hyperflexion of the spine will cause pain. This condition is treated by protection against overflexion by strapping. Activity can be permitted so long as the ligament is protected. Occasionally the ligament will be pulled in two or will be avulsed from the bone and more extensive treatment will be indicated. In this instance immobilization in extension in a brace or with a plaster jacket is in order. If the fragment of the spinous process does not unite, it may be removed. Primary early repair of the ligament would be advisable, but so infrequently is the condition diagnosed in the early stage that this is seldom practical.

Injury to the other ligaments of the back is much more difficult to determine with exactitude. The interspinous ligament is not frequently damaged because it has elastic fibers and is not readily overstretched. However, the articular ligaments around the apophyseal joints are frequently damaged, as is the anterior spinal ligament or the lateral spinal ligaments. Whether or not the ligamentum flavum is damaged by hyperflexion is problematical since it, too, is an elastic structure and probably will allow as much motion without damage as the range of flexion of the back will permit. Diagnosis of these sprains is on the basis of tests bringing stress upon certain areas. In the diagnosis of sprain it should be remembered that passive movements which put stress on the involved ligament will cause pain. For example, sprain of the capsule on the left will cause pain on flexion to the right or on flexion forward.

Treatment of the acute sprain is to place the ligament at complete rest. Unfortunately this is not often done and a chronic sprain ensues. In the acute sprain, muscle spasm is a characteristic symptom. Ideally the patient should be put at bed rest, given muscle relaxants, inductive heat or electric pad until the acute symptoms subside, at which time he should be treated by elastic strapping or corset to protect the area until the ligament is healed. During this time athletics should not be permitted. A sprain is easier to protect than a strain since, if the range of motion is limited, there is no stress on the ligament. For this reason, competition can be allowed much earlier in a sprain of the back than in a strain.

DISLOCATION-SUBLUXATION

Sprain of the lumbar spine rarely goes on to actual dislocation. There may be subluxation, which occurs when the interspinous ligament tears and the articular processes tend to disengage. If this is spontaneously relieved, it should be treated as a sprain. Unilateral dislocation in the lumbar spine is extremely rare and is not a common athletic injury. A frank dislocation of the lumbar spine occurs only after severe violence, such as a fall from a height or motor accident. This is a serious injury. X-ray will reveal the deformity (Fig. 354) and in most cases open reduction will be required. This type of dislocation may cause severe neurological deficit. However, it is not as damaging in the lumbar spine as it is higher because the cord proper does not extend into the lumbar area and so is not primarily involved. The peripheral nerves in the cauda will stand a great deal more trauma than will the substance of the cord.

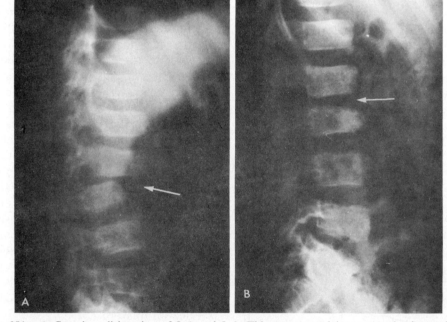

Figure 354. *A*, Complete dislocation of L-2 and L-3. This was treated by open reduction and graft. There were no permanent neurological sequelae. This is possible in spite of the intact lamina because the medullary portion of the cord stops just above this level and the cauda will tolerate much more trauma than will the spinal cord. *B*, Results six months later. The distortion of the body of L-3 may well be due to damage of the epiphysis since the original film does not show any compression here.

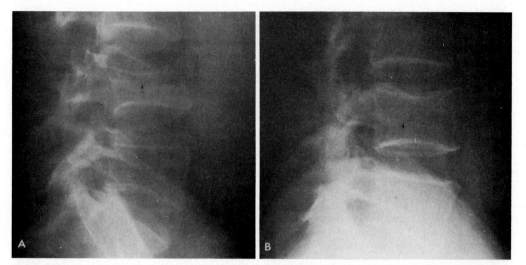

Figure 355. *A*, Severe compression fracture of L-4 following violent jack-knifing. *B*, Eight months later note complete restoration of vertebral height by "jack" decompression.

FRACTURE

Fracture may occur in the body of a lumbar vertebra, a lateral or spinous process, or in some portion of the arch.

Fracture of the Body of the Vertebra

Fracture of the body of the vertebra (Fig. 355) is extremely rare as an athletic injury. It is a major injury and is readily recognized as such. X-ray examination will reveal the deformity and anything beyond minimal deformity should be reduced as indicated above under dorsal spine. Failure to correct the compression may be disabling (Fig. 365). Athletic competition will be limited for many months.

Fracture of the Lateral Process

Fracture of the lateral processes is quite common in athletes. It should be noted that the lumbar vertebrae have spikelike lateral processes, some of which are quite thin or have a narrow neck. These processes are ruptured by two different mechanisms—a direct

blow as a complication of contusion, and violent exertion of the muscle; or by a combination of the two. There is a difference of opinion as to the relative frequency of the two causes since the combination of a blow and exertion often occur simultaneously. However, I think it is quite possible that a direct blow will account for the breaking off of a single lateral process. Fractures of multiple processes are almost always of the avulsion type (Fig. 357). In any event the significance of the fracture is not the broken bone but the muscle injury. The distal fragment frequently separates quite widely and nonunion is often the result. The patient reports a history of a blow on the back by the knee or foot, usually at the time of violent exercise during play. This causes immediate pain in the back which may be quite severe or may be relatively minor. If participation continues, the pain increases and muscles become more spastic. The player's body will be pulled toward the same side. This is more noticeable after a period of rest and then re-initiation of activity. There is localized tenderness over the area of injury. Stretching of the involved side by con-

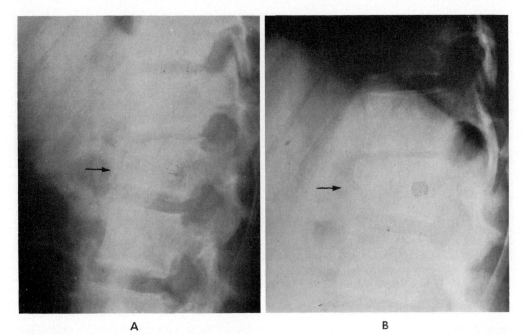

A   B

Figure 356. *A,* Relatively mild compression fracture of the superior portion of the body, of L-1 at eight weeks post-injury. *B,* Note persistent deformity following failure to correct compression. This relatively mild fracture has comparatively severe residual whereas the very severe fracture in Figure 355 is pain-free.

tralateral bending causes pain. Homolateral bending against resistance also is painful and passive forward flexion will cause pain. Active backward flexion will be painful.

Treatment depends almost entirely upon the symptoms present. If the patient is having severe pain and is seriously disabled he should be placed at bed rest with application of cold, followed by heat. In two or three days when the most acute symptoms have subsided (immediately if the primary symptoms are not too severe), some support should be applied to the back. Here again there is a great difference of opinion as to just what the nature of this support should be. I think this depends entirely upon the symptoms. If the patient is having severe pain and marked muscle spasm, a light-weight body jacket will give him good protection. He can wear this ten days or two weeks and then substitute a corset. If the symptoms are not too severe, the back may

be strapped or a corset applied which limits the activity somewhat and gives some degree of support although not as adequately as the cast. Ordinarily the symptoms will subside within three to six weeks. Infrequently in cases of nonunion there will be persistent pain to the point that removal of the fragment becomes necessary.

The player may be allowed to participate in sports just as soon as the back does not hurt him. The pain level is a good indication for continuing or discontinuing the treatment. After recovery there is no need for any restriction of activity even if nonunion of one or more processes is persistent.

Fracture of the Spinous Process

Fracture of the spinous process in the lumbar spine occurs from three different causes. One cause is sharp hyperflexion that pulls off the tip of the

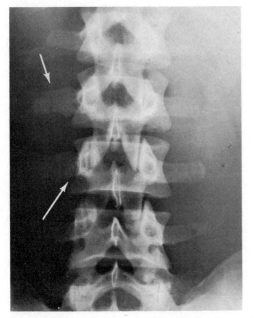

Figure 357. Fractures of transverse processes of the left second and third lumbar vertebrae.

process; another is sharp hyperextension that impinges one process against the other and breaks one or the other. The third cause is a direct blow that mechanically knocks off one of the projecting processes. The condition may ordinarily be diagnosed clinically by the sharp localization of pain, occasionally by the unstable spinous process. It can be confirmed by x-ray made with a technique to visualize the spinous processes (Fig. 358). If there is actual separation of the fragment in the distal 1 inch of the process, a great deal of time and trouble will be saved by removing this fragment since it will be very slow to heal and the case will likely terminate with pain on violent exertion. If the fracture is near the base of the process or in the arch, it will heal much more rapidly and completely, provided the spine is immobilized in extension, preferably by a plaster cast. Athletic competition is interdicted until healing is complete.

Arch Fracture

Any fracture involving the arch of the vertebra is potentially serious because of the danger of neurological involvement. The fracture may be between the articular processes (Fig. 359). It may be through the arch at the base of the process. It may actually be of the articular process. In any event, once the fracture is recognized the patient must be immobilized to permit it to heal since painful function may result if union is imperfect. This is a serious injury which should be treated as such. Athletic competition is forbidden until healing is complete.

NONTRAUMATIC DEFORMITIES OF THE SPINE

KYPHOSIS DORSALIS JUVENILIS (SCHEUERMANN'S DISEASE)

This condition is essentially a disturbance of the growth of the vertebrae. It is often quite extensive, as evidenced

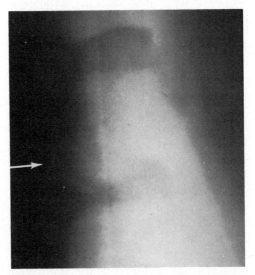

Figure 358. Avulsion fracture of the inferior border of the spinous process of the third lumbar vertebra.

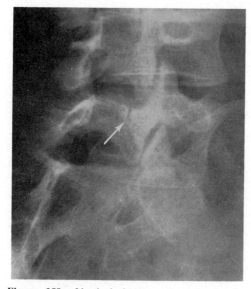

Figure 359. Vertical fracture through the lamina and articular process of L-5 visualized only on this right oblique view.

the absence of pain, the patient may be allowed to participate although he should wear protection against flexion until the bodies are completely reconstituted. I recall one young man who was an ardent baseball player. Toward the end of the course of the involvement, we permitted him to play baseball in a body jacket. He was a catcher and used the cast for a chest protector much to the detriment of the cast but apparently with no bad results to his back (Fig. 361). These cases resemble Perthes' disease in that they cause very little discomfort and yet may give rise to marked deformity (Fig. 362). They occur in a slightly older age group (12 to 15 years) than Perthes' disease and *limiting* activity at this age may be extremely difficult when the patient is not actually having many symptoms. Nevertheless it should be done.

by wedging of many dorsal vertebrae with osteochondrosis of the bodies which often goes on to fragmentation (Figs. 360 and 361). Occasionally only a single vertebra or adjacent ones may be involved and this may cause some confusion in the early stages. There is usually no particular problem in diagnosis. There is no evidence that this condition is actually caused by a single injury. However, it seems quite apparent that malformation of the vertebrae is definitely increased by active or passive forward flexion and by exercise.

The patient should be protected by a hyperextension brace to place the weight back on the arches and articular processes and to take it off the defective portion of the anterior body. The problem here will be with that person who wants to continue athletic competition. Certainly in the active stage of this condition athletics should be banned. As the replacement phase of the condition develops, as evidenced by improved density of the vertebrae and coalescence of the fragmented areas and by

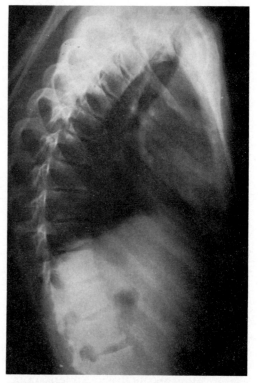

Figure 360. Generalized dorsalis juvenilis epiphysitis. Note wedging of all the dorsal and lumbar vertebrae.

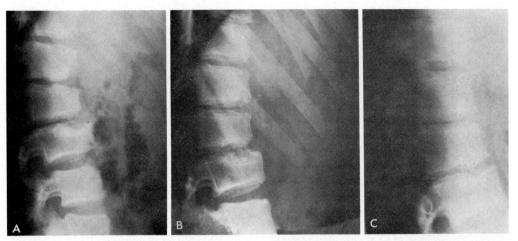

Figure 361. Localized vertebral epiphysitis involving D-12, L-1 and 2. Note characteristic deformity with interference of growth. *A,* The extreme involvement between L-1 and 2 may lead to erroneous diagnosis. *B,* Healing six months later. *C,* Final result six years later shows amazing restoration of architecture with only minimal kyphosis due almost entirely to wedging of L-3. This boy had prolonged protection against anterior weight bearing which I think was the prime factor in his good recovery.

Of more difficulty diagnostically is the localized manifestation of the same condition in which one or two or three of the vertebrae may be involved with quite major changes and yet be essentially pain-free, until an injury calls attention to this area or until the area becomes spontaneously painful. It may be that the injury is entirely coincidental. It should not be confused with an acute fracture. Adequate x-rays will help to differentiate the two. Here again it is necessary to reduce the patient's activity and by serial x-rays determine when the bone is repaired sufficiently to permit the stresses of athletic competition.

One does not add to one's popularity by refusing permission to these young men to participate. Nevertheless a firm stand is vital, particularly if there is any major involvement, since increasing deformity may result in a persistent gibbus.

CONGENITAL DEFORMITIES

Congenital deformities are much more common in the lower back than in the upper, specifically about the fourth and fifth lumbar and the first sacral vertebrae. These deformities are not caused by athletic injuries. However, they often become a problem to the athlete since when recognized following an injury a decision must immediately be made on the advisability of his continuing in athletics and, indeed, on the treatment of the acute condition. The great majority of these conditions do not affect the function of the spine enough to require restriction of activity.

Spina Bifida Occulta

The most common of these deformities is spina bifida occulta in which there is failure of fusion of the arch of one or more of the vertebrae posteriorly (Fig. 363). This is a common finding and is ordinarily of no significance. The player should not be alarmed or be told that he has a dangerous condition of the lower back or that he should be careful the rest of his life. Exceptionally, a wide open spina bifida involving several vertebrae may be of sufficient concern to require the use of additional support or

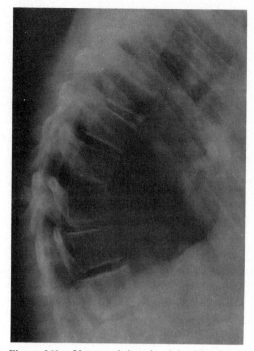

Figure 362. Untreated dorsal epiphysitis of only moderate severity but note extreme deformity.

even the recommendation that some less strenuous activity be followed. A well placed sacral pad may give some reassurance.

Spondylolysis or Spondylolisthesis

Spondylolysis (Fig. 364) is the failure of fusion of the arch of the vertebra, usually between the articular processes. Spondylolisthesis (Fig. 365) is spondylolysis in which there is displacement of the superior vertebra forward on the one below. This laminal defect does, indeed, cause weakness of the spine but to an extremely variable degree. Many persons have spondylolysis or spondylolisthesis all their lives and never know it. However, if the athlete is having trouble in the lower back and spondylolysis is discovered, one may be justified in restricting him to some of the less ac-

tive sports. Athletics basically should not cause serious damage to the spine but he probably will have discomfort to the point that he will not be very effective. After the pain is relieved he should be advised to wear a lumbosacral support or sacroiliac belt during periods of active competition.

In actual spondylolisthesis there is separation at the line of defect, and here again it may be difficult to decide on the proper procedure. If there is sufficient pain, one should seriously consider treatment of the condition rather than interdiction of athletics. However, if the pain occurs only on violent exercise such as football, I think one is justified in discontinuing the football to see how the patient gets along with his condition. If he continues to have pain, treatment should be recommended. The person of 14 or 15 years of age with spondylolisthesis who is already having pain in the back almost inevitably will come to treatment at a later time in spite of any recommendation that he decrease his

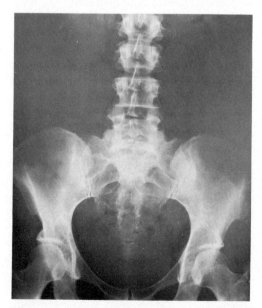

Figure 363. Spina bifida occulta in first sacral vertebra. This is asymptomatic and of no significance.

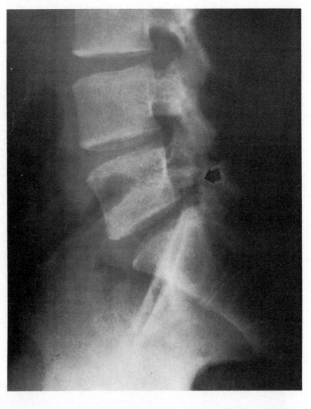

Figure 364. Asymptomatic spondylolysis. Note (arrow) arch defect in the lamina of L-5 but no slipping. No present symptoms.

activities, since degenerative changes will certainly occur as the years pass. It is quite unlikely that he will become pain-free as he gets older. In such a case one cannot assume that simple banning of athletic competition will mean that the person is inactive. If he is an active, energetic type he will occupy himself with an equally strenuous occupation. If he is the indolent type, one questions the advisability of encouraging further indolence to protect a condition that might be remedied surgically.

Variations in Sacral Fusion

As has been noted above, the sacrum originally is made up of five bones which during adolescence fuse into a solid mass. Various anomalous conditions may arise as a part of this process. The lower lumbar vertebra may participate to some extent in the sacral fusion and, indeed, may completely fuse so that there is *sacralization of the fifth lumbar vertebra* (Figs. 366 and 367). This is of no significance activity-wise. If the fusion is incomplete, with one side fusing and the other not, some imbalance may arise in the lower back and occasionally pain will be present. The same can be said here as was said of spondylolisthesis, namely, that a person having pain in his early teens will inevitably have pain when he becomes older. One should therefore proceed to complete the fusion, after which unlimited activity can be permitted. A symptom-free unilateral sacralization is of no significance—and most of the cases are symptom-free. The same is true of *lumbarization of the first sacral vertebra*. If a portion of the sacrum fails to fuse this is of no significance. Certainly the fibrous fusion is extremely firm and highly unlikely to be damaged by any

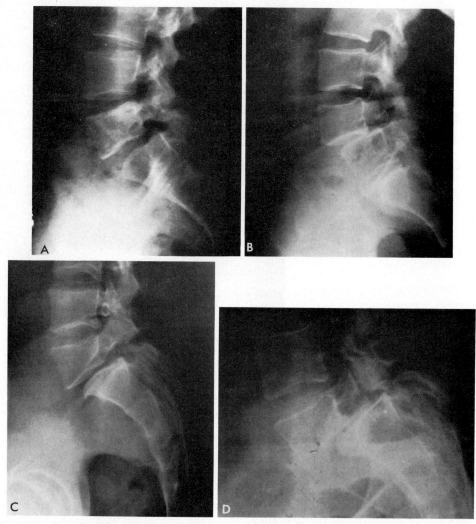

Figure 365.   Spondylolisthesis. Note *A*, Grade I. Again the arch defect in L-5 with mild forward displacement of L-5 on S-1. Backache but no gross disability. *B*, Grade II. Note more forward slipping between L-4 and L-5 with collapse of the intervertebral disc. Definite symptomatic back with restriction of motion, muscle spasm, and curtailment of activities. *C*, Grade III. More extensive slipping combined with a wide separation at the arch defect, and degenerative changes of the disc. Grossly symptomatic. *D*, Grade IV. Vertebra slipped forward over halfway. Severe disability.

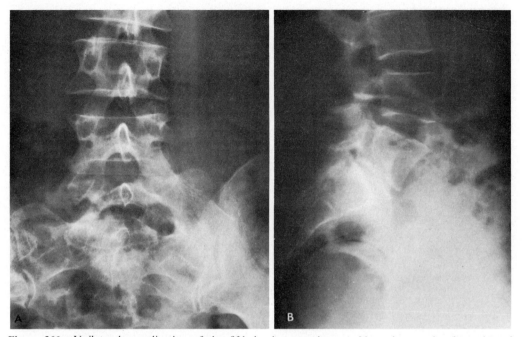

Figure 366. Unilateral sacralization of the fifth lumbar vertebra. *A*, Note the massive formation of sacral ala on the left side with relatively normal transverse process on the right. *B*, Lateral view showing the very narrow disc space and the massive arches.

type of athletic competition. I would not recommend the wearing of a belt or brace or other support. On the other hand, a sprain of the back in which there is a congenital anomaly may be somewhat more resistant to treatment than uncomplicated sprain and protection should be given, not for the congenital anomaly but for the accompanying sprain.

Other Anomalies

Other conditions such as hemivertebrae (Fig. 368), scoliosis (Fig. 369), kyphosis (Fig. 370) and increased lordosis (Fig. 371) must be managed on an individual basis. In many instances, such as extreme lordosis, athletic competition may be valuable from the standpoint of posture. It must be accompanied by instruction in the treatment of the primary condition. The patients must be

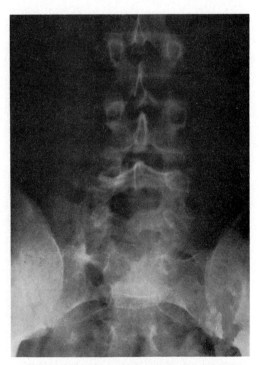

Figure 367. Complete sacralization of L-5.

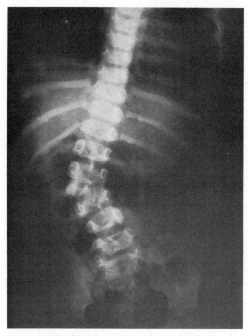

Figure 368. Hemivertebra of the lumbar spine (L-2).

judged symptomatically. The deformity itself is not necessarily disabling if it is not accompanied by signs of secondary involvement such as nerve root pressure and muscle contracture. There is no justification for making a chronic invalid out of a patient because of an x-ray diagnosis of a spinal anomaly.

SPINAL DISC LESIONS

In recent years the diagnosis of disc rupture with attendant nerve root injury has been a major development and consequently must be considered in the treatment of athletes. In my experience this condition has rarely resulted from athletic participation. However, once a ruptured disc is present it tends to be recurrent, and strenuous athletics should be banned until the condition is corrected. The disc is the pad lying be-

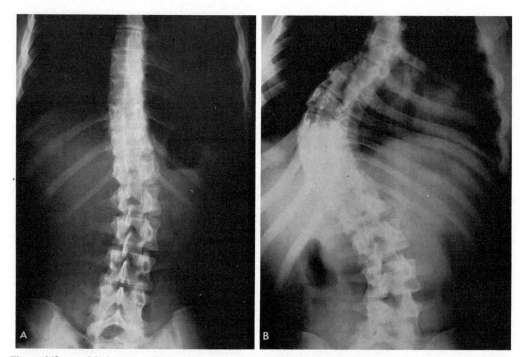

Figure 369. *A,* Moderate scoliosis, asymptomatic. *B,* This asymptomatic scoliosis was found incidentally in a college athlete who had ruptured his cartilage while playing varsity football.

Classic ruptured disc has its origin in a degenerative annulus. The disc commonly ruptures posteriorly owing to the lordosis of the lumbar spine, which causes eccentric weight bearing with an inordinate amount of weight on the back margin of the disc. It is probable that pressure on the disc causes it to rupture or herniate through an area of the annulus already defective. This pressure may be caused by anything that raises the pressure within the disc, such as leaning forward to tie the shoe, but is more likely to be caused by lifting—and particularly lifting in a rather strained position, the same sort of effort that would cause muscular strain. The athlete is not in the common age bracket

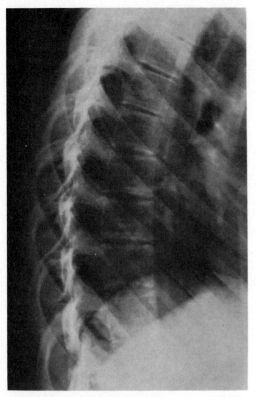

Figure 370. Moderate dorsal kyphosis, probably from asymptomatic mild dorsal epiphysitis although it may be postural.

tween the two vertebrae. The periphery of the pad, the so-called annulus fibrosus, is the firm ligamentous and cartilaginous structure that forms a ring within which is enclosed the softer nucleus pulposus. This arrangement acts as a hydraulic shock absorber between the bodies of the vertebrae. Infrequently the annulus may be subject to damage by excessive motion. Compression of the two vertebrae forcing the bones together puts pressure on the inner mass and causes it to bulge so, theoretically, the disc could rupture. However, the normal annulus is so strong that excessive pressure in a single violent effort usually will break the disc into the body of the vertebra or compress the vertebra rather than rupture the annulus.

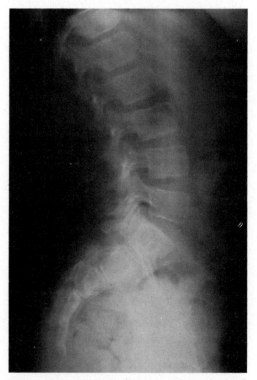

Figure 371. Typical adolescent lordosis in 9 year old boy. The vertebral epiphyses have not yet ossified but these vertebrae are normal for this age. Note that the separate pieces of the sacrum have not yet fused. This condition presents no contraindication to athletics. On the contrary, physical fitness should be encouraged.

for ruptured disc. In addition, his splendid muscular condition takes a good deal of strain off the disc itself.

The classic symptoms will not be reiterated here. One should suspect disc involvement in an injury in which the pain follows the root distribution in the leg and is increased by coughing or sneezing or by raising interspinal pressure by pressure on the jugular veins. The difficult case will be the mild one in which there are few nerve root signs. There is some stiffness in the back but not at a disabling level. Shall this patient be allowed to participate in sports? I think the case must be individualized and some balance struck between the urgency for his participation and the danger of it. If athletic competition will accentuate his discomfort he probably will require definitive treatment anyway, so he likely is doing himself no major harm by participating. Whether or not he is effective is a wholly different thing. Thus, while a ruptured disc must be considered in many conditions of the back, it is not really a major problem in the treatment of athletes.

CHAPTER 16

INJURIES OF THE PELVIS AND HIP

It is convenient to include the pelvis and hip under a single heading, since these areas are closely related anatomically.

ANATOMICAL CONSIDERATIONS

The pelvis is a uniquely devised mechanism designed to transfer the body weight from the single weight-bearing axis of the trunk to the bipolar weight-bearing of the lower extremities (Fig. 351). It is designed to have a whippletree effect. Thus, the spine attaches to the pelvis by a single connection to the sacrum and for stability is anchored in all four directions by various combinations of ligaments and muscles. Through the bony ring of the pelvis the weight is transferred from the spinal column to the two lower extremities so that of necessity the pelvic ring must be intact in order to give stability. The primary function of the pelvis including the bones, joints, ligaments and muscles is this mechanical transfer of weight. A secondary function of the bony pelvis is protection of the pelvic viscera. Enclosed within the pelvis are the bladder,

the female genitalia, the rectum and the great vessels and nerves extending to the lower extremities.

At the lumbosacral level the spinal muscles descend to attach to the sacrum and the wings of the ilia. The hip joint is an extremely stable ball-and-socket joint — stable, that is, from the standpoint of dislocation. However, by virtue of the fact that it is a ball and socket there is no bony restriction of motion in the hip as there is in other joints. The functional stability of the hip depends entirely upon the musculature about the hip. The strong capsule and capsular ligaments maintain the ball within the socket but the stability of the thigh in relation to the pelvis and hence to the trunk is entirely controlled by muscle. There is no stable position in the flail hip as there is, for example, in the flail knee. The knee can be locked in extension by the stabilizing effect of the posterior capsule and collateral ligaments with no muscle action involved. Not so the hip. To effect stability the hip is surrounded by a great mass of muscle which must be adequate to support the trunk in the erect position, and indeed in many other positions. The muscles must also serve to propel the trunk by action

471

of the lower extremities and to give powerful impetus to the lower extremities in relation to the trunk, as in kicking.

The various muscles have wholly different effects as the relative position of the trunk and lower extremities is altered. Careful analysis of the types of force involved will often give a valuable lead as to the injury to be expected.

CONTUSION

Contusions about the pelvis may be of almost any kind or degree since in some areas the pelvic bone is subcutaneous and in other areas is surrounded by masses of muscle. Contusions in general should be managed as is contusion anywhere, depending upon the degree of injury. The local area may be injected with a long-acting anesthetic agent plus hyaluronidase. A compression bandage and cold compresses in the early stage, followed by heat, are useful. Protection against re-injury is by contact pads rather than by strapping.

Muscular contusion frequently involves the buttock and if severe enough may be quite disabling for a period. In a severe contusion with major local symptoms, careful investigation should be made for a possible fracture of the underlying bone. The contusion may result in a deep-seated hematoma which is virtually impossible to diagnose in the early stages. It is not common for a hematoma in the pelvic muscles to progress to myositis ossificans. Occasionally a contusion of the tuberosity of the ischium will cause an ischial bursitis or an ischial periostitis progressing to actual spur formation. Of major importance in contusion is the ruling out of a more serious injury. Subcutaneous hematoma along the crest of the ilium may be extremely tender and require protective padding all season. It can be distin-

guished from deeper injury in that functional movement of the muscles attached to the iliac crest does not cause increased pain.

Because the types of injury to the pelvis vary greatly depending upon the anatomical structure of the area involved, they will be discussed on a regional basis.

INJURIES IN THE VICINITY OF THE ILIAC CREST

Contusion and Strain

A pelvic area that is particularly susceptible to injury is the iliac crest. This area extends from the anterosuperior spine in front over the crest of the pelvic bone (ilium) to the posterosuperior spine in back. Along its outer margin attach the large muscles going to the lower extremities and on its inner margin the group of muscles going to the abdomen and spine (Fig. 372). The area between is largely subcutaneous.

The vast majority of injuries about the pelvic crest are contusions that will respond promptly and well to the simple measures outlined above. A definitive diagnosis should be made at the time of injury to rule out a more serious injury. Too often a more serious injury is detected only after ordinary measures fail to give relief. This results in a delay in definitive treatment for the serious condition that may well prolong morbidity and cause greater permanent disability.

Injury along the pelvic rim may consist of a contusion of the bone of the iliac crest—the so-called hip pointer—a periostitis of the iliac crest, a strain, an avulsion of the muscles attaching to the crest, or other pathology. It is of considerable importance to determine the exact nature of the injury since the treatment, particularly the protective treatment, and also to a considerable ex-

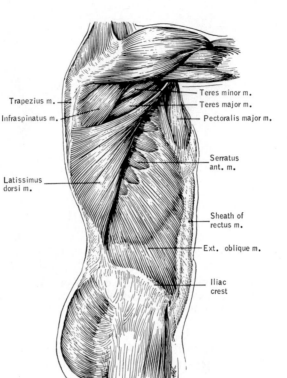

Trapezius m.

Infraspinatus m.

Latissimus dorsi m.

Teres minor m.

Teres major m.

Pectoralis major m.

Serratus ant. m.

Sheath of rectus m.

Ext. oblique m.

Iliac crest

Figure 372. Drawing of iliac crest, subcutaneous but with the hip muscles below and the trunk muscles above. (From Anson, Atlas of Human Anatomy.)

tent the immediate prognosis may depend a great deal upon the muscles involved. The injury frequently damages the attachment of the abdominal muscles along the anterior and inner portion of the iliac crest. This is caused by forceful contraction of the abdominal muscles while the trunk is being forced to the contralateral side. This results in some degree of detachment along the iliac crest, the separation varying from a few fibers to complete detachment of the entire muscle from the bone (Fig. 373).

I recall one case of a high school boy who threw himself in front of an opponent in making a block. He had immediate severe pain along the iliac crest with severe disability. When examined a few hours later he was able to walk only with the hand on the involved side dangling below the knee with the rib cage drawn down into the pelvis. Any effort to straighten him up from this position was strenuously resisted because of severe pain. Palpation revealed extreme tenderness along the entire iliac crest. When we were able to get him to relax a little, a palpable defect was found above the iliac crest. At operation an incision was made completely encircling the iliac crest. There had been complete avulsion of the aponeurotic muscle attachment to the crest of the ilium, so that the attachments of the iliacus and the abdominal muscles remained together but were completely pulled away from the iliac bone. The whole medial crest and interior surface of the ilium were denuded. The damage was easily repaired by placing drill holes along the iliac crest and pulling the detached cap snugly back into position on the crest. The boy had a good recovery and went on to

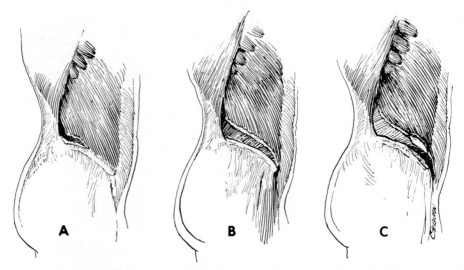

Figure 373. Drawings showing degrees of detachment of the aponeurosis at the iliac crest. *A,* Mild (first degree): a small tear. *B,* Moderate (second degree): an appreciable tear with bare bone exposed. *C,* Severe (third degree): avulsion of the caput.

play varsity collegiate football without disability. This is admittedly an unusual case but illustrates the variation in degree of injury and shows why treatment is so often disappointing.

At examination to determine the type of injury, certain findings are of extreme importance. Tenderness is not particularly diagnostic since tenderness will be noted in both contusion of bone and avulsion of muscle. In contusion, however, contraction of the involved muscle will not cause pain. On the other hand, if the athlete has pain on contracting his abdominal muscles or on flexing to the opposite side, one must assume some degree of damage to the muscle attachment. Similarly, if pain is caused by active abduction or extension of the thigh with the patient lying on his side, one must assume some damage to the gluteal attachments or possibly to the tensor fascia femoris or to the lateral abdominals. Careful check must be made of the muscles that attach in the involved area. Once it has been determined that muscular involvement is present, the next step is to determine its degree. This may be extremely difficult.

If there is complete avulsion, surgical repair should be carried out promptly. Fortunately complete avulsion of the iliac crest seldom occurs. I am sure that it does occur more often than it is diagnosed. A great many of these injuries never actually reach the doctor and are treated by the athlete himself or by the trainer, often without true recognition of the nature of the pathological condition.

If the avulsion is less than complete, treatment should be that of strain. The muscle should be put at rest. In the early stage one should use cold and compression; after 24 hours heat and protection. Since we are assuming some degree of avulsion of the attachment, local treatment may be of considerable value. Any hematoma should be aspirated first, then a long-acting anesthetic agent along with hyaluronidase is injected. Protection must be given to the muscles at the attachment of the iliac crest. Even though the trunk is strapped to hold it toward the involved side, which in itself is difficult, this does not prevent active forceful contraction of the muscle. It simply prevents overstretch. So if there is pain on active use of the abdominal or thigh muscles, a period of inactivity is necessary in order to restore normal function. Rehabilitation should be within the limits of pain and this can be determined most readily by the patient himself. When activity is resumed, strapping of the flank as described in Figure 374 may be undertaken although its accomplishment is quite difficult. Properly applied, this strapping gives considerable restriction of motion. A good plan is to begin the strapping with cross-stretch and progress to long-stretch elastic tape as healing progresses and more activity is permissible. Indeed if applied adequately enough to give good protection against overstretching, it probably will be a material handicap to athletic competition. Contact sports of any kind should not be permitted without very effective protective padding over the iliac crest since the crest will remain extremely sensitive. This protection should be used for the remainder of the season.

A tendency toward recurrence of these lesions is a disheartening factor. I am sure that the majority of them are undertreated rather than overtreated

since they are considered to be simple contusions when they are actually muscular avulsions.

Fracture

Fracture of the *wing of the ilium* is not frequent as an athletic injury. It is usually caused by a direct blow against the wing of the ilium. In most sports in which such a force is likely, the iliac crest is protected by padding to prevent injury to the bone. The most frequent sport in which this occurs is horseback riding, often in the manner described in the illustration (Fig. 375). This, as may be expected, is an extremely painful injury, not only at the time of the blow but in the immediate period after the injury. It will ordinarily be recognized as a serious injury. Examination reveals extreme tenderness along the iliac crest and down onto the wing of the ilium, the area depending upon the extent of the fracture. The patient will usually not permit deep enough palpation that one can actually feel a defect along the rim, although this is occasionally possible. Any attempt at function of the involved

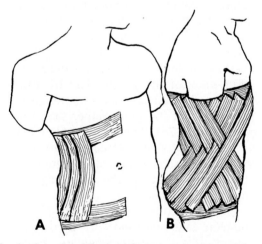

Figure 374. Strapping of flank. The strapping is done with adhesive applied while the patient is in the erect position with the trunk flexed toward the involved side. Broad strips of long-stretch or cross-stretch elastic tape are used. The former stretches on its long axis and allows considerable motion, while the latter stretches on its cross axis and gives more restriction of motion; so the one to be used depends upon the degree of fixation desired. Various methods can be used for application. A good method is by crosshatching the strapping *(B)*, one strip beginning in the region of the substernal notch extending diagonally downward and backward across the anterosuperior spine and over the trochanter to terminate on the back of the thigh, and another beginning in the back, starting at the lateral margin of the opposite lumbar muscle mass and crossing downward over the trochanter to end on the anteromedial thigh. These strips should cross at about the level of the crest. Successive parallel strips extending backward and forward form crosshatching of the adhesive. The crossed strips begin at the trochanter and extend to the lower ribs. For additional support the dressing can be given an underlying foundation of vertical strips as illustrated in *A*. At the completion of the strapping, the tape should be secured by circumferential strips.

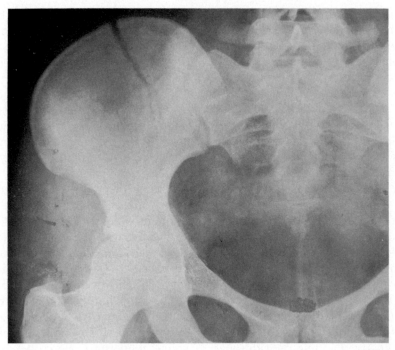

Figure 375. A young woman sustained a linear fracture of the ilium while horseback riding. The horse headed for the stable and turned through a gate so abruptly that the rider bumped the ilium on the center post.

muscles is extremely painful and even involuntary spasm of the abdominal or hip muscles may cause acute distress. It is necessary to have the patient completely relaxed mentally and physically before a definitive examination can be done. If a lesion of this severity is suspected, an x-ray examination should be made. The fracture can be completely overlooked in the ordinary anteroposterior view of the pelvis. The fracture will be well delineated by an anteroposterior view of the ilium rather than the pelvis (Fig. 376). This view is obtained by rotating the pelvis 45 degrees toward the involved side. A lateral view may be obtained by directing the ray along the anterior iliac crest.

This fracture may be treated by complete bed rest, and with a tranquil patient this is usually adequate. Even with some degree of displacement of the fragment, reduction is not necessary.

Reposition would of necessity have to be by open reduction with internal fixation. This is a more formidable procedure than is usually justified. If simple bed rest does not give adequate relief of pain, a pair of plaster pants extending from above the knees to above the rib margin may give substantial relief of discomfort and permit mobility of the patient in bed. A simple corset may suffice or adhesive strapping may relieve the patient. It should be borne in mind that if there is real, measurable displacement of the fragment, a compression dressing with a corset or strapping may increase the pain and in fact increase the displacement. The duration of recumbency will vary widely depending upon the severity of the injury and the equanimity of the patient. Ambulation may be permitted whenever the degree of discomfort permits. It will require six to eight weeks for the fracture to heal, but activity may be permitted as soon as the local reaction subsides and the pain permits.

Another injury in the region of the iliac crest is fracture of the *anterior superior spine of the ilium* (Fig. 377). This fracture is almost always an avulsion fracture, the fragment being pulled off by the sartorius and tensor fasciae femoris attachments. The history is usually of unusual muscular violence in running or jumping — occasionally jumping down from a height. Examination reveals local pain and tenderness at the anterior spine. This can be distinguished from a contusion in this area by the fact that function of the involved muscle attachments is painful and active flexion of the thigh or passive overextension of the thigh will cause pain directly at the area. If one examines the patient early he may be able to palpate a separate fragment of bone which may be 1 inch or more below the location of the attachment at the anterosuperior spine. X-rays should be taken. An anteroposterior view of the ilium rather than of the pelvis may be necessary if the fragment is not to be missed. An avulsion of the tendon may occur without a fragment of bone being displaced.

Treatment of this condition is primarily surgical. If it is diagnosed promptly, surgical correction is relatively atraumatic and not difficult. The fragment can be drawn back into position and fastened by whatever type of internal fixation seems most effective in the individual case. It may vary from a single screw fastening the fragment of bone to the pelvis to direct suture through drill holes. If the avulsion is incomplete or if for some reason surgery is inadvisable, treatment should be by

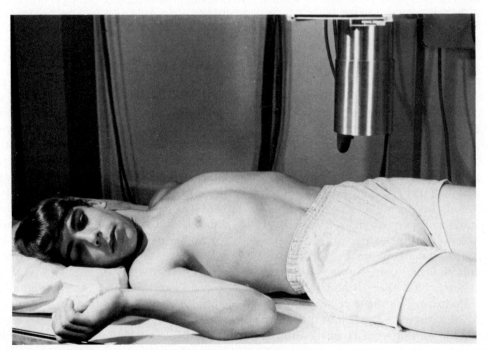

Figure 376. Positioning for x-ray of the wing of the ilium. Place the patient in a supine position. Elevate the unaffected side about 40 or 45 degrees and support with sand bags or angle block. Center the anterior superior iliac spine to the midline of the table and center the cassette to the level of the anterior superior spine. Slightly flex the knees for comfort but keep the hip fully extended. Direct the central ray to the center of the cassette.

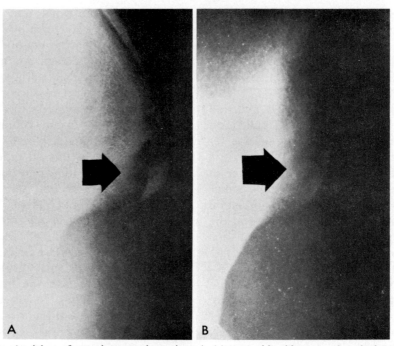

Figure 377. Avulsion of anterior superior spine. A 14 year old athlete was knocked against a wall playing basketball. No symptoms developed until a month later, when he felt something pull while he was running. He continued to have pain for a month before seeking medical attention. *A*, X-ray two months after the injury reveals avulsion of the anterior superior spine of the ilium. Fragment was sutured back through drill holes. *B*, Four months postoperatively the fracture shows good union.

immobilization with the thigh flexed. This can be accomplished by bed rest with the knees elevated or by plaster fixation in the appropriate position. I believe it is more simple and less traumatic to carry out prompt open reduction with definitive fixation than it is to immobilize the patient for the period necessary to permit healing to become complete. If nonsurgical treatment is selected, local measures consist of aspiration of the hematoma, injection with hyaluronidase, compression bandage, cold early, heat after 24 hours.

Following surgical repair, the degree of activity to be permitted will depend upon the security of the internal fixation. If firm fixation is obtained, I prefer to use a short single spica running from the knee on the affected side around the pelvis with the thigh flexed

30 degrees. The patient should be allowed up on crutches within a day or two and rehabilitation promptly commenced. This includes isometric contraction of the involved muscles. At the end of two weeks, the spica is removed. The wound is dressed and if it has properly healed, a spica of elastic adhesive bandage is applied with the patient standing and the thigh and knee slightly flexed by putting the foot on the involved side on a 4 inch block. This permits rehabilitation of the hip joint to proceed. Ordinarily active running should not be permitted short of six weeks and in the case with less secure surgical fixation a longer period may be required.

If at operation the fragment is found to be small or comminuted it should be removed, rather than repaired, and the muscle sutured to the bone. Indeed, there is some argument in favor of routinely removing the fragment and obtaining muscle-to-bone healing rather than waiting for bone-to-bone union. The latter may require considerably longer and may prolong rehabilitation. Unless I can get anatomical reposition and very positive screw fixation, I generally remove the fragment and repair the attachment to the ilium through drill holes.

INJURIES IN THE VICINITY OF THE POSTERIOR SPINES OF THE ILIUM

Injuries to the posterior spines of the ilium are not frequent since the attachments here are such that there is no acute avulsive force applied. The most frequent injury in this vicinity is simple contusion of the posterior superior or inferior spine. While this may be somewhat distressing it is not particularly disabling and responds well to local treatment by heat and other means of physical therapy.

INJURIES IN THE VICINITY OF THE SACRUM AND SACROILIAC JOINTS, INCLUDING THE COCCYX

The sacrum is the keystone of the arch of the pelvis. The two innominate bones are attached to the sacrum at the sacroiliac joints. The sacroiliac joint has extremely irregular contour, the bones fitting together with interdigitations much like the ratchets in the ordinary desk lamp bracket. There is no true articular motion between these two bones but there is articular cartilage and often a synovial lined capsule so it must be classified as a diarthrodial joint (Fig. 378).

Contusion

Contusion in the vicinity of the sacrum and sacroiliac joints is a common injury, so frequent that sacral pads are a required part of the equipment for contact sports. The sacrum itself is largely subcutaneous on its posterior surface, as is the posterior inferior spine of the ilium. A direct blow to the unpro-

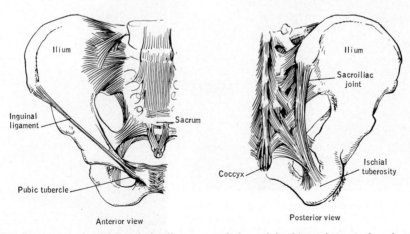

Figure 378. Anteroposterior view of the ligaments of the pelvis. Note the complete investiture of the sacroiliac joints by a continuous band of very heavy ligament. This includes also the ligament attaching the third lumbar vertebra to the ilium. Note that the entire pelvis is firmly bound down with strong ligaments. (From Anson, Atlas of Human Anatomy.)

tected sacrum may cause an extremely painful injury. Examination reveals tenderness over the sacrum which may be diffuse or may be sharply localized on the sacrum or on one of the iliac spines. If the injury appears to be acute, an x-ray should be made since it is not unusual to crack the sacrum or to fracture one of the spines by direct trauma. If fracture can be ruled out, treatment should be by early application of cold and compression followed by heat and support. Actually this injury, while it is quite painful, is not particularly disabling. As long as the sacrum is tender it should be protected against direct contusion.

Fracture

A fracture of the sacrum is usually transverse or stellate in type and will respond quite well to conservative treatment (Fig. 379). This will require a period of bed rest followed by support. Ordinarily a corset will be adequate.

Healing will usually be complete within four weeks but residual tenderness and pain may last another month. If the displacement is gross or if angulation is severe, an orthopaedic consultant should be called. This force is not likely to injure the rectum but a rectal examination should be routine. If blood is encountered, a proctoscopic examination is indicated. One should feel also for irregularities of the inner surface of the sacrum.

Sprain

A sprain of the iliosacral ligaments is possible. It may be of the ligament extending from the posterior projection of the wing of the ilium to the posterior sacrum, or of the ligaments within the pelvis. It should be borne in mind that many of the conditions that used to be called sacroiliac sprain were actually other entities. It was a "wastebasket" term. The sacroiliac ligaments are so strong, particularly in the young athlete,

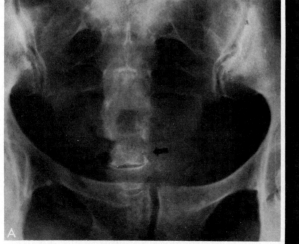
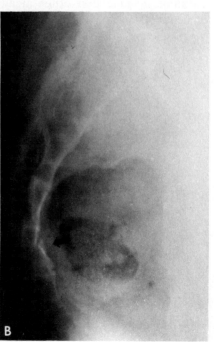

Figure 379. Transverse fracture of sacrum just below the sacroiliac joint, caused by forceful blow against the lower portion of the sacrum. *A,* Anterior view. *B,* Lateral view. This fracture is treated symptomatically. The patient probably would be more comfortable in a sacroiliac support for a few weeks.

that ordinary stresses will cause damage to the lumbosacral ligaments more readily than to the sacroiliac ligaments. One should, therefore, be very wary of the diagnosis of sacroiliac sprain.

Following injury in the vicinity of the sacroiliac joint there will be pain localized about the joint. There also may be pain referred to the groin, hamstrings, or back of the thigh. It will not ordinarily be along the sciatic distribution. If this condition is suspected, great care must be taken to localize the lesion to the sacroiliac joint. Many of the tests that will elicit pain in the sacroiliac joint will also be positive in such conditions as ruptured disc, sciatic neuritis and lumbosacral sprain, so that the mere fact that the tests cause pain is of little significance. The greatest significance is in the location of the pain. In an acute injury this may be extremely difficult to determine accurately. The common tests such as straight leg raising (Fig. 380, *A, B*) which put torsion force on the sacroiliac joint or the similar test of forward flexion of the trunk with the knees straight will cause pain in sacroiliac joint involvement but will also be positive in many other conditions. Some tests are designed to stress the sacroiliac area particularly. The popular Gaenslen test (Fig. 380, *C*), in which the opposite thigh is flexed on the abdomen in order to immobilize the pelvis in forward flexion and then the involved leg is pushed into hyperextension, causes rotatory stress on the sacroiliac joint. Obviously it would also strain other areas, so again the mere positive test is not diagnostic.

Of rather more significance are tests designed to compress or separate the iliac crests (Fig. 380, *E–H*). With the patient lying on his back, simple compression force across the crests will put some stress across the sacroiliac joint. The opposite maneuver of forcing the crests apart can be applied in a thin

individual by locking the heels of the hands against the inner portion of each anterior spine and attempting to separate the spines. A similar test is to have the patient lie on his side with the inferior thigh flexed to 90 degrees to fix the lumbosacral area. Compression downward against the upward iliac crest will throw stress on the sacroiliac joint.

If the sprain is acute, the pain will be relieved by bed rest. Local treatment consists of injection of the tender area with an anesthetic followed by compression made by a constricting elastic adhesive dressing wrapped around the pelvis or by a sacroiliac belt or by a simple corset. Heat will relieve the attendant muscle spasm. As in back injuries, muscle spasm may be relieved by oral antispasmodics. The duration of immobilization in bed depends upon the severity of the injury. The patient may be permitted up as soon as he can get up without pain. If the injury is actually an acute sprain of the ligament, five to six weeks will be needed for the ligament to repair and the area should be carefully protected during this time.

Dislocation

Actual sacroiliac dislocation occurs only as the result of a massive injury that is ordinarily not athletic in origin, although it could occur by being thrown from a horse or similar severe trauma. The treatment will be that of a fractured pelvis which is not within the scope of this work.

Subluxation

Osteopathic physicians have called our attention to the dramatic relief which may be secured by manipulation in the sacroiliac joint. It is probable that in certain circumstances of relaxation of the iliosacral ligaments some of the interdigitations of the joint become caught

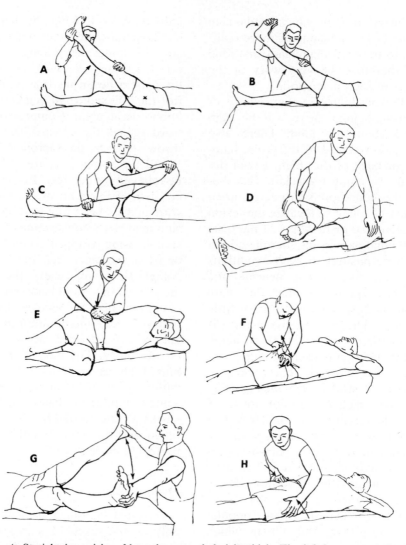

Figure 380. *A*, Straight leg raising. Note the extended right thigh. The left lower extremity is flexed with the knee extended.

B, Straight leg raising test with dorsiflexion of the foot (Lasègue).

C, Thigh flexion test (Gaenslen). Note the right thigh held in extension. It may be dropped off the table in hyperextension while the left thigh is flexed.

D, The heel to knee test. The left pelvis is fixed by the examiner's left hand. With the right heel on the left knee, the right knee is pushed down toward the table.

E, F, G, H, Iliac compression or separation. *E*, Lateral decubitus. With the opposite thigh flexed for stability, the right iliac crest is compressed toward the table. *F*, With the patient supine, the examiner's hands force the iliac crests apart. *G*, With the patient supine, the legs are widely abducted. *H*, Examiner forces crests together.

with a minimal degree of displacement which is undetectable by x-ray. In these cases manipulation may cause them to "snap back into place" and give relief. This happens too frequently to be ignored but I am sure that many times the relief by manipulation either is relief of the muscle tension or is psychic. The

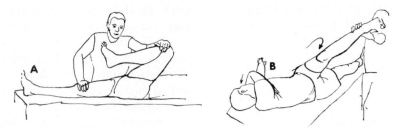

Figure 381. Sacroiliac manipulation. *A,* Forceful flexion of thigh with opposite thigh fixed. *B,* The patient fixes the upper trunk by grasping the edge of the table with the right hand while the left lower extremity is forced up into flexion and adduction, thus rotating the pelvis on the spine.

exact manipulation may vary. One of the most effective maneuvers is the forceful application of the Gaenslen test (Fig. 381, *A*) in which one thigh is sharply flexed and the other hyperextended. Another manipulation (Fig. 381, *B*) is carried out with the patient lying supine on the table. Instruct him to reach over and catch the left edge of the table with the right hand over his left shoulder. The left thigh is then grasped and with the knee in extension the thigh is flexed 45 degrees and then adducted and internally rotated. This rotates the pelvis toward the left. This maneuver can be carried out in either direction. Sometimes it is rewarded by an alarming snap and dramatic relief, but alas, most often with no result at all! Manipulation should not be attempted casually by the uninitiated and by no means under anesthesia. With the patient awake his muscular resistance will usually prevent any actual damage. However, with him relaxed under anesthesia, the leverage applied may cause serious damage to the hip or spine.

As is frequent with ligament injuries there is a tendency toward recurrence, so once the injury has been treated and the patient rehabilitated a well fitting sacroiliac belt should be worn in contact sports for the remainder of the season. It should be emphasized again that before diagnosis of sacroiliac sprain can be made the burden of proof remains with the examiner to show that the condition actually is a sacroiliac sprain and not some other injury.

Coccyx

There will occasionally be injury to the coccyx although this too is not a common injury in sports. It usually occurs by falling in a sitting position or by a blow (inadvertent) from a shoe. While this is an extremely painful injury, it is not especially disabling and usually requires no specific treatment other than local application of heat. The pain may be severe enough to prevent competition for two or three weeks. Local protection is advisable in the nature of a fiber pad, and some degree of constriction helps. Something like a panty girdle will be valuable for this purpose. A suitable pad can be inserted at the appropriate area in the girdle to give local protection. Ordinarily a moderate amount of displacement is of little importance, particularly in the male. The fracture will heal promptly.

There will occasionally be involvement of the sacrococcygeal joint by subluxation or traumatic arthritis. If pain is persistent and disabling, coccygectomy may be justified. Great care must be exercised to be sure that the coccyx is actually the seat of the trouble and that the condition is truly local. I cannot recall having removed a coccyx damaged as a result of athletic injury.

INJURIES IN THE VICINITY OF THE BUTTOCK AND PERINEUM

Contusion

The most common injury to the buttock is from a direct blow. This does not usually cause injury to the skin because of the ample underlying padding. Contusion of the muscle is a common occurrence but usually is of little consequence. In most of the areas of the buttock there is a thick muscle mass with relatively little danger of catching a muscle between two unyielding objects. As a result the condition is usually diffuse without gross hematoma formation in the muscle. A tender, painful muscle mass results which may be uncomfortable but is not actually disabling. The buttock is usually not protected in athletic competition by any padding other than that inherent in the anatomy and so superficial contusion is relatively common here. One should be wary of the condition that appears to be unduly severe or that causes other than local symptoms.

A *contusion of the sciatic nerve* may result in pain in the buttock extending down the back of the thigh into the calf and foot similar to sciatic pain from other causes. This is nonradicular in character and follows the whole distribution of the sciatic nerve rather than that of any single root. Straight leg raising causes pain in the area of the contusion. During the acute period, hyperesthesia of the skin may be evident in the lower portion of the extremity. This contusion is not frequent. The ordinary contusion of the sciatic nerve will require no particular treatment other than protection against stretch. Physical therapy may give considerable relief. A word of caution should be said about inductive heat. If deep therapy

such as short wave diathermy causes increase in the pain it should be promptly discontinued. Sometimes local tension in the nerve will be increased by congestion due to the heat. This does not ordinarily occur with the whirlpool bath or infrared radiation.

Another area of the buttock in which a complication of contusion may arise is over the ischial tuberosity. Here the bone is essentially subcutaneous although it may be protected by an overlying layer of muscle of greater or lesser thickness. A contusion here may cause a *fracture of the tuberosity* in which case there will be severe localized pain. The pain is increased by straight leg raising or by any local pressure. More commonly the result of the blow will be periostitis or fibrositis over the roughened surface of the bone. In other cases there will be involvement of the ischial bursa. It may be impossible in the early stages to distinguish between these conditions. Treatment should be local heat and rest. Usually the symptoms will subside promptly. In the case of periostitis or bursitis there will be persistent pain and extreme local tenderness. In these cases local injection into the area in an attempt to aspirate fluid from the bursa is advisable. If the bursa can be entered, injection of a steroid will often give substantial relief. If not, the area should be infiltrated with a long-acting anesthetic. Indeed, the proper corticoid may be diffused throughout the area, a soluble preparation being preferable to the suspension.

If the injury seems severe or if the symptoms persist, x-ray examination should be made. A simple anteroposterior view of the pelvis may be quite unenlightening and several views or subsequent films may be necessary (Figs. 382 and 383). The injury may occasionally result in spur formation or in calcification within the bursa (Fig. 382). If there is calcification of the bursa and if

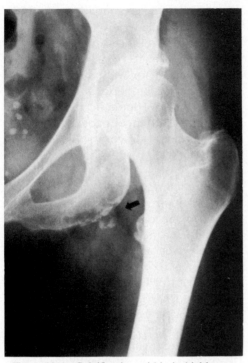

Figure 382. Calcification within ischial bursa.

this does not respond well to aspiration and local injection, surgical excision of the bursa is justified. Usually relief is prompt and complete following surgical excision. If the irritation results in ossification and spur formation which does not respond to treatment and which is constantly disabling, the spurring should be removed surgically. Completely atraumatic technique must be used. Access is readily obtained in this location placing the patient in the lithotomy position with a folded sheet beneath the sacrum. This presents the tuberosity of the ischium in its subcutaneous position. One is able to expose the tuberosity and the ascending ramus of the ischium or whatever area is primarily involved without extensive dissection. If careful attention is paid to hemostasis by proper coagulation, an extremely dry field may be obtained and the exact pathology determined. If there is bursitis, the bursa may

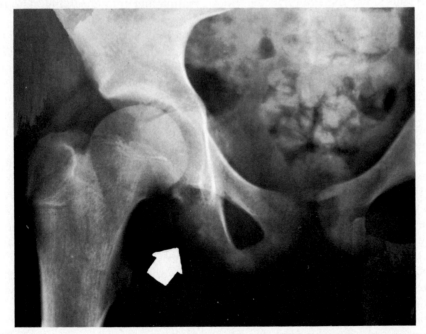

Figure 383. This 14 year old girl fell astraddle the gymnasium rail, receiving a severe perineal contusion, immediate, severe pain and disability with terrific adductor and hamstring spasm. The x-ray was negative. Three weeks post-injury it shows osteomyelitis of the ischium, the result of stagnation of blood from contusion of the bone. A high febrile course began one week post-injury, subsiding under antibiotics. The abscess later required drainage.

be readily removed and the underlying periosteum examined. If on the other hand there is irregularity of the bone or spur formation, the muscle attachments may be stripped away subperiosteally, the bone carefully smoothed off and hemostasis secured with bone wax. The incision need only be as extensive as is required for the lesion encountered.

Occasionally the ascending ramus of the ischium or descending ramus of the pubis will be injured by a direct blow such as a fall astraddle a bar. This may be an extremely painful injury but ordinarily recovery is complete without specific therapy other than local measures. This treatment should depend upon the severity of the condition. Usually cold applications followed by heat and a period at rest will suffice. In the case of serious injury, x-ray study should be made to determine possible fracture. At the time of injury the patient will feel that a major disaster has befallen him since the injury is painful and distressing—and often humiliating. He may try to avoid embarrassment over his ineptitude by appearing to be badly injured.

Injuries to the deeper structures of the perineum hardly fall into the scope of this work since they are very infrequent in athletic pursuits. Probably the most common of them is contusion from falling forcibly on a hard object, with resulting painful hematomata (Fig. 383). In injury of any consequence, careful examination should be made to be sure there is no serious damage to the underlying structures. In the male the cavernous muscles and urethra may be damaged; in the female, the vulva. Suitable consultation should be obtained from a competent urologist or gynecologist particularly if there appears to be subcutaneous bleeding or open laceration. So, also, damage to the anus and rectum may occur. If any question is

present, a rectal examination should be carried out immediately to observe local tenderness, presence of bleeding or even the presence of a palpable defect in the sphincter or wall.

In discussing perineal type injuries, one must not overlook the male genitalia. The almost universal use of the athletic supporter has been very valuable in preventing injury. Contusion is the most common type injury. The penis in its relaxed condition is soft and pliable and is seldom injured by contusion. The testicles, on the contrary, which lack the protection of the abdominal walls, hang relatively free and unprotected and are very subject to injury. Their location between the thighs gives a good deal of protection. Also, the instinctive recoil from a threatened blow serves to render the blow less severe. Nonetheless, the testicular contusion is not uncommon. However, it is not often actually damaging. The immediate pain may be excruciating and thus disabling. The rebound is rapid and disability short.

Trainers have a favorite trick in which the injured person is pulled to a sitting position. The operator grasps his hands in the patient's axillae, lifts him 10 to 12 inches off the field, then drops him hard on his buttocks. Why this is effective is hard to understand. Possibly the pain stimuli from the testicles are short circuited by the new pain stimuli from the drop.

Occasionally bruising may result with swollen, tense and painful scrotum. In this case ice packs for 24 hours followed later by whirlpool, sitz baths, and warm packs are effective. Complete recovery may be expected, although it may be hard to convince the victim of this.

Other types of injuries such as avulsions, lacerations, etc., are very uncommon and obviously will require immediate transportation to a hospital for special care. Skin conditions such as jock itch, excoriation, eczema, and furunculosis will require great care and patience. Cleanliness is imperative with the daily shower, taking care to rinse off all the soap since this in itself may be irritating. Application of some of the bland, lubricating creams will lessen the friction and the discomfort.

Strain

This same ischial area is quite subject to muscle strain (Fig. 384), a common one being strain at the origin of the long head of the biceps and the semitendinosus on the tuberosity of the ischium. This may result in avulsion of the ischial tuberosity, particularly if the epiphysis in this region is not yet closed. It usually occurs as a result of forcible flexion of the hip with the knee extended, as in the leading leg of the hurdler (Fig. 385). Extremely forceful straight leg raising is the same mecha-

nism and throws a heavy pull on the origin of the long head of the biceps. The result may be irritation at the attachment of the muscle or complete avulsion from the bone (Fig. 386). Symptoms are localized pain on pressure over the ischial tuberosity, pain on flexion of the thigh with the knee extended, and pain on active forceful contraction of the biceps muscle. X-ray examination may or may not reveal the nature of the injury.

Treatment is that of avulsion anywhere except that replacement of the avulsed fragment may not be necessary. It should be replaced if the separation is wide and complete. Immobilization of the leg with the knee flexed and avoidance of thigh flexion will usually suffice for protection. In fact, in many instances, simple elimination of forceful activity is enough. If the symptoms are persistent, local injection and physical therapy are of value. A painful nonunion of the fragment may be relieved by

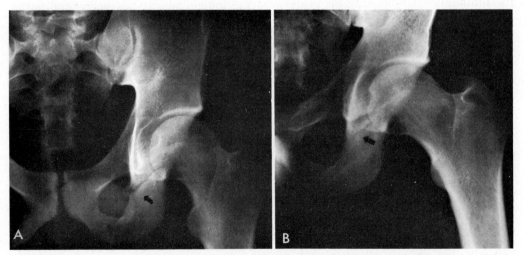

Figure 384. A 21 year old football player faked to the left. He had severe pain and fell as he cut sharply to the right. After a few days local symptoms subsided. Three months later, during a squatting exercise requiring sudden strain, he had a recurrence of the same pain in a more severe form. *A,* X-ray following the second episode showed a stress fracture across the top of the ischium with callus formation. This undoubtedly occurred at the time of the original fall. *B,* Uneventful healing four months later.

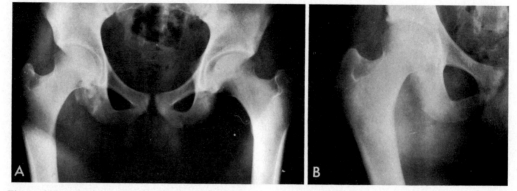

Figure 385. Avulsion of a portion of the ischium by the attachment of the biceps muscle. Following a relatively acute period of two or three weeks, subject had recurrence of pain on running or jumping. The fragment was removed and the muscle sutured to the bed with a good recovery. Recent studies have suggested that even with wide displacement firm fibrous scan may result in a normal hip. Nevertheless, I personally prefer open reduction if the displacement is marked.

  A, Preoperative. *B,* Postoperative.

removal of the fragment although this is seldom necessary. As is true of many avulsions, this one is not compatible with athletic competition. A period of rest from strenuous activity is imperative but under ordinary circumstances there will be no permanent disability. The same surgical technique may be used here as indicated above for ischial bursitis. In some instances, however, the lithotomy position may be inadvisable because it may overstretch the hamstrings. This can usually be minimized by extending the thigh somewhat from the acutely flexed position. The same approach can be utilized with the patient lying prone with a large pillow under the pelvis of the involved side and with the knee flexed.

A straddling injury caused by forceful abduction of the thighs may cause damage to the adductor muscles. They are particularly vulnerable at their attachments to the ischiopubic rami. Following this type of injury the symptoms are readily recognizable since there will be localized tenderness along the subcutaneous edge of the ramus and to the lateral side. The diagnostic test is pain on forceful passive abduction of the thigh and on active adduction against

resistance, each of which causes pain localized at the origin of these muscles along the puboischium. This same force will occasionally cause avulsion of one of the adductors, usually the adductor longus (Fig. 387), in which case the symptoms are more pronounced and there may be a palpable defect between the bone and the muscle belly. I have seen instances in the athlete in which the longus muscle has been ruptured at a distance from the insertion, usually about 2 inches from the attachment of the pelvis. This may simulate a contusion and is often difficult to distinguish from it. If the condition can be recognized, prompt surgical repair of the rupture of the attachment or muscle is indicated. Detachment or rupture may be recognized by the bunching up of the adductor longus muscle a short distance away from the pelvis and by a tender, firm mass which is more noticeable on active adduction of the thigh against resistance. If several weeks have passed, any attempt at repair is doomed to failure because of the inability to get secure enough suture within the muscle substance to overcome the shortening of the muscle. In this instance the condition should be carefully explained to the patient, pointing out that the mass is of no consequence in itself. In most instances the athlete will accept this without insistence on further treatment. Should the pain be persistent and to some extent disabling, late surgery may be justified. At this time the fibromuscular mass should be removed and the remaining muscle belly sutured to the adjoining adductor magnus. An injury of this severity is rather unusual but prompt relief may be obtained by definitive treatment. It is important to point out to the athlete that this treatment will not add to his muscular strength or ability or agility but is simply designed to relieve his pain.

As indicated above, by far the most common injury is a strain at the muscle attachment. In this instance the symptoms are similar to this condition anywhere and are relieved by the same measures. If the patient is seen immediately after the injury there may be some

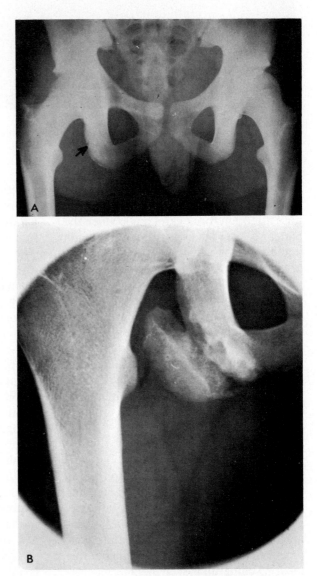

Figure 386. *A*, A high school baseball pitcher who injured his kick-off leg while throwing left-handed. He had pain and soreness but was able to complete the game during which the injury occurred, pitching a one-hitter. Subsequently he was unable to play. Now (eight weeks later) his recovery is proceeding well. The injury represents an avulsion of the attachment of the semitendinosus.

B, An 18 year old boy two years after a skating injury that remained untreated. The x-ray shows tremendous overgrowth of displaced ischial epiphysis. Removal of excess bone and repair of the tendon to the ischium was advised to relieve the symptomatic condition.

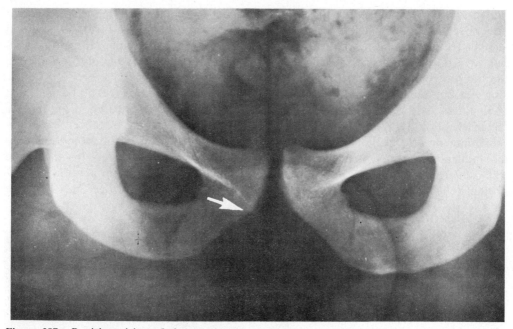

Figure 387. Partial avulsion of the attachment of the adductor longus and gracilis from the pubic ramus. This gave chronic recurrent pain and terminated a player's basketball season. Local injection and physical therapy relieved the symptoms.

virtue in application of cold. Ordinarily the symptoms are not called to the doctor's attention for several days, when the patient is seen because of persistent pain and discomfort. At this time local measures should consist of local injection with long-acting anesthetic and a corticoid preparation, application of heat by sitz baths, whirlpool, diathermy and rest. Injudicious exercise in an attempt to improve the range of abduction will only prolong the symptoms. Constant effort should be made to avoid forcible abduction of the involved thigh (Fig. 388).

Pubic Symphysis

Damage to the pubic symphysis is not frequent except in major accidents involving the pelvis. However, one may get a painful contusion over the subcutaneous anterior surface of the symphysis. This may result in considerable local swelling and even hematoma for-

mation but it is not a dangerous or crippling injury. We have recently seen a girl who fell heavily forward on her mons pubis while ice skating (Fig. 389). The result was the prompt development of a hematoma the size of a small orange which was alarming and distressing to the patient. The actual disability, however, was minimal, the pain being present only on direct pressure. Because of the unsightly swelling, an attempt was made to aspirate it. This was unsuccessful because of infiltration of blood through the fibrofatty pad and ultimately it was necessary for the gynecologist to evacuate the hematoma. This case is mentioned particularly since the condition may seem quite alarming and drastic remedies may appear in order whereas it is a relatively superficial hematoma and ordinarily will respond to the local measures used for hematoma.

In the adolescent the pubic symphysis is not nearly as firmly fixed as it is in the adult and sprain of the liga-

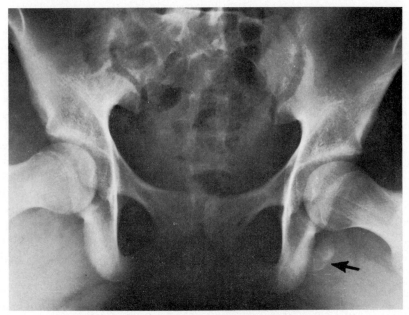

Figure 388.   This 14 year old girl was learning a new dance step when she did an anteroposterior split with immediate, severe pain in the buttock with disability. X-ray revealed complete avulsion of the semitendinosus origin. Treatment by surgical replacement of the fragment resulted in complete recovery.

ments connecting the two pubic bones can occur by forceful abduction of both thighs. This must be distinguished from a contusion which is considerably more common since, in a strain of the pubic ligaments, the force applied is one that separates the pubic bones rather than a direct blow to the local area. The treatment is quite different in the two instances since the treatment in sprain of the pubic ligaments must be designed to hold the pelvic ring together and to prevent wide abduction of the thighs. This can be accomplished by circumferential adhesive strapping or by a well-fitted lumbosacral corset. Early treatment should consist of local injection, application of heat and rest. As with any

sprain, several weeks are required for healing, and protection should be continued for many weeks, particularly if there is participation in any sport that causes tension on these ligaments, such as horseback riding or water skiing. The prognosis is quite favorable if the condition is recognized and treated adequately.

INJURIES IN THE VICINITY OF THE GROIN

Contusion

In this area we find the tunnel formed by the bridging of the anterior pelvis by Poupart's ligament, which

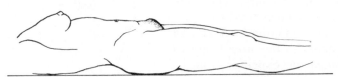

Figure 389.   Injury of the mons pubis by a fall on the ice, with resulting hematoma.

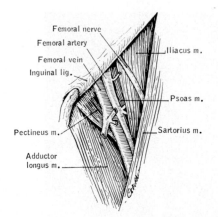

Figure 390. Note compartment formed by the inguinal ligament above, the iliopsoas laterally, adductors medially, the compartment housing the femoral artery, vein and nerve. The sartorius and rectus attach to the anterosuperior spine whereas the adductor muscles attach along the pubic ramus. Note also how the psoas and iliacus blend to form the iliopsoas tendon which attaches to the lesser trochanter of the femur. (From Anson, Atlas of Human Anatomy.)

runs from the pubis across to the anterior superior spine on either side (Fig. 390). Under this ligament pass the vascular sheath, the femoral nerve, the inguinal canal, the cord and some muscle groups, particularly the iliopsoas. A direct blow over this area may cause damage to any of these structures. This is ordinarily not severe but may be relatively painful. It may cause a few minutes or hours of disability, then go on to a good and complete recovery.

Permanent vascular damage after a blow to the groin is infrequent. Traumatic phlebitis and even phlebothrombosis from a direct blow over the femoral vein are possibilities. Trauma to the femoral nerve may cause paresthesia along the front of the thigh which is worrisome to the patient but of little significance from the standpoint of disability. The well-trained athlete has been taught to protect his abdomen and groin by flexion of the thigh so injury in this area is not as frequent as might be expected from its relatively exposed position.

Strain

Muscular strain in this area is relatively frequent, the most frequent being *strain of the iliopsoas tendon*. This may occur at its attachment to the lesser trochanter of the femur or in the musculotendinous junction. It is not caused by a direct blow to the groin but by overactive contraction of the iliopsoas when the thigh is flexed and then forced into extension. The patient complains of severe pain in the groin and holds the thigh in a flexed, adducted and externally rotated position. Any attempt of the examiner to extend or to internally rotate the thigh causes severe pain. So does active contraction of the iliopsoas muscle. Tenderness will be found at the area of the injury. If it is at the lesser trochanteric attachment the tenderness will be below the groin, along the upper anteromedial aspect of the thigh. Careful x-ray study should be made of the lesser trochanter to determine whether there has been an avulsion of the bone (Fig. 391). This is particularly true in the adolescent in

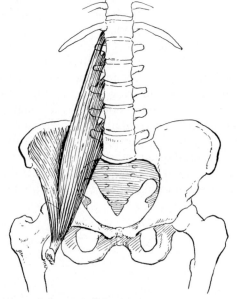

Figure 391. Avulsion of the lesser trochanter.

whom the epiphysis of the lesser trochanter has not united with the shaft. Even if the avulsion is complete surgical repair is rarely indicated. The trochanter reattaches with fibrous union and usually is not painful. Protection should be carried out by immobilization with the thigh flexed and externally rotated. If a painful union occurs, the attachment of the iliopsoas tendon to the lesser tuberosity may be transferred to the anterior femur. If the lesion is incomplete, as it most frequently is, treatment should be by bed rest with the thigh flexed and externally rotated with application of cold compresses in the early stage followed by local heat. After a few days, better determination can be made as to the severity of the injury. Duration of treatment will depend upon the symptoms. This is an extremely disabling condition since any effort to run or jump causes excessive strain on this tendon, with resultant pain. The patient's athletic endeavors must be terminated for whatever period is required for the symptoms to subside, usually several weeks.

Because of the complexity of the various flexors of the hip, it is sometimes difficult to determine whether or not complete avulsion of the tendon has occurred. In case of persistent pain with chronic irritation, treatment by local injection into the tender area may be tried. This area is relatively inaccessible and skillful manipulation of the needle is needed to reach the involved area. The iliopsoas is an important flexor of the thigh and complete recovery is necessary before unrestricted function can be permitted. Strapping that holds the thigh in slight flexion will prevent overstretching of the muscle but does not prevent overactivity and so is relatively ineffectual. Plaster fixation is ordinarily not necessary since the thigh readily assumes the position of flexion which puts the muscle at rest. This position is all too often held even after the lesion has

healed so that troublesome flexion contracture of the thigh may be the result. In order to minimize this danger the patient should be encouraged to extend the thigh actively within the limits of pain several times each day. After the acute symptoms subside a daily period spent lying prone in bed is desirable.

Also susceptible to damage in this area is the abdominal muscle group which attaches along Poupart's ligament. Strain of these muscles must be treated by rest, heat and protection — the same type of treatment necessary for similar injury along the iliac crest. Occasionally there will be a painful strain of the conjoined tendon of the abdominals at the attachment to the pubis at the inner end of Poupart's ligament.

Great care must be taken to eliminate other conditions which may be present in this general area such as hernia, involvement of the spermatic cord, lymphadenitis, and phlebitis, since all of these conditions may well become symptomatic after trauma or overactivity. In case of doubt treatment should be essentially the same except that no injection should be carried out.

INJURIES IN THE VICINITY OF THE TROCHANTER

Contusion

The significant area of contusion in the vicinity of the hip is over the trochanter. In this area the bony trochanter is covered only by the trochanteric bursa, the iliotibial tract and the skin. The tract is separated from the trochanter by the trochanteric bursa, which is a constant structure of considerable size lying beneath the muscle and tendon of the tensor fasciae femoris. Contusion may result in damage to the muscle or to the bursa. The symptoms are the same as in contusion elsewhere and the treatment presents no unusual elements.

A trochanteric *bursitis* may be caused here by a direct blow, by infection or by friction between the adjacent bursal walls. In many instances contusion of the trochanter may result in bursitis and the symptoms will gradually change from those of a contusion to those of involvement of the bursa. In this instance there will be tenderness over the trochanteric area with pain on forcible activity of the thigh. In the course of flexion and extension of the hip or of rotation of the extended thigh, the tensor fasciae femoris slides backward and forward over the trochanter and in the presence of an inflammatory reaction this will cause pain.

On examination there is local tenderness over the bursa often with crepitation on motion. Pain is elicited by adducting the thigh with the knee extended to put the tensor under strain as it passes over the trochanter. In this position, internal and external rotation of the extremity will cause the trochanter to slide back and forth under the tight tensor and pain will be caused on this maneuver which would not be present with a simple contusion.

The so-called snapping hip should be mentioned in this connection. This is due to chronic bursitis with thickening of the bursal walls and spasm of the tensor so that on each step, as the tensor slides back and forth over the trochanter, an audible and palpable snap will occur. This is quite distressing. The condition is much more common in girls, since they have wide pelves and prominent trochanters and the tensor bows over the trochanter at a more acute angle than in the narrower pelvis of the male. X-ray examination is ordinarily of little value although it may occasionally show calcification within the bursa.

Treatment of the acute bursitis is by rest and local heat. Early injection of a local anesthetic into the bursa may give prompt relief. There is a decided tendency toward recurrence and, in the occasional case with chronic recurring bursitis resistant to treatment, excision of the bursa may be necessary. If the chronic bursitis is accompanied by a snapping tensor tendon or by undue tension between the tensor and the trochanter at the time of operation, it will be advisable either to divide the tensor and make suitable repair or to shift it anteriorly or posteriorly. The indication for this operation is extremely uncommon in the male but is relatively frequent in the female although not ordinarily as the result of athletic injury.

The technique for surgery will not be described in detail here other than to say that the whole aim of surgery is to release the tension on the tensor fascia femoris muscle in the iliotibial tract so that it will not be snapping back and forth over the trochanter. This can be done by division of half of the band, transferring it either posteriorly or anteriorly so that on ordinary stride the band does not snap over the trochanter. This is probably preferable to the operation which divides the iliotibial tract, since the tract does have a definite function in the thigh which may be handicapped to some degree by this transection.

Strain

There may be strain of the muscles attaching to the trochanter, particularly the gluteus medius (Fig. 392). This is ordinarily caused by overactivity of the gluteus medius and is usually chronic rather than acute. Symptoms in such a case will be pain on active contraction of the gluteus medius against resistance.

Functional tests are of considerable importance here in finding the exact muscle involved, since active use of the muscle should not cause pain if the in-

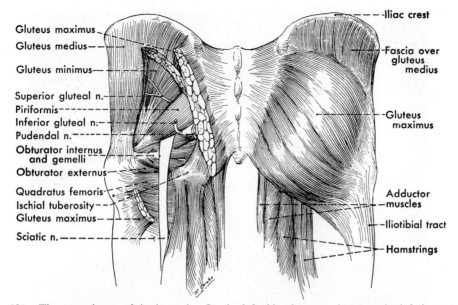

Figure 392. The musculature of the buttocks. On the left side, the space between the inferior gemellus and quadratus femoris is exaggerated so that the insertion of the obturator externus can be shown. (From Anson, Atlas of Human Anatomy.)

volvement is in the bursa alone. To examine the abductors, have the patient lie on his side and actively elevate the leg, putting stress on the gluteus medius and the other adductors. In particular, if this is done against resistance it will be painful. Passive motion through this same arc with the muscles relaxed will be pain-free.

Similarly if it is the external rotators which attach at the back of the trochanter that are involved, pain will be elicited when the thigh is actively externally rotated against resistance, whereas passive external rotation without resistance will not be painful. In order to distinguish injuries to the psoas muscle from other conditions in the groin, flexing the thigh against resistance, particularly flexion and external rotation, will cause pain, whereas passive movement will not. In a similar manner one can determine a suitable test for any muscle which will serve to determine whether the trouble is in the muscle itself or somewhere else. Forced passive motion beyond normal range in any of these directions will cause pain on the opposer. In other words, forcible, passive adduction of the thigh may cause pain in the abductor muscle. Forced internal rotation may cause pain on the external rotator. Forced external rotation may cause pain on the internal rotator, and so forth.

Such contraction will not cause pain if the involvement is of the bursa alone. Similarly, a tendinitis of the rotators of the hip joint attaching along the posterior margin of the trochanter will cause local tenderness at the area of their attachment, with pain on active external rotation or passive forceful internal rotation of the hip. These conditions are treated by local heat, some sort of inductive heat being necessary to reach the area of involvement (diathermy or microtherm). Local injection is relatively simple here and the use of a long-acting local anesthetic plus a suitable

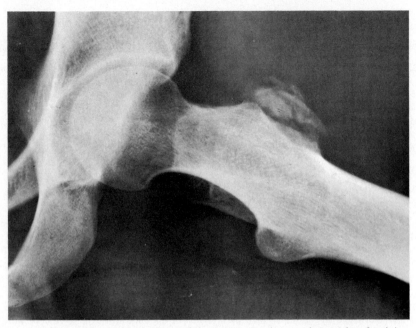

Figure 393. Avulsion of the anterior portion of the greater trochanter six months after injury with nonunion.

corticoid frequently will give very good results.

In the adolescent in whom the greater trochanteric epiphysis is not united with the shaft, an *avulsion* (Figs. 393 and 394), complete or partial, of the trochanteric epiphysis is not infrequent. This is a relatively serious injury and analogous to complete avulsion of the tendon attachment. If the avulsion is incomplete and the epiphyseal plate appears to be only a little bit wide it should be treated by immobilization with the thigh in abduction and slight external rotation. This position is maintained at least six weeks and activity is resumed gradually. If the avulsion is complete it should be treated by surgical replacement and fixation by a long wood screw or similar appliance. The same treatment is advisable if the trochanter is broken and displaced. Following firm internal fixation, support is needed only during the period of wound healing but athletic activity should be eliminated for at least six weeks.

INJURIES TO THE HIP JOINT PROPER

From an orthopaedic standpoint and indeed from the standpoint of the traumatic surgeon, the hip is extremely liable to injury. Fortunately athletic injury to the hip joint is almost a rarity, in contrast to the knee, which is highly vulnerable. Owing to the extremely free motion of the hip joint, sprain of the ligaments of the hip is very uncommon. Strain of the muscles and tendons about the hip has been discussed previously and nothing needs to be added here.

Fracture and Dislocation

Fracture about the hip is unusual in the adolescent and young adult. The bone is exceptionally resilient and the hip is much more likely to dislocate than it is to break. For this reason we may see a *dislocation* of the hip in an athlete although fortunately it is a great rarity.

If it occurs, it is obviously a major injury and should be treated as a medical emergency. The patient is completely disabled at once. He has severe pain in the hip and resists any attempt to manipulate the limb. The extremity is usually held with the thigh internally rotated and adducted with the knee resting above and against its fellow on the opposite side (Fig. 395). The trochanter appears quite prominent. Any attempt to move the thigh from this position of flexion adduction and internal rotation causes severe pain. Diagnosis is confirmed by x-ray and the film should be carefully studied to be sure there is not an accompanying fracture. This is quite infrequent in youth. The posterior acetabular margin, which is so vulnerable in the adult, is seldom broken in the adolescent or young adult.

No attempt should be made to reduce the hip on the field. The patient should be taken immediately for x-ray examination, after which the dislocation must be reduced *under anesthesia* and *at the earliest possible moment.* While these two requirements may seem incompatible they are vital and there is good reason for both. The most important complication of dislocation of the hip is aseptic necrosis of the head of the femur. It has been shown definitely that the frequency and degree of aseptic necrosis of the head varies in direct proportion to the length of time the hip has remained displaced. Even minutes are of vital importance prior to complete reduction. On the other hand, experience has shown that it is virtually impossible to reduce a complete dislocation of the hip without profound relaxation and any effort to do so may cause considerable damage to the vulnerable cartilage of the femoral head.

A third consideration is that it seems unwise to attempt reduction of the dislocated hip until one can be rea-

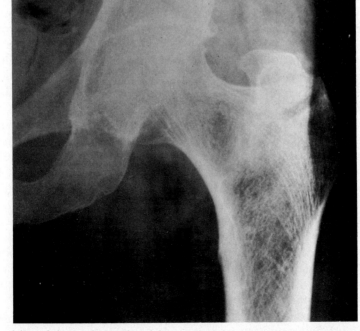

Figure 394. Avulsion of the trochanter by violent, active abduction against resistance. This minimally displaced fragment held without surgery. This is borderline for internal fixation.

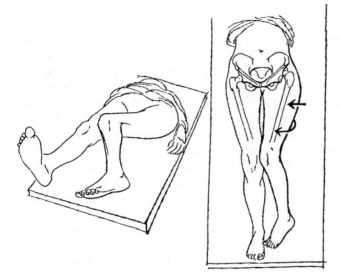

Figure 395. Drawing showing patient with dislocated hip. Note that the leg is shortened, internally rotated, adducted, with tendency to rest the affected foot on top of the opposite foot, with prominence of the greater trochanter laterally. (From DePalma, The Management of Fractures and Dislocations.)

sonably sure there is no other injury such as would be demonstrated by x-ray examination. Clinical examination must be made to determine whether the sciatic nerve has been damaged before and after reduction. It is very distressing to discover a nerve deficit that may or may not have preceded the manipulation. In spite of the patient's discomfort, a few simple movements of the foot will demonstrate an intact nerve. If active motions in plantar flexion, toe flexion and inversion are present, the tibial portion of the nerve is not severed. If the patient can actively dorsiflex and evert the foot, the peroneal division is intact. A rudimentary sensory check may also be made. If the nerve seems completely afunctional and remains so after reduction, an early exploration is advisable since the traumatized area of the nerve may be readily exposed by the posterior approach. On the other hand, if the lesion is incomplete or if the deficit develops gradually, one may safely assume that the injury is a contusion and compression rather than severance. In that case watchful waiting is the best treatment. The deficit may recover in a few days, or a few weeks. If there has

not been definite improvement within three months the sciatic nerve should be explored. During the waiting period it is important to protect drop foot or knee flexion by a suitable brace (Fig. 396). I should like to emphasize that if loss of sciatic function is complete and immediate, surgical exploration must not be delayed more than three weeks.

Following dislocation of the hip it is imperative that the hip be immobilized for sufficient time to permit the capsule to heal. There seems little justification for overly prolonged denial of weight bearing, however. It has been recommended in the past that weight bearing should not be permitted for at least six months in the hope that aseptic necrosis will not develop. Studies have shown conclusively that the die is cast by the time the hip is reduced, that weight bearing itself is not a factor in the development of aseptic necrosis. Immobilization should be continued for four to six weeks and then active rehabilitation encouraged. Active participation in sports should not be permitted for at least three months following a complete dislocation of the hip.

It must be obvious that there are

cases in which the hip dislocation is incomplete and goes unrecognized. The head either does not entirely leave the socket or is spontaneously reduced. The true pathology can be very easily overlooked. The patient usually complains of immediate severe pain at the time of the injury which promptly subsides, and at the time of the examination there may be essentially no positive findings. Explanation for the lack of symptoms rests in the fact that by examination of the hip joint it is very difficult to strain the ligaments of the hip. In the normal hip, subluxation or dislocation cannot occur without laceration of the capsule. This usually occurs posterosuperiorly. This capsular tear is not put under stress by ordinary manipulation of the hip. The significance of this condition is that if one can be reasonably sure subluxation has occurred, the hip should be put at rest for a period of about six to eight weeks in order to permit the capsular tear to repair (Fig. 397). If it does not repair or if it repairs with redundancy, this may well be the cause of repeated episodes of incomplete dislocation of the hip. A diagnosis of incomplete dislocation of the hip is extremely uncommon, especially in the athlete, but it is probable that many such cases are not diagnosed.

In the adolescent with an unfused capital femoral epiphysis there is occasionally a fracture through the epiphyseal plate (Fig. 398). This is a serious injury and requires adequate treatment. The symptoms of this injury, if the displacement is complete, are those of a fracture of the femoral neck. There will be severe pain in the hip, shortening of the extremity, external rotation, and abduction of the thigh. However, the dislocation is frequently not complete and this characteristic position will not be assumed. It possibly may even resemble that of dislocation of the hip, another reason for careful x-ray study before any manipulative measure is carried out. If this is an acute traumatic dislocation of the epiphysis, it should be treated as a fracture of the femoral neck with reduction and internal fixation. If this is to be successful it must be done within days, not weeks. The displaced epiphysis fixes very early to the neck. The force necessary to break it loose and so permit reduction will very likely damage the epiphysis and cause necrosis. Therefore, in *no* case should such force be used.

Special Conditions

A related condition for which one must be on guard is a *slipped capital femoral epiphysis* (Fig. 399). An apparently minor injury may be the precipitating cause of the slipping and careful study should be made in any case of injury about the hip to determine whether there is damage involving the epiphysis or epiphyseal plate. The treatment of slipped femoral epiphysis may be quite different from that of acute epiphyseal fracture. In any of these conditions about the hip, time is of the essence. If the diagnosis is uncertain, consultation should be sought at the earliest possible

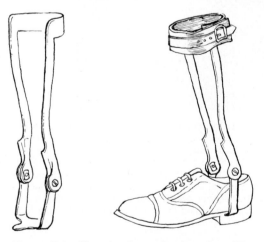

Figure 396. Short leg brace for drop foot. The spring is included in the Klenzak joint.

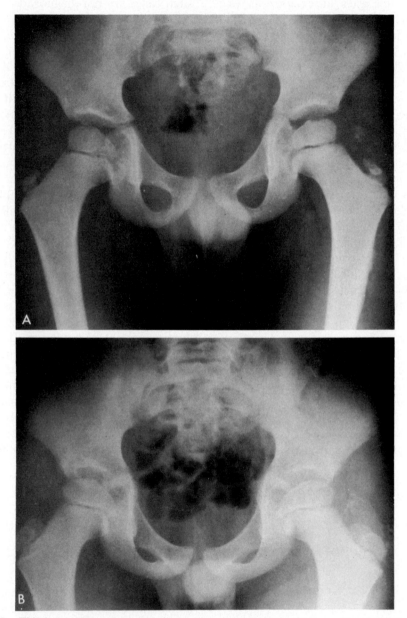

Figure 397. This interesting patient was sent in at the age of four with synovitis of the hip and a history of having had an injury to his hip the year before. It was extremely painful and sore. Perthes' disease seemed one possibility but x-rays at that time were read as negative. He seemed to improve but a year later began to limp again. *A*, X-ray at that time showed calcification within the capsule. No specific treatment was recommended other than to keep it under observation. Six months later the boy's mother called to say he was again having trouble. *B*, X-ray at this time showed increased calcification. The caput looked normal and there was no real derangement of the hip. Inadequate support had resulted in an increase of calcification within the capsule. One year later the calcification looked the same and he had no symptoms. No treatment was recommended.

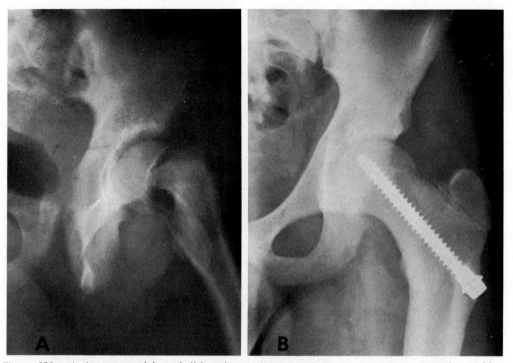

Figure 398. *A*, An acute epiphyseal dislocation analogous to fracture of the neck of the femur. Note that this patient has none of the stigmata of slipped femoral epiphysis.

B, Uneventful healing followed reduction and fixation with a Lorenzo screw. The screw was used to avoid undue trauma to the head which could result from driving in a nail. Multiple threaded pins are probably preferable to the Lorenzo screw. This picture was at one year, but the epiphysis had closed by four months after the fixation.

moment since disaster with loss of function of the hip frequently results from delayed diagnosis.

Slipped capital femoral epiphysis is most likely to happen in the Fröhlich type individual who has excessive deposits of subcutaneous fat together with delay in development of sex characteristics as indicated by the infantile penis and the underdeveloped testicles. In such an individual one's index of suspicion should be extremely high if there is pain in either the hip or knee. Very frequently hip pain is referred to the knee, whereas the knee may be entirely negative. Careful study of the lateral hip x-ray as indicated in Figure 399 will be rewarding since the slip is most often detected in the lateral view. If the slip can be detected at this early stage as

illustrated in Figure 399, adequate internal fixation without manipulation will result in excellent function of the hip. On the other hand if the injury is acute and displacement is more marked and there have been no symptoms prior to this, cautious manipulation may be attempted to reduce the displaced epiphysis in the course of which the hip is rotated into internal rotation and abduction. If this manipulation without force successfully reduces the displacement, the caput should be held by internal fixation with some type of screw, such as Hagey pins, in order to avoid trauma to the femoral head by pounding one of the various types of nails. In this type of individual, namely, the Fröhlich type, prophylactic fixation of the opposite hip by some sort of screw fixation is appropriate

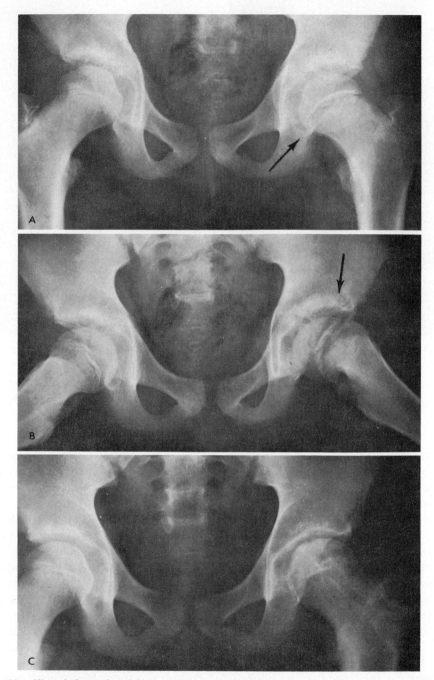

Figure 399. Slipped femoral epiphysis. *A,* In the anteroposterior view the lesion is readily overlooked. *B,* In the lateral view the degree of slipping on the left side is revealed. (Note the osteochondritis dissecans of the acetabular roof on the same side.) *C,* One year after reduction and internal fixation with premature closure of the epiphysis. The osteochondritis dissecans has healed. It is too early to be sure that circulatory changes in the head will not occur, and this area should be observed.

because of the high incidence of bilateral involvement and because prophylactic pinning almost always results in a normal hip, whereas if one waits until the head has slipped off it is very difficult to ever really approach normal again. In any event a youngster with such a problem should be carefully checked by a competent orthopaedist who may be able to prevent extreme and permanent disability in the hip.

Involvement of the acetabulum is not frequent in the athlete. Although chondral fractures can occur along the margin of the acetabulum, it is much more likely that the fragments seen in the x-ray are developmental. Careful study should be made of both hips before diagnosis is made of fracture of the rim of the acetabulum.

Osteochondritis dissecans (Figs. 399, *B,* and 400) is infrequent in the acetabulum or in the femoral head, or at least it is infrequently diagnosed. Even in a joint permitting ready x-ray visualization, such as the knee or ankle, os-

teochondritis dissecans may be extremely difficult to recognize. In the hip it is doubly difficult, not only because of the depth of the joint surrounded by soft tissue but because of the fact that the head is enclosed within the acetabulum and there is superimposition of bone. Special x-ray studies may be required such as stereoscopic pictures or laminograms. If x-ray study shows a specific lesion in the acetabular roof or the femoral head, careful analysis must be made as to whether this is really the cause of this patient's disability. If it is, surgical intervention may be indicated, but in the vast majority of cases non-surgical treatment will result in restoration of the configuration of the acetabulum and the femoral head.

The hip joint is frequently subject to *traumatic synovitis.* It appears that effusion of the hip is more common than is recognized since it is rather difficult to determine whether there is actual distention of the hip capsule by fluid. One infrequently makes the diagnosis of syn-

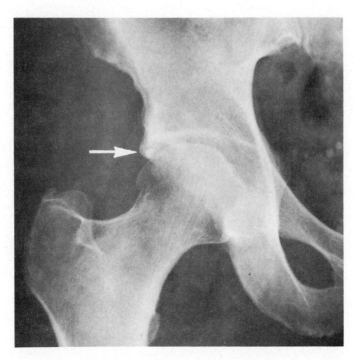

Figure 400. Typical osteochondritis dissecans of superior portion of the acetabulum. The osteocartilaginous fragment is surrounded by a radiolucent area.

ovitis of the hip. This again is probably due to the fact that the hip itself has such freedom of motion that it is not subject to the same forces that damage the knee and ankle. Many cases of limping and undiagnosed painful hips are very probably due to synovitis. In such a case diminution of activity or even complete rest is indicated. This condition may be very distressing because the patient has minimal symptoms, yet the symptoms may persist for a long time. It is hard to keep reassuring the parents that nothing is seriously wrong and that the condition will ultimately subside. If it is persistent and disabling, aspiration of the hip may be rewarding. A culture can be made of the fluid obtained from the hip joint, and if low grade infection is determined by the laboratory report, specific antibiotic treatment may be of considerable benefit. This condition is relatively common in the pre-teenage group and fortunately almost always resolves without any major interference except just careful observation.

CHAPTER 17

INJURIES OF THE THIGH

This chapter covers the thigh proper. Injuries in the vicinity of the knee and hip are discussed under the appropriate heading elsewhere. Anatomically the thigh consists of a single bone completely surrounded by very heavy muscle. One would expect the common injuries to be concerned with the muscle and such is the case. Injuries to the skin are not frequent in the thigh since the skin is well protected by the resilient muscle pad beneath.

CONTUSION

Contusion of the thigh is a frequent injury in contact sports such as football since the thigh often receives the brunt of the collision between participants. The thigh is extremely well suited for this, however, since its thick muscle surrounding smooth bone can absorb a tremendous amount of impact without apparent damage. Ironically, contusion of the muscle is often caused by the edge of the misplaced thigh pad which is designed to protect the anterior part of the thigh from a direct blow. The thigh pad should be firmly strapped in place.

The *symptoms* of contusion of the thigh are much less localized than in the more subcutaneous areas. The patient is usually not disabled at the time of the blow. He is able to continue playing but at the end of the contest complains of aching and soreness within the muscle. There is disability and pain on passive stretching of the muscle involved. By far the most frequent area of involvement is in some portion of the quadriceps, usually the lateralis or intermedius. The rectus is less frequently involved in a contusion since it is protected by the muscles beneath it.

Upon *examination,* diffuse tenderness along the anterior and lateral portion of the thigh may sometimes be accompanied by muscle spasm, elicited by deep palpation. A point of sharply localized tenderness is not commonly present. Partial flexion or extension of the knee is not particularly painful but forced flexion beyond a right angle will cause tension in the swollen muscle fibers and some distress. Active extension of the knee against firm resistance may cause rather minor and undramatic discomfort. Some degree of hematoma is probably present in any contusion of the muscle although the bleeding may be more in the nature of an infiltration in the muscle than of pooled blood. An actual hematoma of the thigh, unless it is quite extensive, can be diagnosed only with extreme difficulty, because it is so deep-seated.

505

Treatment will depend upon the severity of the lesion, and the same principles apply here as in other areas. If there seems to be infiltration of blood or hematoma formation, an attempt at aspiration under aseptic precautions is justifiable. The area is then infiltrated with several ampules of hyaluronidase and a firm pressure bandage is applied. The bandage may be very snug and firm on the thigh of the athlete. If there is some concern about swelling distal to the pressure bandage, the bandage may be started at the toe, run to the knee and then applied with increased pressure above the knee. After the application of the compression bandage the thigh should be carefully packed in ice and the extremity elevated and immobilized by bed rest. Since infiltration of the thigh may be quite extensive, I consider it important to encourage absorption of the blood by local injection of hyaluronidase into the immediate area. Intramuscular injection of an enzyme, 1 cc. for two or three days, is of value. Following this an oral enzyme is used. There is a wide divergence of opinion as to the value of these enzymes since a controlled series is hard to come by and each of us is inclined to judge by his own experience. I believe they help materially and use them freely where blood infiltration is a factor.

Examination the following morning will give good insight into the extent of involvement. If the thigh is tense, swollen and quite painful, immobilization should be continued along with the pressure bandage. After 48 hours, heat should be substituted for cold on the assumption that any active bleeding has stopped and increased circulation is desirable. The degree of immobilization will depend entirely upon the location and extent of the area involved. A good rule of thumb is that no motion should be permitted which is painful. While the patient is in bed simple elastic compression is adequate. When he is allowed to get up one should immobilize the knee by cotton cast or other similar type dressing until the acute stage of the contusion and hematoma has passed.

Rehabilitation is extremely important and should progress as rapidly as possible but within the limits of pain. There is no excuse for forcible stretching of a contused muscle unless muscle healing is complete. On the other hand, the quadriceps muscle normally extends functionally from its resting position so that gentle active flexion of the knee up to the limit of pain does not necessarily put any stress on the injured area and will aid immeasurably in rehabilitation. *There is no place for massage in the early treatment of contusion of a muscle.* The so-called "working it out" or "rubbing it out" simply increases the damage. On the other hand, after healing has progressed for 10 to 14 days massage may be used as a rehabilitative measure, again within the limits of discomfort. A major problem in management is the contusion of lesser extent. The player is anxious to continue his competition and practice and one is hesitant to hold him out when he contends he can use the muscle quite well. Critical judgment is important since a short period of complete inactivity will usually pay dividends in the long run.

MYOSITIS OSSIFICANS

The thigh is particularly prone to myositis ossificans. In my opinion this is due to the fact that the symptoms of muscle injury are often so mild that the player is allowed use of the muscle much beyond the limit set by his injury. This results in chronic irritation in the injured muscle with the reparative response of ossification. Some degree of ossification is extremely frequent and I am sure this is increased by unwise early treatment.

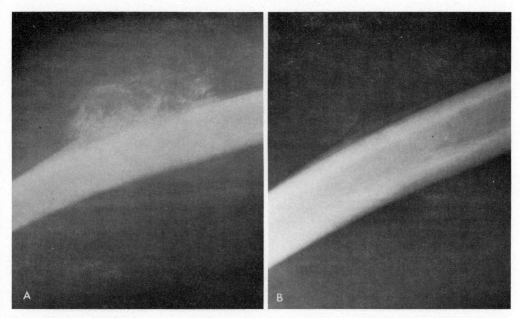

Figure 401. *A,* Ossification in the quadriceps lateralis. *B,* Shows it spontaneously regressed and disappearing. The patient was immobilized for six weeks after which gradually increasing, pain-free exercises were instituted. He had complete recovery.

Treatment. Overenthusiastic massage to "knead out the knotted muscle," forceful passive flexion of the knee, too early active use of the quadriceps, intensive exercise—all are important aggravating factors. Myositis ossificans in the thigh is not necessarily disabling when only a small plaque of bone is present in the muscle. However, it can be and frequently is extremely disabling and the mass may reach an amazing size (Figs. 401 and 402). Once ossification occurs in contusion, the management requires even more patience than before.

Rehabilitation may progress within the limits of pain but manipulation under anesthesia and similar measures are to be condemned (see Chapter 22 on Rehabilitation). *It can be stated unequivocally that early surgical removal of the mass of bone simply invites recurrence and magnifies the extent of the lesion itself and also the extent of disability.* This has been demonstrated too often to require further substantiation

(Fig. 403). If the plaque requires removal because of disability it should be excised only after the lesion is completely mature as demonstrated by clinical findings and x-ray examination. Six months is a minimum and frequently a longer time is needed, particularly if overtreatment has been carried out in the interim. At the proper time, with the proper care, operative excision is extremely gratifying (Figs. 404, 405 and 406).

At operation, an adequate incision that will expose the entire mass to view must be made so that it can be removed without the necessity of scraping, curetting, etc. The mass is not ordinarily covered with periosteum so I do not believe it necessary to carry out sharp dissection leaving the capsule attached to the bone. This does not apply when the parent bone is reached and great care should be taken not to strip the periosteum away from the femur as the mass is detached from the femoral shaft. The location of the lesion will determine the approach and one should fit the ap-

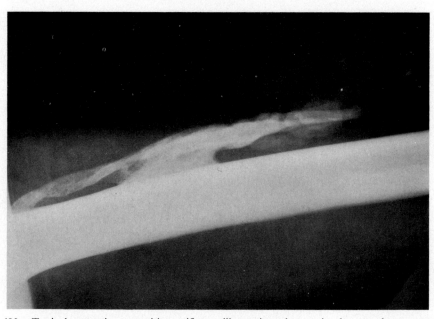

Figure 402. Typical extensive myositis ossificans illustrating plaques in the muscle separated from bone. This case was treated by complete excision of the plaque with some slight recurrence of the mass. This is quite likely to happen in an area which is this extensive.

proach to the lesion, not the lesion to the approach. We recently removed a mass from the anteromedial aspect of the femur (Fig. 407). This was readily removed by an anterior approach whereas it would have been extremely difficult, if not impossible, to handle adequately by the more stereotyped anterolateral approaches. Atraumatic surgery in these conditions is extremely important.

After the incision is made through the skin, meticulous hemostasis is obtained by electrocautery. A very careful atraumatic approach through the intervening muscle mass is important. If it is at all possible, the penetration should be muscle-splitting rather than muscle-dividing. The division of a muscle, if it must be done, should be by sharp dissection obtaining careful hemostasis as the operation proceeds. Care is taken to coagulate only the vessels and not a great deal of the muscle mass. The method of making a small buttonhole

through the muscle and then proceeding to tear it open by so-called blunt dissection is to be condemned. In this method an index finger is placed at each extremity of the wound and the muscle is forcibly pulled apart. This is much more disrupting and traumatic to muscle fibers than is sectioning them with a sharp instrument. It results in many torn blood vessels and muscle fibers, a condition very similar to that occurring at the time of the original contusion to the muscle.

As the bony mass is approached by careful division of the overlying structures there is a temptation, when reaching the mass at one point, to strip the tissues away from it. This temptation must be resisted. The whole purpose of the procedure is to remove the mass of bone in its entirety and leave as little dead space, as little necrotic tissue, and as little infiltrated blood as possible. After the mass is thoroughly exposed it is divided from the femur by a sharp,

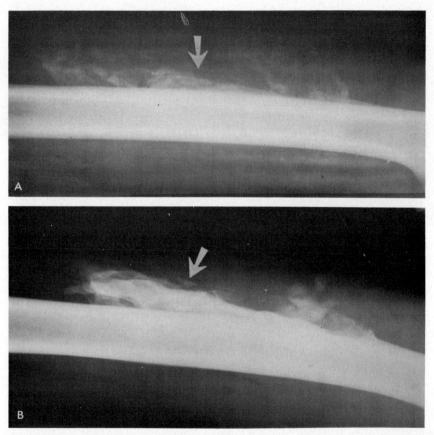

Figure 403. Myositis ossificans. *A*, Preoperative. This mass was obviously immature at the time of the operation which took place only a few months after injury. The surgeon succumbed to the urgings of the player, coach and parents with the result *(B)* that the recurrence was more extensive than the original lesion. These masses must not be disturbed until they are completely mature.

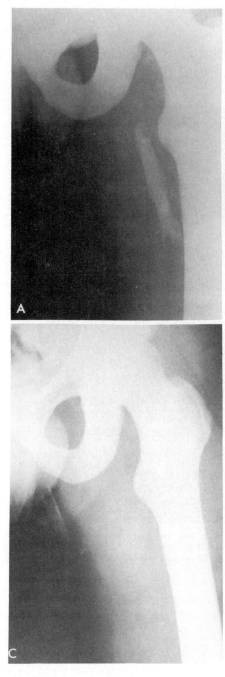

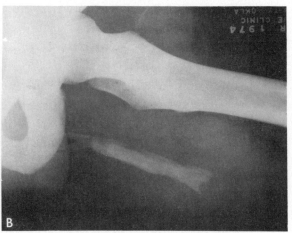

Figure 404. On the first day of spring practice this 19 year old football player, while running, started having pain in the back of the left thigh. This increased in severity so that he had to discontinue running. Further investigation revealed that he had had trouble with both thighs since his sophomore year in high school. He had an injection in the thigh but no other treatment. Examination revealed tenderness along the semitendinosus with a very firm area on the posterior thigh in the upper third. *A*, X-ray reveals the block of bone 9.5 cm. long, 1.5 cm. wide in the hamstrings. The mass appears to be very mature. Note also the mass in the adductor longus which is asymptomatic. *B*, X-ray, lateral view. Surgery revealed the mass to be in the biceps muscle right along its apposition to the semitendinosus. It did not invade the semitendinosus, however. *C*, Four months postoperative. No recurrence of fragment. No change in the fragment in the adductor.

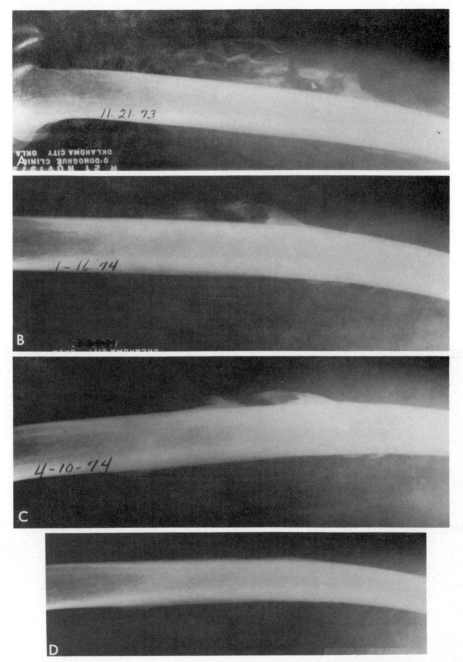

Figure 405. This 17 year old male was hit on the front of the thigh by a football helmet. He had severe pain following this for the next two or three weeks. He continued playing the rest of the game and two more games after the injury. He was told he had a bruised leg. His complaint was enlargement in front of the thigh, limited flexion of the knee, inability to run. Examination showed a large mass which covered the whole front of the middle third of the thigh, knee flexion 90 degrees, forced flexion painful. *A,* X-ray shows the tremendous mass 19 cm. long by 4 cm. deep by 5.5 cm. wide. Since it was only two months post-injury he was advised that the bone was quite immature, that he should definitely limit his activities, and return in two months for recheck. *B,* Two months later note the marked diminution in size of the mass with more definite maturity of bone but poor trabecular pattern. He was advised to wait further. *C,* Three months later (seven months post-injury) showing the mass quite mature, but there was still some of the mass in the muscle which was painful. Excision was carried out at this time. *D,* Two and one-half months postoperative, no recurrence.

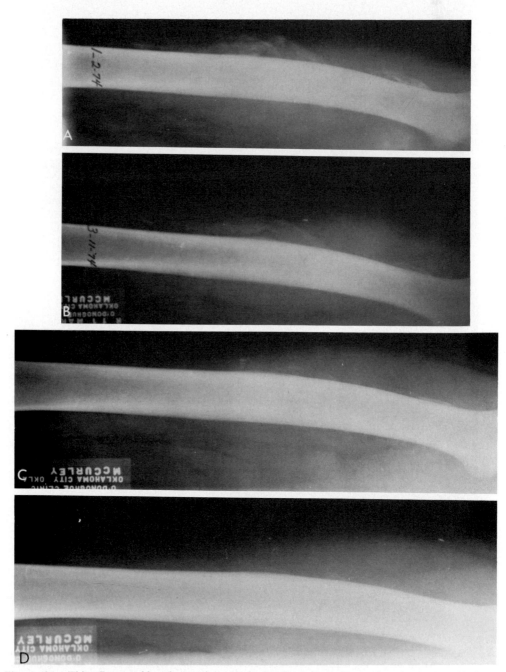

Figure 406.   This 17 year old male was injured playing football three months prior to examination. *A*, X-ray shows the ragged, nonhomogeneous appearance of the new bone. Note especially the smaller involvement proximal to the main mass. He was advised to let the growth mature. *B*, Two months later (five months post-injury) the mass is mature. Note the proximal mass has regressed. He was operated on at this time. The entire mass was resected with careful hemostasis. *C*, X-ray at two months postoperative shows a few remnants of ossification. *D*, X-ray one month later (three months postoperative) shows no remaining ossification. X-rays made later at five months postoperative showed no recurrence.

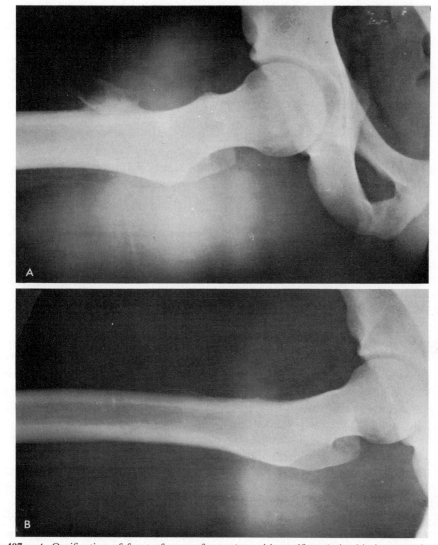

Figure 407. *A*, Ossification of front of upper femur (myositis ossificans), in this instance the result of partial avulsion of the iliopsoas tendon with resulting hematoma and ossification. *B*, Six months postoperative asymptomatic.

curved osteotome, care being taken to leave the femoral surface smooth. In the ordinary case one can readily distinguish the line of division between the recent ossification and the femoral cortex. In the occasional case the ossification may surround the shaft and blend so intimately with the femoral cortex that no line of cleavage can be found. These cases are not ordinarily symptomatic. The femur is simply larger than

normal and surgical removal is not necessary. If attempted, it may only increase the pathology.

After the mass is removed, complete hemostasis should be secured, including the vessels on the femoral surface. As a rule this surface does not bleed but if it does the bleeding can be controlled by judicious application of bone wax. Any shreds of muscle should be carefully clipped away. At the end of the procedure the wound should be dry, clean looking, with well defined margins. Closure is then carried out in layers. If possible the periosteum of the femur is sutured first. The muscle should then be carefully closed in layers, great care being taken not to leave dead space. In placing the sutures it is important that they not constrict large masses of muscle. After closure of the vaginal fascia and the skin, a firm pressure bandage is applied from the toes to the groin. It is my practice to utilize a heavy posterior plaster splint from the toes to the gluteal fold supported by a lateral stirrup running from high on the inner aspect of the thigh under the foot and up to the trochanter laterally (see Fig. 444, page 566). This is bound snugly to the thigh and gives uniform pressure throughout the lower extremity. The patient is placed in bed with the foot elevated. A suitable enzyme is given intramuscularly for three days. An oral enzyme is used post nauseam and continued for five to eight days, depending upon the degree of local reaction.

Active *rehabilitation* is not initiated in the thigh for at least three weeks. This does not interdict isometric contraction of the quadriceps and hamstrings. We urge frequent periods of contraction of the calf and of the other muscles of the leg and foot. Unless the rectus femoris is primarily involved we initiate active physical therapy to the hip on the involved side on the first or second day. It goes without saying that the rest of the muscles of the body are rehabilitated from the onset. The thigh and the wound are inspected at appropriate intervals. At the end of 12 to 14 days the stitches are removed and a long leg walking cast is applied which should be worn for another four weeks so that there has been a total rest period of at least six weeks. This may be continued for a longer period of time if there is still any evidence of reaction in the muscles of the thigh. After removal of the splints at six to eight weeks, graduated active exercises are carefully begun and may need to be continued for three or four months before complete flexion of the knee is obtained. By this time the quadriceps should be of normal size.

Surgery for myositis ossificans of the thigh is not justified unless one is prepared to take the time and the pains required to make the necessarily rigorous regimen a success. This fact must be fully accepted by the surgeon and carefully explained to the player, his parents and the coach so that there can be no misunderstanding as to the time and effort required. Active participation in contact sports cannot be permitted until rehabilitation is complete.

The close resemblance of early myositis ossificans to osteogenic sarcoma has been the cause of constant apprehension and of all too frequent error. In early biopsy the gross pathology in microscopic specimen resembles tumor because of the immature growing bone. A little patience will reveal the different course of the two lesions. Lesions due to myositis ossificans rapidly mature and are sharply delineated as they mature. They do not invade the cortex or the medullary canal. Osteogenic sarcoma or Ewing's tumor is destructive as well as productive and tends to progress rapidly with the destruction becoming more notable as the growth progresses. The malignant tumor may cause fever, malaise, pain and anorexia. The very unfavorable prognosis of even radical treatment of these tumors indicates that one should not panic into a situation of amputation or extensive radiation based on the presence of immature bone. The unfavorable prognosis does not seem to be altered too much by a matter of two or three weeks' observation. In fact, some authorities say treatment is better after a little more maturity of the lesion. Although it may be nerve-racking, in the case of myositis ossificans a period of observation will be rewarded by subsidence of the symptoms and maturity of the lesion, at which time no further treatment may be indicated unless there is a physical mass of bone which will interfere with muscle function later. I must emphasize again the extreme importance of distinguishing myositis ossificans from osteogenic sarcoma. I have personally seen cases which, following biopsy, have been treated radically for osteogenic sarcoma when actually the original lesion was ossification within the muscle. It is almost impossible to distinguish by pathological examination between the early growing bone of a myositis ossificans and the early osteogenesis of a sarcoma of the bone. I have mentioned this again although it has been well covered in Chapter 4 since the majority of these lesions do occur in the thigh.

STRAIN

The muscles of the thigh are subject to the same stresses as muscles in other locations. Actually, these are extreme stresses because of the function of propelling the human body under various degrees of resistance. The strain may be mild, moderate or severe, and the treatment should be gauged accordingly. The mild, or first degree, strain simply will result in a painful muscle because of hemorrhage to a few muscle fibers. This will promptly resolve and result in no disability. Active treatment is really not necessary and the vast majority of these cases never come to the attention of a physician. As in strain anywhere, one must resist the temptation to forcibly massage the muscle and stretch the muscle beyond the pain-free range.

A more severe problem is the moderate, or second degree, strain in which there is definite damage to a segment of the muscle which will definitely reduce the ability of this muscle to function. In this type of case it is important to determine the degree of the tear if possible. Granting that there is not a complete rupture of the muscle, the muscle may be quite severely damaged short of actual rupture. The early treatment should be rest and ice. Resumption of muscle function must be absolutely within the limits of pain. Nothing is to be gained by forcing the painful muscle, since this just increases the spasm. As the acute symptoms subside, the danger point occurs because in a couple of weeks the subjective symptoms may be essentially gone; yet, the muscle will be materially weakened and may well rupture in its next stressful situation. Hence, it is important to decide if there has actually been definite loss of function of a significant percentage of the muscle. It is notable to observe that complete muscle tear is frequently preceded by a less serious injury which has healed inadequately. Since the player wants to resume the very activity which caused the problem in the first place, there is a distressingly large percentage of recurrence under these conditions. Take, for example, the "hamstring pull" so frequent in sprinting in either football, basketball, track, or in fact in any active sport. In this instance, the player, while running, feels a sharp pain in the hamstring muscle somewhere along its course, often sufficient to make him stop running. He goes through the classic stages of pain, muscle spasm, restriction of motion, loss of strength. Yet, his impatience to return to competition means that he does not wait until the muscle actually heals but he simply waits until the symptoms subside. Then he goes back to the same occupation, this time with repeated injuries. That which started out as a relatively minor injury of the muscle may result in complete loss of the season for the player. The only control of this situation is to insist on absolute elimination of stress in this muscle until it is entirely healed. This may be very difficult to do. Painless motion should not cause trouble, so the player can rehabilitate to a certain extent. But when he gets to feeling very good and starts that burst of speed again, the trouble is back and he is back to the doctor with a discouraging recurrence of his disability.

Various measures may serve to reinforce the muscle. Physical therapy in the form of inductive heat is often good. The prevalent habit of strapping the thigh with snugly fitting adhesive seems to help, largely by virtue of the fact that it limits the action of the muscle to some extent. Careful adherence to the principles laid down in the section on Strain (p. 515) will aid in solving this very distressing problem.

MUSCLE RUPTURE

The muscles of the thigh are sometimes ruptured, a particularly susceptible one being the rectus femoris which extends from above the hip to below the knee. The injury often occurs as the result of a forcible blow on the muscle while it is in fixed contraction and the two ends of the muscle are firmly fixed. The muscle mechanism will tolerate considerable stress without rupture. If while the muscle is under maximum stress additional tension is caused by sharp flexion of the knee, the muscle gives way somewhere along its length. This is illustrated by the running athlete as he suddenly reverses the direction of the knee motion from extension to flexion by falling or by having his knee forcibly flexed. The additional force causes the muscle to give way. The most

frequent sites for rupture are at the attachment of the rectus at the hip and to the conjoined tendon above the patella.

If the tear is complete and is recognized early, surgical repair will be quite gratifying. Ordinarily the condition is diagnosed as a contusion or hematoma and it is not until the local swelling and reaction subside that the true nature of the condition becomes apparent. By this time repair may not be possible if the rupture is within the muscle fibers. If there is actual avulsion of the attachment at the anteroinferior spine, it can be repaired even though rather late. Frequently the muscle is torn off the tendon at the junction of the lower and middle third of the thigh or it may be separated at about the level of the lesser trochanter. In either instance the muscle bunches up on contraction and presents a definite tumor mass (Fig. 408). This swelling disappears when the muscle is relaxed. Attempts at repair after several weeks may be very disappointing since it may be impossible to suture the muscle down firmly enough to obtain the additional length required to bring the ends into apposition.

The typical patient will present himself with a painful swollen thigh with rather localized tenderness in the muscle. Following treatment for contusion the soreness will persist and the muscle mass will appear. There may be substantial disability for many weeks. After the local reaction disappears and the nature of the condition is recognized, the surgeon should carefully explain the situation to the patient, assuring him that the rupture will probably cause no actual disability, that the pain and tenderness will completely disappear, but that the bunched-up mass of muscle will remain. He will notice that the muscle of this thigh is different from that of his other thigh. Usually careful explanation of the nature of the condition is satisfactory and the athlete will condition him-

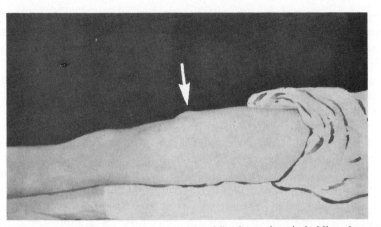

Figure 408. Silhouette view of the front of the thigh while the patient is holding the quadriceps contracted. Arrow indicates bulging mass of the lower end of the rectus resulting from partial avulsion of the rectus attachment to the quadriceps tendon.

self to the asymmetry and is little the worse for his lesion. Occasionally persistent pain will remain, apparently from chronic myositis or constricting fibrosis of the detached muscle ends. In this case careful surgical removal of the detached portion of the muscle eliminates the mass and will relieve the pain (Fig. 409). One can only justify this procedure after very thorough trial of physical therapy and rehabilitation. This type of surgery probably adds no strength to

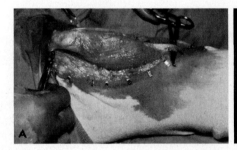

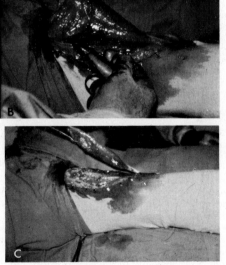

Figure 409. This athlete gave a history of running hard, received "pulled muscle" in the thigh. No treatment was given other than advice to "work it out." He was examined six months after the injury. He had been sent in for Baker's cyst and the notation was that it was a little high. On examination a firm mass was palpable in the posteromedial thigh just above the knee. This mass was nonpulsating and on flexion of the knee against resistance it moved downward and became more prominent. This was accompanied by aching pain. The patient's complaint was that on running hard he had pain of increasing severity in the back of the thigh. At surgery six months post-injury, this mass was found to be a muscle belly with a long tendon below and a spindle-shaped upper end which was attached only by loose areolar tissue (*A*). Further dissection revealed the neurovascular bundle entering the mass in the posterosuperior aspect (*B*). The upper end detached (*C*). Note nerve entering muscle at superior end. The symptoms were caused by traction on the nerve in the neurovascular bundle as the semitendinosus muscle contracted. Muscle was entirely removed, relieving the symptoms.

the thigh but serves only to reduce the muscle mass and to relieve the pain.

This same situation occasionally arises in the adductor muscles, particularly the adductor longus (Fig. 410). The signs will be present at some point between the pubis and the medial condyle of the femur. In this situation, if it is the attachment that is avulsed repair is quite satisfactory. If the tear is within the muscle itself, repair must be carried out within the first two weeks to have much hope for success. This same condition also occurs in the hamstring mus-

cles but avulsion of either origin or attachment is more frequent than tear in the muscle and so is more successfully sutured.

A good deal of acumen is needed to recognize an isolated muscle rupture. This is particularly true when the ruptured muscle is one of several muscles carrying out the same function: for example, the rectus femoris muscle (Fig. 411), one of the adductor muscles, or one of the hamstrings. The telltale sign of bunching up of the muscle because it has lost its attachment is usually well

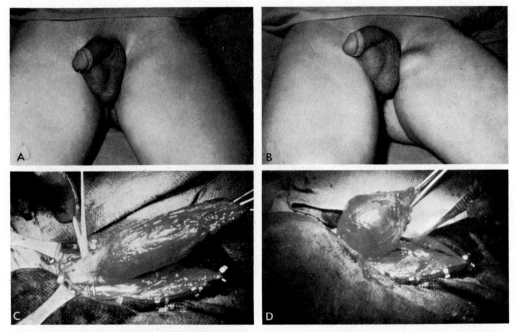

Figure 410. An 18 year old boy was injured at water skiing when his ski turned outward throwing his thigh into forced external rotation–abduction. Severe knifelike pain occurred on the inner side of the thigh with immediate disability. He was treated expectantly with heat and rest after a diagnosis of a ruptured vessel. He was seen four months post-injury because of a firm mass in the upper inner thigh. The mass itself was not painful but varied in size and was disabling because, when the youth would run, the mass would tighten up and strike the testicle. Running was interdicted. On examination there was a soft but firm mass along the adductor muscle just below the pubis extending about 5 inches distally. On contraction of the adductor, this mass would travel upward and become more prominent and more firm. Diagnosis was made of ruptured adductor, either adductor longus or gracilis. Surgery was recommended because of the disability.

A, The muscle at rest. *B,* With the adductor contracted showing impingement against the scrotum. *C,* The muscle dissected out showing complete detachment of the lower end from its femoral attachment and rounding off of the end. Note the tendinous attachment of the avulsed adductor longus with the intact gracilis lying inferior to it.

D, Stimulating the branch of the obturator nerve to the adductor longus. Note contraction of the muscle into the spherical shape suggested in *B.* Uneventful recovery. Early diagnosis and surgical repair might have saved this muscle.

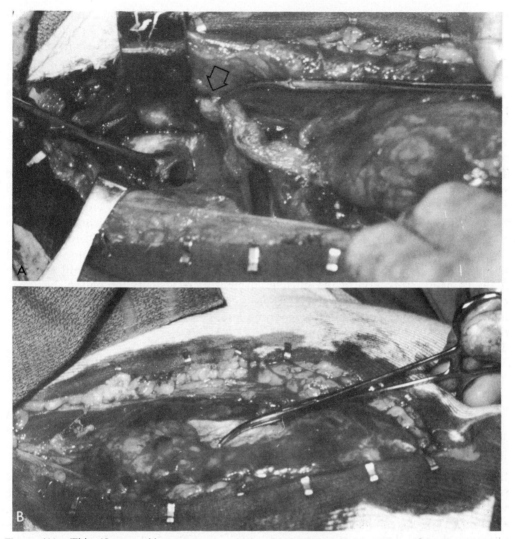

Figure 411. This 40 year old surgeon was playing football with his youngster. ran off the clipped lawn into tall grass, had a knifelike pain in the right groin and fell. Examination revealed local swelling in the groin with severe pain on active flexion of the hip, less severe on passive flexion of the knee. Palpation revealed marked tenderness just in front of the hip with the feeling of a defect above and a nodule below. Midline incision revealed the rectus femoris had been torn off the anterior inferior spine in a "Z" fashion, about half of the tendon tearing off the bone and the other half tearing off the muscle. *A,* Reveals the tendon avulsed from the anterior inferior spine, held in the left hemostat. Arrow, right, indicates the parallel portion of the tendon still attached to the muscle held by long Kelly forceps. *B,* Realignment with side to side apposition of the split tendon.

screened by the associated local swelling during the early stages of the acute injury.

The extremely heavy muscles of the thigh receive tremendous strain in almost any athletic competition. The very fact that the muscle ruptured in a given athlete would suggest excessive strain in the area involved. For this reason athletic competition must be sharply curtailed following such an injury. Certainly during the acute period no active use of the extremity should be permitted. As in so many instances of muscle damage, premature attempts toward strenuous activity can result only in disappointment and prolongation of disability. A minimum of six weeks is needed for the healed tissue to even approach maturity and even at this time the scar is very susceptible to injury. Actually, the best criterion for active use lies in the patient himself, since pain-free activity does not do any harm. The difficulty is that he may go along with ordinary pain-free activity and a sudden burst of exertion may cause reinjury. It would seem advisable to restrict activity sharply for at least six weeks. This is not to say that rehabilitation cannot be proceeding within the limits of pain. Protection of the muscle by padding or strapping is extremely difficult since active contraction rather than passive stretching may cause the damage.

FASCIAL HERNIA

The muscles of the thigh are completely invested in one continuous sheath of fascia—the vaginal fascia of the thigh. Vagina means sheath and this fascial sheath does indeed contain the voluminous muscles in a well-defined envelope. The fascia itself is inelastic but may change shape as the enclosed muscle mass shifts. Therefore, it is not easily torn and a traumatic defect in the fascia of the thigh is not common. It may occur, however, and present itself as a fascial hernia usually along the anterolateral aspect of the thigh where the fascia becomes thinner anterior to the iliotibial band. The ordinary symptoms of fascial hernia may be present. There is a palpable tumor mass, particularly notable when the muscle is relaxed. In some instances, if there is not too much subcutaneous tissue, a linear defect in the fascia may be detected. When the quadriceps muscle is contracted to ex-

tend the knee, the tumor mass will disappear and the defect be less noticeable. If this rent is large enough it probably will be asymptomatic. A small tear may cause some discomfort by pinching of the areolar tissue or fat between the tight edges of the split fascia.

Treatment is usually not necessary. If the symptoms are too severe the condition may be treated surgically by repair of the rent provided the edges are well defined and reparable. If repair of the defect is impossible, relief may be obtained by simply enlarging the slit to a length of 3 or 4 inches. This condition is ordinarily not disabling and treatment can usually be postponed until a convenient time. Usually the patient becomes accustomed to the condition and it becomes asymptomatic.

FRACTURE OF FEMORAL SHAFT

Fracture of the shaft of the femur is a very serious injury but fortunately is not frequent in athletes. The fracture occurs as a result of excessive force, usually rotatory in nature, applied to the lower extremities, and as a rule the ankle, leg or knee will give way before the femur. If the fracture is complete, the disability is immediate and usually there is little difficulty in recognizing the lesion. Incomplete fracture requires an x-ray examination for detection. In the presence of a serious injury to the thigh, the patient should be taken on a stretcher to the hospital and a definitive diagnosis made by x-ray if the fracture is not obvious. For transportation a traction splint is applied, the most useful being a Thomas splint with half ring that rests against the ischial tuberosity, with the traction applied to the foot. For short periods this can be applied by a Jones' hitch (Fig. 412) tied around the ankle and foot and twisted to tighten the

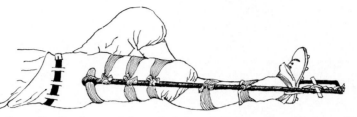

Figure 412. Traction splint for fractured femoral shaft, a half-ring splint with Jones hitch. This type of traction should not be used for a long period and care should be taken to preserve the circulation to the foot.

rope. Great care should be taken not to constrict circulation of the foot for a long time by this apparatus. Treatment of fracture should be instituted at once.

It is not necessary here to define the various methods of *treatment* of fracture of the femur. It will be borne in mind that the athlete is usually a young healthy male, that his healing potential is good and that he is very anxious to be rehabilitated promptly. He will of course lose the current season of competition.

Since this injury has happened to a young person with excellent general health, the very best method may be employed to restore him to normal activity. If open surgery is recommended, it should be balanced against the less hazardous, so-called conservative treatment. If conservative treatment suggests traction for six or eight weeks, it must be demonstrated that this method is better than reduction and cast or open reduction and internal fixation. The ingrown advantage of so-called conservative treatment is not valid in the young athlete. It must be borne in mind that the athlete is usually a young healthy person, that his healing potential is good and that he is very anxious to be rehabilitated promptly.

Rehabilitation is extremely impor-

tant in this type of fracture. The patient should be carefully instructed in exercise of the other extremities and in the use of whatever muscles of the involved extremity are available. If he is treated by traction he can keep the knee mobilized to a considerable degree. If he is placed in a plaster cast, isometric contractions will help, and he should be instructed to contract all the muscle within the cast as by "shrugging" the patella and "setting" the calf. If he is treated by intramedullary fixation and this is successful enough to obviate the necessity for external fixation, rehabilitation can proceed much more rapidly.

One should emphasize again that, although rehabilitation may proceed rapidly, active competition must not be permitted until the fractured femur is solidly united and the muscles of the thigh and calf are as large and strong as those on the other side. The range of the motion in all the joints must be normal. The strain on the fractured femur is magnified tremendously if there is any restriction of flexion of the knee and refracture is certainly a distinct possibility due to the increased leverage. Knee motion must be essentially complete in range before any activity is permitted that could cause forcible flexion of the knee.

CHAPTER 18

INJURIES OF THE KNEE

ANATOMICAL CONSIDERATIONS

The knee is probably the most vulnerable joint of the body from the standpoint of athletic injury. The articular cartilage of the femoral condyle at the lower end of the femur is divided into two areas in its posterior and distal aspect, one the medial condyle and the other the lateral, whereas in front the two become confluent to form the trochlear groove for the patella. While functionally the knee joint is a hinge joint, physiologically it is a gliding joint, the femoral condyle rolling over the saucers of the tibial plateau which are slightly deepened by the semilunar cartilages. The patellofemoral joint particularly is a gliding joint, the patella sliding up and down in the trochlear groove as the knee is flexed and extended. The posterior capsular ligament serves to prevent overextension of the joint and with the knee in complete extension prevents medial or lateral instability (Fig. 439). The lateral ligaments (Fig. 438) prevent lateral motion. The lateral components also help to control rotation of the tibia on the femur. The medial components control slipping between the femur and tibia on the medial side, while the lateral components control the lateral side.

Acting together, they control anterior and posterior displacement of the tibia on the femur. Anteriorly, support is given by the quadriceps mechanism, the tone of which provides constant tension on the ligamentum patellae, no matter what position the knee is in so long as the quadriceps is normal.

The knee is enclosed in a capsule that is very closely applied to the ligaments posteriorly and laterally (Fig. 439). In front it becomes more redundant to permit flexion of the knee. It is tight anteriorly only with the knee in complete flexion. The superior fold of the knee capsule continues into the suprapatellar pouch, the two being divided to a greater or lesser extent by the plica semilunaris. This anterior structure is quite taut with the knee in flexion but becomes quite redundant with the knee in extension. There is a cone-shaped fat pad which fills the gap between the patellar tendon and the joint. This is fastened back to the intercondylar notch by the ligamentum mucosum to give it some degree of fixation. The only intrasynovial structures in the knee are the semilunar cartilages and the popliteus tendon. The cruciate ligaments, the fat pad and all of the other ligaments are extrasynovial.

This anatomically unstable joint is

reinforced mainly by muscular structures. The quadriceps muscles covering the entire front of the thigh converge to attach into the patella, with some of the fibers of the aponeurosis extending medially and laterally as the patellar retinaculum to become continuous with the fascia of the leg. This gives extremely powerful extension to the leg. The anatomical position of the quadriceps is with the knee in extension. The muscle has to be extended from its resting position in order to function as an active knee extensor. The hamstring muscles arise from the back of the femur and the pelvis and extend to below the knee where they attach on either side of the leg. These are powerful flexors of the knee. These muscles contract within their resting length in order to flex the knee. The fact that the internal hamstring tendons sweep around the medial side of the upper tibia to attach in front gives a lateral and rotatory stabilizing component to the hamstrings. They also aid in preventing anterior displacement of the tibia on the femur.

The medial collateral ligament has many divisions, but from the standpoint of function there are essentially two layers. The short fibers run from the femoral condyle to the upper tibial margin and extend forward only to the midlateral line. Posteriorly this blends into the posterior ligament of the knee. The more superficial portion of the medial collateral ligament passes down to attach to the tibia 3 to 4 inches below the upper tibial margin passing under the pes anserinus. It lies under the fascia of the leg. It blends with the deep fibers usually at about the line of the joint. The fact that this attaches well below the tibial margin and anteriorly allows an arc of motion that permits the knee to bend while the ligament remains constantly tense.

The lateral ligamentous support of the knee has been generally misunderstood. True enough, the strong ligamentous band extending from the head of the fibula to the femoral condyle is called the lateral collateral ligament. A brief anatomical consideration would indicate that lateral stability should not depend upon a band from the fibula to the femur. The fibula does not participate in the knee joint and should not be considered as a major supporting factor of the knee. The iliotibial tract is a tremendous factor in stability. As it passes distally from the tensor fascia femoris muscle it becomes the vaginal fascia of the thigh. As it approaches the knee it becomes a very dense fibrous band which attaches to the distal femur through the intermuscular septum. Traversing distally across the knee it attaches to the upper tibial flare at the tubercle of Gerdy. This structure is the true lateral collateral ligament of the knee. Whereas the short capsular fibers on the medial side usually blend with the long fibers of the medial collateral ligament, there is no such arrangement on the lateral side. The short capsular fibers laterally are relatively weak and have no connection to either the iliotibial band or the fibular collateral ligament. They may blend with the short fibular collateral ligament fibers which run from the fibula to the femoral condyle just adjacent to the capsule. The lateral meniscus attaches to these short capsular fibers through the coronary ligament.

With the knee in flexion the femoral condyles are somewhat protected against a direct blow by the patella. The margins are quite vulnerable on either side of the patella, however. A direct blow may damage the articular cartilage of the patella or femur.

The medial and lateral menisci are intrasynovial and serve to deepen somewhat the fossa of the upper plateau of the tibia. They are not for weight bearing but tend to fill the crevice left by the lack of congruity of the arcs of the condyles of the femur and plateau of the tibia. The actual weight bearing is on a relatively small area of the femoral condyle and a similarly small area of the tibial plateau. It should be noted that the menisci have a bony attachment anteriorly and posteriorly, the medial meniscus being "C" shaped and attached well toward the front and well toward the back of the upper surface of the tibia, whereas the lateral meniscus is more "O" shaped and attaches within the two attachments of the medial meniscus.

The anterior cruciate ligament arises from the nonarticular area on top of the tibia in front and extends upward, backward and outward to attach to the medial side of the lateral condyle of the femur well posteriorly in the intercondylar notch. The posterior cruciate ligament, on the other hand, attaches anteriorly in the intercondylar notch on the lateral side of the medial condyle right at the cartilage margin and extends backward, downward and outward, passing over the back edge of the tibia through a well defined groove to attach to the posterior surface of the tibia near the midline.

The popliteus hiatus is an interruption of the short capsular fibers and the coronary ligament formed to permit the passage of the popliteus tendon. The tendon comes forward from the muscle origin on the back of the tibia to attach to the lateral surface of the lower femur just superior to the chondral margin at about the midlateral point.

The entire front of the knee is subcutaneous. In many instances bursae lie between the skin and underlying bone. Posteriorly the gastrocnemius muscle and the hamstring tendons lie between the skin and the underlying bone. The vessels and nerves crossing the popliteal space are well protected by their deep position between the two femoral condyles which project much further posteriorly than anteriorly.

DIFFERENTIAL DIAGNOSIS

The knee joint area presents a real challenge to one who treats its injuries. Anatomically the knee lacks the stability of the hip with its ball and socket or the ankle with the mortise and tenon, each of which gives some degree of bony stability. At the knee joint the socket of the top of the tibia is so minimal that, indeed, the lateral tibial plateau may be flat or even convex. The little buffering by the menisci gives minimal increase in stability since the menisci are unstable themselves. So, the knee must depend largely upon the soft tissue, namely, ligaments, capsule and muscles, aided by the fact that the lower end of the femur is a bipod and one must lift or slide a foot to develop instability. Hence, the extreme importance of making an accurate diagnosis as to the exact nature of the knee injury — doubly so since it is vital that the definitive diagnosis be made early so that treatment can be begun early. Examination must determine two things: what part is injured and how bad it is. The parts that may be injured include:

1. Ligaments
2. Muscle tendon
3. Capsule
4. Meniscus
5. Cartilage
6. Bone
7. Bursae
8. Any combination of these

History

A complete history is vital in order to determine when the injury happened, how it happened, and why it happened. What has been done since the injury? Was the player disabled? Did he come off the field by himself? Was he carried or helped off? Did he continue to play? Did he feel that he was badly hurt? Had anyone straightened out his leg? Did he feel something snap or pop? Did he have severe pain? Was swelling immediate? If so, where was it? Then study his present condition. Did he walk in without support or with crutches? Is the knee still sore? Does it give away or slip? Does motion hurt? Such a complete record should be taken before the knee is actually examined.

Examination

Examination should be done just as soon as the player can get to the place where proper examination can be carried out. A preliminary survey may be done even on the field in order to have some assessment as to the severity of the injury and how the player should be transported. As soon as possible, the player should be taken to the place where his clothes, pads, tape and the like can be removed from both legs. It is better that this is away from a crowd of players, fans and parents. You need to have the injured player's total attention not colored by parents, coaches or teammates. It is always best to examine the opposite knee first. It allays the patient's apprehension and gives the examiner some guide as to the normal of this particular individual.

Observation. First, look at the knee. Observe contusions, swelling, discoloration and especially deformity. Compare one leg's appearance with the other. Is the patella displaced? Is there knock-knee or bowleg? Many times an objective look at the knee may give a real lead as to the pathologic condition (Fig. 413). Position the legs at 90 degree flexion with both feet flat on the table and check the anterior profile. Does the

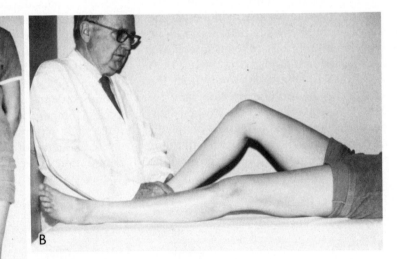

Figure 413. *A*, Standing, front view; note alignment, swelling, and any abnormal appearance. *B*, Examining the leg with the patient supine.

tibia hang backward, suggesting posterior cruciate and posterior capsular redundancy? (Fig. 414.) Is the patellar alignment normal? Note any difference between the injured and the normal leg. With the patient sitting with the legs hanging at 90 degrees over the edge of the table, check the position of the patella in relation to the patellar groove. Is there evidence that the patella angulates and faces laterally rather than straight ahead? Ask the patient to kick the leg up and down from 90 degrees of flexion to complete extension. Observe the path of the patella in the trochlear groove. Does it shift from side to side? Particularly, does it move into a lateral position as it comes toward complete extension? Ask the patient to squat if possible, and determine variation from the normal here (Fig. 415).

Palpation. After observing the extremity, feel it. Note local heat, fluctuation, tension of the skin. Most important of all, locate tenderness exactly. Usually the tenderness will be at the site of the injury, while pain may well be away from this site. Determine if the swelling is actually in the knee. Is it hemarthrosis or effusion or is it in the soft tissues? Careful palpation may indeed give a real lead to the proper diagnosis; for example, palpation of the tibial tuberosity in apophysitis or apophyseal fracture. Tenderness along

the medial edge of the patella may suggest lateral luxation of the patella. The meniscus is likely to be torn where the tenderness is. In ligament injuries tenderness is at the site of the tear. Palpation of a chondral foreign body in the knee may be the only objective clue to its presence when the x-ray is negative and all the physical findings may otherwise be zero.

Manipulation. *Manipulation should not be attempted until observation and palpation have been completed.* Manipulation may be defined as skillful moving with the hands. It should be carried out on the normal knee first. It must be careful and gentle. If you grab the injured leg and shake it around like a terrier does a rat, you not only make a very uncooperative patient but you will get very little useful information. Check active motion first to note pain on motion as from a muscle tendon injury or limitation of motion by a locked meniscus or a foreign body. Check the knee carefully for crepitation under the patella as it is actively flexed and extended. Then add resistance to see if this increases crepitation or pain (Fig. 416). The same is true for chondral damage in other areas of the knee. Compare active and passive motion, since passive motion may demonstrate a range not possible by voluntary contraction of the injured muscle.

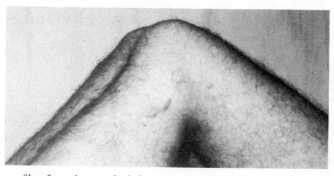

Figure 414. Note profile of two knees; the left (nearer) sags backward compared with the normal right knee, indicating posterior cruciate defect.

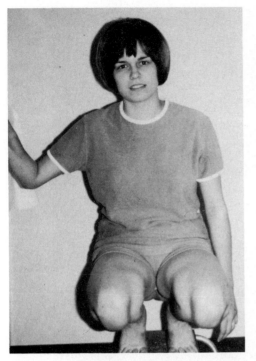

Figure 415. With the patient squatting, note position of patellae, depth of squat, and location of pain.

Examine the patella for tenderness, pain, crepitation or instability as you slide it from side to side (glissement). The apprehension test (Fig. 417) to check for instability of the patella should be done by flexing the knee at 45 degrees with the patient in a supine position. Have someone hold the foot to permit the hamstrings to relax and then force the patella laterally. It may slip off or partially sublux. The patient's apprehension that it may slip off suggests a subluxing or a dislocated patella. Zero response indicates a stable patella. Grade 1 elicits mild anxiety, suggestive of some degree of instability. In Grade 2 there is more marked reaction as the patient moves the leg around, tightening up the muscles. In Grade 3 he grabs the doctor's hands to prevent subluxation. In Grade 4 he takes a swing at the doctor! Note also the "Q" angle formed by the intersection of the line of the quadriceps mechanism to the mid point of the patella and the line from mid patella to the tibial tuberosity (Fig. 469). An increased angle suggests a potential for subluxation (Fig. 470).

Some of the tests for ligaments are as follows: By the "drawer" test (Fig. 450), check the AP motion of the tibia on the femur which suggests damage to the cruciate ligaments. The drawer sign should be checked with the foot at neu-

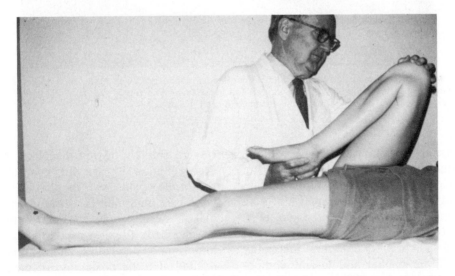

Figure 416. Forced flexion to determine whether there is pain or snapping and where it is.

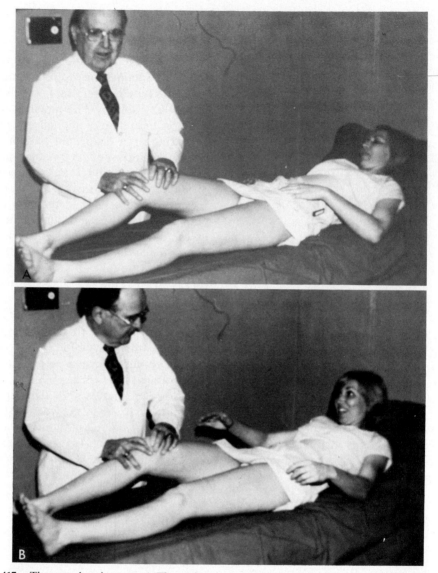

Figure 417. The apprehension test. *A,* The patient is positioned with the knee flexed at 45 degrees. The examiner grasps the patella between the thumb and index finger and forces the patella laterally. *B,* The apprehensive reaction of the patient indicates instability of the patella.

tral, medial rotation, and lateral rotation to determine some possible involvement of the collateral ligaments. Collateral instability should be determined first with the knee in complete extension (Fig. 418). In this position the intact posterior capsule will prevent collateral instability even if the medial and lateral components are damaged. Eliminate the poste-

rior capsule by flexing the knee 30 degrees (Fig. 419). In this position the posterior capsule will not give medial or lateral stability and the defect in the medial or lateral ligamentous elements may be checked. Flexion-rotation tests are important to determine rotatory instability and also the possibility of meniscus damage. One should note the presence

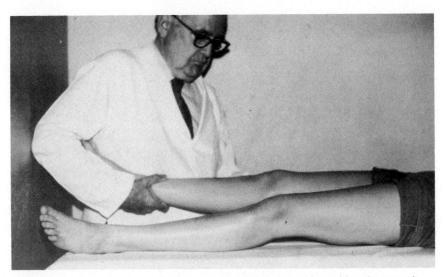

Figure 418. First, check lateral motion with the knee extended. In this position the posterior capsule is tight. Even with the medial collateral ligament gone, the knee will be stable in this position if the posterior capsule is intact.

and location of the pain. If there is snapping or popping, is this constant or transitory? The foot is placed into internal rotation and the flexion test repeated to note variations from the straight position (Fig. 420). The foot is then placed into external rotation and the same tests repeated (Fig. 421).

X-Ray. X-ray examination is an extremely important factor in the diagnosis of any knee injury. It is diagnostic in many conditions and often serves to rule out a suspected lesion. The position of the limb for x-ray is of considerable importance. An "as is" picture may be the most revealing of all. For this pic-

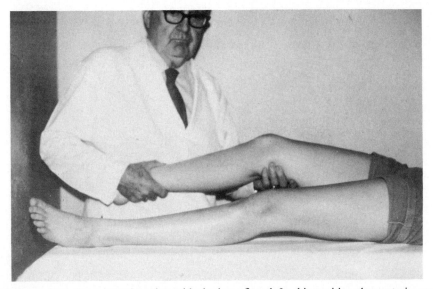

Figure 419. Second, check lateral motion with the knee flexed. In this position the posterior capsule is lax. Instability here indicates medial collateral loss.

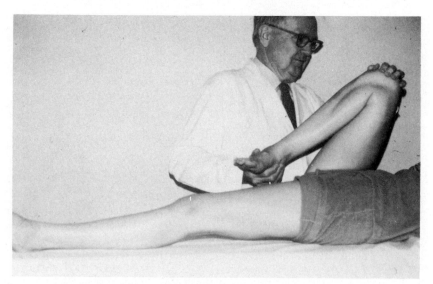

Figure 420.   Forced flexion with the leg internally rotated puts different stress on menisci than straight flexion. Notice snapping and pain and location.

ture, simply place the knee over the x-ray plate without any attempt at positioning the leg or holding the foot. Then snap the picture in this position (Fig. 422). The result may be quite dramatic and also quite revealing in complete or partial dislocation of the knee or in some fractures of the femoral condyles or tibial plateaus (Fig. 524). After this, take "routine" views. I prefer to take a standing AP of both knees if it is feasible, since weight bearing may show things not visible in a supine film. Then take a lateral of each knee. This may reveal an osteochondritis dissecans, osteochondral defects, degenerative

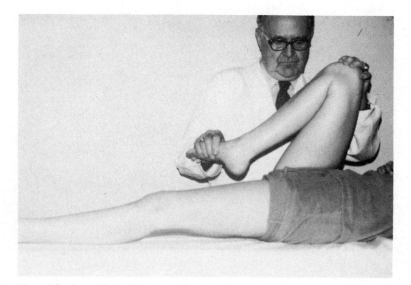

Figure 421.   Forced flexion with the leg externally rotated, the opposite of Figure 420. Note difference in pain or snapping.

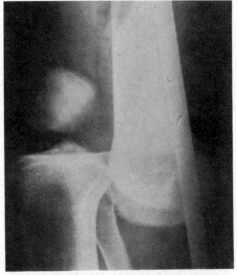

A

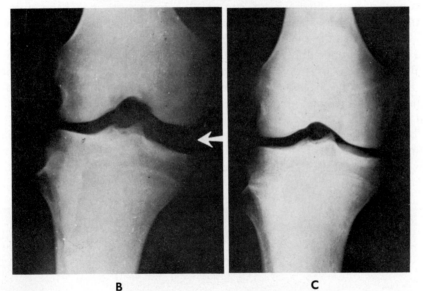

B   C

Figure 422. *A,* "As is" picture showing a complete anterior dislocation of the knee with obvious ligament damage. *B,* "As is" view, *just as significant as A,* showing rupture of the anterior cruciate, medial collateral, and medial posterior capsule. *C,* The "positioned" AP view of the same knee as *B* showing no pathologic change.

changes in the patellofemoral joint, problems of the tibial tuberosity, patellar alta (Fig. 473), and fractures or other injuries to the patella. A silhouette view also should be taken of each patella (Fig. 482). This will help to reveal patellar subluxation, fractures of the patella, either of the bone or of the patellar cartilage, or irregularity of the undersur-

face of the patella. Multiple views may be necessary in case there is any doubt as to the findings on the standard views. It may be necessary to take a right and left oblique view. The oblique views visualize the individual condyles better, particularly in determining damage to the anterior or posterior segment of either condyle. It may be necessary to take a notch view that will show the presence of a foreign body or possible avulsion of the cruciate ligament with a segment of bone.

Only after these views have been made and examined should stress pictures be made (Fig. 423 and 449). The primary function of the stress film is to demonstrate ligament instability. However, it may be a false finding since in the acute injury, if the patient has been examined repeatedly and stress made to determine instability, it may be very difficult for the x-ray technician to hold the knee stressed open while an x-ray is made. There is often a dividend from stress films in that they may reveal some other condition. I have seen patients come in with diagnosis of ruptured medial ligament when there was actually a fracture of the medial femoral condyle or of the upper tibia (Fig. 522). Stress films are also of value in determining how thick the articular cartilage is on the side of the joint that is compressed. As with all other tests, the tests should be done carefully in order not to add damage to a part already injured. For this reason I do not like any of the

mechanical ways of getting stress, since they can exert tremendous forces and may complete an incomplete ligament tear simply by overstress.

A further word about the stress films and ligament instability: I don't think you need stress films to demonstrate ligament instability of the knee. They are helpful in determining whether the instability is medial or lateral, particularly in old cases where the element of acute pain is not present. However, in the acute injury I would accept the findings of a physical examination showing instability of the knee even though the x-ray did not show any actual separation. I would like to emphasize again that the reason for this is that if the knee has been hurt, has been quite painful and has been examined by several people, by the time the x-ray technician gets around to holding the knee open while a picture is made, muscle spasm has taken over and the stress film may be entirely negative, yet there may be obvious clinical instability of the knee.

One should be very critical of x-ray pictures. It is no excuse to later say "it is a poor film so I couldn't see the pa-

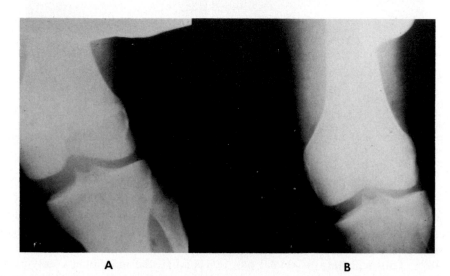

A **B**

Figure 423. Stress films made with the knee flexed *(A)* and with the knee extended *(B)*. Note the markedly greater amount of opening up when the posterior capsule is eliminated in *A*. This indicates major involvement of the medial collateral ligament with a partial tear of the posteromedial capsule.

thology." If the film does not appear to you to satisfactorily demonstrate the area to be surveyed, then have it made again. Nothing is more humiliating than to have someone else make a picture which reveals a pathologic condition that you should have discovered yourself. Demand adequate x-ray pictures.

Arthrography

Arthrography is becoming increasingly popular in the differential diagnosis of knee pathology. Ironically, the doctor who needs it most is likely to utilize it the least and to profit from the result of the study the least. It requires a radiology department with the know-how to make the proper views plus someone, either radiologist or orthopaedist, who can properly interpret the films. This combination is most likely to occur in a situation where many knees are examined. The irony of the situation is that in this circumstance one is least likely to need the added help. Statistical studies are valid only if the conditions are properly controlled. To say that arthrography is 80 per cent correct as confirmed by surgery while clinical examination is only 75 per cent correct becomes valid only by definition of who is doing what. A far different figure will be found between the experienced examiner and the occasional one. I see little excuse for routine arthrography. Not only is it expensive, but it also subjects the patient to another procedure. Even if it is shown that the danger of complication is minimal, it still cannot be a pleasurable experience to the recipient. If the result of arthrography is not going to change your management of that case, I question its relevance. In the problem case it has its place and may be very valuable. If positive, it certainly is comforting to the surgeon who has already decided on arthrotomy. But what

about negative arthrography in the symptomatic patient? One sees patients who have been examined previously and who were advised that since arthrography was negative, nothing was wrong or that nothing could be done. This is small comfort to the patient who knows that something is wrong. A false negative is probably worse than a false positive. In regard to its value of actually localizing the lesion, I say that in most instances a thorough examination of the knee at arthrotomy will discover the occasional mistake in location of the lesion by clinical examination. I certainly do not condemn arthrography. I believe that it should not supplant careful, definitive clinical diagnosis. I examine many arthrographic studies but order them sparingly.

Arthroscopy

Arthroscopy seems to be a more formidable procedure than arthrography. It requires operating room surroundings and usually a general anesthesia, but can be done as an outpatient or ambulatory surgical procedure. However, it may contribute significantly to the preoperative diagnosis. Arthroscopy and arthrography are not duplicating procedures, although a good deal of the information may seem the same. Arthroscopy may be quite definitive in evaluation of lesions of the articular cartilage. It should reveal cruciate ligament conditions well, although the tear screened by synovial covering or the tear posteriorly may be difficult to define. My own experience in arthroscopy has been largely in postoperative evaluation of the progress of articular cartilage lesions treated by various methods, ie., by shaving, trephining and drilling, or by leaving the defect alone. The difficulty here is in advising a somewhat formidable and expensive operation to a person who seems to be progressing nicely. However, if confined to those who are doing poorly it becomes almost worthless as a means of evaluation of the relative merits of a method of treatment. Here, too, one is faced with the prospect of a negative arthroscopic study in a symptomatic patient. The method requires an experienced operator and observer to truly evaluate the pathologic condition. The method is not for the occasional user, but in experienced hands may be quite rewarding.

Details of the techniques of performing arthrography and arthroscopy are not presented, since the use of either requires a more extensive study in technique than is possible here.

CONTUSION

Basically, a contusion about the knee should be treated in the same manner as a contusion in any other location. There are certain characteristics of contusion of the knee joint, however, that deserve more detailed consideration. The knee is a highly vulnerable joint and is particularly liable to contusion either by a fall directly on the front of the knee or by a blow from the side, and one of the major considerations must be the differential diagnosis.

Diagnostically, we identify a contusion by local swelling, local tenderness, ecchymosis and overlying abrasion. Of greater importance, however, are the negative findings, since it is most important to distinguish major injuries from the simple contusions. Thus, an injury along the medial side of the upper tibia may be called a contusion when actually it represents a tear of the tibial attachment of the medial collateral ligament. An injury over the patella may be interpreted as a contusion although there actually has been damage to the quadriceps mechanism in the nature of sprain or strain or even fracture. It is most impor-

tant, therefore, in any given injury to check carefully the function of the underlying structures. Tenderness over the internal condyle of the femur may be simply the result of a blow from an opponent's boot. On the other hand, it may represent a serious injury to the femoral attachment of the medial collateral ligament. Careful attention to detail in examination will largely eliminate this diagnostic hazard. In case of doubt the knee should be treated as if it had received the more serious injury until the actual pathology is evident.

If it is concluded that the injury is a contusion, *treatment* is basically the same whatever area is involved; aspiration for hematoma, local injection with hyaluronidase, cold packs and compression are indicated. In the ordinary contusion, splinting of the part to prevent motion is not necessary. Usually motion itself is not an aggravating element. Athletic participation need not be interdicted since under ordinary circumstances the part can be protected adequately. Protection should be designed to prevent repetition of a direct blow to the injured part. An additional knee pad, a doughnut made of sponge rubber or a plastic guard is ordinarily all that is necessary.

The conditions most likely to be confused with simple contusion are partial tears of the ligament attachments to either the tibia or femur, strain of the attachment of the quadriceps tendon or patellar tendon to the patella, strain of the patellar tendon at its attachment to the patellar tubercle of the tibia, and early apophysitis of the patellar tubercle (Osgood-Schlatter disease, page 662). A direct blow over the patella or femoral condyle may well cause contusion to the synovium with resulting effusion, or may damage the articular cartilage or cause a chondral fracture (Chondral Fracture, page 640). It bears repeating that the injury should be treated as the more serious condition should the diagnosis be in doubt. One should become quite suspicious of the contusion that does not heal promptly. The contusion may be the precursor of a bursitis or tenosynovitis or, more frequently, of hematoma formation with later calcification or ossification.

STRAIN

Injuries to the Muscle-Tendon Unit

The vicinity of the knee is quite susceptible to injuries of the muscle-tendon unit since violent muscular activity is involved in the normal function of this vulnerable joint. A few of the more common strains will be discussed in some detail since they are particularly disabling to the young athlete. (See page 62.)

Quadriceps Mechanism

The quadriceps muscle attaches to the tibia by a succession of different divisions designed to transfer the multiple motors of the quadriceps, namely, the medialis, intermedius, lateralis and rectus, to the anterior tibia. These muscles converge on the patella. Their tendons completely invest the upper portion of the patella and their aponeuroses extend down over the patella to be joined at its distal pole by the patellar tendon, which attaches to the nonarticular extension of the distal pole of the patella. The patellar tendon extends downward to attach to the patellar tubercle of the tibia and fans out over the crest of the tibia below. The stress may be at any point in this mechanism (Fig. 502). It may avulse the quadriceps tendon from the patella; it may strain the medialis attachment along the medial side of the patella; it may damage the lateralis attachment laterally or the rectus

femoris on top. As the force is continued down into the patella it is extended into the upper tibia by the patellar tendon, which runs from the distal pole of the patella to the patellar tubercle of the tibia. The weakest link of this chain may be at any point along this complicated mechanism at any given moment. The injuries to these parts of the unit are essentially the same and require the same basic treatment. The diagnosis is made by local findings—pain, tenderness, swelling—at the site with pain on stress of the quadriceps unit.

Acute Fracture of the Patellar Tubercle

Not to be confused with apophysitis (Osgood-Schlatter disease, page 662) is an acute avulsion fracture of all or a part of the tubercular epiphysis as an acute injury (Fig. 37). In so-called Osgood-Schlatter disease there is usually not a specific, disabling injury that the young person can identify as the initiation of his troubles. He may recall a fall on the knee or an incidence of overexercise, but there is no such acute condition as follows the avulsion. The history of avulsion will be a sudden burst of effort such as high jumping or pole vaulting (Fig. 424). The athlete has severe pain in the knee and the knee collapses and he falls to the ground. He immediately recognizes that he is hurt and cannot extend his knee. The swelling is very local early and is right over the tubercle. If the fracture extends into the joint as it often does, hemarthrosis develops. If not into the knee, the swelling remains local. On examination there is extreme apprehension. The patient is exquisitely tender over the tubercle and cannot or will not actively extend his knee. Passive extension is pain free. Passive flexion is painful. X-ray study is confirmatory. It will show a loose fragment actually pulled away from the tu-

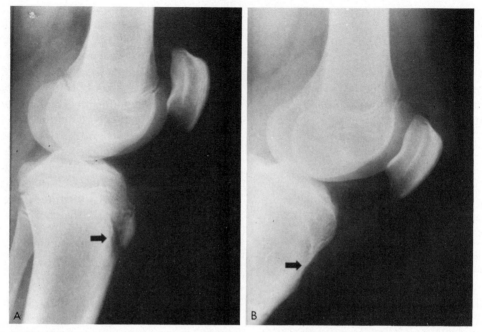

Figure 424. This 15 year old boy was high jumping and felt something give way in his take-off leg. He fell and had immediate swelling, pain localized over the front of the knee distal to the patella, and inability to use his extensors. *A*, X-ray shows the displacement of the recently closed apophysis of the tibia by avulsion of the patellar tendon. *B*, X-ray six months postoperative after removal of the fragment and reattachment of the tendon to the tibia.

bercle rather than show the usual fragmented condition of an apophysitis. This may be just the central portion of the tubercle (Fig. 425) or it may be the whole tubercle even extending into and including the top of the tibia (Fig. 427).

Treatment will depend largely upon your evaluation of the situation. If this is a substantial piece and is obviously displaced, treatment must be surgical. In the case shown in Figure 426, the loose ossicle which had been pulled off the patellar tubercle had folded under and was lying up in the infrapatellar tendon bursa together with a substantial amount of patellar tendon. Other cases, as I have said, may not disturb the attachment of the tendon at all, but the whole tubercle may pull off including the top of the tibia. In this case the fragment should be replaced and held by internal fixation (Fig. 427). Since there is an epiphysis under the tubercle, if the

fragment is the whole central part of the apophyseal side of the epiphysis, it may be better to take the fragment out and repair the tendon rather than to risk fusion of the epiphysis by replacing the fragment and expecting bony union (Fig. 425). In any event the patellar tendon should be securely fixed in order to restore active extension of the knee. In many cases there may be some active extension because the whole tendon may not be avulsed. In most cases there will be difficulty in locking the knee in complete extension, although it may be extended fairly well from 90 degrees to 45 degrees. If, on the other hand, it seems that the fragment is not of major importance and is not grossly displaced, a period of immobilization may permit this to heal, although this is not a very favorable atmosphere for healing because it should be recalled that the fragment is pulled away from the carti-

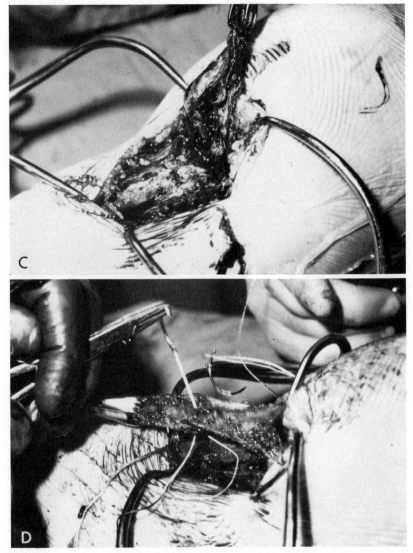

Figure 424 *Continued.* *C,* Surgical view showing in the tenaculum the avulsed patellar tendon reflected upward toward the knee, the raw bed below. *D,* Process of repair, mattress sutures through drill holes suturing this patellar tendon down to the denuded top of the tibia. This boy had a good recovery.

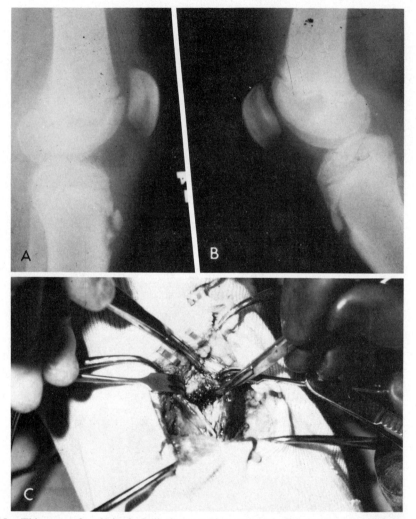

Figure 425.   This young female basketball player made a tremendous leap for a rebound. She fell to the floor with immediate, extreme pain. Complete disability resulted—she would not bend her knee or bear weight on the leg. *A*, X-ray showing the central portion of the epiphysis torn from its bed. *B*, The normal leg for comparison. *C*, Surgical view shows the avulsed patellar tendon with a square block of bone. Lifted up by the hemostat in the light area beneath is the epiphyseal cartilage. The fragment was removed to prevent possible closure of the epiphysis. No growth disturbance was noted.

laginous epiphysis and it may have some difficulty in getting firm union down to the epiphyseal cartilage. I think in the majority of cases an avulsion is better treated by surgical repair. If the epiphysis is open and it is necessary to use internal fixation to hold the fragment down, this should certainly be removed as soon as union is secure in order to have minimal involvement of the circulation and to lessen the danger of epiphyseal fusion.

Knee Flexors

The biceps muscle-tendon unit attaches in the knee area to the fibular head where it bifurcates to interdigitate with the bifid attachment of the fibular collateral ligament. In this area strain must be distinguished from sprain of the ligament since the tenderness is indistinguishable. The key to diagnosis is stress. Active pull of the biceps or passive stretch against the biceps will cause pain in a strain, whereas lateral stress of the leg and the thigh will cause pain in a ligament injury. On the medial side of the knee, hamstring strain may occur at the pes anserinus and may well go on to tenosynovitis or to bursitis in this area. The calf may be strained at the aponeurotic attachment of the gastrocnemius to the posterior capsule or to the femoral condyles. The popliteus may occasionally be strained at its attachment to the femur or in the muscle-tendon junction.

In moderate (second degree) strain there is definite damage to the unit and more or less weakness as a result of this. It is sometimes very difficult to distinguish between the mild injury which really does not require too much treatment on the one hand and the severe injury which requires restoration on the other. In general the symptoms are more severe in moderate than in mild strain, particularly in disturbance of function. For instance if the hamstring muscle is partially torn, it will be ecchymotic and full of blood and very tender and sore. It obviously is a much more serious injury.

As in most of these instances, where the mild condition does not require too much treatment and the severe condition requires repair, the moderate condition requires a good deal of insight to diagnose what exactly has happened. It may easily be confused with a contusion and hematoma, the classic example of this situation occurring in the thigh. Around the knee the most critical areas would probably be at the top of the patella in the quadriceps mechanism or along the muscle-tendon junction in the hamstrings. The importance of the diagnosis is that it requires a substantial period of rest to protect these incomplete tears so that they can heal properly with normal length and without calcification or ossification.

Severe (third degree) or complete strains predicate a complete separation of some component of the muscle-tendon unit. This may be avulsion of the muscle from its origin, rupture of the muscle itself or rupture at any point in the tendon. In the area of the knee these injuries almost always involve the tendon, the exceptions being the popliteus and the gastrocnemius. Even these are usually tendinous ruptures, either in the tendon itself or at the attachment of the tendon to the bone. In severe or complete rupture of the muscle-tendon unit, function is disrupted and the diagnosis can often be made by the bunching up of the involved muscle on active contraction. Localization of the injury can be defined by the area of the tenderness. It may be difficult to diagnose a complete rupture of a muscle in the acute stage (Figs. 428 and 429). Nonetheless it is extremely important, since the time element to initiate treatment is very much more abbreviated in a muscle-tendon injury than in a ligament injury.

Mild and moderate strain of the knee should be treated as indicated in the foregoing, the exact period of treatment depending upon the degree of damage present. The main error here is to assume that the condition is less severe than it actually is. In a mild (first degree) strain treatment is symptomatic; in a moderate (second degree) strain it calls for protection until the lesion heals, whereas in a severe (third degree) strain restoration of the unit is required.

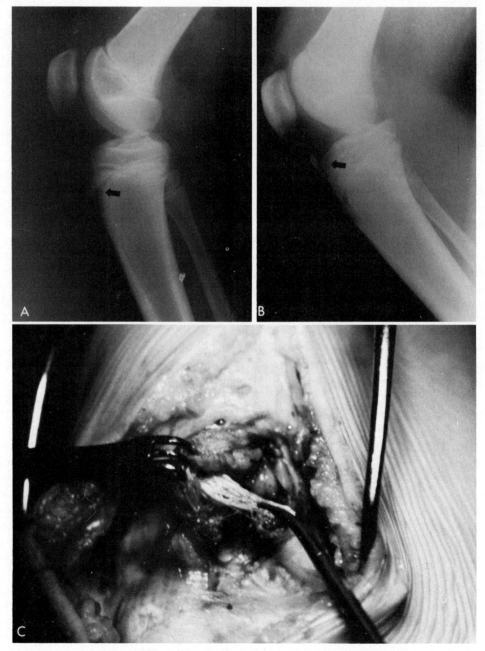

Figure 426. *See legend on opposite page.*

Treatment of moderate (second degree) strain of the knee requires complete rest in order to prevent active function of the muscle involved. In some cases this will require the use of a splint and in others merely the avoidance of strenuous activity. In either case athletic participation is incompatible with proper treatment. Direct therapeutic measures consist of injecting a long-acting local anesthetic into the area. Direct injection into the tendon should be avoided. Use of local heat such as diathermy after 48 hours is in order. Whirlpool baths, hot packs and analgesic balm may all be useful. The treatment of each degree of injury is fundamentally the same and depends upon the amount of damage to the unit.

In the final analysis, for *mild (first degree) strain* a degree of rest is indicated, enough at least to avoid all painful motion lest the acute stress develop into a chronic one. No appreciable weakness is present and disability will be confined to those activities which repeat the stress that caused the condition. So rest, heat and mild exercise are useful; stress is not. Recovery should be prompt and complete.

In a *moderate (second degree) strain* of the tendons about the knee, the knee should be put at complete rest in a splint for a long enough period of time to permit the acute symptoms to subside (three to four weeks). On removal of the splints active motion should be carefully instigated, always within the limits of pain. Complete nonparticipation for an interval long enough to permit definitive treatment may well return the player to active sports. Continued participation in sports may render him quite ineffectual for the season. The danger is in recurrence, since it is difficult to eliminate the cause of the strain if the athlete is not grounded. Once recovery is complete, recurrence need not be anticipated. Straps, wraps and pads will have little effect in preventing re-injury.

In a *severe (third degree) strain* a complete tear of the quadriceps from the patella or an avulsion of a rim of bone requires restoration of the unit by surgery. If the avulsed segment of the patella includes the full thickness of the bone, the fragment should be removed whether it be superior pole, inferior pole, or medial or lateral margins. The tendon may then be sutured to the patella through drill holes with care being taken not to drill through the articular cartilage. If the avulsion is just a skin of bone, it may be replaced in the same

Figure 426.   Six months before I saw him, this 13 year old boy injured his knee playing football. He was seen by an orthopaedist who told him he had Osgood-Schlatter disease, injected the area and applied a cast. *A*, X-ray brought in with the patient shows a loose ossicle at the apophysis. When I saw him six months later he had had persistent pain throughout this time with limited activities. He could not run, play basketball, or do anything else very active. He had pain on hyperflexion of his knee, and pain on extension against resistance. He was tender over the tuberosity of the tibia but also quite tender over the central portion of the patellar tendon. *B*, X-rays made at this time (six months post-injury) reveal a fragment of bone lying apparently under the tendon, possibly in the infrapatellar tendon bursa. This was diagnosed to be the ossicle now missing from the tuberosity but showing up in the tendon above. At surgery, on splitting the tendon we found an area of old granulation tissue at the apophysis where the bed of the fragment was, but the tendon seemed to turn back on itself and pass under the main portion of the tendon into the area of the patellar tendon bursa. *C*, In extracting this tendon, it carried down the loose fragment of bone and cartilage that had been displaced off the apophysis and under the tendon. Removal of the fragment and repair of the tendon gave good results and now, three years postoperative, he is having no problem. This fortifies my opinion that many diagnoses of the so-called Osgood-Schlatter disease or apophysitis of the tendon are really fractures that fail to heal in this particular area because of the avascular tendon on top and the avascular epiphyseal cartilage underneath the fragment.

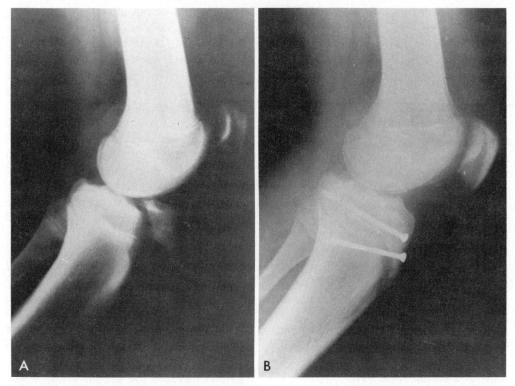

Figure 427. This 15 year old male athlete caught his heel as he took off on a high jump. He had severe pain, fell down, and could not walk or actively extend the knee. Examination at 24 hours showed a badly swollen knee anteriorly with hemarthrosis. The tendon was not palpable. *A*, X-ray showing avulsion of the apophysis extending right up into the joint. Note the high patella. *B*, Postoperative x-ray showing repositioning and internal fixation. No notable growth disturbance, since the epiphyses were closing. The epiphysis seems more vulnerable just before it closes.

manner without removing the thin avulsed layer of bone.

The degree of aftercare depends upon the extent of the rupture and the security of the repair. It will require at least eight weeks to obtain reasonably good union of tendon and bone. With a complete tear of the patellar tendon or the quadriceps tendon, two weeks in a posterior stirrup splint followed by six weeks in a long leg walking cast will be required before rehabilitation can proceed to active resistive exercises. Isometrics can be begun almost at once.

The time in plaster may be shortened by a double bar caliper brace with heel socket. Use of a dial stop at the knee will permit motion earlier and

allow flexion within the limits of tolerance. It will not protect against active resistive motion, however. In the young athlete the brace is not desirable. If the defect is medial or lateral with or without a fragment of bone, the period of immobilization can be much shorter — two weeks in a splint and three weeks in a cast.

Complete rupture of a hamstring tendon is quite rare in athletes. The muscle-tendon junction is much more vulnerable. If a tendon rupture occurs and is recognized, the same treatment as the foregoing is recommended. In no case should competitive athletics be allowed under three months after a complete muscle-tendon rupture.

Rehabilitation

Rehabilitation following any degree of strain is quite different from that of sprain, since in sprain the injured ligament can be protected and active, even stressful motion continued. In strain, the injury is to the motor unit itself so that active contraction of the unit must be carefully controlled until the healing is complete.

Calcification or Ossification

Calcification after strain about the knee usually follows chronic strain with repetitive injury. Ossification usually occurs after acute injury. Calcification is most common at the attachment of the patellar tendon to the tubercle of the tibia. Treatment is the same as for chronic strain—rest, heat and local injection. It may be necessary to immobilize the knee in splints or a walking cast. Serial injections of a long-acting local anesthetic plus a corticoid around the area may be valuable. If injection gives complete relief it need not be repeated. However, if symptoms begin to recur after 7 to 10 days, the injection should be repeated and then again if necessary up to three or four times. Injection must not be made into the tendon. This treatment is much more effective if accompanied by immobilization and physical therapy. Occasionally ossification may have to be removed surgically. If this involves detaching any tendon, the appropriate degree of protective immobilization must be carried out since the lesion may well recur.

Dislocation of the patella is another relatively common cause of damage to the muscle-tendon unit at the knee because of the frequent involvement of the quadriceps medialis attachment to the patella. (For details of this see page 600.)

It is worth emphasizing again that one should spare no effort to make a specific diagnosis in these conditions about the knee. Proper diagnosis is the antecedent to proper treatment. Watchful waiting is usually "watchful neglect!"

BURSITIS

It was noted in the general discussion of bursae that many of them are relatively constant while many others are adventitious. As a basic concept, a bursa develops in order to permit friction-free motion between contiguous moving parts. There is a wealth of bursae about the knee (Fig. 430) and a detailed anatomical description of them all is not pertinent here. With a few exceptions only those which are consistent in their formation and are particularly prone to involvement in the athlete will be discussed.

BURSITIS ON THE ANTERIOR ASPECT OF THE KNEE

Prepatellar Bursa

Anteriorly the bursa most commonly involved is the prepatellar (Fig. 430). This bursal sac lies between the skin and the anterior surface of the patella and serves to permit free sliding of the relatively thin skin over the underlying subcutaneous bone. This bursa is particularly susceptible to damage by direct trauma, as by falling on the flexed knee. Whereas in its normal state this bursa is somewhat smaller than the underlying patella, it may reach amazing size when its sac is distended. Involvement of this bursa may be acute or chronic.

Acute Prepatellar Bursitis. Acute involvement will usually begin as an area of tenderness, reddening and inflammation directly over the kneecap. The skin becomes red and warm and sensitive to touch. If the knee is examined very early, snowball crepitation

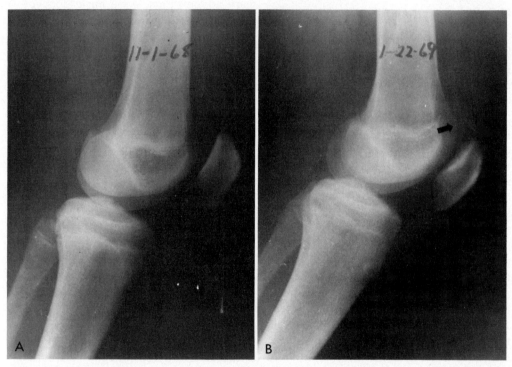

Figure 428.   This 16 year old male, while convalescing from knee surgery following a football injury, fell down the stairs, injuring his knee. He had gross swelling. X-ray was made *(A)*, which did not show avulsion of bone but did show some upward tilting of the proximal end of the patella when compared with the normal opposite knee *(F)*. Successive pictures show *(B)* early ossification in the quadriceps tendon three months post-injury.

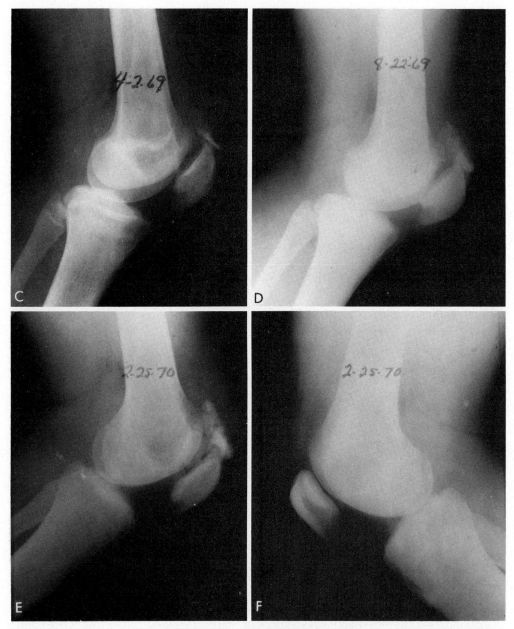

Figure 428 *Continued.*   *C*, Six months post-injury, note the massive ossification. *D*, Ten months post-injury, continued ossification. *E*, Sixteen months post-injury, at which time he was examined here. Meantime he had continued to try to run and play, without success. Examination revealed the tremendously large mass of patella. He complained on flexion and extension. He also complained that the patella tried to slip sideways when he tried to cut. Poorly developed medialis. Marked atrophy of the whole quadriceps. It would be difficult to remove this mass of bone without destroying the quadriceps tendon mechanism. Early repair of this avulsion of the quadriceps tendon probably would have prevented this result.

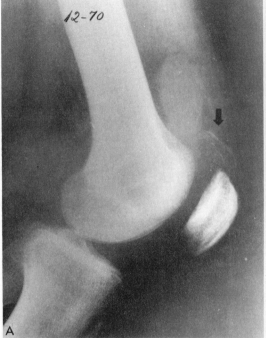

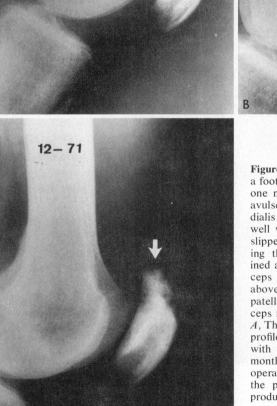

Figure 429. This 18 year old male suffered a football injury that required surgical repair one month later consisting of repair of the avulsed attachment of the quadriceps medialis to the femur. He was progressing very well when at two months postoperative he slipped in a wet shower and fell, hyperflexing the knee. At this time he was examined and had obvious damage to his quadriceps mechanism. He had a palpable defect above, with the rectus detached from the patella. He was operated on and the quadriceps mechanism was attached to the patella. *A*, The original radiograph showed a phantom profile of the superior border of the patella with the patella somewhat low. *B*, Four months postoperative. *C*, One year postoperative showing the union of the rectus to the patella with a lot of exogenous bone produced but with excellent function.

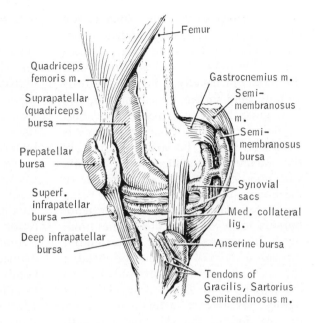

Figure 430. The bursae about the knee. Medial aspect.

Quadriceps femoris m.

Suprapatellar (quadriceps) bursa

Prepatellar bursa

Superf. infrapatellar bursa

Deep infrapatellar bursa

Femur

Gastrocnemius m.

Semi-membranosus m.

Semi-membranosus bursa

Synovial sacs

Med. collateral lig.

Anserine bursa

Tendons of Gracilis, Sartorius Semitendinosus m.

can often be elicited between the walls of the bursa as the skin is moved over the patella. This inflammation progresses rapidly to the formation of effusion so that there is tense, hot swelling localized directly over the patella (Fig. 431). Ordinary motion of the knee is pain free, but flexion to the point of skin tension will cause pain. This condition can be readily distinguished from involvement of the knee joint by its definite localization in front of the patella.

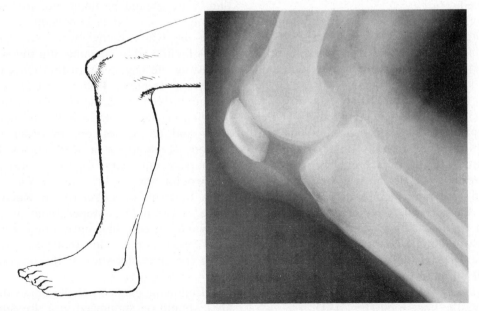

Figure 431. Prepatellar bursitis of the patella in its normal position with swelling between patella and skin.

Treatment in the acute stage is that of any acute inflammatory reaction. Immobilization of the knee in a posterior splint (Fig. 444, *A*) and a warm saline dressing will usually suffice. If there is definite fluid in the sac, aspiration will distinguish between gross pus and bursal fluid. A culture of the fluid, if any is obtained, should be made. Ordinarily the inflammation will subside quickly with only a slight residual thickening of the lining, the period of disability being only a few days. It is unusual for acute bursitis to go on to acute suppuration, but if this occurs drainage is carried out through a short (4 cm.) incision through the skin on either side parallel to the patella about 1 cm. away from its border. Great care is taken to restrict the incision to the skin and bursa to avoid any possibility of opening into the knee joint. Through-and-through rubber tissue drainage together with moderate pressure and continuation of the hot pack will suffice in most local situations. A broad-spectrum antibiotic is given until definite sensitivity of the organism to a specific antibiotic can be determined.

Following acute bursitis, adequate protective padding over the knee should be used since recurrence is a strong possibility owing to the extremely vulnerable location of the bursa.

Chronic Prepatellar Bursitis. A much more frequent involvement of the prepatellar bursa is chronic bursitis. This may develop as a sequel to repeated attacks of acute bursitis but is more likely to be the result of repeated mild traumata which cause thickening of the bursal wall, oversecretion of fluid and gradual filling of the bursal sac. Early examination of the knee will be unrewarding, the only finding being the well outlined discrete sac of fluid very obviously subcutaneous. It does not involve the knee joint (Fig. 431).

Treatment at this stage should consist of aspiration of the fluid, injection of a corticoid and a firm pressure dressing. Since the condition is not disabling, and since a pressure dressing is not consistent with active sports participation, it is unusual for the player to seek or accept this particular plan of treatment. Usually the condition is allowed to continue and, as he falls repeatedly or kneels on the distended bursa, pressure on its wall causes it to stretch and the sac to expand. A bursa which actually is much smaller in diameter than the patella may distend to cover the whole anterior surface of the knee, not infrequently reaching 15 to 20 cm. in diameter. It presents itself as a loose, floppy, fluctuant tumor mass causing symptoms largely by its very bulk (Fig. 432). Once a bursa has reached this stage no treatment short of surgical excision is adequate. Surgical excision is relatively simple, a transverse incision being made slightly above the midline of the patella and extending from 8 to 15 cm., depending upon the size of the bursa. The bursa is carefully dissected out. This is particularly difficult directly over the patella where the skin is very thin. Care should be taken not to buttonhole the skin. It is important to remove the whole lining of the sac and this is facilitated by opening into the sac and using the finger within the bursa to determine its limits. Following excision it is advisable to tack the skin to the underlying fascia over the patellar retinaculum and the quadriceps in order to prevent development of dead spaces. If the bursa is quite large the two angles of the wound should be drained for 48 hours by strips of rubber tissue. Recurrence of the fluid postoperatively is to be avoided if possible, since an adventitious bursa may develop that may have all of the characteristics of the original one.

Following excision of the bursa the knee should be supported in a dressing such as the cotton cast (Fig. 433) in order to prevent excess motion between

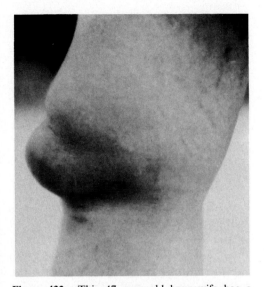

Figure 432. This 47 year old housewife has a prepatellar bursitis of 10 months' standing. Picture shows the very localized, discrete, swollen bursa. This was treated by excision of the prepatellar bursa with excellent results. Many times, particularly in the athlete, the bursa is much flatter than this because it has been subjected to repeated trauma and so spreads the bursal wall out until it sometimes may be 15 to 20 cm. in diameter.

the skin and patella until such time as the space is completely obliterated. This usually requires about four weeks. It is important that the knee be inspected at frequent intervals during the early post-operative period since any fluid that accumulates must be promptly aspirated. It is discouraging to the surgeon, and I dare say even more to the patient, to have the bursa recur. Those most likely to recur are the large ones. For this reason it is recommended that the bursa should be removed as soon as it can be definitely determined that irreversible chronic bursitis is present. The removal of a small, sharply localized bursa is relatively simple and very effectual whereas some of the larger ones may present a major problem.

I recall a case of a football player who insisted on playing without knee pads. He carried his prepatellar bursitis through an entire season, being treated only by repeated aspirations and some

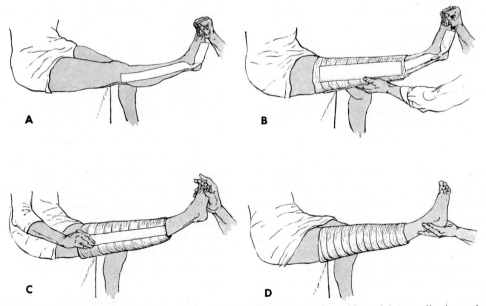

Figure 433. Cotton cast. *A,* The leg is shaved from the knee to the ankle and 8-cm. adhesive strip is applied to either side. *B,* The knee is wrapped in regular sheet wadding, usually five or six rolls, slightly longer than the length of the yucca board. A moistened yucca board splint is applied on either side and posteriorly, centering at the knee. *C,* Yucca board splints have been wrapped snugly in place with 8-cm. gauze. The two adhesive strips are pulled back firmly over the ends of the two lateral boards. *D,* The finished cotton cast, the adhesive strips having been wrapped down snugly with gauze and the whole protected by spiral 2½-cm. adhesive tape.

feeble attempt at pressure. At one time over a quart of fluid was removed from the bursa. At operation it was found to be of tremendous size, extending as high as midthigh and down to about 10 cm. above the ankle. The player was cured by surgical excision of the sac (which could hardly be called a bursa) and suture of the skin to the underlying fascia. In spite of care at the original operation there was a small area of recurrence which required a second excision. The player had remarkably little disability even during the period of extreme distention of the sac. One of the complaints was a sloshing up and down of the contained fluid as he ran.

Characteristically the wall of an extremely expanded bursa will upon examination present the picture of a very chronic synovitis, usually without villous thickening. It has a shiny, almost plastic appearance interspersed with areas of petechiae the size of the end of the finger. The superficial appearance of these areas is similar to that of psoriasis on the skin. The pathological report has uniformly been "chronic synovial inflammation." During the chronic stage of this noninflammatory type of bursitis it may be necessary to aspirate the sac repeatedly, continue pressure bandages and allow participation until a more convenient time for surgical removal. However, if the sac is widely distended it is not desirable to permit competitive athletics for the reasons noted above. In carrying out aspiration it must be remembered that the sac is just beneath the skin and great care should be taken that the aspirating needle does not inadvertently penetrate into the knee joint. This is particularly important if there is an acute inflammation, in which case also the accident is much more likely to happen since there will be edema, tension and considerable inelasticity of the tissue. Prepatellar bursitis treated nonsurgically is prone to recur; hence, adequate padding of the knee is mandatory in order to prevent direct trauma over the patella. After surgical excision also, even though there appears to be complete cure, it is wise to insist that a player wear knee pads whenever he is engaged in competitive or contact sports.

Infrapatellar Tendon Bursa
(Deep Infrapatellar Bursa)

The infrapatellar tendon bursa lies behind the patellar tendon and in front of the infrapatellar fat pad (Fig. 430). It does not ordinarily communicate with the knee joint, being separated from the knee by the fat pad. The etiology of infrapatellar bursitis is quite different from that of prepatellar bursitis. The prepatellar bursa is frequently traumatized by a direct blow upon the hard patella which makes up its floor, whereas the infrapatellar bursa is not particularly subject to direct trauma since it lies behind the thick patellar tendon and in front of the soft fat pad. Occasionally the lower part of the bursa, which extends down over the front of the upper end of the tibia, may be traumatized but inflammation of this bursa is ordinarily due to friction between the patellar tendon and structures behind it (upper tibia and fat pad), the result of overactivity.

The *symptoms* are usually pain on complete passive flexion and on active complete extension of the knee. Tenderness surrounds the patellar tendon and is particularly notable under its edges. If the tendon is picked up between the thumb and forefinger and the thumb and forefinger are permitted to slip behind it, direct pressure will cause pain.

Diagnosis. Infrapatellar bursitis must, if possible, be distinguished from involvement of the infrapatellar fat pad which lies directly behind it. In inflammation of the bursa which has proceeded to the point of fluid formation, it may be possible to demonstrate fluid in the sac lying directly behind the patellar tendon, which bulges out on either side. Pressure on one side will cause it to bulge out on the other. Similarly, flexion of the knee will cause the patellar tendon to compress the sac and make it balloon out on either side. Inflammation of the infrapatellar fat pad, on the other hand, will seem to be deeper, more posterior. Passive extension of the knee should be pain-free in infrapatellar tendon bursitis, whereas if the fat pad is inflamed and swollen, complete passive extension may be impossible or will cause pain. Complete flexion of the knee will cause pain in either instance. An attempt at aspiration may be quite rewarding if it is positive. The needle should be slipped along just under the patellar tendon. Once it enters the fat pad, all is lost and the aspiration will be negative. A negative aspiration attempt does not rule out infrapatellar tendon bursitis. One distressing symptom of both conditions is the sharp twinge of pain on pendulum extension of the knee which is particularly distressing to the place kicker, since in completing this kick there is snap extension of the knee, whereas in the punt or ordinary running there is much less of this particular motion. If the involvement in infrapatellar bursitis is severe enough it will seriously interfere with active motion of the knee, particularly in extremes in either flexion or extension. The condition must also be distinguished from apophysitis of the patellar tubercle (page 662). In this condition the pain and tenderness are more specifically in the tendon or in the patellar tubercle. However, the same clinical tests will cause discomfort, namely, extension of the knee against resistance, overflexion of the knee, and direct pressure over the area.

The *treatment* of infrapatellar bursitis is that of bursitis anywhere. In the early stages local heat and splinting of the knee in extension will reduce the inflammation. Aspiration of the bursa with removal of any fluid encountered, followed by injection of a corticoid, is particularly effective if done early. If effusion is recurrent and resistant to local treatment the bursa may readily be excised, incision being made usually on the inner side of the patellar tendon. The bursa can usually be removed entirely through the single incision. If the bursal mass should appear to be more extensive laterally, incision may be made on the outer side of the patellar tendon. Following careful removal of the entire bursal sac, the fat pad is sutured to the back of the patellar tendon to obliterate the dead space. The knee is splinted in extension with a type of dressing that gives both immobilization and compression (cotton cast). The dressing must be maintained for at least three weeks.

Suprapatellar Tubercle Bursa (Superficial Infrapatellar Bursa)

Another bursa on the anterior aspect of the knee that may become symptomatic lies between the skin and patellar tubercle of the tibia (Figs. 430 and 434). This is not a consistent bursa nor is it frequently involved. In a young individual there may be some difficulty in distinguishing inflammation of this bursa from early apophysitis of the patellar tubercle (Osgood-Schlatter disease). Indeed, many of these cases of apophysitis of the patellar tubercle which have apparently been relieved by local injection may well have been involvement of this pretibial bursa.

Symptoms of involvement of this bursa are sharply localized pain and tenderness directly over the patellar tubercle. They vary from those of infrapatellar bursitis in that active function of the knee does not cause pain since the

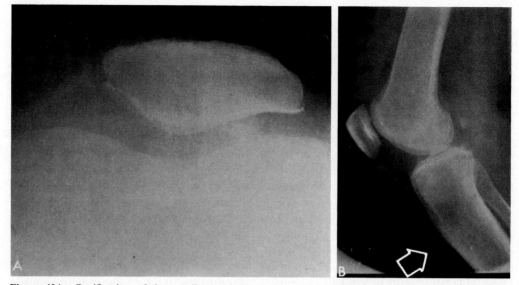

Figure 434. Ossification of the patellar tendon attachment. *A,* Silhouette view of patella, apparently showing an osteochondritic fragment in the joint. *B,* Lateral view showing the calcification in the patellar tendon attachment. Although in the silhouette view this appeared to be under the patella, it was actually some 10 cm. away. This illustrates the value of very careful interpretation of the film. The fact that this fragment did not show under the patella in the lateral view was suggestive. (Note the normal fabella, a sesamoid bone lying within the gastrocnemius and articulating with the femoral condyle.)

attachment of the patellar tendon is not involved. In the acute type, local inflammation will be the characteristic finding. I have yet to see an extensive collection of fluid in this bursa.

Since active function of the knee is not affected, protection against direct trauma is the most pertinent point in prevention of recurrence. Following local treatment there is no particular indication for immobilization of the knee, hence the importance of distinguishing this condition from patellar tubercle apophysitis, strain of the patellar tendon attachment, infrapatellar bursitis and other neighboring conditions which do require immobilization and do cause disability.

BURSITIS ON THE MEDIAL ASPECT OF THE KNEE

Anserine Bursa

Another bursa consistently present but not so frequently involved is the an-

serine bursa (Fig. 430). While this bursa may have the usual variants and may be single or multiple, it ordinarily lies between the aponeurosis of the attachment of the internal hamstrings (pes anserinus) and of the long fibers of the medial collateral ligament and the underlying anteromedial face of the upper end of the tibia (Fig. 430). Under normal circumstances the pes anserinus and the long fibers of the collateral ligament attach to the anterior border of the tibia some 3 inches below the superior articular surface. The bursa serves to separate these freely sliding portions of the tendon from the periosteum of the tibia and the medial collateral ligament. Bursitis in this area is typically of the friction type, although it may be initiated by an external blow impinging the bursa against the hard tibia beneath. The resulting congestion and inflammation cause the same reaction that occurs in tenosynovitis or any friction bursitis.

Original *symptoms* are pain from

the contusion, which is persistent and rather sharply localized. Symptoms are aggravated by flexion and extension of the knee. Since the symptoms will be located on the upper anteromedial face of the tibia, they may be confused with those of injury to the medial collateral ligament. However, they are quite distinguishable under careful examination, the tenderness being located not at the attachment of the tendon and ligament but under their unattached portion. Crepitation, if elicitable, is diagnostic.

Treatment is application of local heat and immobilization of the knee. Recovery can be expedited by injection of a corticoid into the bursa. While this condition may be quite acute it seldom causes suppuration. In fact, I have never seen a case of acute suppuration in this bursa. The involvement does tend to be chronic, particularly if full activity is allowed too early. Protective pads against contusion are of little value, since real protection requires elimination of motion of the knee joint and so will demand nonparticipation in athletics. One is seldom able successfully to aspirate fluid from this bursa or see fluid develop to the point that it could be demonstrated as fluctuation. I think one explanation of this is the tension that exists between the tendon and ligament structures and the tibia, allowing for no redundant fold of bursa that can be filled with fluid.

Other Bursae

Other bursae may be present in this area but are not frequently involved. Further posterior on the medial side is the semimembranosus bursa (Fig. 430) lying between the attachment of the semimembranosus muscle to the upper tibia and medial capsule of the joint. This position is slightly posterior to the midline of the tibia and extends about 1 inch below its upper end. Further poste-

rior is the gastrocnemius bursa lying between the tendon of origin of the medial head of the gastrocnemius and semimembranosus tendon. There may also be bursae between the tendons of the semimembranosus and semitendinosus and gracilis. All of these are subject to involvement, the symptoms depending upon the location and the degree of involvement. Inflammation of the semimembranosus bursa may be confused with damage to the medial collateral ligament but is distinguished by the fact that tension on the medial collateral ligament does not cause increase in pain. The tenderness is distinctly over the semimembranosus tendon just short of its attachment.

BURSITIS ON THE POSTERIOR ASPECT OF THE KNEE

Baker's Cyst

Posteriorly, the most common involvement in athletes is the so-called Baker's cyst. The confusion which so frequently accompanies the use of eponyms is certainly evident here since the term "Baker's cyst" has been extended to include almost any synovial hernia or bursitis involving the posterior aspect of the knee.

One type of "Baker's cyst" is bursitis of the semimembranosus or of the medial gastrocnemius bursa (Figs. 430 and 435), a bursa which lies between the medial head of the gastrocnemius and semimembranosus tendon. Involvement of the bursa causes expansion of its wall, usually posteriorly since there is no particular obstruction to its expansion in this direction. It presents itself as a large soft tumor mass in the popliteal space. The appearance of the mass is usually preceded by a varying period of chronic, aching type pain in the back of the knee. Since the bursa frequently communicates with the knee, often by a

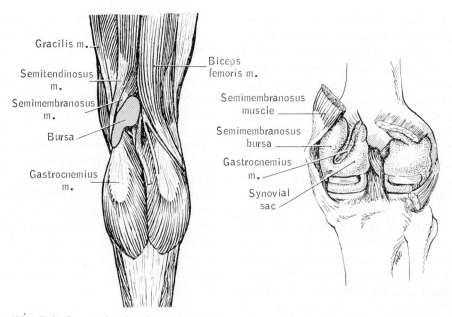

Figure 435. Baker's cyst showing the semimembranosus bursa lying between the semimembranosus and medial head of the gastrocnemius. The actual enlargement of the sac may be palpable at any level. If it protrudes proximally, it will appear in the midline. If it protrudes in its distal portion, it will appear medial to the midline. The medial gastrocnemius bursa (not labeled) lies under the tendon.

valvelike arrangement, the swelling may come and go and present great difficulty diagnostically. As a consequence of the valvelike connection with the knee joint, sufficient fluid may collect to make a sizable tumor. This fluid then concentrates to the characteristic jell contained in a synovial hernia. Later as a result of trauma or other cause it may be discharged into the knee, where the concentrated fluid becomes an irritative factor and causes synovitis. We frequently have found a to-and-fro connection between the knee and bursa so that increased fluid in the knee will distend the bursa and, as the knee recovers, the bursal fluid may remain only to be discharged back into the knee and cause recurrence of the joint effusion. It has been my observation that this bursal involvement is frequently the result of chronic trauma and is too often related to posterior damage of the medial meniscus to be entirely coincidental. Whether the trauma actually opens up

the space between the bursa and knee or causes exudation of fluid that discharges into the bursa rather than into the suprapatellar pouch varies with the individual case. The patient with semimembranosus bursal cyst, therefore, may present himself with a perfectly benign, asymptomatic swelling back of the knee or he may have swelling incidental to internal derangement or to chronic synovitis of the knee. So it can be seen that in this one entity, namely, the involvement of the medial gastrocnemius bursa and semimembranosus bursa, there may be several different conditions that can be called Baker's cyst.

So also may Baker's cyst be the result of a synovial hernia off one of the tendon sheaths, specifically, the semitendinosus. Add to this the fact that the cyst may also result from a true synovial hernia from the back of the joint due to a defect or degeneration in the posterior capsule similar to the formation of a ganglion anywhere and we have several different etiological conditions giving the same terminal diagnosis. One should if at all possible avoid the eponym "Baker's cyst" and be more specific in the diagnosis, since specificity of diagnosis will aid in treatment.

Diagnosis. This condition must be distinguished from other tumor masses, such as aneurysm of the popliteal artery, arterial venous fistula or soft tissue tumor. Occasionally wholly benign conditions may present a confusing picture. I well recall my humiliation at confidently exposing the mass of a "Baker's cyst" only to find that in this singularly well muscled individual the "cyst" was an unusually low lying belly of the semimembranosus muscle. The only pathologic finding in this instance was a preoperatively diagnosed posterior tear of the medial meniscus. As a rule, these conditions present no emergency and time and patience will permit diagnosis. If it is necessary to operate upon the knee for some other cause, as in the case mentioned above, exploration of this area cannot be condemned since a second operation may thus be avoided. On the other hand, one would be quite chagrined to operate under a primary diagnosis of Baker's cyst and find only overredundant fat or overdeveloped muscle.

Treatment. If the pathology is that of a synovial hernia off the joint, then dissecting out the mass and carefully closing the defect into the knee joint will ordinarily institute a cure. If it is an involvement of the bursa with an open connection into the knee joint, removal of the bursa must include careful suture of the defect in the joint capsule. If it is a result of involvement of the medial meniscus, removal of the Baker's cyst or of the medial meniscus alone will be disappointing. On many occasions we have been able to demonstrate the opening extending into the bursa back of the knee in the course of exposing the posterior compartment for complete removal of the medial meniscus.

If the Baker's cyst is primarily an irritative bursitis of the bursa lying between the semimembranosus and gastrocnemius, removal of the bursa should be followed by careful suture of the semimembranosus to the gastrocnemius, thus eliminating the irritative friction point between these two muscles. I have done this on many occasions and have yet to see any untoward symptoms as the result of suturing these structures together.

If this discussion of treatment for Baker's cyst seems somewhat confusing it is because of the heterogeneous group of conditions that are lumped together under this name. Carefully analyzed it will be seen that the treatment recommended is the treatment for the basic underlying condition. If bursitis, excision of the bursa. If hernia of the joint or tendon, repair of the hernia. If a defect in the posterior capsule or medial meniscus, appropriate treatment for the underlying lesion. In this situation, as in many others, the proper treatment will depend upon accurate diagnosis. In many instances this diagnosis may not be made preoperatively and one must be alert at operation to determine if at all possible the basic underlying pathologic condition so that he can remove the condition as well as the symptoms.

Following surgical correction it is advisable to hold the knee in compression immobilization (Fig. 433) for at least four weeks. As in synovial hernia or ganglion elsewhere, recurrence may be prevented by adequate repair. If the condition is a true bursitis, recurrence may be prevented by permitting complete healing of the structures involved. In my hands nonsurgical management of these swellings in the back of the knee has not been satisfactory. I have occasionally aspirated the mass for diagnostic purposes and at other times have seen the tumor disappear spontaneously but have been dissatisfied with treatment by aspiration, local injection and immobilization.

BURSITIS ON THE LATERAL ASPECT OF THE KNEE

Bursae About the Head of the Fibula

On the lateral aspect of the knee are several bursae, any one of which may cause symptoms. The most common are bursae about the upper end of the fibula. A rather consistent bursa, the bicipital, lies between the fibular collateral ligament and the biceps tendon just adjacent to the fibular attachment. Since each of these strong, fibrous structures splits to encompass the other, there may be several bursae in this area to permit active motion between them.

Diagnostically, inflammation of these bursae may present a considerable problem since they are consistent in neither size nor location. Characteristically the pain is proximal to the head of the fibula with tenderness around the fibular collateral ligament and the biceps. However, the same findings may be present in a strain of the biceps tendon or a sprain of the fibular collateral ligament. In many instances it is impossible to distinguish between these conditions and in other instances they coexist. Only in the unusual case does synovial effusion develop in sufficient amount to permit palpation of a fluctuant mass. However, local swelling in this area, even though it may be diffuse, is much more common in bursitis than it is in the other conditions commonly found here. Thickening of the bursal wall plus effusion with local irritation may become severe enough to cause pressure on the peroneal nerve as it winds around the back of the fibular head. Symptoms are

of pain along the distribution of the nerve; on occasion an actual peroneal palsy develops. Bursitis in this location is not commonly prone to calcification. The presence of a hard, calcified mass contained within the constricting walls of the bursa may be exceedingly painful and may indeed cause pressure on the nerve. In case of unexplained peroneal neuritis one should suspect bursitis about the head of the fibula.

Treatment of bursitis in this area is local heat, rest and local injection. It should be noted that this treatment is similar to that of strain or sprain and in many cases one may not have distinguished between these conditions. This is particularly likely since active motion of the knee will cause pain in all of them. Strictly speaking, active flexion against resistance should hurt more in a strain or tenosynovitis of the biceps tendon than it should in a true bursitis, whereas direct pressure or passive extension of the knee might be expected to be more painful in bursitis. Bursal pain may also be elicited by activity within a range of motion that does not cause strain on the tendon. It should be realized that these are more impressions than diagnostic certainties. Involvement in this area may be particularly disheartening since it is exceedingly prone to recur because of the previously mentioned anatomical relationships with two bifid attachments interdigitating with each other to make multiple friction points.

If pyogenic bursitis develops it should be treated appropriately for the infection. If the response to antibiotic therapy is not reasonably prompt, the best definitive treatment for pyogenic bursitis is early drainage with identification of the organism and institution of specific antibiotic therapy. If one succumbs to the temptation to treat the condition by antibiotics alone it is very apt to terminate in excessive thickening of the bursal walls and painful scar formation even if the acute infection subsides. It is much more likely to go on to chronic suppurative involvement with a long period of disability. If calcification develops in the early stages it may respond to aspiration and injection with a corticoid, whereas in the later stages it must be surgically removed. I recall one instance in which exceedingly distressing peroneal pain had been attributed to many other things including psychoneurosis. The patient, a woman, had a very large calcifying bursitis and at operation the peroneal nerve was found to be tightly stretched over the firm, solid mass of the bursa full of calcium. Excision of the bursa and saline neurolysis of the nerve gave prompt and complete relief (Fig. 436).

Popliteal Bursa

A little higher up on the fibular collateral ligament a bursa will be found lying between the popliteus tendon and the fibular collateral ligament slightly above the line of the knee joint. Another relatively consistent bursa lies upon the lateral head of the gastrocnemius located slightly behind the biceps tendon. Any of these lateral bursae may connect with the knee joint, particularly the one between the lateral condyle of the femur and tendon of the popliteus and the one between the popliteus and fibular collateral ligament. In this area, too, a specific diagnosis may present great difficulty because of the variety of structures which present a similarity of symptoms. It has been said that the popliteus muscle is the overlooked structure of the knee since its lesions are so infrequently diagnosed. Differentiation between popliteal bursitis, popliteal tenosynovitis, strain of the popliteus muscle or tendon, and involvement of the adjacent bursae is difficult. It is sufficient to state that treatment of the lateral aspect of the knee is local treat-

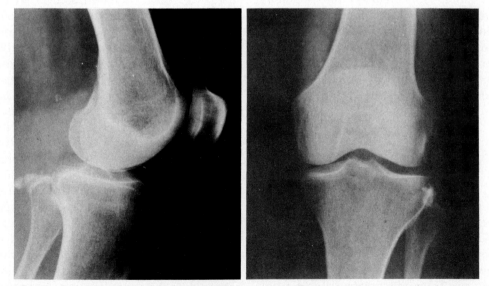

Figure 436. Calcification of bursa about the fibular head with nerve involvement. This patient developed soreness around the outer side of the knee which was attributable to increased activity. The pain gradually became more intense and lancinating in character down the peroneal nerve distribution. Physical examination revealed inability to straighten the knee with peroneal nerve pain on attempting to straighten it, and palpable tumor in the vicinity of the head and biceps tendon. X-ray revealed calcification in the bicipital bursa. Excision of the mass resulted in dramatic relief with uneventful recovery.

ment of the tender area: injection, local heat, and protection against any motion that causes pain. This whole lateral complex of lateral meniscus, fibular collateral ligament, popliteus muscle and biceps tendon may present well-nigh insuperable obstacles to diagnosis. Fortunately, as has been mentioned, the basic treatment is essentially the same in the incipient case and the more advanced cases will present more specific diagnostic points.

Other Bursae

As one proceeds posteriorly he encounters the *lateral gastrocnemius bursa* lying between the condyle of the femur and the lateral head of the gastrocnemius. Involvement of this bursa is infrequently diagnosed. As to its frequency or whether it occurs as part of another pathological symptom complex I have no information. I have never been able to diagnose inflammation of the *bursa lying beneath the popliteus muscle,* since in acute conditions it is indistinguishable from other conditions in the back of the popliteal space and in chronic conditions I have never seen it sufficiently distended with fluid to provide a clue.

SPRAIN

It must be remembered that a ligament is a fibrous structure designed to prevent abnormal motion of a joint. Any injury to a ligament caused by abnormal motion may be defined as a sprain. It should be obvious, then, that a sprain can vary from a complete dislocation of a joint with total loss of integrity of the ligament at one extreme to a slight tearing of a few isolated fibers with no loss of function at the other. Properly it

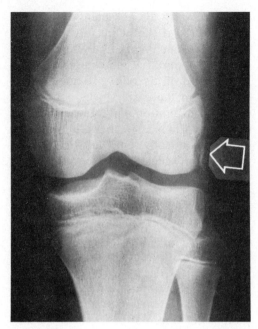

Figure 437. Acute avulsion of fibular collateral ligament from the femur with a flake of bone.

should include avulsion of the ligament from bone with or without a small fragment of bone (sprain-fracture) (Fig. 437), partial avulsion of the ligament from the bone, or tearing of the ligament within its substance either transversely, obliquely or longitudinally. In the last instance the ligament will be elongated although it may appear to be intact. The function of the ligament depends not only upon its strength but upon its length, and a ligament that is elongated does not carry out its function of preventing abnormal motion of the joint. Since we are primarily concerned clinically with the function of the ligament, it matters little in what way but a great deal to what extent this function is disturbed. It is apparent that the severity of the injury is of much more significance than the exact location or type of the tear. It follows that the determination of the degree of loss of function of the involved ligament at the earliest possible moment is of prime importance.

Ligamentous Anatomy of the Knee

The anatomical drawings (Figs. 438 and 439) will serve as a review of the ligamentous structures of the knee. The knee consists essentially of two long bones meeting end to end without benefit of either the deep ball and socket of the hip or the mortise and tenon of the ankle. The bony stability of the knee derives solely from the fact that the femur is a bipod with two separate distal condyles, and lateral instability will be present only when one or the other foot of the femur can be lifted from the tibia. This bipod provides lateral stability with much less demand upon ligament strength than would be necessary if there were but a single condyle. Nonetheless, real stability of the joint depends in major degree upon the intri-cately designed and ingeniously arranged ligaments of the knee.

The **lateral ligaments** (Fig. 438) and the **posterior ligament** (or capsule) (Fig. 439) actually are a part of the great investiture of the joint by ligamentous structures which are massive and very strong on each side and posteriorly but which become thinned in front to permit motion of the joint. These ligaments are supported and their strength greatly augmented by the **cruciate ligaments** (Fig. 438) which are very strong, fan-shaped structures, each twisted on itself to permit motion but to provide maximum stability. The anterior cruciate ligament arising anteromedially from the tibial plateau in front of the tibial spines extends backward, upward and outward to attach to the femur posterolaterally in the intercondylar notch. While it has

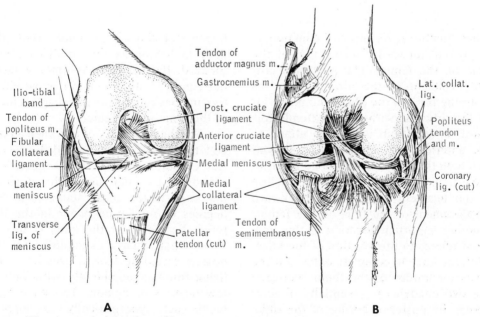

Figure 438. Anatomical drawings of knee.

A, Anterior view. Patellar tendon is sectioned and the patella reflected upward. Knee flexed. Note that the cruciate ligament rises in front of anterior tibial spine, not from it. Note also that the medial meniscus is firmly attached to the medial collateral ligament.

B, Posterior view, knee extended. Note that the posterior ligament has been removed. The two layers of the medial collateral ligament are shown diagrammatically, also the tibial portion of the lateral collateral ligament. The posterior cruciate ligament rises behind the tibia, not on its upper surface. Observe the femoral attachment of the anterior cruciate ligament at the back of the notch.

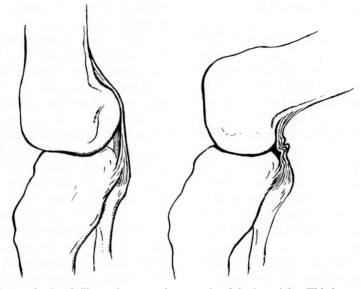

Figure 439. Anatomic sketch illustrating posterior capsule of the knee joint. This is an extremely dense fibrous structure attaching above the condyles clear across the back of the femur extra-articularly. It attaches below the knee all the way across the tibia and onto the fibula. This structure is tight in extension *(left)*, at which time it adds materially to the stability of the knee in all directions except flexion. It is an extremely positive check ligament to prevent overextension. With the knee flexed *(right)*, the ligament becomes redundant, so that it no longer has any stabilizing effect in any direction.

other functions, its primary function is to prevent forward displacement of the tibia on the femur. The posterior cruciate ligament, on the other hand, arises from the back of the tibia, well posterior to the articular surface. It extends forward, upward and inward to attach to the anterior edge of the intercondylar notch on the medial side just adjacent to the articular margin. A primary function of this ligament is to prevent backward displacement of the tibia on the femur. Another important function of this ligament relates to the position of the knee. With the knee in complete extension the posterior border of the femur between the two condyles is essentially directly above the posterior border of the tibia. So in complete extension the posterior cruciate ligament runs vertically from the back of the femur on the lateral side of the medial femoral condyle almost directly downward to the back of the tibia. This gives a very firm check to

hyperextension of the knee. With the knee in flexion as the condyles rotate forward, the ligament assumes a more horizontal position and so is most effective in checking backward displacement of the tibia on the femur.

All the ligaments of the knee—both collaterals, the cruciates and the posterior capsule—are taut in complete extension of the knee and in this position the knee is the most stable. Varying degrees of relaxation occur in the different ligaments as the knee is flexed. This is particularly exemplified by the posterior capsule which loses its stabilizing function completely with only a few degrees of flexion. The knee ligaments act synergistically to support each other in preventing abnormal mobility of the knee while at the same time permitting normal motion. Functionally the knee joint is a hinge joint although anatomically the motion is much more complicated than this. The ligaments of the joint are designed to prevent abnormal lateral motion, abnormal rotatory motion and abnormal forward and backward displacement of tibia on femur. The heavy posterior ligament serves to prevent overextension of the joint. The anatomy of the menisci will be described later in this chapter.

The ligaments, while providing good stability, are not strong enough to withstand the great stresses on the knee without active cooperation from the various supporting muscles. The ligaments must be considered as a first line of defense. Note the complete knee instability of the flail leg following polio in which the muscle support is lost and the ligaments soon stretch.

Etiology

Sprain of the knee is caused by an abnormal motion of the joint that throws stress on the ligament or ligaments designed to prevent this motion. Forced motion beyond this normal limit will result in some degree of injury to the ligament primarily involved. This motion may be in any direction—adduction or abduction, overextension, internal or external rotation, forward or backward displacement—or almost any combination of these. Certain particular combinations are more frequent than others.

Although frequently it is not obtainable, detailed knowledge of the manner of injury can be of great importance since it may indicate the type of ligament damage and so permit early, definitive treatment. In the classic athletic injury of the knee, the foot is fixed to the ground, the thigh rotates inward and the leg outward, the knee is forced inward toward the opposite leg and the stress is primarily received on the ligaments on the inner side of the knee. It is generally caused by the familiar lateral blocking or by the "cut-back" motion of the running athlete, when the foot is forced into external rotation and stress is exerted against the medial collateral ligament of the knee, the superficial layer of which takes the strain first. As this stretches, tears or gives way, the force reaches the deep layer, to which is attached the medial meniscus. If the force continues, the anterior cruciate receives the stress and it, too, may fail. In severe injuries, the posterior cruciate may also give way. We would expect in injuries of this causation to find sprain of the medial collateral and anterior cruciate ligaments and damage to the medial meniscus ("The Unhappy Triad") (Figs. 440, 441, 442). Obviously, the injury may stop at any point in this progression of events. In a similar manner the adduction and internal rotation type of injury places the stress against the lateral ligaments of the knee, the lateral cartilage, and the anterior and posterior cruciate (Fig 443). If either medial or lateral stress is continued or if stress occurs with the knee extended, the corresponding part of the posterior capsular ligament will give way. Similarly, hyperextension of the knee throws initial tension on the posterior ligament of the joint, followed by stress against the cruciate ligaments and the posterior part of the two collaterals if the hyperextension continues. Direct forward motion of the tibia on the femur will injure the anterior cruciate while the opposite motion will damage the posterior cruciate. Many different varieties of stress may cause damage to the knee ligaments. If the stress of the medial side is primarily rotatory with less abduction force, one may find injury to the short capsular fibers (the deep layer) and to the anterior cruciate ligament, or to either alone, with the long fibers of the medial collateral ligament left intact. The severity of this injury may be difficult to determine since ordinary lateral stress will not reveal instability, yet the injury may be quite major. Aspiration of gross

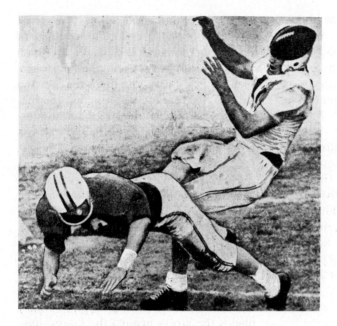

Figure 440. Photograph illustrating the forces causing "The Unhappy Triad," namely, sprain of the medial collateral and anterior cruciate ligaments and damage to the medial meniscus. (Permission to print granted by The Miami Herald, Miami, Florida.)

blood after what appears to be a relatively nondisabling injury should raise your index of suspicion that there has been some serious internal damage.

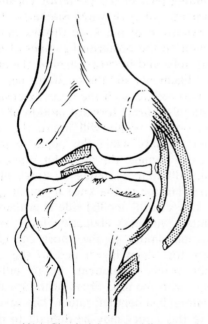

Figure 441. Classic injury resulting from forces shown in Figure 440. Note superficial layer and deep layer of medial collateral ligament torn near tibial attachment. Medial meniscus is ruptured and anterior cruciate ligament has torn completely.

Diagnosis

Diagnosis begins with a general evaluation of the situation. Did it seem to be a serious injury? Was the player immediately disabled, or was he able to keep going? Did he himself feel that he had received a serious injury? Was he able to leave the field under his own power, or was he carried? Was he suffering extreme pain, or was it relatively mild? This general evaluation is subject to further modification following examination but is often of considerable importance in determining the severity of the injury. Following this an early, careful and complete physical examination of the joint is of great importance. The earlier this can be done the better, since factors can often be determined then which become obscure after pain and swelling screen the symptoms. Note whether tenderness is at the joint line, above the joint, or below. Check the knee carefully for abnormal mobility in any direction, including rotation, lateral motion, anterior and posterior motion of the tibia on the femur. Observe the degree and the rapidity of swelling. Investigate whether the knee was actually

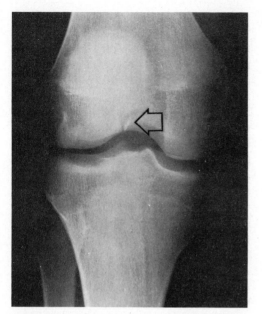

Figure 442. "Unhappy triad." Classic injury with the medial collateral off the tibia, the anterior cruciate pulled off the femur with a fragment of bone. This is very favorable for cruciate repair.

locked at the time of the injury, and whether it is actually locked at the time of the examination. All of these findings are of extreme importance if they are

obtained in the early stage before swelling, apprehension and pain obscure the true pathology. Often, in this initial examination, a definitive diagnosis can be made, not only as to the location but as to the extent of a ligament injury. (For further discussion of diagnosis, see page 524.)

A summary of diagnosis appears in Table 18–1.

For purposes of diagnosis and treatment, the various ligament injuries may be classified according to their severity into three general groups—mild (first degree), moderate (second degree) and severe (third degree) (Table 18–2).

Mild (First Degree) Ligament Sprain

In a mild ligament injury (Table 18–3), there has been some tear in the ligament fibers but its strength has not been particularly impaired. There has been some degree of damage, either within the ligament itself or at one of its attachments. The *symptoms* of such a

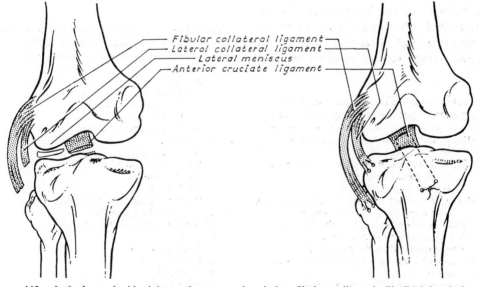

Fibular collateral ligament
Lateral collateral ligament
Lateral meniscus
Anterior cruciate ligament

Figure 443. *Left,* Lateral side injury, the succession being fibular collateral, iliotibial band, lateral meniscus, anterior cruciate. The biceps tendon may or may not be avulsed, depending on the level of the injury. *Right,* Note the iliotibial band repaired to the tibia through drill holes, the fibular collateral ligament to the fibula through drill holes. The anterior cruciate is shown held by drill holes from the anteromedial face of the tibia. (O'Donoghue, D. H.: J. Bone & Joint Surg. *32–A*:735.)

Table 18–1.   The Diagnosis of Knee
Ligament Injury

Demands early, careful, meticulous examination
Note particularly:
1. Apparent severity of injury
2. Degree of disability
3. Restriction or pain on normal motion
4. Presence of abnormal motion
5. Location and extent of tenderness
6. Amount and rapidity of the swelling
7. Location of swelling — intra- or extrasynovial
8. Deformity, either present or reported
9. Locking?

---

tear are tenderness at the site of the tear, pain on active use of the knee, local swelling at the site of the injury and pain on forced motion or on attempt to duplicate the motion which caused the tear. Negative findings of significance are no instability, no blood in the joint or infiltrated through the tissues, no effusion, no locking and no pain on normal motion.

If the injury is indubitably mild — and fortunately the great majority of ligament injuries fall into this classification — *treatment* is symptomatic and can be based on the premise that the strength of the ligament is actually unimpaired. Prolonged and extensive treatment is not necessary; in fact, the injured person seldom reaches the doc-

Table 18–2.   Classification of Knee
Ligament Injury According to Severity

A. Mild (first degree) — A few fibers of the
      ligament damaged
      No actual loss of strength of the ligament
      Little treatment necessary
      Treatment is symptomatic.
B. Moderate (second degree) — A definite tear in
      some component of the ligament
      Definite loss of strength of the ligament
      No wide separation of the fibers
      Treatment is primarily protective
C. Severe (third degree) — Ligament torn clear
      across
      Complete loss of ligament function
      Potentially wide separation of the fragments
      Treatment: Restoration of ligament
      continuity

tor and practically never the specialist. The basis of treatment is, first, protection against further injury and, second, reduction of local reaction. Immediate application of a pressure bandage with an ice pack will minimize local swelling. These are the cases in which apparently dramatic results may be obtained by local treatment. Application of cold pack, use of so-called "ice cup" for massage or ethyl chloride spray will tend to reduce the vascular spasm and will add comfort as well as reduce swelling when the degree of injury is quite local. Local anesthesia inserted into the injured area will reduce pain and vessel spasm. Injection of hyaluronidase into the hematoma will speed absorption and reduce swelling and ecchymosis. Protective wrapping will permit prompt resumption of activity. Complete immobilization is neither necessary nor desirable. The patient may be rapidly rehabilitated without danger. *Warning!* Since the diagnosis may not be entirely certain at the time of injury, the player should not be permitted to participate in

Table 18–3.   Symptoms and Treatment of
Mild (First Degree) Knee Sprain

---

1. Symptoms
    a. Positive
        (1) Tender at site of tear
        (2) Pain on abnormal stress
        (3) Local swelling
        (4) Pain on forced motion
    b. Negative
        (1) No instability
        (2) No blood in joint
        (3) No effusion
        (4) No locking
        (5) No pain on normal motion
2. Treatment — Symptomatic
    (Designed to relieve discomfort)
    a. Rest
    b. Local injection
    c. Compression
    d. Cold early
    e. Heat later
    f. Early, active use
    g. *No* immobilization
    h. Early activity permissible

sports immediately if a local anesthetic has been injected. The injection may screen his symptoms and permit re-injury.

Moderate (Second Degree) Ligament Sprain

In moderate ligament injury (Table 18–4), it is postulated that the ligament has been partially torn. This group actually includes most of the sprains that require extensive treatment, ranging from a slight tear to tears with only a few intact fibers remaining. The strength of the ligament is impaired to a greater or lesser degree. The *symptoms* here are very similar in pattern to those of mild injury but are greater in degree, one group shading imperceptibly into the other. The positive findings are: pain in the knee; tenderness at the site of the injury; disability of a greater degree than in the mild type; swelling at first localized at the area of damage, later

---

Table 18–4. Symptoms and Treatment of Moderate (Second Degree) Knee Sprain

---

1. Symptoms
   a. Positive
      (1) Immediate disability to some extent
      (2) Swelling at first localized, later within the joint
      (3) Pain in and about the knee
      (4) Pain on lateral or rotatory motion of the knee
      (5) Local tenderness at the point of injury
      (6) Locking may or may not be present
   b. Negative
      No abnormal mobility in any direction
2. Treatment—Protective
   a. Complete bed rest with elevation of the leg
   b. Aspiration
   c. Injection, local anesthetic plus hyaluronidase
   d. Compression—Cotton cast or elastic bandage
   e. Cold—Ice pack applied directly over compression bandage for 12 to 36 hours
   f. Later, heat (after 36 hours)
   g. Protection by long leg stirrup splints, to long leg cast, to cotton cast, to taping
   h. Rehabilitation

---

spreading to a diffuse swelling of the joint; fluid or blood in the joint; pain on reproduction of the force and direction of the injury. There may or may not be locking due to meniscus damage. The findings *not present* in a moderate injury are excess lateral motion and increased anteroposterior slipping of tibia on femur with the knee flexed (positive drawer sign). These latter two tests and rotatory tests each indicate complete loss of function of a ligament permitting abnormal motion and are not positive if the ligament is only partially severed.

Treatment is protective and is based upon the premise that there has actually been a significant damage to the ligament with weakening of its structure and considerable loss, or at least potential loss, of function. Therefore, treatment must be more comprehensive than in the mild group and the emphasis is on protection from further injury. A firm compression bandage should be used and ice pack applied. Aspiration of the local hematoma or of the knee joint following injection of a local anesthetic is carried out. Hyaluronidase is valuable if hemorrhage is recent and not in the joint. Since the exact degree of injury may not be readily apparent, one must protect the joint against further insult as long as symptoms persist. Bleeding is reduced by immediate compression with elastic bandage and application of ice. Later, plaster splints (Fig. 444), graduating to long leg cast, then to cotton cast (Fig. 433) to adhesive strapping (Fig. 445) and finally to elastic wrap, as symptoms permit, will serve to promote healing and prevent further injury. If fluid in the joint persists, aspiration should be repeated as often as is necessary. Protection must be maintained and insisted upon long after symptoms disappear. Contact participation should not be permitted without firm adhesive strapping (Fig. 445) which serves to protect the ligaments of the knee better than any

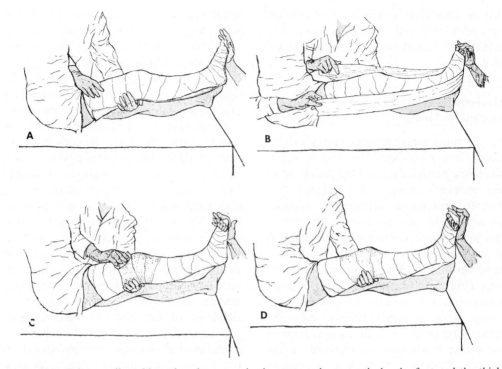

Figure 444. Stirrup splints. Note that the extremity is supported constantly by the foot and the thigh, permitting the tibia to drop backward and relax the anterior cruciate. *A*, A heavy posterior splint is applied first, wrapped with gauze and allowed to harden a little. *B*, The lateral splint is then applied and wrapped with gauze. After this has set, a single layer of sheet wadding is wrapped 15 cm. above to 15 cm. below the knee, and this is covered with a single roll of 15-cm. plaster (*C*). *D*, The completed splint. The circular plaster roll *C* is applied only during the postanesthesia stage in the operative case. It is not used routinely. The same type of splint may be used from below the knee to the toes if it is not necessary to immobilize the knee. This, of course, is not effective in any knee injury.

available type of compression knee bandage or short brace.

Several years ago our prime emphasis was placed on the treatment of the complete ligament tear. It is generally recognized by those treating knee injuries that the complete tear should be surgically repaired or, if not repaired, it should at least be protected for ten to twelve weeks in order for healing to occur. My own experiments have shown that in the dog a complete tear will require 12 to 14 weeks before it becomes firmly united. Similarly, a ligament which is cut half way in two will require at least eight weeks before it becomes mature and approaches its original strength.

New emphasis must be placed on the treatment of the partial ligament

tear, the second degree or moderate injury. This condition may be very well treated in the early stages by protection in a splint, pressure, compression, ice bag and so forth. In two or three weeks the acute symptoms have subsided and the patient becomes relatively asymptomatic. At this time the ligament is no stronger than it was the day of the injury. The symptoms have disappeared but the ligament is not healed. The player returns to the game and re-injures his knee. The same cycle may be repeated three or four times during the season. At the season's end the knee injury which had caused no instability initially has terminated in complete instability of the involved ligament. This instability is recognized too late for primary repair, and reconstruction now becomes necessary. One must be extremely wary of accepting subsidence of clinical symptoms as a sign that there has been healing of the ligament. If activity is permitted too early, a moderate sprain may develop into a complete one. The physician must recognize that healing requires time. Function and stress before this time has elapsed results in re-injury from minor trauma. *It will take as long for the ligament to heal as it would for a fracture of similar degree.*

It is difficult to state positively just how comprehensive treatment should be in a given case but it is quite apparent that the sprain which causes only moderate damage will not require as extensive or as prolonged treatment as one that is more severe. As a general rule, compression and ice pack should be continued for several hours or even longer if the swelling is severe. Use of one of the enzyme preparations systemically may be of value—for the first 24 hours intramuscularly, then orally for a few days. With discontinuance of the

compression bandage and ice pack, decision should be made as to whether the injury was severe enough to require plaster splints from groin to toes or some type of coaptation splint (such as the cotton cast) from midthigh to midcalf. If the ligament is actually torn, at least eight to ten weeks will be required for complete healing and there should be an additional period of protection by strapping. Here again the degree of the damage will be the governing factor, since if the greater part of the ligament is intact, the ligament remaining may serve to protect the injured portion, while if the defect is a major one a longer period of external protection will be indicated to prevent re-injury. The posterior and stirrup long leg splints may be worn for seven to ten days and then be replaced by a long leg walking cast (Fig. 446) for several weeks. This may be followed by short splints and later by an elastic bandage, particularly if swelling or effusion persists. It merits repeating that the knee capsule should not be permitted to remain distended over a long period of

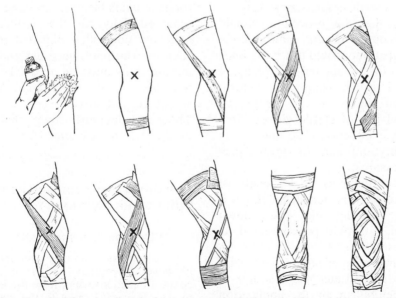

Figure 445. A method for strapping the knee to support the lateral collateral ligaments. The crisscross straps should cross in the midline. Maximum support for this dressing is directly medially and laterally.

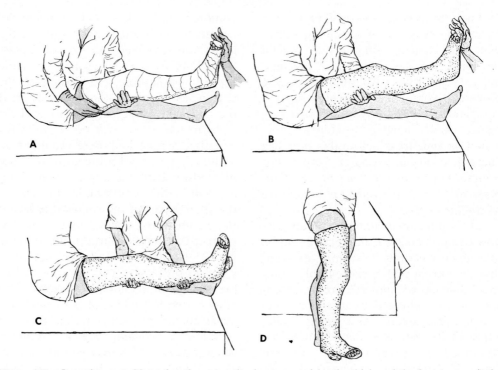

Figure 446. Long leg cast. Note that the extremity is supported by the thigh and the foot to permit the tibia to drop backward to relax the anterior cruciate. *A,* Posterior plaster slab. *B,* The completed cast with the foot in slight eversion, the ankle neutral, the knee at 20 degrees. *C,* The heel. *D,* Standing position. Note that the patient should have a shoe with heel of equal height on the good leg to balance the pelvis.

time and that aspiration should be repeated as frequently and for as long as necessary. Worth emphasizing again is the caution that this procedure should be carried out with the same aseptic technique that one would use if the knee joint were to be opened surgically. I prefer a thorough soap (hexachlorophene) and water scrub, protective draping and use of sterile gloves. One need not fear infection if he anticipates its possibility and takes the proper preventive measures.

Opinions differ as to the length of time the ice pack is beneficial. Since it diminishes bleeding and slows down metabolism, it should be continued as long as these two ends are desirable. In the ordinary case bleeding will stop after a few hours. Later it is desirable to increase metabolism by the application of local heat by means of an electric

pad, diathermy or hot bath. If a well-equipped and well-controlled training room is available, the dressing may be removed daily for the application of heat and controlled physical measures such as whirlpool, massage and careful motion. This must be under the protective eye of a qualified trainer. A typical set of rehabilitative exercises follows. There are obviously many that can be used (Also, see Chapter 22.)

REHABILITATIVE EXERCISES TO THE LOWER EXTREMITY

O'Donoghue Orthopaedic Clinic

Each of the following exercises should be done deliberately and to a particular count. In each instance, raise the leg slowly to the count of 3, hold to the count of 3, lower to the count of 3 and rest. Repeat this series ten times. Rest. Repeat this through three series of ten times each, 30 times total. The exercise should be repeated two or three times a day, depending upon your tolerance. Whenever you are able to complete this series of 30, add weight and start a new series, gradually adding weight as your strength improves. Build this weight up to 25 pounds if possible. Chart your daily progress and record it. Continue this until the involved thigh is (a) as large as the normal side, (b) as strong as the normal side and (c) normal motion is reached.

The following exercises should be done as indicated above, starting while the leg is still in the cast.

1. Lying on the back, raise the leg up with the knee straight and not flexing.

2. Lie on the unaffected side. Raise the leg up with the knee straight.

3. Lie face down. Raise the leg up with the knee straight.

(N.B. In each instance, increase weight as indicated above.)

4. After removal of fixation and sitting with the leg hanging and the knee at a right angle, go through the series of exercises with spring resistance or weight. If there is ligament damage, a spring or system of pulleys and weights is preferred to hanging the weight on the foot.

5. Lie face down with weight on the foot, flex the leg to vertical through the same series.

Exercises 1, 2 and 3 should be begun immediately postoperatively, or even started preoperatively. Exercises 4 and 5 should be done after removal of the cast and should not be done if there is synovitis with effusion.

Active physical therapy, increasingly active use, protective strapping and reeducation are all of importance. Injudicious overuse or too early return to physical activity will interfere with prompt and complete recovery. Reduction of pain and swelling by local injection must not be permitted to cover up the true nature of the injury since active stress must not be allowed until healing is complete. Ordinarily complete recovery should be expected, with no residual disability in the joint if treatment is adequate (Fig. 447). After complete healing there is no justification for limiting the

activity of the patient. It is the unusual or the untreated case that has permanent disability from a moderate sprain. "Once a sprain always a sprain" is an excuse to screen inadequate treatment.

Severe Ligament Sprain

In severe ligament injuries (Table 18–5), the *diagnosis* is based on the premise that one or more of the major ligaments of the knee are completely torn loose from their attachment, or torn through their substance. The mechanism of this injury is that previously mentioned, namely, forcing the knee through a wide range of abnormal motion beyond the tolerance of the ligament. Symptoms in this type of injury are much more severe. There is immediate disability, usually severe. There is the feeling that the knee has given way or dislocated. There is often extreme pain at the time of injury. Examination and evaluation reveal early disability, giving way of the knee joint, severe pain in the knee or leg, blood in the joint, blood infiltrating through the tissues (Fig. 448), and local swelling first at the site of injury and very rapidly into the knee itself. Confirmatory stress x-rays (Fig. 449) show abnormal lateral motion at the knee joint. Locking may or may not be present. While the above symptoms and signs strongly suggest a complete ligament avulsion, *the one single confirmatory finding is instability.* One should be able to demonstrate by his examination loss of function of one or more ligaments of the knee. It should be noted also that a torn ligament, particularly a cruciate, may be present without the signs of major injury indicated above. (See page 561.)

Increased abduction of the tibia with the knee in complete extension means loss of the medial collateral, anterior cruciate, and at least part of the posterior ligament (Fig. 449,*A*). A knee

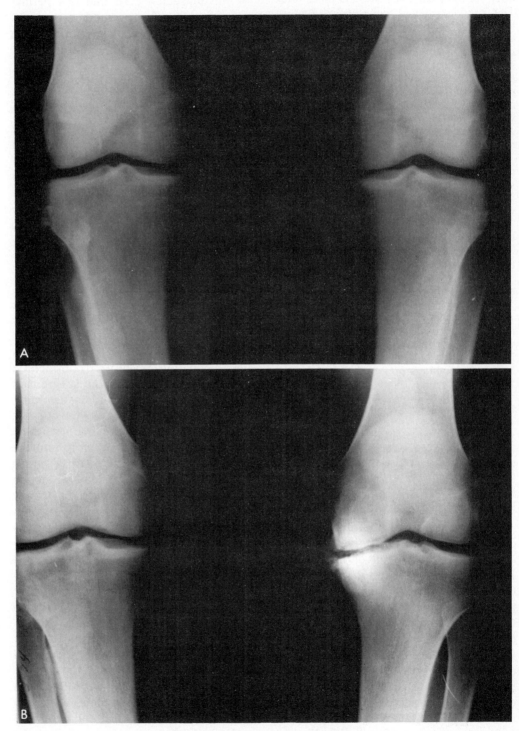

Figure 447. *See legend on opposite page.*

Table 18–5. Symptoms and Treatment of Severe Knee Sprain

1. Symptoms
   a. Immediate disability, usually severe; patient apprehensive
   b. Knee "gives way" on attempt at weight bearing, particularly with flexion
   c. Severe pain
   d. Blood infiltrated in tissues but may collect in joint
   e. Marked swelling, first local, later diffuse about the knee
   f. Pain on stress (lateral, rotatory, anteroposterior)
   g. *Abnormal mobility.*
   h. Positive stress x-ray
2. Treatment (Designed to restore continuity of the ligament)
   a. Surgical treatment should be given if at all possible
      (1) Make prompt diagnosis and decision as to surgery
      (2) Operate as soon as feasible
      (3) Repair each torn ligament
   b. Nonsurgical (not desirable)
      Same as for moderate sprain, but longer protection

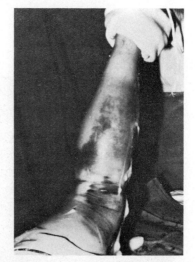

Figure 448. Appearance of leg 48 hours after injury with avulsion of posterior cruciate and posterior capsule from the tibia. Note extreme swelling, ecchymosis and hematoma formation.

that is stable in extension but not at 30 degrees indicates that the medial or lateral collateral is gone but the posterior ligament is intact. Increased anterior-posterior mobility of the flexed tibia (90 degrees) on the femur indicates anterior or posterior cruciate ligament damage (drawer sign, Fig. 450). The importance of these findings cannot be overemphasized. If surgery is indicated for some other reason, such as a locked knee or a knee with positive lateral instability and questionable anterior-posterior instability, the cruciate ligament can be checked at the time of the operation. Appropriate measures can be taken for repair at that time without the necessity of a preliminary diagnostic anesthetic. In doubtful cases it is justifiable to induce anesthesia for diagnosis. Stress films are not always necessary to confirm instability but they should always be taken to demonstrate other pathology. Instability may be posterior or anterior and a stress film may be necessary to demonstrate which it is, although physical examination will usually reveal it (Figs. 451 and 452).

Diagnosis must be early and be definitive in order to permit the proper decision as to treatment. If one waits

Figure 447. This patient was first seen for his left knee at age 27 in 1970. He was originally hurt the previous Fall and missed two games. He was hurt again one month later and has had several injuries since. Examination showed medial collateral and posterior cruciate instability. Note in view *A* the right and left knees showing apparently very little difference between them with essentially no degenerative change. He declined treatment. *B,* Four years later, his instability having continued, note the very gross involvement of the medial side of the joint. This is a good illustration of the fact that instability does lead to degenerative changes. Osteotomy and debridement was recommended. The patient was then 31 years old. Reduction of his instability by surgical reconstruction would probably have lessened or stopped his degenerative change.

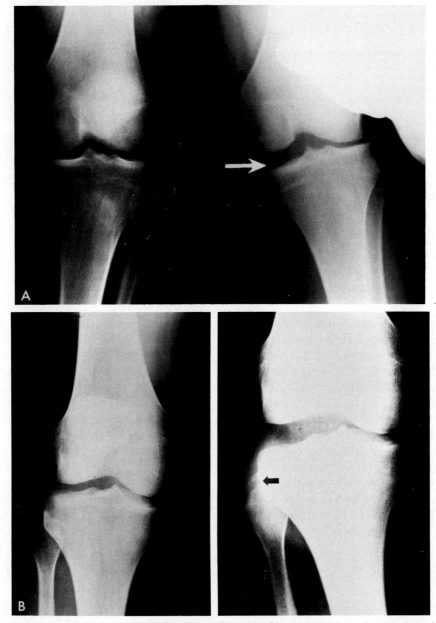

Figure 449. *A*, X-ray of injury to medial collateral ligament of knee. *Left*, Neutral anteroposterior view; *right*, position of abduction of leg on thigh; arrow indicates increased tibiofemoral joint space.

B, X-ray illustrating damage to lateral collateral ligament. *Left*, Neutral anteroposterior view of knee; *right*, stress film showing rupture of fibular collateral and iliotibial band. Arrow indicates avulsion of tip of fibula.

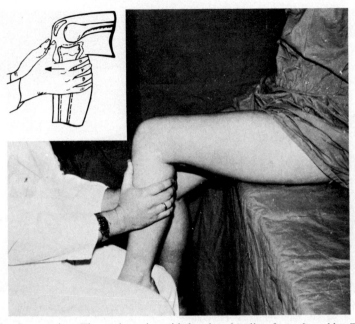

Figure 450. The drawer sign. The patient sits with her leg dangling from the table. The examiner is seated in front of her with the foot clasped between his knees, hands as shown. Forward pressure will demonstrate anterior cruciate instability; backward pressure, posterior cruciate instability. This motion should be made by slow, steady pull rather than by a succession of jerks, which will be painful to the injured knee. The inset shows a positive anterior drawer sign, the tibia sliding forward and downward in relation to the normal position.

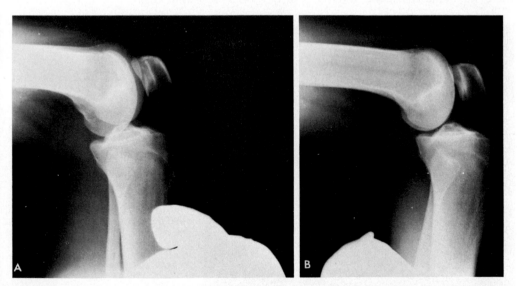

Figure 451. Fifteen-year-old female fell while doing acrobatics and twisted her knee. She had a torn anterior cruciate ligament with injury to medial collateral ligament and medial meniscus. *A*, Lateral with posterior stress—negative. *B*, Lateral with anterior stress shows tibia far forward, indicating loss of the anterior cruciate ligament.

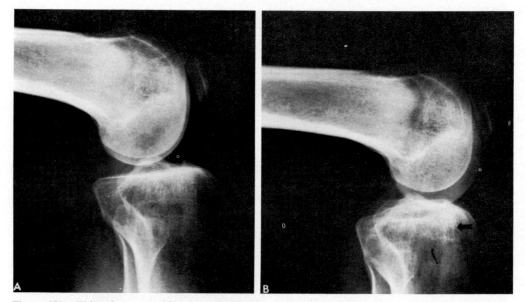

Figure 452. Thirty-four-year old male sustained hyperextension and valgus strain to the knee joint when he fell a distance of six feet. Had lateral collateral and posterior cruciate instability. *A*, Anterior stress—negative. *B*, Posterior stress shows marked posterior displacement. No anterior instability was present. Indicates loss of posterior cruciate ligament.

three or four weeks until swelling and pain subside, instability becomes quite obvious. In the meantime the optimum time for treatment has passed. While instability is necessary to confirm complete ligament tear, one must be sure that the instability is actually due to the ligament and not to a related injury to the bone which has given the *impression* of instability of the knee while, in fact, the ligaments are actually intact (Figs. 453, 519 and 522).

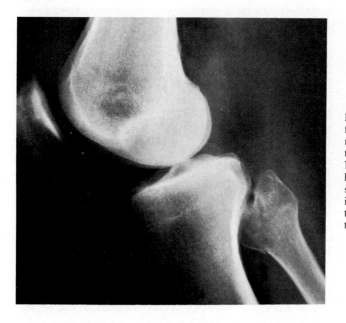

Figure 453. Patient injured knee falling off a horse and landing on a rock. Came in with diagnosis of ruptured fibular collateral ligament. Note fracture-dislocation of fibular head with instability of the fibula simulating ligament injury. This is an illustration of the danger of assuming that the ligament is torn just because there is instability.

Treatment. Treatment poses the question: Why is it essential that diagnosis should be made definitively and at once? The answer is basic in our approach to the problem of treatment. If all ligament injuries are to be treated by modifications of the same basic method, it may indeed be of academic interest only to define the exact pathology. It is agreed that certain basic measures are of value in the treatment of an injured knee ligament. We have seen that aspiration, local injection, compression, ice packs, immobilization, protection and rehabilitation are utilized to a greater or lesser degree, depending upon the severity of the injury. Under such a concept, whether the sprain be moderate or severe, treatment will require only some variation of the extent to which these measures are utilized.

Obviously, if there is no effusion, aspiration will not be necessary. If effusion is recurrent, aspiration will need to be repeated. If the injury is mild, compression may well be the only protection applied, and soon be discarded. If swelling persists, so must compression bandaging whether it be elastic wrap or cotton cast. If symptoms subside promptly, no protection by splint or cast is necessary. On the other hand, if symptoms remain severe, a cylinder for eight weeks may be required. The same concept applies to rehabilitation which can be perfunctory in the injury requiring only brief treatment but must be extensive if prolonged protection has been required.

Why, then, do we demand "careful, tender but meticulously complete examination" of every sprain of the knee? If the treatment is to be the same whatever the injury, why not initiate this treatment first and then decide as we go along just how extensively the injury must be treated? Severity could be judged by the manner in which the condition responds to therapy.

Such specious reasoning, by appearing reasonable on the surface, insidiously undermines one's actual understanding of the condition which he is treating. It is easy to see how the habit of treating these injuries "by feel" rather than by diagnosis becomes fixed. If one is called upon to examine a knee injury and responds by directing that it be "packed in ice" until morning, the next time the trainer or team physician encounters this injury, he will "pack it in ice" himself. Indeed, if the treatment is to be standardized into a certain pattern, he is perfectly correct in doing so.

Many of us have found through years of observation that nonsurgical treatment is not always the best treatment. We may differ substantially on how frequently surgery is indicated and how complete it must be but most would agree that many cases will require surgical treatment.

We have been able to show that early operation (within two weeks) is distinctly more favorable than late operation (Fig. 454 and Table 18–6). In a series of 80 cases of knee ligament operations the vital factor governing the degree of recovery was not the severity of the injury, the location of the tear or the age of the patient. It was the time of the operation. Almost without exception the patient who was operated upon within two weeks obtained a better end result than the patient with a comparable injury operated upon later. Indeed, a more satisfactory result was obtained in the severe case treated by early operation than in the milder case in which operation was late.

So if we grant these two premises, namely, that some cases need surgery and that early surgery is better than late, it follows that the decision whether to operate or not must be based on early, thorough, careful examination, under anesthesia if necessary. We must not treat all knee injuries alike if we are to

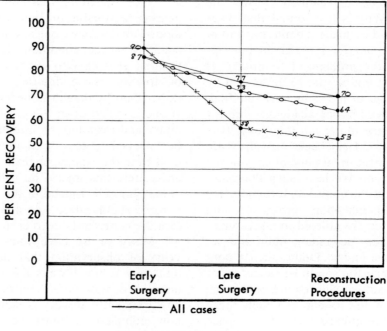

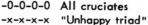

——— All cases

-0-0-0-0 All cruciates
-x-x-x-x "Unhappy triad"

Figure 454. Showing end results of operations on ligaments of the knee. Note the time of operation, which is most important. (From The Journal of Bone and Joint Surgery, Vol. 37A.)

treat them the best way. Attention to the exact diagnosis must be an integral part of the management of any knee ligament injury.

These injuries provide a classic example of the importance of the precepts mentioned in the Introduction, which must be constantly kept in mind. The goal of treatment must be 100 per cent recovery. The best treatment must be selected rather than the most convenient treatment. The decision must be entirely objective without consideration of extraneous influences. Above all, treatment must be prompt. A definitive decision as to the proper treatment must be made at the earliest possible moment.

Table 18–6. Follow-up Chart of 80 Knee Ligament Operations
(Comparison by Age Groups)

	EARLY SURGERY	LATE SURGERY	RECONSTRUCTION PROCEDURES	TOTAL
Under 20 years				
No. of Cases	21	12	12	45
Grade	89 (average)	75 (average)	66 (average)	79 (average)
Over 20 years				
No. of Cases	23	8	4	35
Grade	84 (average)	78 (average)	60 (average)	80 (average)

Note that the result was essentially the same whether they were under 20 or over 20. There were consistently poor results from surgery delayed over two weeks. In this table "early" is under two weeks, "late" is two to six weeks.

(From The Journal of Bone and Joint Surgery, Vol. 37A.)

Once the diagnosis of a complete ligament tear has been made, the method of treatment must be elected. It will not suffice to try so-called conservative treatment first and then proceed to surgery. Early surgical repair yields so much better and surer results than late repair or reconstruction that surgery must not be reserved for only those cases in which conservative treatment has failed. Modern anesthesia, operating room asepsis, highly skilled personnel and antibiotics have minimized the hazards to the degree that in the well run hospital with a competent surgical team, open surgery can confidently take its place alongside nonsurgical measures. In the absence of complicating factors, the management chosen must be that which will give the best chance of complete recovery in the shortest time.

I believe that, when one can demonstrate complete severance of any single ligament or of any combination of ligaments of the knee, surgical repair is mandatory. The repair should include not only one ligament but all ligaments involved. It makes little sense to repair the collateral ligament and ignore the cruciate because it "adds to the severity of the operation" or is "too difficult" or "may not be essential." The cruciates are not vestigial. One has only to examine the splendid mechanism of the anterior cruciate, to note its size, to check its strength, to recognize its vital structure, in order to realize that it is not an evolutionary misfit ready for the discard. The cruciates play a living, vibrant part in that ingenious mechanism that is the knee. We may argue about their exact function but be assured they have a major one.

Even though we agree that the many interlocking ligaments of the knee act as a physiological unit and that a portion of this unit may be spared without great disaster, we must acknowledge that the knee without the cruciate is ac-

tually or potentially less than normal. Each of the various ligaments adds strength to the stability of the knee. One might make a comparison to the television aerial; one row of guy wires may be removed and the structure may not fall, but it may well collapse in the next high wind. The cruciate should be repaired since in no other way may a normal knee joint be attained.

I examine many knees in which the only detectable complaint is cruciate instability. These patients seek surgical reconstruction because to them the condition is materially disabling. This in itself is evidence that the cruciate in a given case may be vital for adequate function.

Late cruciate reconstruction is highly speculative and should be done when the stakes are high, as for example in a professional baseball player who is unable to play because of anterior-posterior instability or when the degree of anterior-posterior instability is actually disabling or when the instability is such that late degenerative changes may be expected. Early cruciate repair is highly successful and should be done as a matter of course. The operation, which is not unduly technical, is within the capabilities of any competent orthopaedist who properly prepares himself in the necessary technique.

In certain cases the ligament may heal spontaneously. This is particularly true of tears of the collateral ligaments. The real danger is in our inability to determine short of surgery which case will heal with normal length and which will not. At operation I have actually found the tibial end of the medial collateral lying in the joint underneath the medial meniscus (Fig. 455). I have seen the ligament torn with the ends disengaged and retracted an inch or more (Fig. 456). I have located the femoral attachment of the medial collateral ligament lying in the joint on top of the meniscus

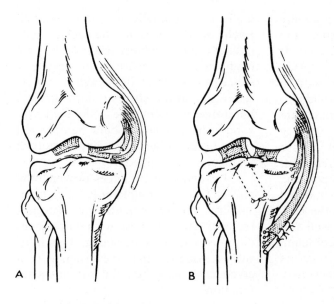

Figure 455. Both cruciates off tibia. Tibial end of medial collateral under medial meniscus. Tendon widely separated. (From The Journal of Bone and Joint Surgery, Vol. 32A.)

(Fig. 457); also the femoral end of the anterior cruciate lying over the lateral meniscus (Fig. 458). There are many other such situations which are unredeemable except by surgery. Anyone who has actually seen these or similar lesions at operation becomes very skeptical of the uniformly good results reported from nonsurgical treatment.

The results of surgical treatment recommend it. In 80 consecutive cases of ligament injuries,* early repair gave results in approximately 90 per cent of cases (over 90 per cent in athletes), regardless of the severity of the injury. It was demonstrated that the promptness of the operation and the completeness of the repair were much more important

*O'Donoghue, Don H.: An Analysis of End Results of Surgical Treatment of Major Injuries to the Ligaments of the Knee. J. Bone & Joint Surg., 37A:1–13 (Jan.), 1955.

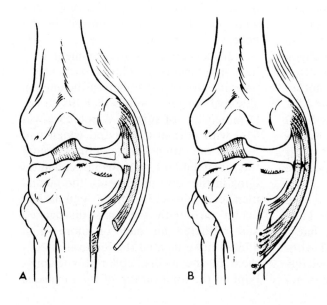

Figure 456. Tendon and medial ligament widely separated from the lower attachment. (From The Journal of Bone and Joint Surgery, Vol. 32A.)

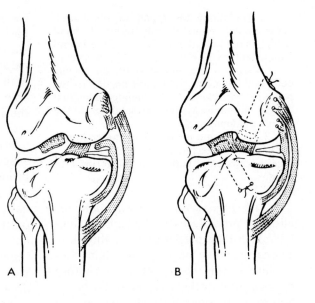

Figure 457. Anterior cruciate torn from tibia. Posterior cruciate torn from femur. Medial collateral torn from femur and lying on top of medial meniscus. (From The Journal of Bone and Joint Surgery, Vol. 32A.)

than the nature or severity of the injury; failure of cruciate repair was the most common single cause of permanent disability in knee ligament injuries; and repair of the cruciates was highly successful early but very unpredictable late.

OPERATIVE TECHNIQUE

I will attempt in this section to indicate some of the more common surgical procedures for ligament repair, and to describe in detail those which I personally prefer. The exact pathology encountered may have many variants but the diagnoses nevertheless fall into more or less definite categories. The procedures may be grouped as follows on the basis of the diagnosis:

1. Technique for repair of the medial collateral, the medial portion of the posterior ligament, the anterior and/or posterior cruciate ligament, medial meniscus, medial hamstring tendons.

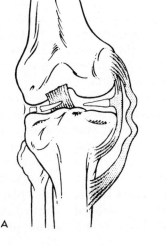
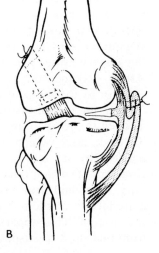

Figure 458. Anterior cruciate avulsed from femur and lying on top of lateral meniscus. (From The Journal of Bone and Joint Surgery. Vol. 32A.)

2. Technique for repair of the lateral components, namely, the iliotibial band (which is actually the strongest of the lateral components, and is similar to the deep capsular fibers on the medial side), the fibular collateral ligament, the lateral portion of the posterior capsule and the cruciate ligaments; the lateral meniscus; the peroneal nerve; the biceps tendon.

3. Technique for repair of the posterior components — the posterior approach for either the posterior capsule or posterior cruciate.

The *preoperative preparation* for all these procedures is the same, namely, meticulous preparation of the skin. In the presence of a specific skin contamination this begins 48 hours before the operation, otherwise 12 to 24 hours before. If the operation must be delayed because of inability to obtain a hospital bed or for some other reason (such as irritative abrasions, cuts, etc.), we provide the patient with a hexachlorophene soap and instruct him to scrub his knee vigorously with very heavy lather at least ten minutes twice a day. If there is a lesion on the skin, it must have healed as completely as possible. However, we sometimes plan our incision to avoid an abrasion on the skin rather than postpone an operation unduly. Infected skin is a definite contraindication to surgical treatment.

The leg is carefully shaved from the toes to the groin in the immediate preoperative period, in the surgical suite. We prefer shaving the leg just before the surgery rather than the night before. After shaving, the patient is taken directly to the surgical amphitheater.

On the day of operation the patient is taken to the operating room and anesthetized, after which the leg is suspended by a foot-holding apparatus (Fig. 459, *A*) which relieves the nurse or other individual from holding the heavy extremity throughout the period of the preparation. This apparatus is modified from that used to suspend fluids from a carrier and consists of a rather broad base with a vertical telescoping upright surmounted by a strong hook. The apparatus is placed on the operating table with the base beneath the pad. A suitable loop is thrown around the foot and the leg is suspended as high as it will conveniently go (preferably at least 45 degrees from horizontal). Use of the suspension frame is more difficult in the prone position than in the supine but still is easier than holding the leg manually. The tourniquet is applied as high on the thigh as possible, because one is never sure of the extent of incision required. The tourniquet is fastened with adhesive so that it will not roll down the cone-shaped thigh. Employment of the leg holder permits the nurse to use both hands in the preparation and encourages a full length scrub time.

With the leg suspended in the apparatus, the surgical preparation is carried out with Betadine scrub (8 min.), followed by Betadine solution (2 min.), the preparer wearing sterile gloves and using both hands with compresses to work up a very generous lather. Scrub is continued for a total of eight minutes by the clock (Fig. 459). It does not include the foot. It is my belief that when the foot is included in the preparation, an inordinate amount of time is spent in cleaning the toenails and foot whereas, if the foot is draped out, the entire preparation may be concentrated about the knee. At the conclusion of the preparation the foot is grasped by the preparer and removed from the suspension apparatus (Fig. 459, *D*). The leg is held elevated at all times to help drain the blood from the extremity. Over the foot is rolled a combination of stockinette and plastic stocking (Fig. 459) which will extend from the toes well up to above the knee. This stockinette, plus the plastic, is impervious so it can be rolled directly over the unprepped foot and up the leg. Meanwhile a barrier

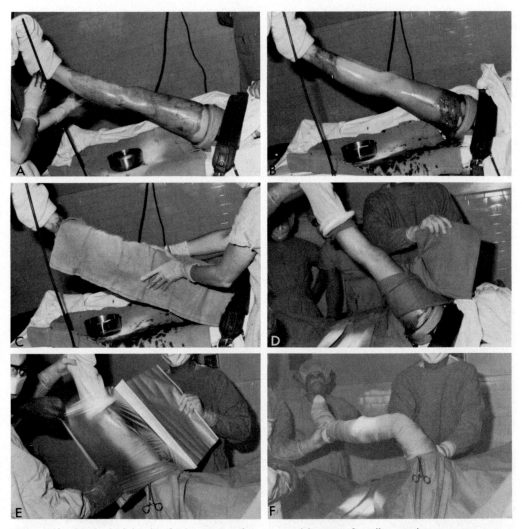

Figure 459. Method of draping for knee operation not requiring use of sterile tourniquet.

A, Notice leg suspended from suitable suspension apparatus to permit use of both hands in the scrub. The Betadine prep does not reach the tourniquet, nor does it reach the unsterile stockinette over the foot. Scrub lasts eight minutes. (We now use Betadine scrub for the preliminary wash, followed by Betadine solution instead of the Ioprep and alcohol. See text.)

B, Note cuff of Betadine prep at each end to assure that the prep does not reach contaminated skin.

C, Betadine solution blotted with double sterile towel by preparer.

D, Draping. Note the sterile towel wrapped around the leg just above the ankle at the junction of the prep and the foot to prevent any of the Betadine from oozing through the doubled sterile stockinetting which is applied over the foot and up the leg. Note the folded towel around the top of the prep. Note two double fan sheets which will be clamped around the folded towel.

E, Steri-drape folded around the exposed, prepared area.

F, Leg wrapped firmly with 15-cm. elastic bandage, knee flexed and tourniquet inflated.

We now use barrier stockinette plus plastic instead of stockinette.

sheet is placed on the table beneath the leg and up under the thigh. A folded towel is wrapped around the tourniquet and held securely with a towel clamp.

At this point a double fan sheet is placed under the leg and pulled up to the level of the top edge of the barrier sheet while the assistant holds the leg in an elevated position. A second double fan is placed on top of the double fan under the leg and not fanned out until a third double fan is placed on the thigh above the knee. The inferior edge of the upper sheet is clamped to the superior edge of the second double fan which is placed beneath the leg. At this time the plastic and stockinette covering is pulled up over the sheets so that it completely covers the thigh and the draping sheets. The leg is held elevated all during this time. The combination plastic-stockinette sleeve is then split over the top of the knee, the edges are retracted

to either side, and the steri-drape is pulled over this so the area of the surgery is exposed with only the steri-drape covering it. Then the leg is wrapped with an elastic bandage from the toes to the upper thigh. The pneumatic tourniquet is then inflated and the time carefully noted. From the moment of application of the tourniquet no unnecessary delays can be tolerated since the tourniquet time becomes all-important.

In certain instances when we need to reach a higher point on the thigh, such as in reconstruction operations or

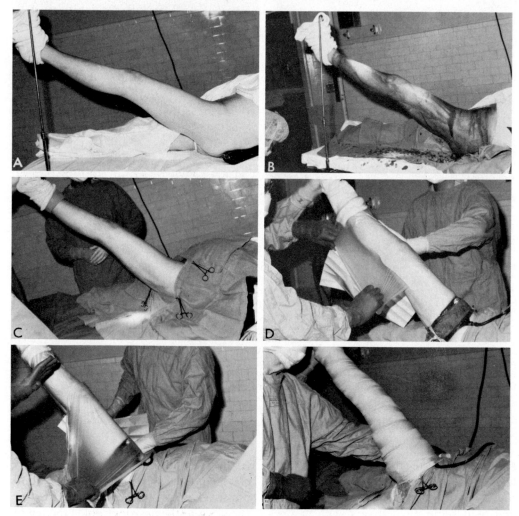

Figure 460.   *See legend on opposite page.*

muscular conditions of the thigh, we use the sterile tourniquet as indicated in Fig. 460.

1. Technique for Repair of the Medial Collateral, the Medial Portion of the Posterior Ligament, the Anterior or Posterior Cruciate Ligament

Exposure for Definition of the Pathology. A sweeping anteromedial incision is made beginning above the level of the superior pole of the patella (Fig. 461). It extends downward and forward toward the middle of the medial border of the patella, then is continued downward along the anteromedial aspect of the joint paralleling, and 2 cm. medial to, the patella and the patellar tendon. At the level of the patellar tubercle of the tibia it curves backward to end at

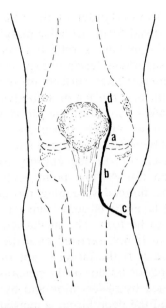

Figure 461. Medial incision for repair of the medial collateral ligament. Any part of this incision may be used. *a, b,* The portion of incision utilized for medial meniscectomy. It may be extended to *d* to further explore the knee joint or treat the patella, and extended down to *c* for repair of the medial collateral ligament.

Figure 460. Method of draping for knee operation requiring use of sterile tourniquet.

Leg is suspended for prep when it is necessary to use a sterile tourniquet. The purpose of the sterile tourniquet is to permit a much greater visualization of the entire leg, as is required in osteotomy for angular deformity, and also to provide a wider range of incision, such as in ligament reconstruction requiring exposure of the iliotibial tract.

A, Note the double sterile stockinette which has been placed over the extremity up as high as the hip following a shave, including pubis, and a soap and water prep the night before. This is rolled down and the leg is suspended from the foot. Note the sand bag under the upper portion of the buttock which permits the prep to extend under the buttock. The prep should also extend up on the thigh, including the groin and the lower abdomen as illustrated in *B.*

B, Eight-minute scrub of leg and thigh does not include the foot. If the foot is included an undue amount of time is spent in preparing the foot and the toes—time which could be better spent scrubbing around the knee. Note that the buttock rests on a sand bag so that the buttock is suspended away from the table and the Betadine is spread around the complete buttock. The towels underneath the leg are sterile. Care is taken not to touch the stocking covering the foot nor any of the unsterile drape at the top.

C, After the Betadine has been removed by a 2-minute scrub with Betadine solution, the prep nurse releases the foot and removes the standard. A surgical assistant has rolled a sterile double stockinette over the foot. Just above the ankle a towel has been wrapped around the leg, and the stockinette is rolled over this to prevent a seeping of contaminated preparation fluid through the stockinette. Note the squaring of sterile towels around the top of the thigh. The extremity is ready for application of the sterile tourniquet.

D, Fan sheet is placed under the leg as high as the sterile towels at the buttock and another fan sheet above, and these are clamped around the thigh. Second lap sheet is placed under the leg and not fanned. Steri-drape is now applied to cover the leg, from the stockinette at the bottom to over the tourniquet above.

E, The second piece of steri-drape is pulled over the upper thigh including the tourniquet.

F, The whole leg wrapped with an Ace bandage for exsanguination, and the tourniquet is inflated. Also split barrier drape is wrapped around upper leg and split steri-drape to exclude genitalia.

We no longer use double stockinette over the foot as a "preliminary day before prep," so the foot is fastened into the apparatus without the stockinetting. See text.

the posterior border of the tibia about 8 cm. distal to its articular margin. The medial skin flap is reflected backward along superficial fascia to expose the entire anteromedial surface of the tibia, the joint and the femoral condylar area (Fig. 462, *A*). All of the blood vessels and nerves in the subcutaneous area should be reflected with the flap, leaving the fascia of the leg entirely exposed with no fat. At this point ecchymosis may be noticed spreading through the fascial layer. It is quite unusual for the fascia to be torn. The medial collateral ligament is not exposed until the fascia is divided. If the fascia is not ruptured the superior border of the pes anserinus is defined by observation and by palpation and the deep fascia is incised along this line, care being taken not to cut through into the long fibers of the medial collateral ligament which are immediately beneath. On reflecting this fascia the long fibers of the medial collateral ligament will be seen passing under the pes anserinus beginning at about the midmedial line of the tibia and extending well back behind its posterior margin. At this point the area of the tear in the long fibers may be defined. If it is obscure, rocking the leg open may serve to develop the defective area.

The incision is now carried through the patellar retinaculum along the edge of the patella and the edge of the patellar tendon, just below the patellar tubercle. An instrument then can be passed beneath the superficial portion of the ligament in order to better demonstrate the area of the damage. The tear is defined usually either at the tibial attachment or just above this but below the line of the joint, and the superficial layer is reflected proximally with the fascia to expose the deep layer. In many instances the superficial layer may be reflected as a separate layer to a point above the line of the joint. At other times the superficial and deep layers will blend just below the joint. As this layer has been detached and folded backward, the deep layer is exposed (Fig. 462, *B*). This layer must be inspected entirely across the line of the joint from front to back. Again rocking the tibia may give a clue as to the site of the tear. This tear is readily seen if the operation is done before healing begins.

Frequently, the ligament will be torn in an irregular fashion. A commonly found tear begins at the mid-medial line on the tibia attachment of the deep layer and extends backward 2 to 5 cm. and then vertically upward across the joint and posteromedially across the femoral attachment. Another lesion frequently seen is a tear of the deep layer from its tibial attachment all the way posteriorly to include the medial one-third of the posterior ligament. In other instances the ligament may tear at the joint line and the meniscus may be split, the upper part going with the femur, the lower with the tibia. Usually the ligament will not give way from the midline forward since the medial ligament becomes very thin here to permit flexion of the knee and so has enough redundancy to permit the knee to "open up."

It is advisable at this stage to enter the knee by an incision through the synovium along the medial parapatellar line. In some instances this incision may be required to open the joint in order to specifically define the area of the tear, which sometimes can be better demonstrated from within out than from without in. At this point the deep layer of the medial ligament is reflected away from the tear. In other words, if the tear is along the tibial margin it is reflected upward. If the tear is along the femoral margin it is reflected downward. This gives ready access to the medial meniscus, which should be removed routinely to permit shortening of the medial collateral ligament. This is particularly necessary if the detachment is from the tibia below the meniscus. An effort is made to leave about 2 mm. of the cartilage intact to the medial ligament since it provides a very firm area through which to place the plicating sutures.

After this exposure is made the knee can readily be examined (Fig. 462, C). If the anterior cruciate ligament is torn, the knee will open up more widely and the pathology of the cruciate ligament may readily be determined. The posterior cruciate ligament should also be carefully examined.

If the anterior cruciate ligament is torn from or near the femur, it may be repaired by mattress sutures placed through two drill holes extending from the lateral epicondylar ridge into the posterior part of the intercondylar notch on the medial side of the lateral condyle. These holes are best made with a smooth pin the size of a guide wire for hip nailing (2.38 mm.). Guide pins are much better than twist drills since they damage the bone less, make less bone crumbs, and are in no danger of breaking. The holes should be placed at least 12.7 mm. apart where they exit into the notch and they should be as far posterior as possible. If the knee will open up, particularly if a smooth wire is used, the drill hole may be made from within outward for more accurate placement of the drill holes within the knee. It may be necessary to use a sleeve on the 2.38 mm. guide wire. Two 1–0 cotton sutures, one blue and one white, are passed through the posterior hole into the knee with the aid of a ligature passer made out of a fine wire with a knurled handle (Fig. 463). A curved needle holder and a stout, small (15.88 mm.) "knee needle" are used to separately mattress each thread into the torn stump of the cruciate ligament, care being taken to spread the ligament out at least 12.7 to 19 mm. rather than to pull it all together

to one point. The suture is then pulled out through the second drill hole by means of a ligature carrier with a loop of thread to pull the two thread ends through. With this type of equipment the holes can be made very much smaller and thus will be less traumatic. The sutures are placed while the knee still can be opened up since this facilitates suturing into the cruciate ligament. It can readily be done with the knee entirely stable but the drill holes must then be made from outside into the knee.

If the cruciate is torn off the tibial attachment, drill holes are made from the anteromedial face of the tibia up into the tibial origin of the cruciate ligament on the superior surface of the tibia. This is considerably easier than the other repair. Similar plication is done within the stump of the cruciate. If it is torn in the middle I frequently will make drill holes in both bones, pick up the tibial stump through femoral drill holes and the femoral stump through tibial drill holes. I believe this, as a rule, is more successful than direct suture although we sometimes utilize the latter, too. The important consideration is to get good contact of the torn ends. These sutures are placed but not tied. If the ligament is found to be redundant but not obviously torn, the most effective way to shorten it is to detach it completely from its tibial attachment preferably with a scale of bone. If parallel drill holes are made through the upper tibia, as described in the foregoing, the ligament may be advanced forward to get the proper degree of tension. Sutures on the epicondylar ridge should be extrasynovial. None of these procedures is formidable, and with proper tools should add no more than 15 to 20 minutes to the operative time. After the placing of these sutures, they are not tied until the medial ligament repair is completed, the leg is positioned at 20 to 30 degree flexion and the wounds are ready to close.

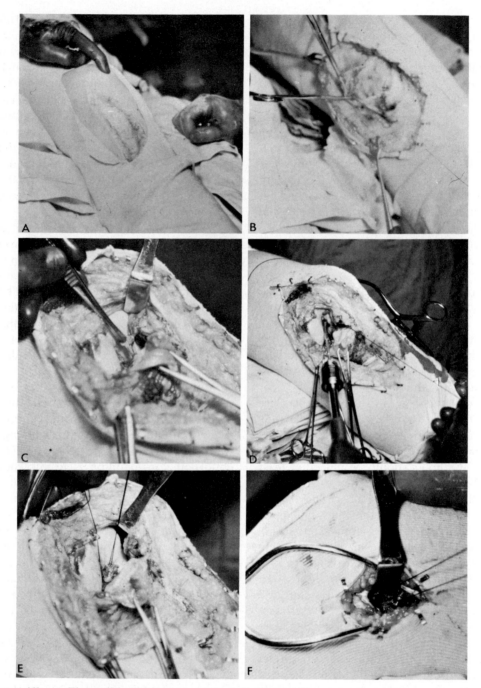

Figure 462. *A,* The medial utility incision as drawn in Figure 461.

B, Incision has been made through the patellar retinaculum and the superficial layer of the medial collateral ligament reflected upward in the tenaculum, revealing the joint line with irregular laceration of the deep layer of the medial collateral ligament which in this instance is torn off the femoral attachment.

C, The medial incision, the superficial layer of the ligament reflected upward, the deep layer reflected downward, the Russian forceps holding the anterior cruciate ligament which is torn off the femur.

D, The medial incision. A 3-mm. drill protected with a short sleeve (a 2.38-mm. guide wire is preferred) is drilled through the back of the intercondylar notch to emerge on the lateral epicondylar ridge. Two parallel holes are made. If the knee will not open up sufficiently to approach from within-out, the drill holes can be made from without-in. It is important to get the holes as far back in the notch as possible.

E, Two sutures engaging the torn femoral attachment of the anterior cruciate ligament.

F, The lateral incision along the epicondylar ridge showing the two #0 cotton sutures as they exit on the lateral side of the femur.

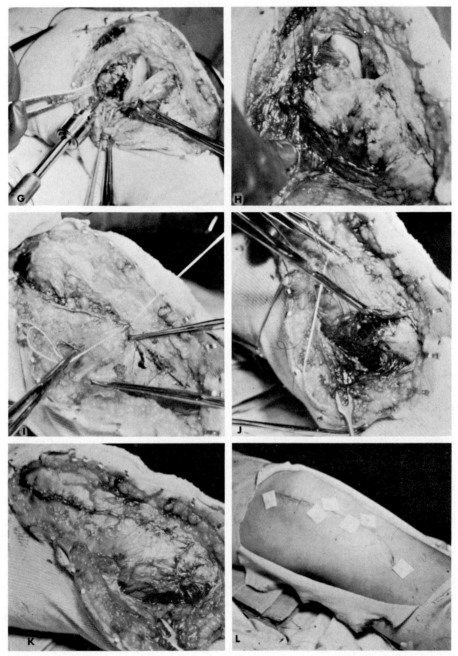

Figure 462 *Continued.*

   G, The medial incision. Drill holes are placed in the denuded medial femoral condyle through which #0 cotton mattress sutures are placed to hold the proximal end of the deep layer of the medial collateral ligament.

   H, The deep layer is ligated to the lower femur by #0 cotton mattress sutures.

   I, A heavy #1 cotton stay suture is placed at the anterior edge of the reflected medial collateral ligament and is pulled snugly forward. This is about the level of the patellar tubercle.

   J, A #0 cotton mattress suture placed through the periosteum of the tibia beneath the pes anserinus.

   K, The superficial ligament is sutured into position.

   L, Wound closed with subcuticular wire and/or Steri-Strips.

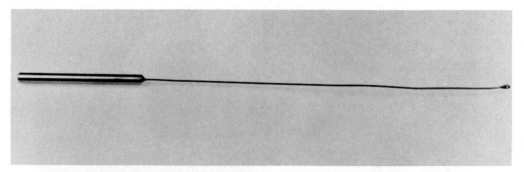

Figure 463. Ligature passer. The diameter of the eye must be less than 2.38 mm.

Repair of the Medial Collateral Ligament. The immediate repair of the deep layer of the collateral ligament may be by one of several methods. If there is a direct tear in the ligament with two well-defined margins, simple suture will suffice, with imbrication if feasible. If the ligament is avulsed from the bone, the best method of repair consists of a series of three or four superficial drill holes about 1 cm. apart at the site of the attachment to the tibial margin or femoral condyle (Fig. 462, *G*), as the case may be. Suitable suture (No. 0 cotton) is passed through the ligament into one drill hole out of an adjacent drill hole, and back through the ligament. When all of these have been placed the knee is positioned at about 20 to 30 degrees of flexion with the leg internally rotated, and all ligatures are tied (Fig. 462, *H*). As a rule, the superficial layer can be repaired by simple suture to its bed, overlapping the edges (Fig. 462, *J*) if possible. If this is not possible, a similar procedure may be carried out by drill holes at the level desired.

In the collateral repair every effort should be made to obtain maximum shortening of the ligament, and its tibial attachment should be pulled forward as far as is possible (Fig. 462, *I*). All loose tags are carefully sutured down (Fig. 462, *K*).

Repair of the Posterior Capsular Ligament. With a rupture of both layers of the medial collateral ligament and one or both cruciate ligaments there is, as a rule, damage to the posterior capsular ligament. Frequently the posterior capsule will simply split all the way around to the midline. At other times it will be pulled away from the tibia. It is seldom pulled off from the femoral attachment since it blends together with and is very firmly secured along the gastrocnemius muscle origin. Care must be taken not to overlook the posterior capsular tear just because the synovial fold seems intact. Although the two blend very closely together in the posterior capsule, it is possible to have a tear of the capsule proper without an obvious rent in the synovium.

Since the posterior capsule does play a large role in the stability of the knee in general, both in preventing overextension and in stabilizing the knee in extension, it is vitally important that it be repaired. It is not adequate to assume that the ends will fall together. We recently did a delayed reconstruction on a young man who had such a tear in the posterior capsule which in spite of six months elapsing had not healed at all.

With the knee flexed at 30 degrees it is easy to pull the capsule together and make the sutures quite snug. To carry out this repair we use the same smooth guide wire. The drill hole is started in the front of the tibia about 1 cm. below the articular margin and 1 cm. medial to the patellar tendon. This hole is drilled parallel to the top of the tibia and is drilled from front to back to exit at exactly the same point posteriorly; that is, about 1 cm. below the top of the tibia. With the medial collateral ligament torn and the posterior capsule torn, access can easily be obtained to this area. It expedites the procedure and adds materially to the accuracy of the drilling if a power drill is used. It is imperative that this drill have a variable speed because the hole should be drilled slowly so that the bone will not become eburnated. Three or four holes are made about 1 cm. apart, paralleling the first hole, and they are drilled from front to back, so that there may be three or four holes which would permit two or three mattress sutures. This depends to a considerable degree on the extent of the tear posteriorly. With the use of the ligature carrier, as previously described—and it is important that this small carrier be used—a loop of suture is passed from front to back. A loop of No. 0 cotton blue suture and one No. 0 white suture is passed through this loop and as the ligature carrier is pulled out it pulls one end of the blue and the white cotton thread through the tibia and out the hole in front. A curved needle holder and a trocar needle the same size as the one which is used in the cruciate ligament is then used to mattress the suture through the posterior capsule with the mattress loop being placed in such a way that it is behind the ligament. This pulls the ligament flush against the back of the bone. If the posterior tear is a direct one, it can be sutured by apposition sutures with the knot placed outside the capsule. It is vital that the posteromedial "corner" be snugly secured since this is very important for stability of the knee.

From this point onward the procedure is similar for the different types of incision and has already been described. I will discuss the postoperative handling of the extremity at the end of this section. All apparent bleeding points are coagulated and the wound is closed. Sutures used are cotton 4-0 for the synovium, 2-0 for the retinaculum, 1-0 for the ligaments, 4-0 collagen or cotton for the subcutaneous tissues and No. 32 subcuticular wire and/or Steri-Strips for the skin. Color coding with blue and white sutures being used for the front to back ligatures and for the cruciate is simply a way of making it much easier to identify the sutures. It is not necessary but expedites the procedure.

Repair of the Posterior Cruciate Ligament Through an Anteromedial Incision. (See also 3. Technique for Repair of the Posterior Components, page 592.) If the posterior cruciate ligament has been avulsed from the tibia and additionally the medial collateral ligament has ruptured, repair will frequently be possible from in front. A drill hole starts in front of the tibia about 1 cm. distal to the articular margin and proceeds directly backward, paralleling the articular surface to emerge posteriorly at the midline near the attachment of the posterior cruciate ligament. These are similar to the drill holes made for the repair of the posterior capsule and if the posterior capsule is torn both structures can be repaired through the same holes. It is important that the most lateral hole be located in the midline in order to keep the posterior cruciate ligament toward the midline. A similar drill hole is passed parallel to and about 1 cm. medial to the first. The suture can be passed with a suitable ligature carrier from front to back to emerge posteriorly. This suture is then placed in the knee needle and, since the knee will open up well, it is possible with some patience to plicate the ligature through the detached portion of the posterior cruciate ligament. The needle is then removed and a suture is again threaded in the ligature carrier and pulled out through the second hole to be tied in front of the tibia after the other portion of the repair has been completed (Fig. 455). It is important here also to use two sutures, one blue and one white, to make two mattress sutures of 1-0 cotton. Then, too, if one or the other of the sutures breaks when being tied, the remaining one can be used rather than requiring the whole knee to be opened again to replace the suture.

Repair of the posterior cruciate that has been torn off the femur is very easy through the anteromedial incision (Fig. 461). The medial femoral condyle is already exposed. We simply denude an area extrasynovially along the medial epicondylar ridge and direct the drill holes from this area almost directly lateralward to emerge at the chondral margin in the front of the knee on the lateral side of the medial condyle of the femur. To put it another way, the drill hole emerges on the medial side of the intercondylar notch as far forward as possible. A similar drill hole is made 1 cm. away, paralleling the first one. The two ligatures can be readily passed through this hole, plicated through the stump of the posterior cruciate and back out on the medial condylar margin where each is tied.

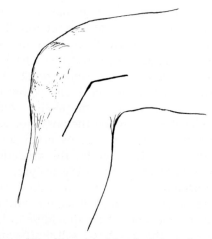

Figure 464. Lateral incision for approach to the knee joint. This incision parallels the iliotibial band to within a fingerbreadth of the patella and then parallels the patellar tendon. This permits the iliotibial band to be split and reflected backward, giving good access to the lateral compartment. It must be extended downward and backward below the fibular head for lateral ligament repair or for treatment of peroneal nerve injury.

2. Technique for Repair of the Lateral Components

With the patient lying on his back with a sandbag under the buttock on the involved side to hold the thigh in internal rotation, the same meticulous preparation and draping are carried out as indicated above. The incision begins at the level of the superior pole of the patella and about 1 cm. lateral to its lateral margin (Fig. 464). It proceeds distally at this distance from the patella and pa-

tellar tendon to the level of the patellar tubercle of the tibia, then swings downward and backward to terminate at the level of the fibular shaft about 2 cm. from its proximal end. The posterior flap is reflected backward to expose the lateral aspect of the knee, care being taken to take all the subcutaneous tissue with the skin flap.

Careful investigation is now made to determine the nature and degree of the injury. The upper end of the fibula should be carefully examined to see if there has been avulsion of the combined attachment of the biceps tendon and fibular collateral ligament. If the lesion is in this vicinity or if the fibular collateral ligament is avulsed from its femoral attachment, the flap should be resected far enough so that the peroneal nerve may be examined and suitably protected either by leaving it under observation in its normal course or by dissecting it free and protecting it with a rubber drain retractor. My personal preference is not to strip out the nerve unless this is necessary because of nerve injury. The attachment of the iliotibial band to the tibia should be carefully inspected. Frequently it will be found to be avulsed. The iliotibial band actually is analogous to the superficial layer of the medial collateral ligament. It becomes a ligament of the knee because of its firm attachment to the femoral condyle through the intermuscular septum so that the section of the band from the femur to the tibia is a lateral tibial collateral ligament. One may easily overlook a rupture of the intermuscular septum which binds the iliotibial tract to its femoral attachment. It is important to be sure this is intact. This can readily be done as the operation proceeds by passing an instrument or a finger under the iliotibial band to see if the intermuscular septum is holding it down to the femur.

After the nature of the lesion is defined the knee should then be opened along the line of the skin incision (lateral parapatellar) and the lateral meniscus carefully explored. If the knee will open up readily on the lateral side, this exploration is relatively easy. At the same time the popliteus tendon should be inspected. If there is serious ligament injury on the lateral side, it is advisable to remove the lateral cartilage for the same reason we remove the medial one on the opposite side, namely, to permit more positive plication of the ligaments. The cruciate ligaments may be inspected from this incision and suitable repair carried out as noted on page 583.

From this incision it is easy to make the drill holes to repair the anterior cruciate to the femur without a separate incision. If the anterior cruciate is avulsed from the tibia there is no necessity for making a medial incision. Drill holes can be made from the lateral plateau forward, inward and upward to emerge on the medial side of the extra-articular portion of the superior tibial surface and a suitable suture passed through these two holes as indicated above. If it is necessary to repair the posterior cruciate to the femur, a separate incision on the medial side will be necessary to permit drill holes to be passed through the medial femoral condyle and into the medial side of the intercondylar notch just at its anterior edge. If the posterior cruciate is detached from the tibia, a similar procedure can be carried out as indicated above for the medial repair, provided the lateral components are badly torn.

After the sutures for repair of the cruciate ligaments have been passed, one then proceeds to the lateral repair. It should be emphasized that replacement of the fibular collateral ligament is in itself not adequate in lateral ligament rupture, since usually far greater damage is present. The same technique is used to repair the posterior capsule as on the medial side, the posterior capsule being pulled downward to the back of the tibia with every effort made to get it as tight as possible with the knee flexed about 30 degrees. Similar repair of the fibular collateral ligament is made, either of the femoral attachment to the femur or of the fibular attachment to the fibula. The latter frequently includes the biceps tendon attachment which must also be replaced. The tibial attachment of the iliotibial band should be carefully replaced even if this requires drill holes along the tibial margin. If the iliotibial band is detached from the femur, this should be carefully repaired. If necessary, the band can be divided and sutured down to the femur. After all the sutures are placed the knee is positioned at about 30 degrees of flexion and all sutures tied. The leg is not permitted to externally rotate to beyond neutral while the thigh is kept in internal rotation by the sandbag under the buttock as the ligatures are tied. Closure is then carried out by usual methods.

3. Technique for Repair of the Posterior Components

The patient is positioned face downward with the entire leg exposed and protected by a steri-drape as previously illustrated. During a portion of the operation a folded sheet may be placed under the knee to hold it in complete extension. The sheet may be moved beneath the foot to flex the knee when this is necessary to facilitate the operation. The incision begins about 8 cm. above the popliteal fold over the semitendinosus tendon, extends distally along the semitendinosus tendon to the level of the popliteal fold and then swings sharply laterally across the fold to the bicipital tendon and down the calf for about 8 cm. along the posterolateral surface (Fig. 465). This curvilinear incision has no sharp angles and as it proceeds transversely across the back of the knee is slightly oblique.

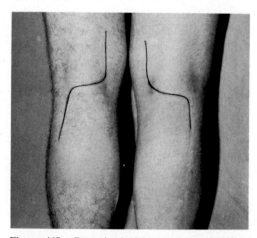

Figure 465. Posterior incision. Note general line of incision. This can be extended proximally or distally or a shorter segment of it may be used. Two important points are that the vertical portion above the knee should be medial and parallel the semitendinosus tendon; the transverse portion should cross the skin folds behind the knee with rounded rather than right angle corners. The vertical portion parallels the biceps tendon just slightly medial to it.

The posterior approach is utilized for repair of the posterior cruciate ligament when avulsed from the tibia and for repair of the posterior ligament of the joint which occurs as a result of hyperextension of the knee. The posterior ligament may be avulsed from the femoral attachment above the femoral condyles but more frequently it is torn from the tibia. In this instance the whole attachment is peeled off the tibia as a cuff, leaving the upper end of the tibia denuded. It usually includes the posterior cruciate ligament. While the posterior portion of the meniscus can be exposed by this incision, the approach is not a proper one for entering the posterior compartment to remove a foreign body or to complete removal of the posterior horn of either meniscus.

The popliteal fascia is exposed by reflecting both skin flaps. The classic landmark in this area is the posterior cutaneous nerve of the calf which uniformly lies beneath the fascia centering between the two heads of the gastrocnemius. The fascia may be split along the line of this nerve proximally as far as the fascial termination above the knee joint, where the nerve will be found to join with the tibial nerve. Following the tibial nerve proximally one may locate the peroneal as it comes off to the lateral side and extends down the lateral side of the popliteal space. This exposure is facilitated by the use of a tourniquet but care should be taken to clamp and coagulate or ligate any vessel which may be damaged in the area. The tibial nerve is located posterior (and so superficial) to the artery and vein so that it may be followed down across the posterior space to the bifurcation of the two heads of the gastrocnemius. It is ordinarily not necessary to dissect out the peroneal nerve so long as it is located and adequately protected. Since the peroneal nerve has a firm attachment, it is relatively immobile and will not tolerate forceful retraction, particularly toward the medial side. After these structures are located, careful dissection deeper into the space will reveal the popliteal artery and vein. These can be retracted toward the lateral side, which will expose the medial head of the gastrocnemius. The geniculate vessels crossing behind the knee in the popliteal space may be sacrificed as necessary, depending upon the pathologic findings.

Having defined the medial head of the gastrocnemius by retracting the vessels and nerves laterally, the tendinous attachment of the medial head of the gastrocnemius to the femur is divided, leaving 1.3 cm. attached to the femur for re-suture. It is extremely important that the approach be made from the medial side for, by sectioning the medial head of the gastrocnemius, the whole neurovascular bundle may be retracted laterally. The tibial nerve has much more retractability than the peroneal and it is not as satisfactory to remove the lateral head of the gastrocnemius in an attempt to enter the area between the peroneal and tibial nerves.

By this division and retraction of the medial head of the gastrocnemius and the vessels and nerves laterally, the posterior capsule of the joint is exposed. The posterior ligament of the joint is revealed and the pathology here may be defined. If the posterior ligament has been avulsed from the tibia by hyperextension of the knee, a very heavy, firm rim of ligament will be found with a free distal margin extending transversely across the lower portion of the popliteal space. This can be lifted up by a suitable instrument and the posterior surface of the tibia will be found to be denuded. In most cases the posterior cruciate ligament is included with this avulsed posterior capsule. If not, it may be readily examined by reflecting the capsule or cuff proximally to inspect the posterior part of the knee. If the poste-

rior capsule itself seems to be intact or possibly only stretched, access to the posterior cruciate may be obtained by a vertical incision in the midline extending from the level of the femoral condyles to a point below the upper end of the tibia. By retracting the margins of the capsular incision the posterior cruciate is exposed as it arises behind the tibia on its posterior surface and courses upward, forward and inward to attach to the lateral margin of the medial femoral condyle anteriorly.

The posterior ligament of the joint actually is made up of many structures but usually it is torn en masse so that separate repair of each of these structures is not necessary. If it is necessary to carry out isolated repair of the posterior cruciate ligament, the exact procedure will depend upon the nature of the tear. If the avulsion is from the tibia, suitable drill holes are made in the back of the tibia and sutures are passed through the drill holes and mattressed into the end of the ligament. This is a favorable type of repair. At this point the knee should be flexed to facilitate relaxation of the tissues in the popliteal space. If the tear in the posterior cruciate is anterior, it will be necessary to make a second incision on the medial aspect of the lower thigh in order to expose the subcutaneous border of the medial femoral condyle and permit drill holes to be made into the intercondylar notch as indicated above. Although this seems quite formidable, it can readily be accomplished from the two incisions. Sutures are passed through the drill hole in the femur with a suitable ligature carrier and recovered in the posterior incision as they emerge in the notch. They are then plicated through the posterior cruciate and passed back out through the second drill hole. As tension is put on this suture it replaces the posterior cruciate ligament against its attachment to the femur. If the posterior capsule is torn directly across, it may be repaired by direct suture. If torn away from the femur it also may be repaired by suture to the attachment of the gastrocnemius. A certain amount of ingenuity may be necessary, depending upon the pathologic findings.

I would like to emphasize that one cannot count on simple flexion of the knee to approximate the separate edges of the torn capsule. A recent case illustrates this very well. When the knee was hyperextended the denuded part of the tibia was exposed, the whole posterior ligament and posterior cruciate ligament being torn away like a cuff. As the knee was flexed, this cuff did not slide down over the end of the tibia. Rather, it buckled into the back of the joint so that even if union had occurred it would have been with considerable redundancy of the ligaments. It is possible that with an intact posterior cruciate the torn posterior capsule might well heal spontaneously by simple flexion of the knee. As in the case of other complete ligament tears about the knee, however, there is no means of ascertaining short of operation the exact nature of the lesion. Hence, surgical repair offers a much better overall prognosis. Granted, there are instances in which a good result is obtained by nonsurgical measures following complete rupture, yet the percentage of these good results is substantially less than with surgical repair because of those cases which obviously cannot return to normal without the latter.

After all the ligatures are placed, the knee should be positioned at about 30 degrees of flexion and all the sutures tied. Closure is remarkably easy in this posterior approach. The gastrocnemius head is sutured back to its tendinous attachment. No other deep sutures are necessary since, as the popliteal fascia is closed, the whole area is snugly pulled together.

Postoperative Care

After closure of the skin, the management of the extremity varies according to the type of repair which has been made. Up to this time the leg has been positioned on the table at about 25 to 30 degrees of flexion with the foot in internal rotation for medial repair, or neutral for lateral or posterior repair. If there has been damage to the anterior cruciate ligament, the extremity must be supported above the knee and the upper end of the leg be permitted to drop backward. Two attendants hold the leg by the thigh and by the foot (Fig. 444). This position is maintained until the dressing is completed. If in addition to the cruciate the medial collateral ligament is torn, the lower leg should be internally rotated in relationship to the femur and held in this position until the external fixation is secure. If on the other hand the posterior cruciate ligament is involved, the support should be behind the calf rather than the thigh in order to hold the leg forward and relax the tension on the posterior cruciate ligament. If both cruciate ligaments have been torn, a neutral position will be held by maintaining support under both calf and thigh. These measures are extremely important since the simple weight of the leg may be enough to pull out the rather insecure suturing through the cruciate ligament. If the combination is anterior cruciate and lateral collateral, the leg should be supported by the thigh and foot and with the leg in neutral rotation. If it is posterior cruciate and posterior capsule and the incision is posterior, a heavy posterior plaster slab may be applied to the leg in the prone position extending from the gluteal fold to the toes and the lateral stirrup applied after this has set.

After this careful positioning of the extremity by the attendants, the knee is wrapped in sterile sheet wadding. We prefer to use Sof-Rol at the top of the thigh since it does not fray out so badly. A posterior slab is placed from the gluteal fold to the toes (Fig. 444, *A*). In whatever way the leg is held, the foot must be placed in the weight-bearing position, namely, slight eversion and zero dorsal flexion. The plaster slab is wrapped in place with 8-cm. gauze bandage and then supported by a lateral stirrup running from the perineum to the trochanter (Fig. 444, *B*). This is firmly wrapped in place with gauze.

At this point we have completed the stirrup splint (Fig. 444, *C*). However, the patient is usually an active athlete and in order to obviate the possibility of his flexing his knee abruptly through the opening in front of the splint as he awakens following the procedure, a single roll of sheet wadding is wrapped around the knee from 15 cm. above the knee to 15 cm. below. Directly over this is wrapped a single roll of 15 cm. plaster of Paris bandage (Fig. 444, *D*). If the repair has been posterior and by a posterior approach, the splint may be applied with the patient lying on his face. Preferably the very heavy posterior splint is applied and permitted to set. Then the patient is turned on his back for completion of the dressing. The advantage of this type of stirrup splint is that, as swelling occurs, it may be readily opened. As swelling regresses it may be tightened again.

By the time the patient is well awake that evening the plaster circular bandage is removed. If there is any doubt concerning the swelling, the entire dressing is split from the toes to the groin and the splint rewrapped. The dressing must not be split over the knee only. If swelling is severe enough to suggest an effusion or hemarthrosis, the dressing is removed under surgical precautions with the surgeon wearing cap, mask and sterile gloves and the knee is aspirated. This dressing is left for about two weeks, at which time under ordinary circumstances the size of the leg will be static. The dressing is then removed and the stitches are taken out and a lightweight, long leg plaster cast is applied with the knee flexed 15 to 20 degrees (Fig. 446). The leg should be supported in exactly the same manner for application of this cast as for application of the original dressing since union of the ligament is quite insecure at the end of two weeks. This plaster cast is worn for four to six weeks. Frequently a walking heel is used if the repair seems stable and if the patient is reasonably agile. He may use the heel for weight bearing but is advised to continue his crutches. At the end of four weeks in the solid cast (six weeks postoperative) it may be removed and a cotton cast (Fig. 433) applied. Aspiration is repeated as often as it is indicated. This splint is removed in two weeks (eight weeks postoperative) and an elastic bandage utilized as indicated. If effusion persists, repeated aspiration and injection may be done. Most cases do not require even one aspiration.

For *rehabilitation,* quadriceps setting and straight leg raising of both legs are encouraged from the first day (page 568). The patient is in a wheel chair at 24 to 48 hours after the operation. He should be able to actively raise the leg, splint and all, by 72 hours and to walk on crutches in two to four days. Weight bearing is not permitted, however. After the solid cast is applied (two weeks postoperative) he may walk with crutches on a walking heel if progress is good. In the meantime, exercise of all other available muscles is encouraged. (See chapter on Rehabilitation.)

After the cotton cast is applied at six weeks (postoperative) the patient is urged to walk, gradually discarding his crutches. He is to continue his exercises. Two weeks later (eight weeks postoperative) the cotton cast is removed and quadriceps rehabilitation continues until the circumference of both thighs is equal. The actual level of activity varies much with the individual patient. The agile, wiry person of relatively light weight may be allowed more freedom than the heavy lumbering giant whose ligaments are normally relaxed. Progressive resistive exercise in which the knee is flexed and extended should not be initiated if effusion or swelling is marked.

Running is permitted if synovitis is not marked. No contact is allowed until four months and not then if the quadriceps is not completely rehabilitated. The knee must be thoroughly taped for every competition or every practice session.

Naturally, each case must be strictly individualized as to both type of repair and postoperative management. A patient with a good, tight repair with intact ligament fibers can be permitted considerable liberty. Some patients need to be pushed in their rehabilitation (for example compensation cases and females) and the period of immobilization may be shortened. Other patients must be curbed (for example, 16 to 18 year old athletes) and their knees will require a full eight weeks of protection. The elastic bandage should be discarded early in the timorous and retained as a reminder in the overbold. If effusion persists, the usual treatment for effusion is followed — namely, aspiration repeated as needed with injection of a corticoid and use of an elastic bandage — as long as moderate effusion persists. Some synovitis will ordinarily be present until essentially normal motion is recovered. In an occasional case there will be some difficulty in obtaining normal motion. This is made more probable by the fact that we suture each ligament as snugly as possible with the knee placed in the most relaxed position for that ligament. I would rather have some restriction of motion than any instabili-

ty. Unfortunately the converse is more often true, more patients having persistent instability than limitation of motion.

If limitation of motion is intractable one may, after four months, under Pentothal anesthesia, carefully and slowly manipulate the knee to increase the range of flexion. Such a manipulation may require 40 to 60 minutes and good judgment is necessary to prevent injury. Manipulation must be followed by active physical therapy in order to maintain the motion obtained.

Such a regimen carefully followed with early examination, prompt decision and complete repair of all torn ligaments, followed by conscientious rehabilitation, will give increasingly gratifying results in the treatment of major injuries to the ligaments of the knee.

In our series of cases, 80 per cent of the patients are under 25 years of age (Fig. 466), 60 per cent under 20 years of age. Since so many of these injuries occur in young people, we must try particularly to obtain the best possible recovery of function in the shortest time.

Following an injury to the ligaments of the knee, the question will arise as to whether or not the player should be allowed to compete in contact sports. The answer must depend entirely upon the individual circumstances. There is no reason why patients with *mild* (first degree) and *moderate* (second degree) sprains should not recover completely and be as strong as ever provided they had proper management at the time of injury. Obviously, for one reason or another, complete recovery in other cases will not always be attained. In these cases the decision must be made as to whether or not the remaining ligament function is adequate to withstand the rigors of athletic competition. The same decision must be made following an injury that has been treated surgically. If the operation was early and adequate ligament

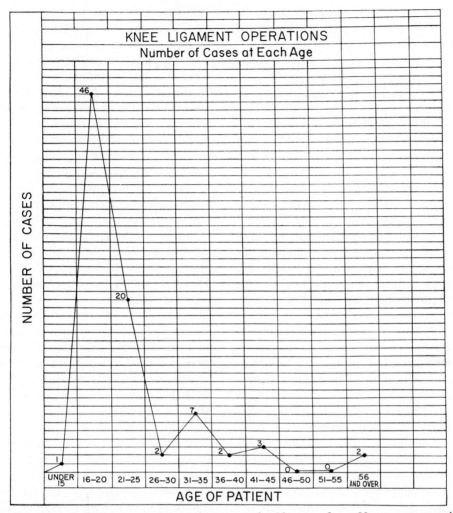

Figure 466. Note that 60 per cent of the patients are under 20 years of age; 80 per cent are under 25. (O'Donoghue, D. H.: J. Bone & Joint Surg. *37–A*:4.)

repair was carried out, the player may usually expect a normally functioning knee. But if complete rehabilitation is not obtainable, the vital decision must be made as to what level of athletic attainment should be permitted. If athletics have been an incidental factor in his life and competition is not truly important to him, he may want to abandon contact sports for fear the injury will be repeated. This might happen even though good recovery had been ob-

tained. We have seen many players return to competitive athletics with no apparent impairment following major injuries. The point I would like to make in this discussion is that one must not be casual one way or the other. The case must be carefully studied and a considered opinion given since this matter is of considerable importance to the persons most closely concerned. If chronic irritation persists with recurring synovitis, if there is slight instability, if there is pain on stress, these factors must be considered in advising the player on his athletic future.

OSSIFICATION OR CALCIFICATION

There is a distinct difference between calcification through the knee and ossification. Calcification as a rule is a sign of degenerative change and weakens the ligament. It has no function in the repair. Ossification is the laying down of mature bone in the ligament which in some circumstances may give increased strength to the ligament although it may also interfere with full range of motion. These conditions are not common about the knee but they do occur and may leave distressing sequelae. As with ossification elsewhere, I believe that one of its major causes is repeated irritation around the joint following infiltration of blood from an injury. In my experience, I have not seen gross ossification following early surgical repair of a knee ligament. I have seen it on many occasions after non-operated sprains, but it would be unfair to assume that surgical evacuation of the hematoma would have prevented ossification. It is my impression that ossification is more frequent following late operation that disrupts the organization of blood after it is well advanced (Fig. 467). This certainly has not been the rule, however, since in most cases ossification does not occur.

A moderate degree of ossification in the medial collateral ligament may not be troublesome. Major symptoms develop from ossification in the part of the ligament that glides back and forth over the condyle of the femur or the upper end of the tibia. Ossification here actually seems to give more trouble than ossification in the ligament attachment itself which we see occasionally following a moderate sprain.

Treatment. A nodule of ossification that causes persistent symptoms may be removed, but one should be particularly wary at removing the bone when it is not symptomatic. A good test is the injection of a local anesthetic around the area to determine whether it relieves the pain. In removing the bony plaque, great care should be taken to split the ligament fibers longitudinally, even if more than one split is necessary to get all of the bone out. Transverse section offers extreme difficulty in repair and will necessitate another long period of immobilization, whereas if the ligament is divided along the line of its fibers a couple of weeks will be ample. There is a tendency to examine a patient, to take an x-ray which shows some ossification and to recommend removal of the bone without any real analysis of the symptoms. Disappointment will usually result since there are, indeed, many areas of spurring in the body that cause no symptoms whatever. Many cases diagnosed by x-ray as bone fragments in the back of the knee have been referred to us for removal when actually the finding was a normal fabella that was perfectly innocent of any symptoms. Ossification of the lateral collateral ligament is infrequent. Ossification of the posterior ligament occurs but is usually not symptomatic since this ligament does not slide directly over the condylar surface. Whereas ossification is relatively common to some degree, calcification is not. We are more likely to see calcification within the ligaments themselves than along the bone.

PELLEGRINI-STIEDA DISEASE

A condition commonly called Pellegrini-Stieda disease consists of the

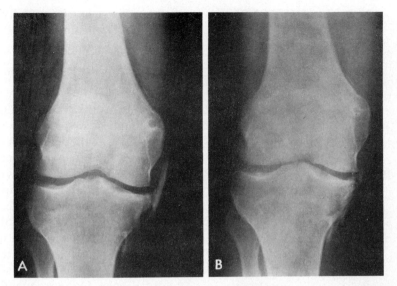

Figure 467. This 19 year old athlete with major injury to the knee was seen 24 hours after injury. He had tremendous swelling of the knee in the popliteal area extending down into the calf with obvious severance of the medial collateral ligament. Any attempt to straighten the knee beyond 60 degrees caused immediate pallor of the foot and cessation of arterial pulsation for a period of minutes. Because of the extreme swelling, he was treated expectantly by aspiration of the hematoma, aspiration of the knee, elevation, ice pack, etc. He was operated on ten days subsequent to the injury. The medial collateral ligament was avulsed from the tibia including the sartorius and semitendinosus; the posterior ligament was detached clear around to the midline; the posterior cruciate was torn off the medial femoral condyle; the anterior cruciate off the femur. There was excessive hemorrhage into the popliteal space with gross blood clot which was evacuated. He had good stability following ligament repair but developed tremendous ossification. This was later excised. Now a surgeon, the patient still has restriction of motion of the knee. Before the ossification was removed he could not flex the knee 90 degrees. Three years postoperative he had 15-degree restriction of flexion with a completely stable knee. This injury occurred almost 20 years ago. In a similar case I would now recommend immediate exploration of the popliteal space with evacuation of the hematoma and ligation or repair of whatever circulatory damage had been done.

    A, Three years after the injury.

    B, Three years after operation for bone removal. No attempt was made to remove the bone at the lower end of the ligaments, since this was not symptomatic.

formation of a plaque of calcium or bone along the medial femoral condyle in the vicinity of the adductor tubercle, separated from the tibia by a band of radiolucency (Fig. 468). It is in some instances a reaction to a sprain in which there has been a forcible detachment of the medial collateral ligament at its attachment to the femoral condyle, and in other instances to partial avulsion of the adductor longus tendon. The symptoms are of sprain of the knee with tenderness high on the condyle in the one case and of adductor strain in the other. The presence of the mass is not necessarily of any consequence, the signifi-

cant factor being the degree of pain. Frequently the area remains painful even after the injury has healed.

Treatment. In some instances removal of the plaque is necessary. A word of warning is in order, however. If the surgeon is too eager and removes the mass before it is entirely mature, it will simply form again. If it is necessary to remove it, great care should be taken that there is no interference with the attachment of the ligament to the femur. In a preponderance of cases removal of the plaque will not be necessary since the condition may mature and become quite inert with the passage of time.

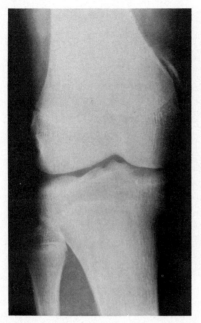

Figure 468. Typical Pellegrini-Stieda disease caused by partial avulsion of the adductor muscle from the adductor tubercle of the femur and ossification within the hematoma. This particular case was persistently painful and the ossification was removed. This ossification is not within the medial collateral ligament. Early treatment here should have been protection against abduction or any adduction stress, together with local measures.

DISLOCATION

Dislocations of the knee are the end result of a severe sprain, since in order for any portion of a normal knee joint to dislocate, certain groups of ligaments must be disrupted. Two basic dislocations of the knee occurring in athletic competition are the *patellofemoral dislocations* and *tibiofemoral dislocations*. In each instance we speak of the femur as being the stable bone with the other bone being displaced in relationship to it.

PATELLAR DISLOCATIONS

Patellar dislocations may be classified as acute or recurrent. Recurrent dislocations may be subdivided into congenital and acquired.

Recurrent Dislocation of the Patella

Basically the true congenital dislocation implies an actual and constant dislocation of the patella usually laterally over the femoral condyle. This condition if fully developed will more or less interdict athletic participation and need not be emphasized here. Of much greater importance is the dislocation that occurs infrequently and under certain circumstances. It may be due to repeated episodes of acute dislocation in a normal knee. Quite frequently there is no true congenital dislocation; but there are certain physical characteristics that predispose to and set the stage for subluxation or luxation. One predisposing anatomical condition is an abnormally acute angle between the axis of the patellar tendon and the axis of the quadriceps mechanism, the so-called Q angle (Fig. 469). If the patellar tendon tends to angulate sharply laterally to reach its tibial attachment, this combined with the fact that the quadriceps mechanism tends to angulate medially at the knee results in an increased angle (Fig. 470) between the patellar tendon and the long axis of the quadriceps so that, as the quadriceps muscle is contracted, there is a tendency for this angle to straighten by slipping of the patella laterally. This action may be inhibited by the prominence of the lateral femoral condyle anteriorly, but the general tendency is for the patella to slide laterally with each forceful extension of the knee. The female with her wide pelvis (Fig. 480) and internally angulated femora is thus much more prone to patellar subluxation or dislocation than the male. A similar situation arises in a person with knock-knee. A dislocated patella in a bowlegged individual is quite uncommon since in such a person the axis of the patellar tendon and quadriceps is esentially parallel. However, in some bowlegged individuals this bow is part of internal torsion of the femur so that the femoral condyles are rotated toward the midline. Such a person often has an associated external rotation of the tibia in order to straighten the long axis of the leg. In this instance the "Q angle" may be markedly more acute as the patellar tendon moves from the internally rotated patella down to the externally rotated patellar tubercle.

One may, therefore, expect recurrent

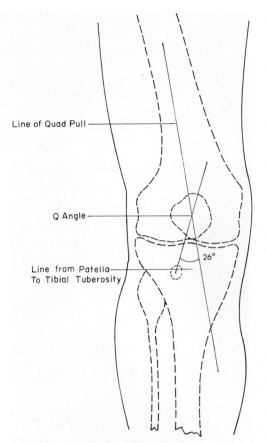

Line of Quad Pull

Q Angle

Line from Patella
To Tibial Tuberosity

26°

Figure 470. This figure shows an increase of the "Q" angle which indicates a more lateral position of the tibial tuberosity. This predisposes to dislocation or lateral luxation of the patella.

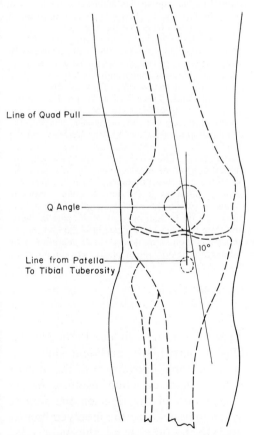

Line of Quad Pull

Q Angle

Line from Patella
To Tibial Tuberosity

10°

Figure 469. The Q angle is the angle formed by two intersecting lines. One is the line of the quadriceps pull, extending down the thigh to mid-patella; the other is a line from the middle of the patella to the center of the tibial tuberosity. The angle illustrated is within normal limits.

dislocation of the patella in a person with a wide pelvis, knock-knee and a relatively flat lateral femoral condyle. This recurring dislocation may arise gradually with the patella subluxating laterally, stretching the medial portion of the patellar retinaculum until the patella finally slips off either as a result of a relatively minor blow on its medial side or from a violent contraction of the quadriceps (Fig. 471, *A*). Ordinarily in the initial instance the patella simply snaps off, slips right back on and there are few, if any, residual symptoms. The patient may describe his knee as having "given way." He may actually have fallen since his proprioceptive mecha-

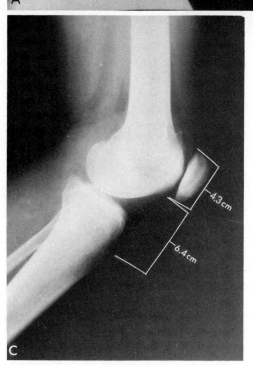

Figure 471. This 17 year old girl seven weeks before was playing basketball when she came down hard on the left leg, twisting the knee and falling to the floor. She had severe pain and swelling, and could not extend her knee. Her history was that she had had recurrent episodes with the knee before this acute injury where something "seemed to be slipping" and the knee would be quite painful. She had the feeling that the knee cap slipped to the side. It has been very much worse since the last injury. She cannot squat or go up or down stairs, and feels that the knee cap slips off to the side. Examination in the sitting position revealed the patellae seem to have a normal relationship. She gets a lateral shift as the patella comes to complete extension, much more severe on the left. As a matter of fact, it slips off every time she extends the knee. There was a 4+ positive apprehension test (see Fig. 417). *A*, Normally positioned silhouette view of the patella* showing the patella slipping sideways and the fragment off the patella, indicating a recent tear of the medial retinaculum. *B*, The Hughston view* showing the dramatic level of displacement in this position. Note the fragment remaining in essentially the same position as it did in the other silhouette (View A) while the medial margin of the patella moves away. *C*, Lateral view of the patella showing the patellar index 6.4 cm. to 4.3 cm., a definite amount. (See Fig. 473 for discussion of patellar index.) Note also that the patella is above Blumenstadt's line even though the picture is made at 45 degrees flexion rather than at 30 degrees flexion. If it were moved up to 30 degrees flexion, the disparity between the distal pole of the patella and the Blumenstadt's line would be more marked. (See Fig. 473 for discussion of Blumenstadt's line.)

*For discussion of x-ray techniques, see Figures 482 and 483.

nism has warned him of the impending dislocation and relaxed the knee to prevent it.

On examination, findings may be entirely negative. One must carefully distinguish between the giving way incident to catching of the meniscus or foreign body and the giving way caused by impending or actual subluxation of the patella. Many a knee has been subjected to meniscectomy when the "giv-

ing way" was actually due to the patella. This is particularly pertinent since the same "cutting" movement of the athlete as he changes direction results in external rotation of the tibia on the femur, which may displace the involved meniscus. On the other hand, this same relationship with the femur rotating in and the tibia rotating out sets the scene for slipping the patella off laterally. One must always suspect patellar subluxation in the knee which for unaccountable reason to the patient simply gives away. In fact, a well-developed patellar subluxation and ultimate dislocation may occur with no actual tearing of the retinaculum. This patient soon learns that his activities must be curtailed and presents himself for treatment only when the recurrence becomes so frequent that it interferes with his ordinary activity. Surgical measures designed for correction of this condition must be carried out if the disability justifies them.

Treatment. One must carefully analyze the characteristics of the injured extremity. Frequently what appears to be a recurrent dislocation of the patella may actually be one of repeated episodes of acute dislocation with no anatomical predisposition. This is particularly likely since the most commonly accepted treatment for the acutely dislocated patella at the present time is nonsurgical. After replacement of the dislocated bone the torn edges of the patellar retinaculum remain more or less widely separated. After healing, this inevitably results in a relaxed medial retinaculum so that as the knee flexes the patella does not receive as much pull medially as it does laterally and any additional force applied to the patella on the medial side will snap it over the lateral condylar ridge. This may occur as repeated episodes of subluxation with only an occasional complete dislocation. One must be on the alert, therefore, when examining a patient with such a history to determine whether or not there is actually a congenital (Fig. 472) or developmental defect since the remedial measures may be quite different in the two conditions.

If the anatomical characteristics are normal, all that may be necessary will be medial plication of the patellar retinaculum usually accompanied by division of the lateral patellar retinaculum and

quad lateralis attachment, particularly if the condition has persisted over a long period of time. If on the other hand the angle of the patellar ligament is faulty, any of the capsuloplasty operations will give disappointing results since the predisposing cause is still present. Many procedures have been designed to correct the basic anatomic condition causing recurrent displacement. One may expect excellent results from any of them if the proper indication for it is present. Once successful correction is carried out, activity need not ordinarily be restricted. I recall a figure skater with bilateral recurrent dislocation of the patella symptomatic to the point that she had to give up her skating. Following transference of the tibial attachment of the patellar tendon medially and capsuloplasty of the knee she returned to her skating without further handicap. This particular patient was in her early 20's and one knee required almost a year for complete rehabilitation. I mention this to deprecate the all-too-prevalent tendency to warn a person that he must permanently decrease his activity when carefully designed treatment may permit normal use.

As has been indicated above, transference of the patellar tendon has very many different techniques recommended. I have tried most of these techniques in the course of treating the dislocating patella. The one which for me is the most satisfactory is as follows: A medial parapatellar incision is made beginning at the superior border of the patella following along the medial margin of the patella, swinging over to parallel the patellar tendon down to the patellar tubercle, or tuberosity of the tibia, then curving medially to expose the medial face of the upper tibia. This skin flap is reflected to the lateral side. The lateral retinaculum is defined and incised beginning at the level of the top of the patella or maybe slightly above,

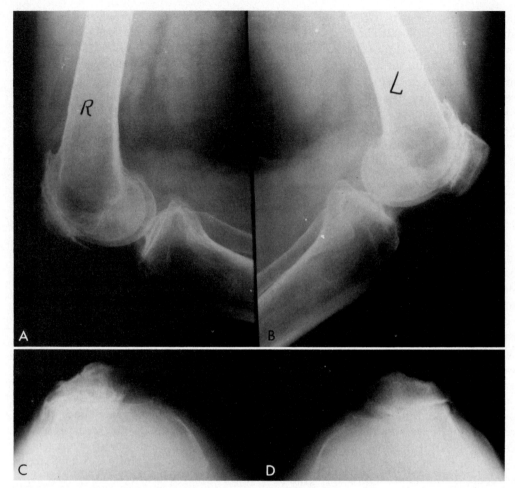

Figure 472. This 76 year old female says her knee caps have been dislocating ever since her childhood, now very much more severe. They do not actually dislocate, just slip sideways. She uses a cane so that she does not fall. Patellectomy may possibly be indicated if the symptoms are severe enough. *A* and *B* show the right and left patellae with very extensive osteoarthritis. *C* and *D* are the silhouette views (see Fig. 482). Treatment at an early stage would possibly have prevented this serious disability.

depending upon the degree of tightness, advancing along the lateral border of the patella, and down along the lateral margin of the patellar tendon to the tuberosity. The tuberosity in most instances is found to be displaced laterally with an increased Q angle (Fig. 470). Definition should have been made as to whether or not patellar alta is present by using the patellar tendon–patella index and also the oblique cortical line extending across the femoral condyle (Blumenstadt's) to estimate just about how high the patella is situated (Fig. 473). A block of bone is then outlined 2 cm. wide and 4 cm. long beginning about 1 cm. above the attachment of the patellar tendon to the tibial tubercle so that there is a block of bone about 1 cm. long and about 2 cm. wide, as a tongue, above the attachment. The saw cut is then continued down to about 4 cm. below the proximal transverse line, at which point an oblique cut is made extending at a 45 degree angle to make a "sled runner" toe on the block (Fig.

474). The block is then excised with the tendon attachment intact. The distal cortical part can be rather thin because its cortical bone is strong. The proximal cancellous part is thicker since it is very easy to break off the proximal extension which is the key to the block.

The block with the tendon attached should be carefully removed so as not to break off the proximal extension. The patellar tendon is separated from the fat pad. The tendon and patella are re-flected proximally to expose the under-side of the patella. Now whatever is necessary can be done to the patella whether this be a chondroplasty by shaving, by trephining and drilling, by facetectomy, or whatever seems indi-cated for the pathologic condition found.

Once the patella has been taken care of, it is then necessary to determine how far the patellar tendon should be transferred distally and how far me-

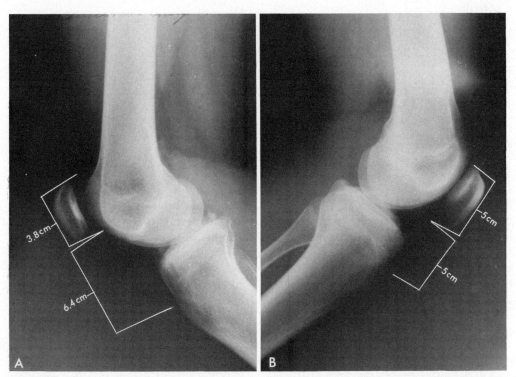

Figure 473. There has always been considerable concern about just how one defines patellar alta. Where should the patella normally be and how can one judge it? A simple way was recommended by Blumen-stadt some time ago. He reported that with the knee at about 30 degrees flexion, the distal end of the pa-tella ought to be at the level of the oblique cortical line extending across the femoral condyles. More recently popularized is the patellar index; for this, take a measurement of the length of the patella, then a measurement of the distance from the distal tip of the patella to the dimple on the top of the patellar tubercle of the tibia. If the distance from the patella to the tubercle is over 1 cm. greater than the length of the patella, this would suggest patellar alta. The more the difference, the more the alta. This index can be made in essentially any position of flexion as long as the patellar tendon is tight. Therefore, the same film could permit both criteria (Blumenstadt line and patellar index) to be used. Obviously, neither of these tests is entirely accurate. Often in determining the patellar index it is difficult to determine just exactly where the dimple is on the patellar tubercle, and sometimes it does not seem to be present at all; so, it comes down to the fact that you just have to evaluate whether you think the patella is high and the pa-tellar tendon is long. These two tests do help.

A, Case demonstrating the patella situated higher than normal. *B,* Normal position of the patella.

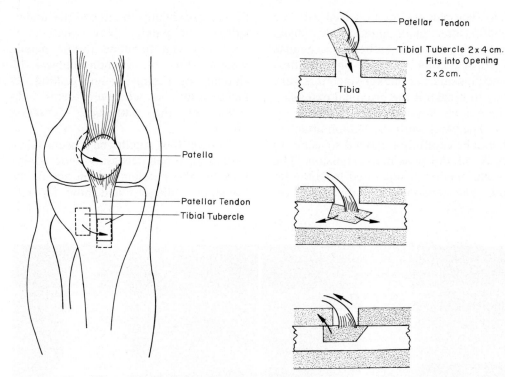

Figure 474.   Technique for transference of patellar tendon. See text.

dially. The medial displacement is determined by trial and error by simply holding the block against the proximal tibial face at different spots and flexing the knee. The tendon attachment should not be advanced distally unless there is a definite confirmable patellar alta, else the patella will be pulled down too far toward the tibia (Figs. 475, 476 and 477). The general plan followed is that if the patellar alta is in the range of 2 cm., advancement would be made perhaps 1 cm. It should be remembered in cutting the window that the length of the block that is above the tendon attachment will be undermined under the tibial cortex. If the extension is 1 cm., you lose 1 cm. of advancement by virtue of the proximal 1 cm. of the block being slipped proximally. The hole in the tibial face is made the same width as the bony block, roughly half its length, so that the hole will be approximately 2 cm. square. The

cancellous bone is cut out in this window to permit the block to be inserted as illustrated in Figure 474. The distal end of the block is inserted in the hole and passed down along the medullary canal of the tibia far enough to permit the proximal end to be dropped into the hole, after which the knee is flexed and the proximal end of the block slides up into the excavation which has been made proximal to the proximal end of the cavity made for the transference and locks there. The block in this way is completely strong and requires no healing to be secure.

The knee can be flexed completely to test the position to get some idea how much you need to imbricate the medial side, or advance the medialis, or release the lateral side in order that this patella will glide freely in the groove without tending to slip laterally. Once it is locked in, you can pack cancellous bone around the block although this is not necessary. It may leave somewhat less of an open space. The defect where the block was removed is covered with a thin layer of bone wax. The block removed in preparation for the transplant is not placed in the hole left at the tubercle. The closure continues by imbrication of the medial retinaculum to whatever extent is necessary, including advancement of the medialis. The lateral retinaculum is left open, this gap being filled by transferring the fat pad to fill the lateral hole even if it is necessary to completely free it from its previous bed. We have noticed no difficulty when this has been done, except in two cases where young female patients noticed that the fat pad was more lateral than normal.

In this type of repair we keep the patient in either long leg stirrup splints or coaptation splints for 2 weeks, permitting ambulation as soon as the patient is able, in 1 or 2 days. At the end of 2 weeks remove the splints and test the function, test the range of motion, and then put the knee in either a long leg walking cast or long leg cylinder for approximately another 2 weeks with full weight bearing, straight leg raising and further exercises for the knee (page 568). At the end of 4 weeks the external fixation can be removed and the patient is advised to walk on crutches until obtaining 90 degrees of flexion. We recommend straight leg raising and active exercises from the first postoperative day, since the block is entirely secure at that time.

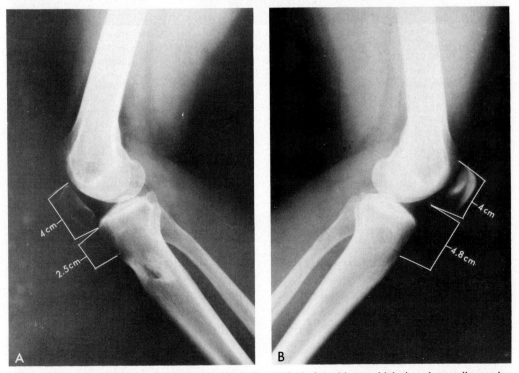

Figure 475.   This 35 year old female had surgery 18 months before this, at which time the patellar tendon was transferred too far distally. *A*, X-ray, postoperative, showing patellar baja and actually an articulation between the patella and the top of the tibia, the index being 2.5 cm. to 4 cm. This was treated by patellectomy, since the patella was too badly damaged to salvage. *B*, X-ray of the opposite knee shows she does not have a patellar baja, the index being 4.8 cm. to 4 cm. (For discussion of patellar index, see Fig. 473.)

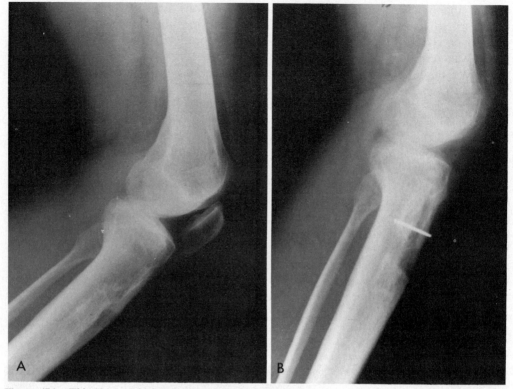

Figure 476. This 29 year old female was operated on at age 16 with transfer of the patellar tubercle distally. The tubercle was actually transferred 4 cm. distally, which pulled the patella down below the top of the tibia as shown in *A*. She has had recurring episodes of subluxation and dislocation of this left patella ever since. She cannot flex the knee more than 90 degrees. Examination at age 29 reveals gross subpatellar crepitation. At this time patellectomy and advancement of the tendon proximally were done. *B*, X-ray at three months postoperative showing the block transferred 2 cm. proximally. At six months postoperative the knee was doing well except it popped a lot. Mild extensor lag. She could actively extend to zero.

We have been gradually shortening the time of immobilization, depending upon the disposition of the patient and the condition of the surgical wound. If the knee is not swollen, the wound is healing well and the patient is quite responsible, we have on occasion left the fixation off at 2 weeks rather than holding it for 4 weeks. I do not believe this is advisable unless the knee can be flexed at 2 weeks approximately 90 degrees.

Admittedly there are many other techniques which may be equally adequate. In my own experience I have been able to mobilize the knee much quicker with this method, since there is nothing that needs to heal except the trauma of the operation and of the skin flap. The transfer is secure once it is locked in.

It should be noted that this type of advancement should be done only when the epiphyses are closed or essentially closed. There not only is a hazard of premature closing of the anterior part of the tibial epiphysis, causing a recurvation, but the more pertinent fact that if you transfer the tubercle below the upper tibial epiphysis, as the leg grows the tubercle will grow farther and farther distally until in some instances the

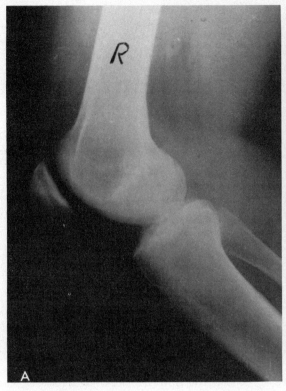

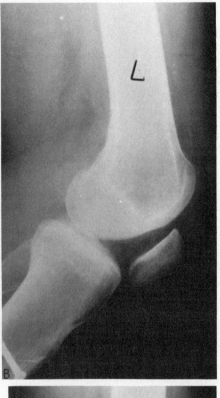

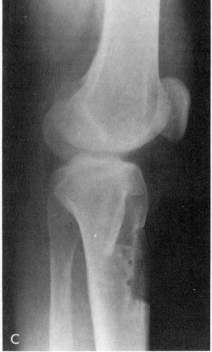

Figure 477. This 29 year old doctor's wife has had recurrent subluxing patella since age 15 when she was active in ballet. There had been gradually increasing episodes until she was operated on at age 27 – "Houser" procedure – with very long rehabilitation. When she actively extended she could extend her knee to 45 degrees. She would have to assist it by this point and then could extend on up to zero. The same thing occurred with the knee flexed. The patella slipped out of the groove at 45 degrees and then it would flex further. Increasing pain and disability. *A*, Lateral view of the right "good" knee. *B*, Lateral view of the left knee showing downward displacement of the patella. *C*, Postoperative film after replacing the patellar tendon attachment medially and shortening of the patellar tendon. Marked improvement with no subsequent dislocation.

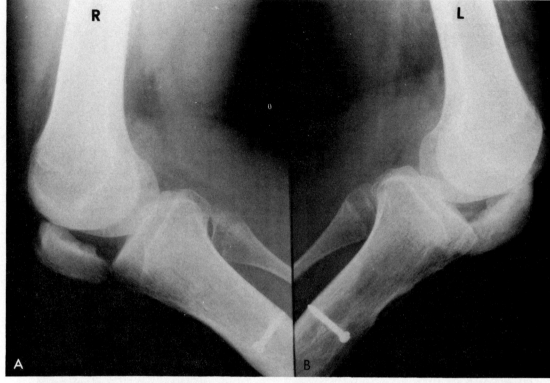

Figure 478.   This 16 year old male was operated on at age 12, with bilateral patellar tendon transference distal to the proximal tibial epiphysis. As the leg continued to grow, the block that was below the epiphysis moved down the leg in relationship to the knee and pulled the patella down so that, *A*, the patella on the right knee was at the top of the tibia and, *B*, on the left the patella was well below the level of the top of the tibia. At age 16 he has severe symptoms with swelling, pain, weakness, snapping and extension lag, which lately are much more severe. When he tries to extend his left leg he has to lift it with his hand while the patella slips back into the groove. Treated by patellectomy and shortening of the extensor mechanism. This figure illustrates the result from transference of the tubercle below the growing epiphyseal plate.

patella will be dragged down to or below the level of the top of the tibia (Fig. 478).

While particular techniques are not to be described here, I should emphasize again that the technique must be matched to the case. One must not try to match his case to a predetermined or stereotyped procedure. If patellar alignment is at fault, it must be corrected. Capsulorrhaphy by release laterally and plication medially will certainly fail in this case. On the other hand, a patellar tendon attachment transfer is contraindicated if this alignment is normal. One must not transfer the tendon or the tubercle below the upper tibial epiphysis

if growth is not complete. In the young person some other means must be used rather than tubercle transference. Plastic operations in the patellar tendon or the quadriceps tendon or in both may be effective. Transference of the attachment must be accompanied by release of the lateral retinaculum or the quad lateralis attachment since alignment cannot be corrected otherwise. Careful attention to the under surface of the patella is a "must" since chondral damage is the rule in recurrent dislocation. There may also be damage to the cartilage on the lateral condyle. Recurrent dislocation of the patella may be very distressing to the athlete, particularly if it goes unrecognized. Many unsuccessful meniscectomies have been done because of an unrecognized subluxation of the patella. Correction of this underlying condition, if done before irreparable chondral damage, should result in the return of the player to active competition.

Acute Dislocation of the Patella

While acute dislocations of the patella may occur with no predisposing anatomical condition, certain factors do predispose to this injury. Thus, a shallow patellar groove, an abnormal patella, an abnormally positioned patella, a laterally displaced patellar tendon attachment or some combination of these conditions is often present. The mechanics of the injury is as follows. As the person turns away from the externally rotating leg with the knee flexed, a violent contraction of the quadriceps may put intolerable stress on the medial retinaculum. The quad medialis is at a disadvantage and the retinaculum tears, permitting the patella to snap over the lateral condyle. If the knee remains flexed, the deformity will persist and the patella will lie against the outer side of the lateral condyle. If the leg is extended either spontaneously by the patient or by someone else, the patella will usually slip back in place.

On initial examination the patient will be in severe pain with the knee flexed, the tibia apparently abducted. He resists any attempt to manipulate the knee.

Careful examination makes the *diagnosis* obvious, if the patella is unreduced, since it will be found to be riding lateral to the lateral condyle of the femur. Much more frequently the dislocation is spontaneously reduced as the knee extends so that the patient will give a story of an injury accompanied by severe pain and often describes the knee as having been "dislocated" and then having slipped back into place. It should be noted that this history is quite similar to that obtained from injury to the medial collateral ligament and not too different from that of an acute meniscus tear with locking spontaneously reduced. In describing the dislocation, the patient will often state that the distal end of the femur has displaced medially and is quite prominent in this position. This is explained by the fact that as the patella slips off, the anterior contour of the knee changes, and with the leg in external rotation and somewhat abducted, the medial femoral condyle becomes very prominent. The patient will describe the displacement as being medial where actually the patellar displacement is lateral.

If examination is done quite early there may be a palpable defect along the medial border of the patella with exquisite tenderness along the medial edge of this bone. The patient is extremely apprehensive of any attempt to push the patella laterally and will cry out and try to restrain the examiner's hand, particularly if manipulation is accompanied by a gesture toward flexing the knee (Fig. 417). If examination is delayed, the knee joint will be filled with fluid and there will be diffuse swelling, more severe anteriorly whereas in the case of a medial collateral tear it will be toward the medial side. On palpation of the knee one finds tenderness around the medial border of the patella with pain on flexion of the knee, which is pathognomonic. The negative findings are of considerable importance since there will be neither tenderness along the collateral ligaments nor pain on lateral motion of the tibia on the femur with the knee either extended or flexed. The patient who has had an acute patellar dislocation will permit a careful and considerate examiner to flex the knee a few degrees and externally rotate and abduct the tibia on the femur with no complaint, whereas in the acute case of medial collateral or indeed meniscus injuries this will not be possible. If hours elapse before the examination is carried out, the findings become less specific since muscle spasm tends to immobilize the knee, swelling becomes diffuse and tension within the capsule causes diffuse pain about the knee.

The lesion in acute dislocation is a rupture of the medial portion of the patellar retinaculum, which may be complete and may include a portion or all of the attachment of the vastus medialis. In fact, the vastus aponeurosis and patellar retinaculum may be peeled away from the medial border of the patella, leaving it bare or actually tearing off a portion of the bone (Fig. 484). Or the patellar retinaculum will split, much as a piece of cloth is torn, with the jagged tear extending anywhere along the medial aspect of the knee from the anterior

edge of the deep layer of the medial collateral ligament to the patella.

X-ray is important (Fig. 479). Careful study of films may reveal an avulsion fracture or provide a clue particularly in regard to the general contour of bone, the anteroposterior view (Fig. 480) showing the increased tibiofemoral angle which predisposes to dislocation, and the silhouette view (Figs. 481, 482 and 483) showing the shallow patellar groove. More specifically, the latter may show the fragmentation along the medial border of the patella where there has been an avulsion of the ligament retinaculum (Fig. 484).

Treatment. The treatment of acute dislocation of the patella in the athlete is surgical. One has only to see the damage to tissues to realize that there can be no real substitute for accurate repositioning of the torn fibers and adequate repair. Research work is confirming more and more the conclusions that we have reached clinically, namely,

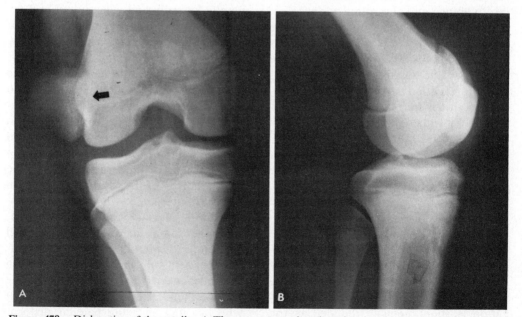

Figure 479. Dislocation of the patella. *A,* The anteroposterior view showing the patella locked laterally. *B,* The straight lateral view with significant overriding of the patella and femur, indicating there must be dislocation.

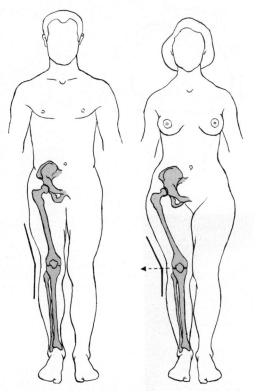

Figure 480. Note that with the broader pelvis in the female, it is necessary for the femur to come inward at an increased angle in order to make the distal end of the condyles parallel with the ground. The quadriceps, patella and patellar tendon make an angle centered at the patella. As the quadriceps contracts, this angle tends to straighten, which forces the patella laterally.

lesion being essentially subcutaneous. With proper precautions in a well-conditioned athlete, it should pose no undue hazard. The reward will be a prompt and complete recovery.

Since the acceptable treatment is surgical, the general management is consistent with this concept. After a careful examination and diagnosis, a compression bandage is applied and ice is used together with fixation of the knee until the operation can be carried out. The ideal time for surgical repair is immediately or at least as soon as proper preparation can be made. While a day or two delay does not completely preclude a good result, increasing experience indicates that there is no time like the present for surgical treatment of the ordinary acute injury. Ideally it is best treated the day it happens, but in no instance later than the following morning provided there is no contraindication to surgery.

The operative technique will vary with the pathologic findings. As a general rule, a curved incision is made in the medial parapatellar area, beginning at the upper pole of the patella about 1 cm. medial to it, extending along the border of the patella and paralleling the patellar tendon. On retraction of the skin edges the patellar retinaculum can be visualized and the nature of the damage ascertained. The incision may need to be extended higher if the vastus medialis has been avulsed, or swung lower and somewhat posteriorly if the medial flap must be reflected to expose the retinaculum further toward the inner side. Usually the capsule of the knee will be torn open. The joint should be carefully inspected, particularly the undersurface of the patella and the lateral edge of the lateral femoral condyle. An osteochondral fracture may be present in either location (Fig. 485). If there is a chondral fracture or chondromalacia it should be carefully treated by chondrec-

that ligament or tendon heals by ligament or tendon if good apposition is secured, whereas a gap that must be bridged in the healing process is likely to remain inadequate inelastic scar. I have seen separations of 2 to 3 cm. along the patellar retinaculum following acute dislocation with no tendency for the split fibers to fall spontaneously into apposition. Indeed, even slight flexion of the knee tends to force them further apart, the only acceptable position being complete extension or indeed hyperextension of the knee. This cannot or at least should not be tolerated for the length of time required for tissue repair. The operation is relatively simple, the

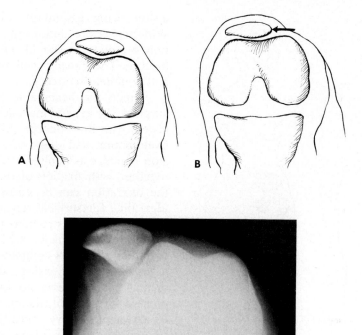

Figure 481. *A*, Normal silhouette view of the patella. Note that the patella seats well in the groove with configuration between the undersurface of the patella and the femoral condyles. The lateral edge of the groove serves to help hold the patella in its normal position. *B*, Shallow groove with flat patella. The lateral buttress is lost, predisposing to dislocation. *C*, Silhouette radiograph of acute complete dislocation of the patella. Note the relatively shallow groove but the sharply peaked patella. (For positioning of silhouette view, see Fig. 482.)

tomy or other measures, the exact technique depending upon the severity of the condition. One may suspect chondromalacia in a knee with a dislocated patella since the tendency for the patella to slide laterally on extension of the knee may be quite traumatic to the cartilage over a period of time. Malacia along the medial and superior facets of the patella is quite common and should be corrected at the time of operation. Treatment of the dislocation itself is relatively simple. By appropriate suture the defect is closed. If one is unable to suture to the edge of the patella, drill

holes may be made along the edge of bone, carefully avoiding penetrating the patellar cartilage. Fixation is readily obtained in this manner. The lateral retinaculum and lateralis attachment along the margin of the patella should be incised if it is at all tight as the knee flexes.

Postoperatively the leg is placed in long leg posterior and lateral stirrup splints with the knee slightly flexed (10 to 15 degrees) for seven to ten days, at which time the sutures are removed and the knee is further protected against flexion by an appropriate cast with or without weight bearing, depending upon the individual case. Healing will be prompt. The long leg cast can be removed after another three weeks to be followed by a fourth week in a cotton cast (total six weeks) while activity is gradually increased and the customary rehabilitative measures are initiated. A word of caution should be said. If the patient has the anatomical characteristics that predispose to recurrent dislocation, these should be carefully analyzed and a definite plan of management instituted. Either his activity should be sharply curtailed or reconstructive measures should be carried out to reduce the tendency toward lateral slipping. This is particularly important if there has been damage to the patella. One should have no hesitation in recommending transference of the patellar tendon attachment from the lateral to the medial aspect of the tibia in such a case, since without it recurrent trouble in later life is almost inevitable, even though athletic activities are curtailed. If the anatomical alignment is normal and no predisposing characteristics are manifest, further protection after the completion of healing is not indicated. In this instance there should be no more predilection for trouble than there would be following a broken tibia, for example.

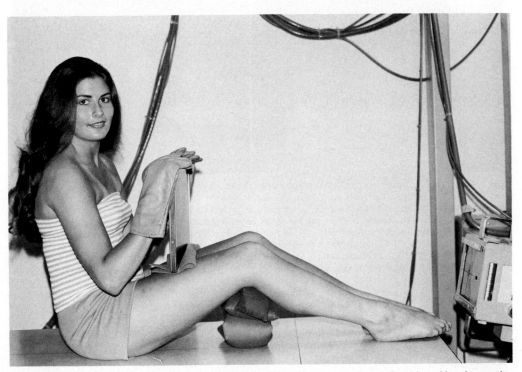

Figure 482. Silhouette of the patella ("Sunrise View"). With the patient seated on the table, elevate the knees and support them with sand bags until the femur and tibia form an angle of about 45 degrees. Have the patient hold the cassette in a vertical position about 30 cm. proximal to the patellae. Direct the central ray to the patellofemoral joint space, forming about an 80 degree angle with the cassette. The angle of the knees and central ray may be varied according to the patient's tolerance. A centering light aids in directing the central ray just beneath the patellae. A piece of art foam may be used to anchor the cassette if necessary. Both patellae, for comparison, are visualized on the film.

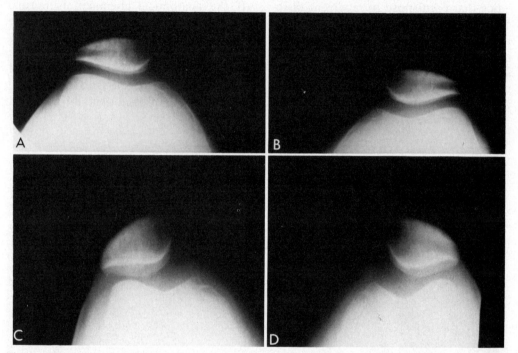

Figure 483. This figure shows the comparison between the Hughston view versus the normal silhouette. This 34 year old female had a history of recurring trouble with her patellae as far back as she can remember. *A* and *B*, the silhouette views, could be interpreted as having some lateral subluxation of the left patella *(A)*, since the lateral edge of the patella is beyond the lateral edge of the trochlear groove, particularly as compared with the right side *(B)*. In the Hughston view, *C* and *D*, there is definite tilting apparent on both patellae. I would interpret the Hughston view on the right *(D)* as being negative. However, if the left one *(C)* was not available for comparison, the right one might be considered to be tilted abnormally. I think one has to determine a normal in order to have a basis for accurate judgment of the Hughston view.

See Figure 482 for x-ray positioning of the silhouette view. The Hughston view is made with the patient prone with the plate lying under the knees, the knees flexed to about 60 degrees, and the tube paralleling the tibia.

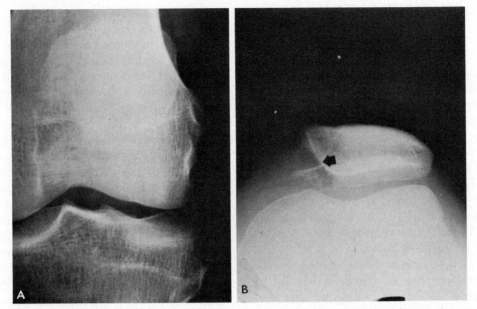

Figure 484. Patellar dislocation with avulsion of patellar tendon and medial retinaculum. *A*, Anteroposterior view showing dislocation. *B*, Silhouette view. Arrow indicates avulsed retinaculum. Note also the shallow patellar groove which tends to predispose to dislocation.

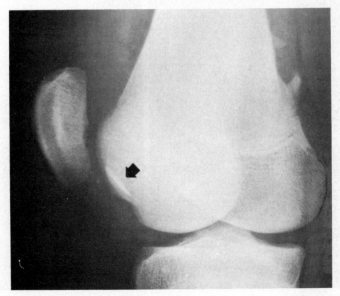

Figure 485. Acute dislocation of the patella in the oblique view with chondral fracture of the undersurface of the patella. Note the fragment lying just behind the femoral condyle slightly distal to the lower pole of the patella. Note also the defect on the underside of the patella. At operation an acute fracture with a fresh bleeding bed under the patella was found. The hooklike processes on the medial epicondylar ridge are a normal variant. This is the type of trauma that can cause apparent "patellar malacia" if unrecognized early.

TIBIOFEMORAL
DISLOCATION

There seems to be general agreement that a recognizable complete dislocation of the knee is a rare injury. The recorded diagnosis seems to depend upon the dislocation persisting until it can be examined in the hospital by physical examination and by x-ray study. Very few patients do reach the hospital with a dislocation unreduced. A New York hospital reported only 2 cases out of 20,000 admissions; one in Philadelphia reported only 2 cases out of 140,000 admissions. I think this gives a very inaccurate picture of the actual number of cases in which the knee is dislocated. Certainly many of the cases are reduced spontaneously or

at the scene and are never documented as dislocations (Figs. 486 and 487). The statements that "my knee slipped out of joint" or "my leg was off to the side and someone pulled it back straight" tend to be discounted and considered to be meniscus slipping.

I see many old cases for consideration of reconstruction in which both cruciates, often both collaterals, and both sides of the posterior capsule are grossly unstable, some of them with peroneal nerve injury. This is not the place to document these cases in detail, but a relatively casual review of our cases that have required two-stage medial collateral, lateral collateral, and both cruciate reconstructions were determined, probably by careful history taking, to have actually had a disloca-

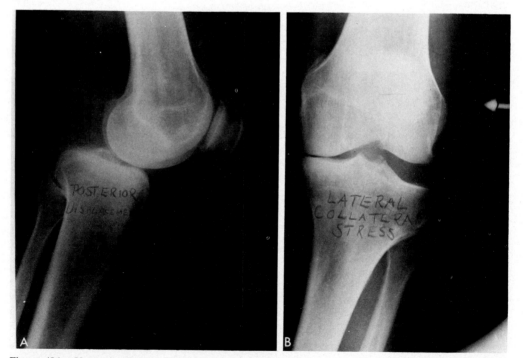

Figure 486. X-ray showing late dislocation of the tibia posteriorly. This was a football injury, with gross swelling and complication of circulation to the foot and to the peroneal nerve. The x-ray many months later showed posterior displacement of the tibia on the femur and complete lateral instability. This was a posterolateral dislocation of the knee sparing the medial components. At reconstructive surgery the patient had absent posterior and anterior cruciate ligaments with complete lateral side instability. *A*, Posterior displacement. *B*, Showing lateral and cruciate ligament damage.

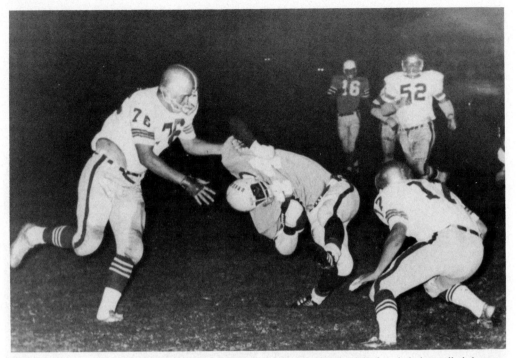

Figure 487. This 17 year old high school player with his weight on the right foot is being pulled the same direction so that his right knee is bent at 90 degrees. In this position the knee is completely dislocated. The medial side was completely torn with damage to the posterior capsule and both cruciates. The position was corrected on the field, which is proper. He had complete disruption of the anterior and posterior cruciate, the medial collateral, and medial posterior capsule. The lateral side was largely spared. Nerve and blood supply were undamaged.

tion (Fig. 488). I mention this for two reasons: first, to state that this injury is not all that rare, and second, to point out that in a severe knee injury one must always be on the alert for vascular damage whether or not there is an actual recorded dislocation.

Complete tibiofemoral dislocation is also very rarely recognized in the athlete. There is some separation of the tibia from the femur in any complete tear of the collateral ligaments. Usually this subluxation is spontaneously reduced and by the time the patient is examined it appears to be what it indeed is, a ligament injury. In some instances the displacement is so complete that it does not reduce spontaneously. At other times a frank dislocation has been noted before it is reduced by a fellow

player or some other individual on the field. With a history of complete dislocation one should investigate very carefully to determine whether it actually was tibiofemoral in character. A dislocation of the patella or indeed a dislocation of a meniscus with temporary locking may quite often be interpreted by the player himself as a dislocation of the knee.

The tibiofemoral displacement may be in any direction and determination of this direction has important bearing on the surgical approach. Knee dislocations are classified according to the position of the tibia in relation to the femur. Hence:

1. Anterior Dislocation—the most common

2. Posterior Dislocation

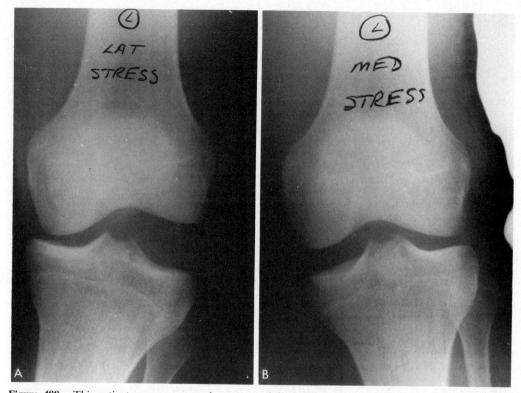

Figure 488.   This patient was seen several years post-injury. He reportedly had a dislocation of the knee which was treated by reduction and cast; several days later bilateral meniscectomy was done with repair of the medial collateral, lateral collateral and both cruciates. Without subsequent injury he had increasing instability of the lateral side. We recommended and carried out lateral side, anterior and posterior cruciate ligament reconstruction, with marked improvement. *A*, Lateral stress x-ray several months post-injury shows wide opening of the lateral side, indicating the lateral collateral and both cruciates were completely afunctional, which I think confirms the fact that he did have a dislocated knee. *B*, Medial stress x-ray. Note the medial slipping of the tibia on the femur, indicating redundancy of the medial structures as well.

3. Lateral Dislocation
4. Medial Dislocation
5. Rotatory Dislocation

Anterior Dislocation

The mechanism of injury has been much discussed in relation to the type. Thus, hyperextension will cause anterior dislocation. Since hyperextension is a common injury, this is the most common type of dislocation. In this condition the force angulates the tibia forward until first the posterior capsule tears, then the anterior cruciate, then the posterior cruciate. Usually the me-dial and collateral components are damaged but they are not necessarily completely disrupted for the tibia to slip forward on the femur. As the overextension continues, the tibia slides forward and locks there (Fig. 489). This overextension may place intolerable stress on the popliteal artery, which is well tethered above and below the popliteal space. The artery is stretched and often large segments of the artery will show multiple ruptures, contusions and gross edema. This may require resection of such a large section of artery that direct suture is not possible. The intima of the artery may rupture while the outside wall may seem intact. Hence, delayed thrombosis may develop to trap the unwary.

Posterior Dislocation

Posterior dislocation cannot occur by overflexion. The force here is a direct force applied to the front of the tibia with the knee semiflexed (Fig. 490). The tibia is driven backward, the posterior cruciate and posterior capsule rupture. Almost always one or both of the lateral components must give way and there is a rotatory component, lateral to spare the medial ligament and medial to spare the lateral ligament. We are speaking now of movement of the tibia on the femur.

The vascular injury here is usually a frank rupture of popliteal artery in the popliteal space. Suture is often feasible here. The peroneal nerve is usually spared.

The ligament injury is the posterior capsule, posterior cruciate, medial and lateral collateral ligaments.

Lateral Dislocation

Lateral dislocation is caused by a force driving the leg into wide abduction on the thigh. The medial collateral components, the medial posterior capsule, the anterior and posterior cruciate ligaments give way and the tibia slips laterally off the femur without serious damage to the lateral components, although they may also be torn (Figs. 490 and 491).

Vascular injuries are not frequent in this type of dislocation although damage may occur if the dislocation is gross. The neurovascular bundle can move lat-

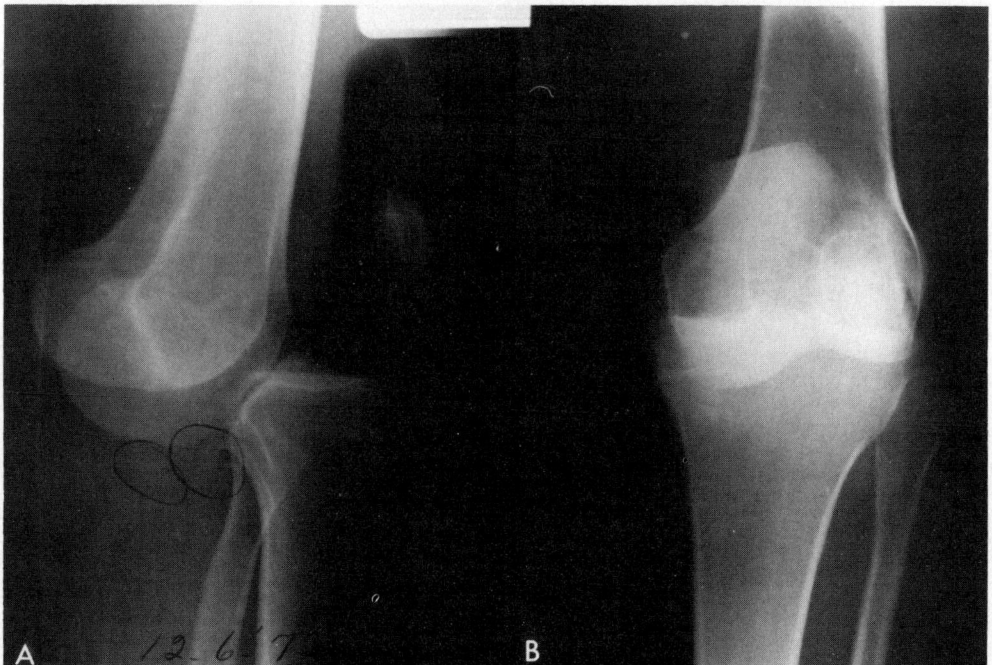

Figure 489. This patient was struck from the rear by a car, receiving compound anterior dislocation of his knee. Both cruciate ligaments were torn. He was treated elsewhere by early repair which was successful except for residual posterior instability. *A*, Lateral view showing the anterior displacement. *B*, Showing superposition of the tibia and femur. Late reconstruction was required for the posterior instability.

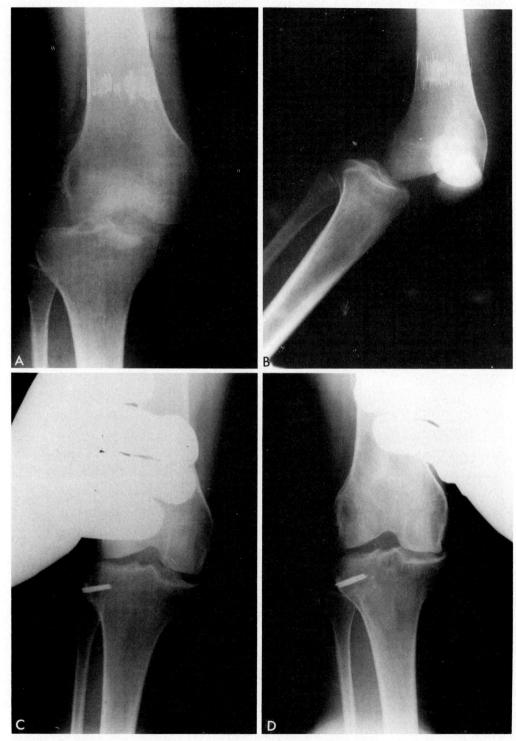

Figure 490. *See legend on the opposite page.*

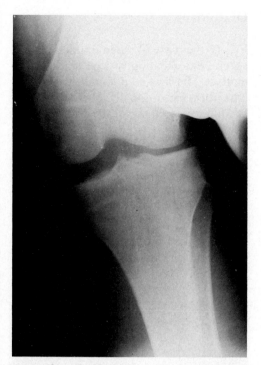

Figure 491. Football injury with the player having been hit on the lateral side of the knee, forcing the femur inward and the tibia outward, causing a lateral displacement of the tibia on the femur. Six months post-injury he had complete medial and anterior instability, which was reconstructed. X-ray shows the stress film indicating the medial and anterior instability. Note the lateral subluxation of the tibia on the femoral condyle.

erally with much more freedom than medially. Hence, it is more often spared.

The ligament injury here is the medial collateral, medial posterior capsule, anterior cruciate, posterior cruciate, with lateral injury less likely although it may occur if there has been very major trauma.

Medial Dislocation

Medial dislocation is caused by a force driving the lower leg medially, a force not commonly present in athletic injuries. Striking the lower leg from directly laterally, as for instance a car striking a pedestrian from the side, angulates the tibia medially and the tibia slides medially on the femur with rupture of the lateral components, the two cruciates and the posterior capsule (Fig. 492). The medial components may strip away from the femur and so not be ruptured. This medial dislocation is quite uncommon. Peroneal injury is often present.

Rotatory Dislocation

In posterolateral dislocation the force is anteromedial rotation of the femur on the tibia when the foot is fixed and the tibia dislocates posterolaterally off the lateral condyle (Figs. 490 and 493). The medial components may be spared as the rotation point is on the medial tibial plateau. The cruciate ligaments are often torn, particularly the posterior cruciate. With extreme continuation of this force the medial condyle may burst through the medial capsule in front and be trapped there. This type of dislocation usually requires open reduction.

In posteromedial dislocation the opposite is true. The rotation is on the lateral plateau of the tibia, the foot being rotated inward and the thigh outward so that the tibia displaces backward off the

Figure 490. This 19 year old girl was involved in an automobile accident two years before. Complete posterior or posterolateral dislocation of the right knee. Critical general condition with ruptured spleen, etc. The dislocation was reduced under anesthetic; nothing else was done. Several weeks later she was operated on and the ruptured quadriceps tendon was repaired with a little suturing on the medial side. At 10 months postoperative she was operated on again with meniscectomy and attempt to repair the posterior capsule. Three months later the dislocation was reduced but there was gross medial and lateral instability. Treatment here was by medial side reconstruction followed by lateral side reconstruction and reconstruction of the anterior cruciate. *A*, The lateral dislocation of the tibia on the femur. *B*, Showing the posterolateral displacement. *C*, Medial stress and, *D*, lateral stress at four years post-reconstruction. Excellent stability with essentially no complaint of the knee, but note severe degenerative changes.

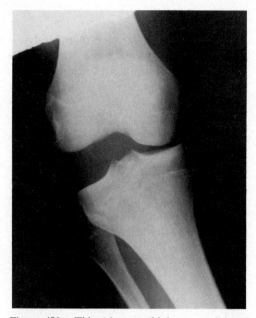

Figure 492. This 16 year old boy was injured playing football the night before when he was struck on the lower leg, forcing the leg medially. It appeared to be off to the side, and was straightened on the field. My examination revealed gross lateral instability with the whole lateral side of the knee completely absent in flexion or in extension. X-ray shows the gross lateral instability even with the knee in extension. At surgery everything was torn off laterally, including the peroneal nerve, both cruciates, lateral collateral, popliteus and biceps. The medial side was ecchymotic and swollen but apparently stable. His immediate postoperative course was satisfactory. At four months postoperative the knee is laterally stable in extension and flexion; no anteroposterior instability; 3+ effusion; flexion to 130 degrees. Excellent result so far.

femoral condyle. In this instance the damage is largely medial; anterior and posterior cruciate; medial posterior capsule.

In any of these various positions other injuries may occur. The menisci are usually damaged, often completely loose. There may be chondral fractures, avulsion of the gastrocnemius attachment, rupture of the patellar tendon, fracture of a condyle or of the patella. There may be damage to the blood vessels and nerves about the knee which may take precedence over all else.

DIAGNOSIS

If the case is seen immediately a careful examination will be highly informative. The first step should be to evaluate the circulation to the foot and the second to determine the state of the nerve supply. It is extremely important to know whether or not there has been immediate loss of innervation to any part of the foot. Late paralysis will suggest pressure intrinsic or extrinsic on the nerve and may well require different management than would early paralysis. The peroneal nerve is particularly vulnerable in dislocations.

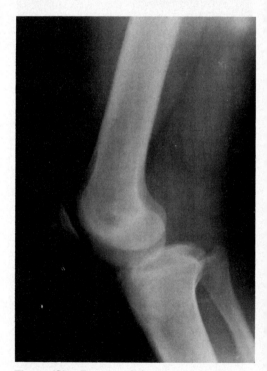

Figure 493. Rotatory dislocation caused by the foot being caught in a power take-off. Note residual posterior dislocation. At surgery both cruciate ligaments were torn and de-rotated. The posterior cruciate was torn off the femur, the anterior cruciate was torn off the tibia, the posterior capsule was torn, the iliotibial band was torn off the tibia, the biceps and fibular collateral were pulled off the fibula. Following subacute repair, 17 days, he obtained good stability, since the two cruciate ligaments were torn off the bone rather than by their fibers.

After the preliminary survey of the condition of the leg and foot, attention is directed to the knee. Careful inspection will reveal any persistent deformity and its direction, thus providing a valuable guide to the pathology of the injury. If the deformity has been reduced either spontaneously or manually before the examination, it may be possible at this early date to determine the degree of instability of the knee. This examination should be extremely careful, taking particular pains not to reproduce the dislocation. I remember one instance in which the patient had a complete dislocation of the knee that was spontaneously reduced and re-dislocated three times before x-ray films were made that showed the complete dislocation (Fig. 422, A). Obviously, re-dislocation is a serious hazard and should be assiduously guarded against. After examination and some definition of the degree of pathology, measures for treatment should be promptly initiated.

PRIMARY TREATMENT

There may seem to be some disparity of opinion as to the treatment of acute dislocation of the knee. Actually, however, there is a surprising agreement on the basics of treatment. All agree that the primary consideration in knee ligament dislocation is the circulation to the leg. Soft tissue injury or fractures must give way to a serious consideration of the viability of the circulation. The essentials of treatment generally accepted are:

1. immediate reduction;
2. evaluation of circulation;
3. arteriogram;
4. open surgery for vascular damage.

Reduction. There can be no doubt and it has been well documented by many that early, in fact immediate, reduction is the very first priority. The

end result may depend entirely upon this factor. Hence, reduction should be and ordinarily can be done at the scene. A prior knowledge of the force applied will help but is not essential. Careful, gentle traction in the line of the extremity will usually suffice to slip the tibia back under the femur. The more complete the disruption, the easier the reduction. If the femoral condyle is locked over the front of the tibia, simple extension of the leg will usually dislodge it. If not, flexion of the leg with forward pull on the calf will accomplish reduction. Usually this can be done under vocal analgesia, namely, calm reassurance and gentle encouragement.

In lateral or posterior positions it may be necessary to gently rock the tibia while continuing traction. Gentleness is the key to success. The longer the dislocation continues, the harder reduction becomes as muscle spasm fixes the displacement. Strenuous manipulation is never justified.

If the dislocation cannot be reduced without anesthesia, the emergency becomes more urgent and the patient must be rushed to the emergency room, preferably where definitive treatment can begin. If undue delay of several hours is necessary to accomplish this, the patient should be taken first to the nearest available place in order to reduce the dislocation. The only justification for x-rays showing the deformity is if they can be snapped while other necessary arrangements are being made, such as calling the doctor, giving the anesthetic, and so on. If atraumatic reduction cannot be carried out without anesthesia, anesthesia should be given. A spinal may be done because it may help circulation. If reduction cannot be carried out by gentle manipulation under anesthesia, open reduction must accompany inspection of the vessels.

Circulation. Circulation is the first priority after reduction! If the foot has been pale, cold and pulseless before reduction, this should promptly disappear and a flush is noted if the circulation is adequate. The dorsalis pedis and the posterior tibial pulse should return at once. The coolness disappears to be replaced by local warmth as circulation returns to the capillaries. Danger signs are:

1. absent or diminished pulses;
2. continued pallor;
3. diminished sensation;
4. continued coolness.

One must not be misled, however, by questionable warmth on top of the foot. The top of the foot may be warm and the circulation quite inadequate. Simple absence of the pulses on this foot which are present on the other side is sufficient justification for exploration of the artery.

Watchful waiting here is disastrous. An arteriogram is helpful although some say it may cause local irritation. If there is any doubt about the adequacy of the circulation, operation should be carried out. The following procedures are in general order of preference (see posterior approach to the knee, page 592):

1. Direct end to end anastomosis seems most successful, but one must be able to approximate the artery ends without tension.

2. Resection to normal artery and replacement by a reverse vein graft from the opposite saphenous vein has had considerable success and many prefer this to any artificial prosthesis.

3. Replacement by artificial prosthesis.

4. *Simple ligation is disastrous.* The leg will not ordinarily survive rapid loss of the popliteal artery.

After the dislocation is reduced, the extremity must be protected while further definitive treatment is considered. A posterior slab is best since it can be nonconstrictive and it does permit observation. If there has been evidence of

circulatory disturbance which has not required surgery, a suitable waiting period should ensue, 24 to 48 hours, depending upon the condition of the leg. If surgical repair of the vessel has been necessary, the same conditions prevail. Constant observation must be made and reported to the responsible doctor. A few hours' delay from 2:00 A.M. until "morning" may be fatal for the leg. The same rules apply here. The appropriate surgeon should be on the alert and if there is any doubt the vessel should be explored.

TREATMENT OF THE INJURED LIGAMENTS

Treatment of the knee injury includes the following:

1. reduction;
2. splinting;
3. observation (24–48–72 hours);
4. surgical repair of each torn ligament;
5. postoperative immobilization (8 weeks plus);
6. rehabilitation.

Although the treatment to this point has been generally accepted, there has been difference of opinion as to the treatment of the injured ligaments. My position is quite clear. If there is evidence that any ligament is completely torn and if the leg is safe for surgery, I think this ligament should be repaired at the time when there seems to be no doubt about the adequacy of the circulation. Although ligaments are better repaired at once, the elapsed time interval is not that important up to 7 to 10 days or even a little later if absolutely necessary. The pendulum seems to have swung toward repair of all torn ligaments. It has been documented many times that ligaments repair the best if they are placed end to end and immobilized until they heal. One only needs to see the inside of a dislocated knee to be impressed with the virtual impossibility of complete spontaneous repair. Indeed, I have seen the posterior capsule invaginated into the joint, the medial collateral ligament often lying on top of the tibia, and various other combinations that seem impossible to recover by closed treatment.

Surgical correction should be done at the earliest safe moment, hopefully from 48 hours to 10 days. If the patient has been operated on for vein graft or arterial repair, I think one should wait at least 48 hours and preferably 72 hours to be sure the vessel is patent. This could also be confirmed by an arteriogram. Since immobilization must be continued for eight weeks from the day of the surgery, undue delay in initiating the surgery increases the total period of immobilization and so increases the time of rehabilitation.

If surgery is necessary for arterial damage, I would take advantage of this incision to get some evaluation of the location of the various injuries. This would help in the selection of the best approach for repair of the ligaments. If the posterior capsule is torn with the posterior cruciate off the tibia, I would quickly repair this if it did not require further dissection or trauma. I would not make another incision or unduly enlarge the one made for the vascular repair. Needless to say, if secondary operation is done one must wait until the first surgery is adequately dry.

Certainly in the athlete the treatment of dislocation of the knee is surgical and adequate repair requires all the skill one can muster. True enough there have been cases treated nonsurgically with recovery of a useful degree of function of the knee, but I have never known of one so treated to end with anything approaching *normal* function. Immediate measures are as for any ligament injury of the knee. Following examination, aspiration of blood and injection of hyaluronidase and the application of a pressure bandage with ice are imperative. Then, without fail, the whole extremity must be protected by adequate splinting since irreparable damage may be done to the leg by careless handling. The patient should not walk from the field with assistance or be carried, leg dangling, with his arms over another player's shoulders. He should be tightly splinted manually, placed on a stretcher and not moved from the stretcher until proper support is applied to the knee.

I cannot emphasize too strongly the vital importance of the circulation to the leg and foot. The popliteal vessels are well tethered in the popliteal space and do not tolerate much stretching. The injury may be to the arteries or to the veins. The artery may rupture, permitting excessive bleeding and intolerable pressure in this area with compression of the veins and the nerves. Venous bleeding will be less dramatic and more readily controlled by pressure.

A normal pulse in the early stages of the injury does not preclude arterial injury since the intima may be damaged with no damage to the arterial wall. This may not be visible even on surgical examination of the outside of the vessel wall. The damaged intima encourages mural thrombus formation along the injured area. As the thrombus develops it may completely obliterate arterial circulation. If there is *any* doubt about the integrity of the circulation, definitive surgery for repair of the ligaments should be delayed. If there is a serious question as to whether or not vascular exploration should be done, it should be done. Several days' delay in definitive treatment of the ligaments is a cheap price to pay for an intact circulation. Vacillation about the condition of the circulation, however, should not permit unnecessarily long postponement of any necessary surgical treatment.

After reassurance that the circulation is safe, plans are made for definitive treatment even though the first consideration is for the circulation of the leg. This should not be interpreted as meaning that repair should "wait until the swelling goes down." It simply means that one should assure himself of the adequacy of the circulation of the foot, since if this is not adequate and does not respond to paravertebral sympathetic block and similar measures, the first step may well be exploration of the popliteal space. Rupture of the popliteal artery or vein is a distinct possibility. If it is necessary to explore posteriorly and if the circulation is not too disturbed, some degree of posterior repair may be carried out at this time. Repair of the posterior cruciate and posterior capsule may be feasible as part of this procedure. If the circulation of the extremity is intact, then a choice must be made between an approach to the knee from the medial or from the lateral side. This choice will depend upon where the major damage is suspected. One may obtain surprisingly good access to almost all parts of a badly torn knee with an incision on one side only. I have been able to repair the posterior cruciate to the tibia, the posterior capsule to the tibia, the anterior cruciate to the femur, and the medial collateral ligament to the femur and tibia, together with medial and lateral meniscectomy, all through a medial approach since the knee can be very carefully opened up in these circumstances to permit placement of sutures which can be tied after the joint is reduced and positioned. Tourniquet time must be carefully guarded, 90 minutes maximum. Indeed, much of the closure may be carried out after the tourniquet is removed. Removal of the tourniquet before closure has the added advantage of permitting control of bleeding. It is good for one's peace of mind to know that no major

vessel is the cause of the postoperative swelling which is almost inevitable. The whole procedure may be done without tourniquet if deemed advisable. This does make for a long and tedious surgical experience and use of a tourniquet is usually proper.

Following a suitable period of recovery from the initial injury and the reparative surgery, a second operation may be carried out if necessary. If the peroneal nerve has been primarily damaged it should be explored and repaired within a relatively early period, say within two weeks. There is a degree of urgency of treatment of each of these structures and the priority is definitely in the following order: (1) circulatory embarrassment, (2) damage to the cruciate ligaments, (3) collateral ligament damage and (4) neurological deficit. Justification for this timing is quite evident with a little consideration. After the circulation I give second priority to the cruciates because the success of cruciate ligament repair varies inversely with the elapsed time after injury. It must be done within the first two weeks and the sooner the better.

A dislocation of the knee is an extremely serious injury. This is not sufficient justification for a negative approach to the problem, since the dislocation need not necessarily terminate in a major disability. Time is of the very essence. The patient should be placed promptly in the hands of the specialist who will carry out the definitive treatment.

A recent personal experience is unique in so far as my information is concerned, consisting of complete anterior dislocation of the tibia on the femur, bilaterally. The 19 year old male was involved in an automobile accident with multiple bruises but major injury to his lower extremities. He arrived at the hospital with both lower extremities dislocated at the knee joint. In Figure 494,

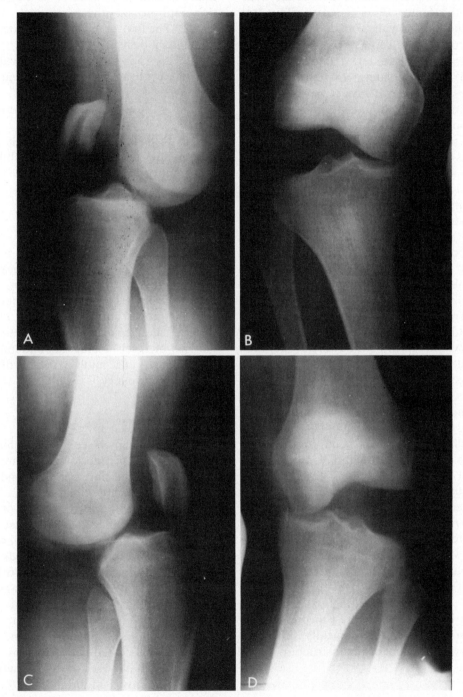

Figure 494. The case which is described on page 628 of the text. *A*, Right knee showing complete anterior dislocation of the tibia on the femur. *B*, The stress film made with basically no force shows medial subluxation of the tibia on the femoral condyle as well as wide open lateral side. *C*, The left knee showing essentially the same pathologic condition as the right knee. *D*, The stress film showing even more medial shift of the leg.

A shows anterior dislocation of the tibia on the femur. *B* is a stress film after reduction showing complete lateral side disruption. *C* shows complete anterior dislocation of the left tibia on the femur and complete lateral disruption in the stress film in *D*. X-rays were made while waiting for the anesthesiologist. The dislocated knees were reduced under anesthetic. Arteriograms of both extremities showed no disturbance of the vascular system. The patient was immobilized and observed overnight, then sent to me. With intact circulation 60 hours post-injury, the left leg was operated on and complete disruption of the lateral side found; the anterior and posterior cruciate ligaments were off the femur; the gastrocnemius was off the femur; the biceps and fibular collateral were off the fibula; the iliotibial band was off the tibia; the peroneal nerve was torn. Five days later the same findings were found on the opposite knee. Surgical repair in each instance was by repair of the cruciates to the femur, the gastrocnemius to the femur, the biceps and fibular collateral to the fibula, the iliotibial band to the tibia. Ten weeks postoperative the patient still had good stability. Delayed nerve suture was carried out. This case is unusual in that the patient reached the hospital with both knees dislocated. In spite of this long time interval there was no vascular disturbance at any time although there was complete peroneal palsy.

A partial dislocation or subluxation has been amply covered in our discussion of sprain. A chronically subluxing knee is a ligament reconstruction problem.

SUMMARY

1. Many more dislocations actually occur than are diagnosed.

2. Any grossly unstable knee after injury should be considered as a dislocation until proved otherwise.

3. The first priority for treatment is circulatory damage.

4. As soon as possible surgical repair of torn ligaments should be carried out.

5. All torn ligaments should be repaired.

6. Rehabilitation is extremely important and should start at once while in the splint or cast.

MENISCUS INJURY

Another common condition is injury to the menisci. This injury goes hand in glove with ligament sprain. The general structural anatomy of the menisci is well known but it is well to recall certain significant differences between the two menisci in order to understand the damage one may expect from a given type of injury.

Medial Meniscus

The medial meniscus is "C" shaped (Fig. 495, *A*). Its anterior attachment is on the top of the tibia near the midline and in front of the tibial spines. The posterior attachment is on the top of the tibia behind the spines. In each case the attachment is relatively near the periphery of the tibia so that the two ends are quite widely separated from each other. The meniscus is attached by means of the coronary ligament (which has its origin around the top of the tibia) to the medial collateral ligament and hence to the tibia. This attachment is firm and while it does allow a little play there is no very extensive motion permitted in the normal medial meniscus.

In sprain of the medial collateral ligament, the tibia and femur tend to separate on the medial side and stress is applied in the area of the attachment of

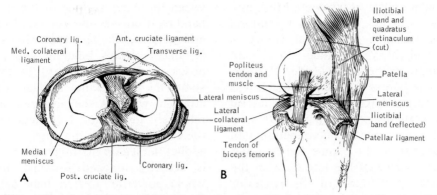

Figure 495. *A*, Drawing of the top of the tibia showing the menisci and the coronary ligament. *B*, Drawing showing attachment of lateral meniscus to tensor fascia femoris which is frequently noted.

the meniscus to the medial ligament. The cartilage may be forced to accompany either the femur or the tibia, depending upon the location of the ligament injury. Since the structure of the meniscus does not allow much bending stress, it will tear transversely or more commonly split around its periphery. If the tear is actually in the attachment to the ligament, it may heal. If it is within the substance of the meniscus it will not. In my experience meniscus injury accompanies repeated sprains to the knee more frequently than it does the initial single sprain. I know of no way to determine in an acute injury whether or not the meniscus is torn unless the knee is actually locked. If the knee is locked and the ligaments appear to be stable and the episode is the first, one may be justified in attempting to reduce the displacement by careful manipulation or by traction. If the meniscus has been detached at its periphery, this attachment may then heal. This possibility is much more likely if the meniscus has slipped into the knee and locked and then immediately unlocked. Such an incident occurs where the player hurts the knee and it is forcibly extended manually immediately following the injury and the meniscus snaps back in place. My own opinion is that if the knee actually locks even once the knee should be operated

upon, the meniscus examined and, if torn, removed. However, I have no particular argument with the surgeon who prefers to wait for the second episode. There is nothing to be gained by waiting for repeated episodes of locking, and bragging of them by the patient cannot be condoned. We have been able to show that locking of the knee has a definitely deleterious effect upon the articular cartilage, not only on the condyles of the femur and tibia but more particularly on the patella. Careful explanation to the patient of the undesirable effects of the locking episodes will ordinarily convince him that he had better have his knee operated upon early with the prospect of an excellent result than postpone operation until malacia has become advanced.

Lateral Meniscus

Whereas the medial meniscus is "C" shaped with widely separated anterior and posterior attachments, the lateral meniscus is almost "O" shaped (Fig. 495, *A*), its anterior and posterior attachments being deep in the tibial notch and very close to each other. In many instances they are continuous with each other. The coronary ligament usually is much less firm and is more redundant. This meniscus is not attached to the fibular collateral ligament. More motion is normally possible in the lateral meniscus than in the medial. Injury to the lateral side of the knee is less common than to the medial side. Furthermore, the lateral meniscus is much less likely to be damaged by acute lateral stress so that it is not frequent to see a lateral meniscus tear in conjunction with an acute sprain of the knee. On the other hand, by virtue of the looseness of the meniscus, particularly in its posterior portion, it is quite vulnerable to chronic damage so that it is more likely to be hurt by chronic overflexion of the knee. Frequently the damage comes on insidiously as a result of squatting with the heel against the buttock for long intervals on frequent occasions. I have been so impressed with the vulnerability of the lateral meniscus because of redundancy of its posterior one-third that I do not recommend deep knee bends or the so-called duck waddle as conditioning exercises. As the knee moves into complete flexion, the back of the meniscus may be caught between the impinging femoral condyle and tibial plateau and thrust forward, much as one would pinch an apple seed between his finger tips. This strains the posterior peripheral attachment until the meniscus may actually snap in front of the femoral condyle and finally progress to the typical bucket handle position and lie within the notch in front of and medial to the lateral articular condyle of the femur.

Although as a general rule the attachments of the lateral meniscus to the other lateral components of the knee are much less firm than is the case with the medial meniscus, this is not always true. In many instances there is a very firm attachment of the anterolateral section of the lateral meniscus to the iliotibial band. I have noted this to be almost always the case in partial or complete discoid menisci. Indeed, one often cannot distinguish a line of separation be-

tween the inner surface of the iliotibial band as it crosses the knee and the lateral margin of the lateral meniscus. This is almost always bilateral and predisposes markedly to injury. In this instance the front of the cartilage is firmly attached whereas the posterior part is relatively loose. As a consequence of this firm fixation, as the stress occurs to adduct the leg on the thigh, the cartilage is actually dragged forward and its whole posterior portion may catch in front of the femoral condyle. This anatomical variant has real significance in the fact that the lateral compartment is extremely difficult to expose until the cartilage is separated from the iliotibial band (Fig. 495, B).

DIAGNOSIS

If one never makes the diagnosis of meniscus injury until the knee has undergone repeated locking he is overlooking many torn menisci! The diagnosis of meniscus injury may be made by history alone and it is extremely important that the history be carefully and objectively taken. It is not wise to put words in the patient's mouth. If he gives a definite, detailed and reliable history of locking of the knee, one may assume meniscus damage until he can prove it to be otherwise. More difficult is the case of chronic knee trouble with recurrent effusion and recurring periods of disability but with no locking or "giving way." One suspects meniscus damage. In this instance a very careful examination will be of extreme value. There is usually tenderness along the joint line in the damaged area. This may be posterior as a result of posterior tearing, or it may be midlateral or in front. The examiner should familiarize himself with the various manipulations that put stress on each meniscus. There are many manipulations described such as McMurray, Ashly, and so forth. None of these are specific but many of them may be quite confirmatory, and combined with other symptoms they can aid in the diagnosis. Pain, sharply localized, during these various tests may be as diagnostic as the click. The McMurray test is carried out with the patient supine; some others with the patient prone. With the knee semiflexed, lateral stress will usually cause pain in acute injuries but not as consistently in chronic meniscus damage. There is usually pain on rotatory stress. With the knee flexed, the calf is grasped firmly and the leg rotated laterally and medially. Pain will frequently be noted at the exact site of the injury to the meniscus. One should at least be able to determine which side of the knee is involved. Another test which I think is quite valuable is carried out with the patient supine. The knee is placed in complete flexion and then hyperflexed to determine whether this causes pain and where the pain is located. Many cases of posterior tear will give a definite cartilage click on this maneuver. In fact, this maneuver may actually cause the cartilage to slip forward and the knee to be locked. In this same completely flexed position the foot is turned into external rotation and the knee flexed and extended a few degrees. The leg is then placed in internal rotation and the knee flexed and extended. Consistent clicking in these tests must be considered significant. Another similar test is conducted with the patient in a supine position. Bring the leg to complete extension while palpating the joint with the leg either externally or internally rotated. A similar test can be done with the patient standing and squatting, with the leg either turned in or turned out. In the final analysis, the knee that stubbornly resists conservative treatment and in which meniscus damage is suspected justifies arthrotomy. This is not to say that every painful knee should be operated upon for meniscus damage. The weight of the evidence must point toward meniscus damage to justify surgery under this preoperative diagnosis.

TREATMENT

I have previously stated that if the knee locks this in itself is justification for surgical treatment. The locking may be due to meniscus damage, or to a foreign body in the joint, displaced osteochondritis dissecans, and so on. One must be particularly wary of pseudolocking in which the patient cannot extend the knee completely and feels that his knee is locked. If this is several hours subsequent to the injury, hamstring spasm may well prevent complete extension since the painful knee tends to flex and will resist extension. There are certain clues which help to distinguish between the types of locking. One is the history in which the patient has definite recollection that he immediately could not extend the knee. This is valid reason to conclude that it is probably actually locked. This is confirmed if the pain on extension is in the location of the meniscus. If, however, the patient is uncertain as to when he could not extend his knee because he actually did not try it and if on attempt to extend his complaint is posterior in the hamstring area, one would assume that the loss of motion is probably due to hamstring spasm and not bona fide blocking from internal derangement. At arthrotomy one must be prepared to treat whatever lesion is found. If the knee locks, some presumptive cause must be found if the operation is to be successful. Removing a normal meniscus will not stop the knee from locking! (See Fig. 496.)

Some general principles referable to surgery are important. There is no

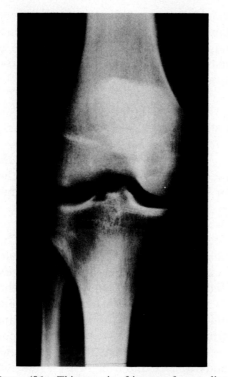

Figure 496. This case is of interest from a diagnostic standpoint. The boy had an abduction injury to the leg with symptoms of medial meniscus pathology. He actually did have a bucket-handle fracture of the medial meniscus. Survey x-rays revealed a tumor in the femoral condyle. It proved to be a benign chondroblastoma. In this instance the solid tumor was an incidental finding. Treatment of the tumor designed to improve the condition of the knee would have failed. The tumor was removed at a second operation.

justification for removing a normal meniscus just because one has diagnosed meniscus damage preoperatively. It is true that the front of the meniscus upon examination may appear to be normal but there may be posterior damage that cannot be determined from in front; nonetheless it is pretty drastic to detach the anterior end of the meniscus in order to determine whether its posterior portion is torn. A better procedure is to enter the knee behind the medial collateral ligament to permit inspection of the posterior part of the meniscus. As stated, the removal of a normal menis-

cus is unjustifiable, and particularly so because it does not eliminate the cause of the trouble in the knee. If upon inspection no abnormality is found in either meniscus, the knee must be carefully explored for other lesions to account for the symptoms. These may or may not be remediable but are not helped by removing a normal meniscus.

A question that must be answered is, "What constitutes a 'normal' meniscus?" This is an area in which surgical experience counts heavily. I have no hesitation in removing a meniscus that is yellow and sclerotic or in which there is redundancy of one or the other attachments although there may be no obvious tear. However, I would feel extremely uneasy about removing a sclerotic meniscus in a knee in which there is a history of locking or giving way since certainly a sclerotic meniscus could not be expected to cause these symptoms. Frequently at arthrotomy there will be found a rather marked redundancy of the fat pad, the posterior margin of which may appear grossly sclerotic. This can be symptomatic, usually causing pain on forced or rapid extension of the knee as in place kicking. However, once again I would feel quite uneasy about simply trimming away the fat pad unless I could assure myself that there is no other pathologic condition in the knee. Fat pad symptoms should be around the pad and are elicited by pressure on this area.

I realize that this is vast oversimplification of the meniscus problem but would like to state a few of my own convictions.

1. A locking knee should be operated upon regardless of freedom from symptoms in the intervals between episodes.

2. Authentic "giving way" of the knee may be almost as significant of meniscus damage as is locking.

3. The most constant symptom of

meniscus damage is tenderness located at the site of the damage.

4. A careful history suggestive of meniscus damage supported by pertinent findings justifies arthrotomy provided there is real disability of the knee. If the symptoms are so mild as to cause no effusion, instability or actual disability from pain, arthrotomy may be postponed since the knee is not undergoing deterioration because of delay.

Technique for Medial Meniscectomy

The patient is placed in the supine position (Fig. 459) and given the usual meticulous preparation of the skin. The leg is draped and steri-drape is used. The footpiece (Fig. 497, *A*) of the table is then dropped to permit the leg to dangle off the table at a 90 degree angle. The surgeon drapes a double fan sheet around his body extending from his waist to the floor. He is seated at the foot of the table with the patient's foot between his knees. I prefer a straight incision (Fig. 497, *B*) which begins about 1 cm. proximal to the lower pole of the patella and 0.5 cm. medial to the patellar tendon and proceeds parallel to the patellar tendon to terminate just proximal to the patellar tubercle. This is actually the central portion of the anteromedial incision which we use for knee ligament repair (Fig. 461). The patellar retinaculum is split along the line of the incision and the synovium is opened. At this point the knee is carefully lavaged (Fig. 497, *C*) with warm sterile saline plus an antibiotic, particularly if blood is encountered. Through this short incision, a surprisingly good exploration of the knee can be carried out. The anterior attachment of the medial meniscus is examined. The anterior cruciate is checked. The posterior cruciate is noted. The knee is extended and the undersurface of the patella inspected by lifting it up with a toothed retractor and also by palpation with the finger.

Should there be attendant damage, particularly involvement of the lower end of the patella, the incision is extended proximally at this time to permit better exposure. It is not necessary to enlarge this incision in order to carry out adequate repair of the anterior cruciate ligament. If there is damage to the collateral ligament which should be repaired, the incision is extended distally.

The meniscus is now carefully examined. If it is possible to spring the knee open on the medial side, the entire cartilage may be visible. This is the exception rather than the rule. The periphery of the cartilage may be palpated with a blunt Kelly forceps to determine whether there is a defect in the coronary ligament attachment or a split in the cartilage. I have devised a "feeler" for this purpose which is a small rod curved in the arc of the femoral condyle with a 1 cm. right-angled blunt hook at its end (Fig. 498). The hook is to avoid any possibility that the point of the forceps will be forced through the coronary ligament rather than hooked into a defect. Anterior examination will ordinarily determine whether there has been damage to the meniscus. If the feeler hooks in the split in the cartilage or in its attachment, we assume the presence of a posterior tear. With the knee flexed at 90 degrees, it is possible that the feeler may catch in a fold of synovium. This danger is obviated by bringing the knee to an extended position, at which time the synovium in back of the joint is taut and there is no recess in which the feeler may catch. We routinely carry out this maneuver in case the meniscectomy is going to depend upon the impression that there is a posterior tear by use of the feeler. Very often the feeler can be hooked into the torn meniscus either from the top or from underneath and ac-

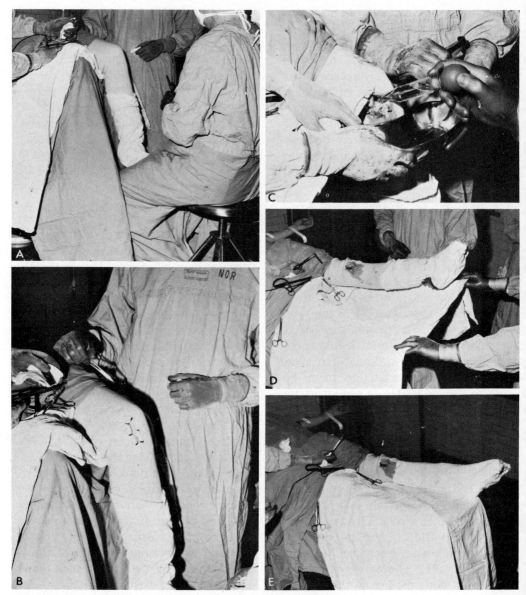

Figure 497. The author's general set-up for medial meniscus surgery.

A, The leg is prepared and draped as shown in Figure 460, using steri-drape. (These pictures show sterile stockinetting which we previously used.) Note the knee flexed to 90 degrees with the foot caught between the operator's knees. The surgeon is draped with an extra double fan wrapped around as a skirt. Note the white double fan lying under the knee and not fanned out.

B, The short incision which is actually the central part of the general utility incision on the medial side of the knee (Fig. 461). This incision can be extended upward if it is desirable to expose the undersurface of the patella, downward if it is necessary to repair the medial ligament.

C, At the beginning and termination of the operation the knee is thoroughly lavaged with warm saline plus an antibiotic. The basin which catches the return flow will reveal many bits of foreign material which would be best out of the knee.

D, As the anesthetist extends the end of the table, the double fan which has been lying under the knee is extended out over the end of the table, thus covering the whole end of the table which has been proximate to the floor.

E, Position for exploration of the patella or any other procedure needed with the knee extended. The skin and capsular incisions are more readily closed with the knee in extension.

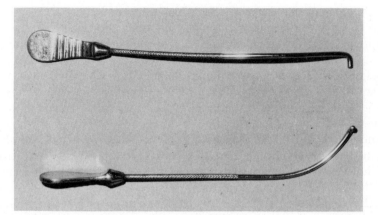

Figure 498. Anteroposterior and lateral views of the "cartilage feeler." Note the curve corresponding to the curve of the upper end of the tibia and the short, blunt hook at the end. This can be deceptive if it is allowed to turn as it goes into the posterior compartment and then catches in the synovial sac, but it is a useful adjunct in the exploration. This synovial fold, which may catch the feeler in the flexed position, is eliminated as the knee is extended so that the catch should be confirmed by extending the knee and repeating the test.

tually pulled forward between the tibia and femur to demonstrate how redundant it really is. If the anterior part of the cartilage is friable, ecchymotic and redundant, we assume that the meniscus has been damaged somewhere. A very common finding in meniscus pathology is a greater or lesser triangular-shaped overgrowth of synovium extending over the femoral condyle at just about the area where the anterior segment of the meniscus would impinge (Fig. 499). This finding is surprisingly consistent, and it often gives one a feeling of comfort to find this condition as he opens the knee expecting to find meniscus pathology. If this examination leads to the conclusion that the cartilage is pathological, it is removed as follows:

The anterior bony attachment is separated from the upper end of the tibia and the periphery of the cartilage is carefully divided from the coronary ligament as far back as convenient with the ordinary scalpel. At this point traction forward on the cartilage will confirm posterior damage. A cartilage knife or meniscotome is utilized to divide the meniscus from the coronary ligament as

far back as possible. This instrument must be exceedingly sharp and care must be taken that it follows the contour of the tibial rim, not the femoral condyle. If this instrument does not pass

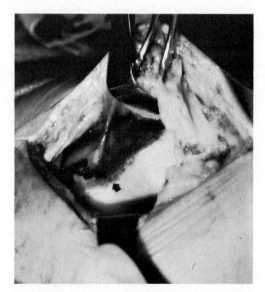

Figure 499. Acute meniscus injury (two weeks), uncomplicated. Note the inflamed synovium growing out over the medial femoral condyle. Arrow indicates the fold of synovium with the invasive edge going over the normal appearing femoral condylar cartilage. Bucket-handle meniscus plus pannus. No other pathology.

readily it should not be forced since damage can be done to the femoral condyle, the upper end of the tibia, the medial collateral ligament or the posterior cruciate ligament by unwise instrumentation. When the straight, very sharp meniscotome is used, great care should be taken in making the dissection. The meniscotome is intended to be a dissector, not a guillotine. It should be held as you would hold a pen or pencil and not grasped in the fist. The crossbar on the handle of the meniscotome is not intended for pushing with the heel of the hand. It simply indicates where the blade is. Dissection should be carried out alternately above and below the meniscus at about a 30 degree angle. It is seldom advisable to push it around vertically.

At this point traction forward will tend to slide the cartilage under the femoral condyle. If it is detached peripherally posteriorly it will slide over into the notch. More frequently it slides part way over. Then, rather than dragging it over into the notch, which leaves the posterior attachment folded over, it is better to use the meniscus as a spreader. If you can hold it between the tibia and the femur it will permit the passage of the thin meniscotome posteriorly to complete the separation of the meniscus from the posterior capsule. A very thin straight meniscotome is used to divide the bony attachment, with care being taken to get all of the meniscus. The operation to this point has all been done through the anterior incision which means that the pathologic characteristics were determined from in front, that the cartilage was readily divided by a meniscotome, that we removed all of the meniscus when we detached the posterior bony attachment. Failing any of these things, exposure of the posterior compartment of the knee must be made. This may be done in one of two ways. The anterior

skin incision can be extended as for the ligament approach and the medial skin flap reflected subcutaneously. The posterior margin of the medial collateral ligament can be palpated as the curve of the tibial plateau swings posteriorly and a vertical split is made along the line of its fibers. Dividing through the synovium will give access to the posterior compartment. This same area may be reached by making a short vertical incision through the skin paralleling the ligament fibers just at the posterior edge of the medial collateral ligament. The posterior ligament is relaxed in this flexed position and the posterior compartment can be readily visualized through this exposure. If no pathologic signs were present in front, the cartilage is particularly examined for them posteriorly. If we find no signs of damage to the cartilage it is not removed. If the removal from in front left a posterior tag or if the cartilage did not readily separate, we complete the meniscectomy posteriorly. Careful examination of this space is carried out to make sure there is no other damaged tissue. The posterior cruciate ligament can be palpated readily. The posterior femoral condyle can be inspected as can the upper end of the tibia. The wound is now thoroughly flushed with the saline and antibiotic solution and closed in layers, 4-0 cotton in the synovium, 2-0 cotton in the ligament, 4-0 cotton in the subcutaneous tissue, No. 32 subcuticular wire for the skin.

Attention is next redirected to the anterior portion of the incision. The operative wound is thoroughly lavaged and the fat pad inspected. Any other morbid changes are noted and treated. If the patella is normal, the incision is then closed similarly to the posterior one. If it is necessary to treat the undersurface of the patella, the knee is then extended. the end of the table raised and draped as indicated (Fig. 497, *D*) and appropriate chondroplasty of the patella carried out by trephine and drilling (see page 672), shaving, or partial or complete patellectomy as the case may be. At the conclusion of the operation a cotton cast (Fig. 433) is applied and the tourniquet removed.

Technique for Lateral Meniscectomy

The lateral compartment is more difficult to expose than the medial. The leg is prepared and positioned as indicated above. The incision I prefer at present has a horizontal and a vertical component. The horizontal limb begins about 3 cm. proximal to the lower end of the patella and level with it, extends straight forward along the line of the iliotibial tract to the edge of the patellar tendon and then parallels the edge of the patellar tendon to the tubercle of the tibia (Fig. 464). The decussating fibers of the iliotibial band, which swing forward to attach to the margin of the patella, are split parallel to the incision as far down as the patellar tendon. This permits the iliotibial band to be reflected backward without impairing its strength. The fat pad is troublesome but is incised to expose the knee. Electrocoagulation is used to seal obvious vessels. The lateral meniscus is now visualized. It is usually considerably more redundant than the medial. The same general rules are applied laterally as medially. There is one notable difference, however. This is in respect to the popliteal hiatus. There is normally a defect in the coronary ligament at the midlateral line of the meniscus through which the popliteus tendon traverses. One must not be misled into interpreting this as a tear. There is frequently a tear, sometimes difficult to detect, of the meniscus attachment from the popliteal hiatus back to the posterior meniscal attachment. If the cartilage is found by anterior inspec-

tion to be pathological, it should be detached in front and pulled forward, whereupon the posterior characteristics can be readily determined. If the anterior part appears to be completely normal, a second incision must be made similar to that on the medial side, the approach being just behind the fibular collateral ligament and in front of the popliteus tendon. This is somewhat more difficult than on the medial side since one encounters the popliteus tendon as it crosses the back of the knee laterally and care should be taken not to damage it. I cannot emphasize too strongly the fact that excision of the meniscus should be a delicate dissection. There is no necessity to drag the meniscus out. It is undesirable to use a curved meniscotome and slice around the back of the joint in order to cut the posterior portion of the coronary ligament. All of these maneuvers result in damage to other parts of the knee with a corresponding delay in recovery and the possibility of permanent damage. The instruments must be very sharp, and one must resist the temptation to force the knife.

Postoperative Care

The postoperative care really should begin prior to the surgery. The patient should be instructed to walk with crutches and taught to walk with a normal weight bearing gait. He is handed an excercise sheet (see page 568) which spells out in considerable detail just exactly what exercises should be done and when they should be initiated. I like to have the patient practice straight leg raising before the surgery and so know exactly what to do when he starts straight leg raising in the splint.

Our postoperative care for meniscus injury is as follows: A cotton cast is applied and the tourniquet removed. An elastic bandage is placed from the toes to the bottom of the cotton cast. Rehabilitation is started immediately. The patient is expected to raise his leg that night; to exercise all of his muscles the next morning; be up in a chair the first postoperative day, be up on crutches with direct weight bearing the second postoperative day. Weight bearing without crutches is discouraged, however, because of the tendency to lurch and so strain the knee laterally. Since the cotton cast loosens up in a few days, the elastic bandage is removed from the foot and wrapped around the dressing.

The patient is allowed to go home in a few days and in instructed to rewrap the elastic bandage over the cotton cast every few days to keep it snug. When he reports back two weeks after the operation, the cotton cast and stitches are removed. If there is effusion the knee is aspirated, and an elastic bandage provided. If there is no effusion, rehabilitation is continued. At this point no effort is made to force motion of the knee other than by the patient's voluntary effort. In the uncomplicated case recovery is rapid. Aspiration is repeated as often as indicated by effusion. It usually is not necessary at all. Athletic participation will be permitted as soon as the range of motion is normal and the strength of the operated leg is equal to that of the good leg. This may be at four weeks or may be later depending upon the many factors that influence recovery, such as the duration of symptoms prior to the operation, the degree of synovitis of the knee, and postoperative bleeding or effusion. We have specific exercises which are recommended for rehabilitation after operations on the knee, and in the case of meniscectomy they may be started on the night of the surgery. They are first done with a splint on. This does not move the knee. In the occasional case where there has been previous synovitis or where there

were complications of other conditions of the knee with synovitis with effusion, isotonic exercises should not be done. Actually walking does little damage to inflamed synovium, but stair climbing, running and squatting do. We do not allow any exercises which bend the knee to be initiated if there is painful synovitis or extensive effusion. I would like to emphasize again that persistent effusion is contributed to by irritation of an already irritated joint. Therefore, I urge the patient not to do knee flexing exercises with the foot loaded since this tends to force the synovial membranes together and increase effusion. He may, however, rapidly increase his isometric exercises done with the knee straight. (See also Chapter 22.)

CHONDRAL AND OSTEOCHONDRAL FRACTURE

A chondral fracture is a fracture involving the articular cartilage and is particularly prevalent at the knee owing to the direct stresses and strains applied to the knee joint. A chondral fracture may be extremely difficult to diagnose and in many instances may be determined only after arthrotomy of the knee. If there is no fragment of underlying bone involved, the x-ray will be entirely negative. The reader is strongly urged to refer to Chapter 4, page 103 for a more complete discussion of this very interesting and distressing and often frustrating condition.

The *diagnosis* must rest on history and clinical symptoms. If the fracture is complete and if a piece of cartilage is loose in the knee the symptoms will be those of a foreign body within the joint. While this fracture may be quite difficult to distinguish from a tear of one of the menisci or from osteochondritis dissecans, early differentiation is somewhat academic since in any case arthrotomy is indicated. Many chondral fractures go completely unrecognized, particularly when they are incomplete so that the fragment is not actually dislodged. I feel quite sure that many cases of osteo-chondritis dissecans are in fact initiated by fractures of the cartilage. The most vulnerable areas in the joint are, first, the patella, and second, the two femoral condyles. The patella is particularly vul-nerable because it is so common for the athlete to fall upon the flexed knee. The result may be a contusion to the articu-lar cartilage, an actual fissuring of the cartilage, or in other circumstances a complete chondral facture with a piece of cartilage separated from the bone (Figs. 500 and 501).

The symptoms are those of damage to the undersurface of the patella, i.e., pain on flexion and extension, particu-larly against resistance, and pain on manual pressure of the patella against the femoral condyle, particularly on "rubbing" the patella against the condy-lar groove with the knee in complete ex-tension (glissement). Such a fracture may cause actual catching or locking of

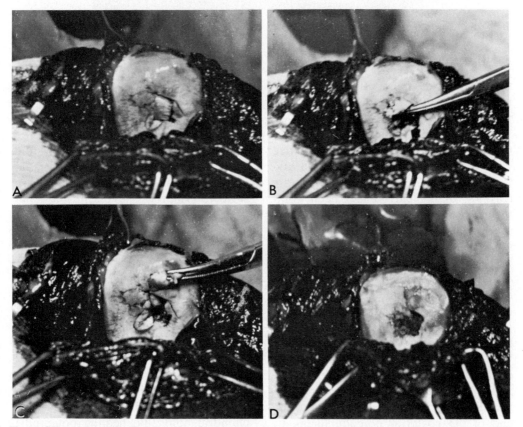

Figure 500.   Acute chondral fracture of the patella with negative x-ray. The patient had a history of fall-ing on the flexed knee with more than the usual amount of symptoms including hemarthrosis. Surgery revealed *(A)* acute chondral fracture of the patella with multiple fragments of cartilage. Definitely not degenerative. *B,* The fragments may be lifted up, revealing the hemorrhagic bleeding bone beneath an acute injury. *C,* Further removal of the fragments and, *D,* fragments all removed and the vascular bed of the bone exposed. Note the apparently normal cartilage surrounding the defect with no evidence of fibrillation or malacia. This would later have been described as a typical osteochondritis dissecans or chondromalacia, either of which would have been wrong. This patient went on to a good recovery with no patellar symptoms at present.

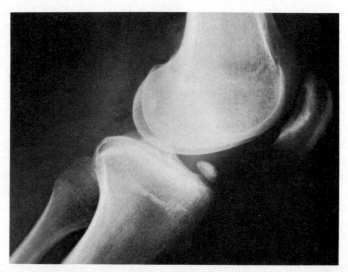

Figure 501. This is a case similar to that of Figure 500 seen much later. Note the typical osteochondritic fragment. Note also the defect under the patella.

the knee by an interruption of the normal glide pattern of the patella in the patellar groove.

I recently operated on a case diagnosed as intrinsic injury to the knee with chondromalacia of the patella and was surprised to find two-thirds of the cartilage of the patella had been completely broken away and could be lifted up from its bed as a flap, exposing raw bone beneath. Another frequent chondral injury is an avulsion type fracture of the cartilage and bone along the lateral margin of the medial femoral condyle at the femoral attachment of the posterior cruciate ligament (Fig. 528). I have seen many cases at operation which had been diagnosed as osteochondritis dissecans of the medial femoral condyle, in which the loose body was actually attached to the anterior end of the posterior cruciate ligament. Some have been encountered in which the chondral body was completely free except for the fact that it was still attached to the posterior cruciate ligament. These are, in my opinion, chondral factures rather than osteochondritis dissecans.

The primary diagnostic problem of chondral fracture will be to differentiate it from other intrinsic conditions of the knee. It should be suspected if there is persistent pain and persistent dysfunction around an otherwise normal-appearing patella. This is particularly true if acute symptoms have followed immediately upon an injury. The orthopaedist will see these patients relatively late since they are usually treated for a contusion or a sprain and the question of chondral fracture may arise only after the knee has failed to respond to ordinary therapeutic measures.

Proper *treatment* depends largely upon a proper diagnosis. If there is definitely a subchondral facture it is possible that protective immobilization will permit it to heal. However, if the cartilage itself is broken without subchondral bone, the healing potential is so poor that it probably will not heal in any event. As a rule the exact condition is not previously diagnosed and one must be prepared to carry out whatever definitive measure is indicated at the time of the arthrotomy of the knee.

Where a fragment of cartilage with

some subchondral bone has been torn away, including a portion of the posterior cruciate attachment, the treatment is removal of this fragment and suture of the posterior cruciate to the cartilage bed through drill holes. This will successfully restore posterior cruciate integrity. In other cases in which the amount of cruciate ligament involved has been relatively small, I have simply sutured the torn ligament to its uninvolved portion. The loose fragment of bone and cartilage should be removed in any event and appropriate measures carried out to minimize the potential damage to the mechanism of the knee. Most of the young patients tolerate partial chondrectomy very well. One may smooth off the margins of the bed either on the patella or on the femoral condyle and expect a considerable degree of filling in as healing proceeds. If the lesion is relatively localized and surrounded by healthy appearing cartilage, it is much better to treat it by trephine and drilling (see page 672) than by chondral shaving since trephining does not extend the area involved in the lesion. Indeed, in many cases the fossa has pretty well smoothed itself out before arthrotomy has been accepted by the patient. I am extremely loath to sacrifice the patella in a young athlete. I would oppose even more the use of a metallic prosthesis since in either case the femoral condyle is exposed to considerable direct trauma. The small metallic prosthesis serves to concentrate the force in a small area and is potentially more dangerous than any direct trauma to the condyle protected by the quadriceps aponeurosis only, after removal of the patella.

FRACTURE

Fracture about the knee is not a frequent injury in the young athlete. The ordinary fracture is treated in the same manner as a similar fracture in any other patient, bearing in mind the general principles for treatment of the athlete particularly in reference to prompt diagnosis with the aid of x-ray. The aphorism in fracture treatment that "the nearer the joint the more perfect the reduction" is doubly true in the knee since the normally functioning knee joint will not tolerate any gross irregularity of its articular surfaces. This discussion will be confined to the treatment of those fractures about the knee which are more common to the athlete.

Fracture of the Patella

Fracture of the patella occurs in athletes but is not as common as chondral fracture of the patella. Fractures of either the upper (Fig. 502, *A*) or lower pole (Fig. 502, *B*) or along the medial or lateral margin (Figs. 502, *C* and 503) usually are actually either strain fractures or sprain fractures and should be treated as such by removal of the fragment of bone and suture of the ligament or tendon to the patella. This should be done promptly and a perfectly functioning knee may be expected. It should be emphasized here that there is little place for bone repair in the treatment of fracture of the patella and I can think of few circumstances justifying the securing of bone-to-bone apposition and waiting for patellar union. The exception is in the incomplete fracture or possibly in the linear fracture extending from upper to lower pole. One should particularly suspect chondral fracture to accompany stellate fracture of the patella without displacement. It is not wise to carry out patellectomy in the athlete if it can be avoided since complete patellectomy is not compatible with such strenuous sport as soccer, football and the like, not because of failure of the quadriceps mechanism but because of the extreme vulnerability of the femoral condyles

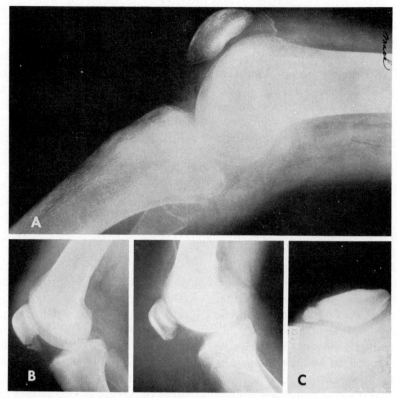

Figure 502. *A*, Avulsed quadriceps tendon and fragment from superior pole of patella. The shell of bone makes the diagnosis simple but the lesion is really a tendon avulsion rather than a fractured patella. Treatment by repair of the quadriceps to the patella.

   B, Avulsion fracture of lower pole of patella. In effect, a rupture of the tendon. Note that after removal of the fragments and repair of the tendon to the patella, there is essentially normal appearing patella remaining.

   C, Fracture of lateral margin of the patella by a direct blow. This should be treated by removal of the fragment and suture of the lateral retinaculum to the patella.

after removal of the patella. I would be even more fearful of permitting athletic participation following replacement of the patella by metallic prosthesis since this concentrates the force and in my opinion is more dangerous than complete patellectomy.

   Fracture of the patella by direct contusion is not infrequent. The fracture usually involves the lateral portion of the patella since the bone is thinner in this area (Fig. 504). This fracture differs from the avulsion type in which the fragment is torn away by the tendon or the fragment. The avulsion fracture is usually on the medial side and occurs as the patella is forced laterally. It also

differs from the explosive type fracture caused by a forceful blow against the patella with the quadriceps in violent contraction, such as occurs when the knee hits the dashboard in a car accident. The contusion fracture is due to a sharp blow in a relatively localized area, as is sometimes received by a baseball fielder. As he is squatted down with his knees flexed, the ball caroms to one side and hits directly on the patella. This same force may cause chondral damage. A typical example of this fracture is illustrated in Figure 502, *C*. The silhouette view made its diagnosis much easier since the small fragment is difficult to visualize in the anteroposterior view

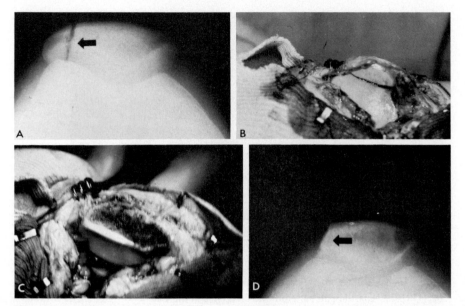

Figure 503.   Patient fell directly on the flexed knee, fracturing the patella. *A*, Preoperative radiograph. *B*, Operative picture showing linear fracture across the medial one fourth of the patella. *C*, Operative picture showing the fracture and the patella after the removal of the fragment. *D*, Postoperative radiograph after fragment was removed (facetectomy).

unless the x-ray is particularly good (see Fig. 482). This condition is treated by removal of the fragment and suture of the retinaculum to the patella. Uneventful recovery should be expected. At the time of repair the undersurface of the patella and the cartilage of the patellar groove should be carefully inspected for possible chondral damage.

Care should be taken not to confuse the *bipartite* or *tripartite patella* with acute injury (Fig. 505). The partite patella is usually bilateral and symmetrical, and is asymptomatic. Careful examination will demonstrate that the symptoms are not in the area of the anomaly. It should be borne in mind, however, that it is possible for the quadriceps lateralis to avulse or partially avulse the separate piece, in which event the condition will become symptomatic. This ordinarily will respond well to rest and protection. If the symptoms persist, one is justified in removing the piece and suturing the tendon to the patella. This condition is quite analogous to avulsion of the accessory navicular in the foot. In

both instances there is an underlying congenital anomaly on which is superimposed an acute injury.

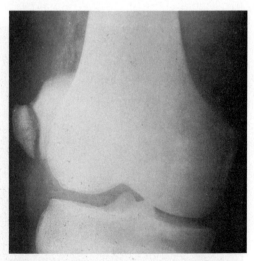

Figure 504.   This professional baseball player received a sharp blow on the knee with a baseball, had immediate swelling, pain and discomfort. He was treated for contusion. On examination some weeks later, the oblique view shows the fracture which had been overlooked in the anteroposterior and lateral views. The silhouette view (as in Fig. 502, *C*) would demonstrate this even better.

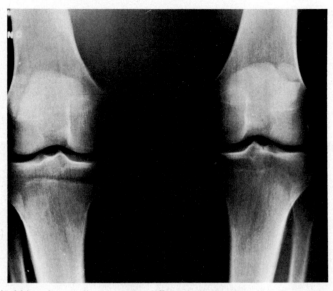

Figure 505.   Typical bipartite patella. Note the difference in the two sides, but general location is same. Also note definite rounded off line between the fragments. This is not an acute fracture. However, this fragment may be avulsed or partially avulsed and become symptomatic.

Avulsion Fracture

The *avulsion fracture of the upper tibia* (Fig. 506) is basically an avulsion of the anterior cruciate ligament and should be treated as such, the main emphasis being placed on the restoration of the anterior cruciate ligament to its normal length and function. Only in the exceptional case can this be done nonsurgically. I much prefer to expose the

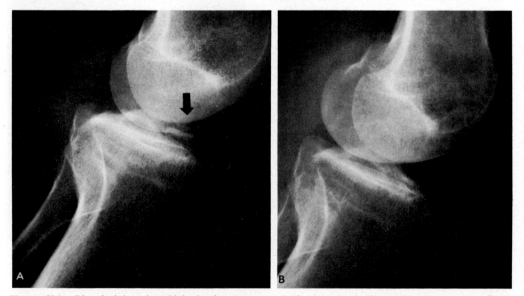

Figure 506.   Bicycle injury in which the foot was caught in the wheel. The child was thrown off the bicycle. *A,* Illustrates avulsion of the top of the tibia by anterior cruciate. Note the tibial spines are intact, since the cruciate does not attach there. *B,* After replacement and suture. No anteroposterior instability.

knee anteromedially, examine it carefully for other lesions and then carry out whatever measures will best restore the function of the anterior cruciate. The occasional "locking" caused by a displaced fragment obviously demands reduction of the fragment. If there is a large fragment involving a portion of the articular cartilage on either side, it should be replaced and held in its bed by a transfixion screw or by sutures passed through parallel drill holes running from in front of the tibia to the bed of the fragment and thence mattressed through the fragment. The sutures must be carefully placed so that the drill holes coincide in the fragment and in its bed or else the fragment will not be perfectly reduced.

If the fragment is relatively small or comminuted it should be removed and the cruciate ligament pulled down into the defect and firmly sutured, in which instance it will heal less rapidly than it will if the bone is replaced (Fig. 507). There is little purpose in leaving a small, thin fragment subject to necrosis. On the other hand, when the fragment is large and makes up a substantial portion of the upper tibia, as is frequently the case in younger persons, it should be preserved in the manner described. Normal function of the knee will not tolerate gross unreduced displacement of the superior surface of the tibia.

Avulsion fracture of the distal end of the patella. Some degree of injury commonly occurs, the so-called jumper's knee, where there is some damage to the tendon attachment at the distal pole of the patella. A similar type injury is avulsion of a tip of bone from the distal pole of the patella. Sometimes the tendon will be partially avulsed, tak-

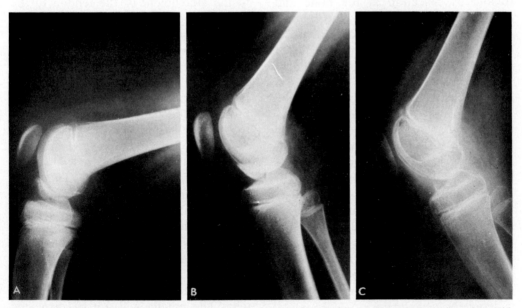

Figure 507. This 9 year old girl fell from a bicycle, injuring her right knee. The doctor made x-rays, told her she had a "bone sliver" and told her to keep it at rest for two weeks. No support. No other treatment.

A, The acute injury showing a large fragment of the upper tibia avulsed by the anterior cruciate.

B, Four months later, the fragment in the same position. Film made with the knee at its maximum extension. Range of motion, 30 degrees.

C, Two months after removal of the fragment, some recurrence of the ossification. This knee has had very extensive physical therapy, active and passive motion. Range now (nine months post-injury — five months postoperative) is 20 to 90 degrees. This disability could have been prevented by early adequate treatment.

ing a shell of bone with it which fills in and makes a prominence at the distal pole of the patella (Fig. 510). Ossification in this area is likely to be diminished by proper immobilization to permit the area to heal without irritation. Continuation of chronic irritation lays down a deposit of bone which may become quite extensive. This is not like the deposit of calcium in the tendon which is a degenerative change and which will be out in the substance of the tendon. The bone usually forms contiguous to the patella. Occasionally there will actually be a piece of bone pulled off, resulting in fracture. On other occasions it will heal without bone formation. Sometimes it does heal with bone formation, making a rather extensive addition to the distal end of the patella as illustrated in Figure 510, C.

If there is fracture of the distal pole of the patella with separation, it is best treated by resection of the bone and repair of the tendon to the patella through drill holes. Actually, even if there is a relatively substantial piece of bone avulsed by the patellar tendon, it is probably better to take the fragment out and sew the tendon to the parent patella since fracture of the patella is notoriously slow to heal and sometimes will go on to a painful nonunion (Fig. 510, A). If the bone in the tendon is not painful, of course, it requires no treatment. Sometimes there is pain even though there is apparent union and in some instances it is justifiable to detach the tendon and take out the exogenous bone. However, this is a pretty major procedure from the standpoint of morbidity and should not be done unless it is definitely necessary.

Avulsion fracture of the patellar tubercle of the tibia may occur. Diagnosis can readily be made by location of pain and tenderness and disturbance of the quadriceps mechanism. It should be confirmed by x-ray. The most important consideration is the function of the tendon rather than the fragment of displaced bone. The tendon should be replaced surgically. If the bone fragment is small or comminuted it should be removed and the tendon repaired to its bed. If large it may be handled by repositioning of the fragment and internal fixation preferably by a transfixion screw (Fig. 508). If the epiphyses are open, care must be taken not to close them.

There may also be *avulsion at the superior pole of the patella,* in which instance the quadriceps attachment is pulled away from the patella with or without a shell of the patellar bone. In incomplete avulsion the mechanism of injury is a powerful contraction of the quadriceps while the leg is being forcibly flexed. This is, in fact, a strain type injury and as the forces are arrested there may be greater or lesser damage to the attachment of the tendon to the upper pole of the patella. This will cause pain on active function of the quadriceps but will not interfere with extension of the knee otherwise. The incomplete injury is treated by protection, local injection and local heat. The degree of protection depends upon the extent of the damage.

If the force is severe enough, the whole quadriceps aponeurosis may be detached from the patella. This is a painful injury. Examination will reveal swelling about the upper end of the patella with tenderness along its superior margin. The patient will be unable to actively extend the knee completely. When he contracts the quadriceps a palpable defect may be felt above the patella. The patella will not be displaced downward since there is no muscular mechanism attaching to the patella from below and its distance from the tibia will remain constant whether the knee is flexed or extended. X-ray may be of diagnostic value since often a shell of

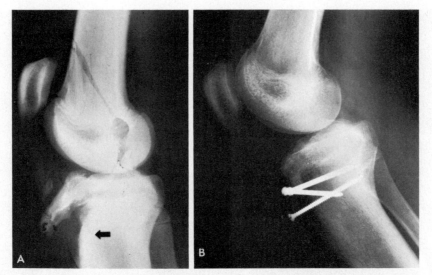

Figure 508. Boy injured while high jumping. This leg was not in contact with the ground. *A*, Showing avulsion by violent contraction of the muscle, which pulled off the patellar tubercle and the anterior one third of the upper surface of the tibia. *B*, Two months post-repair showing good healing. He went on to a good and complete recovery.

bone may be avulsed (Figs. 509 and 510). Treatment should be surgical repair with snug suture of the aponeurosis to the patella through drill holes. I recall one case in an older man in which he caught his heel on a step as he descended a stairway. Both of his knees flexed sharply and in a violent effort to regain his equilibrium he detached the quadriceps from the patella on both knees. Uneventful recovery followed surgical repair.

Major fractures about the knee are not particularly frequent as athletic injuries and are readily recognized by the accompanying major disability and by confirmatory x-ray. One should be particularly alert to the *associated ligament injuries*. Avulsion of the collateral ligament with a fragment of bone from the tibial plateau or femoral condyle is in reality a ligament injury and should be treated as such (Figs. 511 and 512). One must be aware that when a small fragment of bone has been pulled off the condyle the probabilities are that the ligament is attached to it (Fig. 513). One

must not assume that it is a chip fracture. For example, if the tip of the fibula is broken one should suspect avulsion of the biceps (Fig. 449, *B*) and/or the fibular collateral ligament.

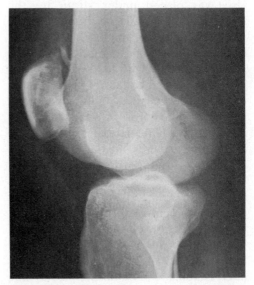

Figure 509. Flexion injury of the knee with avulsion of the quadriceps tendon attachment from upper pole of the patella. Surgery revealed the whole quadriceps tendon pulled off the patella.

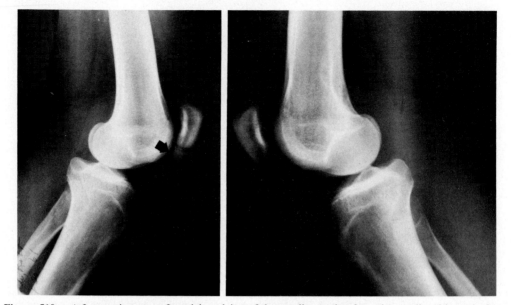

Figure 510.   *A*, Interesting case of partial avulsion of the patellar tendon from the patella with marked ossification and painful nonunion. The exogenous bone was removed and the patellar tendon repaired to the patella. *B*, Opposite patella for comparison. This is not a fractured patella but a tendon avulsion.

If the lateral table of the tibia is compressed, one should examine very carefully to determine the function of the medial collateral ligament which also was placed under strain by the force which caused the fracture (Fig. 514). The mechanism of this injury is force applied to the lateral side of the knee, very likely with the knee in extension. The medial collateral ligament and the posterior capsule hold the knee stable in this position and the relatively sharp edge of the lateral femoral condyle rotates slightly medially and drives into the central portion of the lateral tibial plateau. This force may split the edge of the plateau out laterally, may depress the central portion or cause any type of fracture of the upper tibia or, indeed, may snub off a portion of the femoral condyle. The same force, however, is being applied on the medial side of the knee. These fractures ordinarily occur in older people in whom the ligament is ordinarily stronger than the bone. In a young person there may be ligament damage as well. In the case which occurs with the knee slightly flexed the force is accepted mostly on the rounded portion of the condyle and no lateral bony damage occurs and the ligament tears on the medial side. If the leg is in extension with the support by the posterior capsule, the medial ligament holds for a period long enough that the bone breaks. If the force is continued on the femoral condyle, further compressing the tibia, the ligament may give way. We have, therefore, injuries on both sides of the knee, either one of which may be easily overlooked.

In checking a case with obvious medial collateral ligament damage, one should inspect the x-ray carefully to see whether there is some compression of the lateral plateau. Similarly, if the lateral plateau is compressed it is necessary to eliminate medial collateral ligament avulsion. The test of gross instability may be quite misleading be-

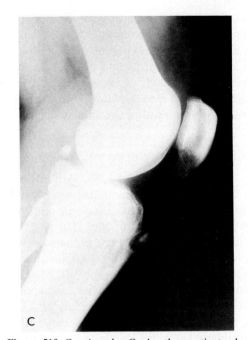

C

Figure 510 *Continued. C,* Another patient who had had previous trouble at the distal pole of the patella which in the last few months had subsided. Notice he has an old apophysitis with an ossicle in the patellar tendon which is now symptomatic. Following resection of this ossicle from the tendon and a suitable period of rehabilitation, the patient returned to his ordinary activity. This simply illustrates that the deposit of bone, not calcium, at the distal pole of the patella may not be symptomatic if there is union between this exogenous bone and the patella.

by whatever method is most effective in a particular case.

Fracture of the Head of the Fibula

While, strictly speaking, fracture of the head of the fibula is not an injury to the knee, it does sometimes become a diagnostic problem (Fig. 453). The head of the fibula may be broken by a direct blow in which there is an ordinary comminuted type fracture without gross displacement. Any fracture below the head, actually involving the neck, should cast immediate suspicion on the ankle joint rather than the knee. If the fracture is of the head of the bone one should determine particularly whether or not there is any displacement and check for involvement of the peroneal nerve as well as the biceps tendon and external collateral ligament. If the fracture involves the ligament and tendon attachments, treatment must be much

cause either of these conditions alone will give instability of the knee with the leg going into more abduction than normal. Stress x-ray will in this instance be of great value since it will show whether or not the medial margin of the joint opens up (Fig. 515). It is extremely disappointing to fix the tibial plateau and find an unstable knee resulting from medial ligament damage. It will be equally disappointing to make a skillful repair of the medial collateral ligament, only to find that bony damage on the opposite side has impaired the result. The true importance of the treatment of fractures about the knee must be to obtain complete restoration of normal function

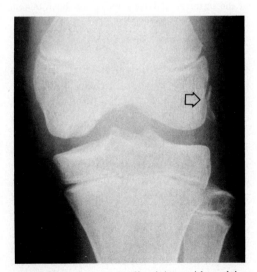

Figure 511. Acute wrestling injury with avulsion of the popliteus tendon attachment from the femur with a relatively large fragment of bone. This was the only injury. Uneventful recovery following repair. The osteochondritis dissecans was an incidental finding, was asymptomatic and was not demonstrable surgically.

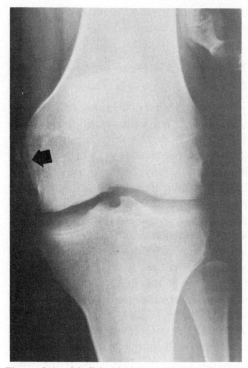

Figure 512. Medial side injury. This is an avulsion of the femoral attachment of the medial collateral ligament. Notice this is definitely below the adductor tubercle. The medial joint space is somewhat wider than the lateral. This is likely to heal with a painful prominence and some redundancy of the ligament. Advise removal of the fragment and repair of the ligament to the fracture bed.

more extensive than if it were simply a direct trauma type fracture of the bone.

There may occasionally be a *dislocation of the fibula from the tibia* (Fig. 516). Here, again, one should immediately suspect a twisting force with resultant damage to the ankle joint. The condition, however, may be localized at the knee and have been caused by direct trauma against the fibular head, knocking it away by tearing the relatively weak superior tibiofibular ligaments. In such an instance replacement should be accurate and, if there is any tendency whatever toward instability of the fibula, it may be fixed by internal fixation with a transfixion screw through the fibula into the upper end of the tibia. This

screw should be removed as soon as ligament healing is complete. Use of internal fixation will expedite rehabilitation. Careful attention should be paid to possible involvement of the peroneal nerve since it is in a very vulnerable location as it crosses around the fibular neck.

Epiphyseal Fractures

A word should be said about epiphyseal fractures about the knee since they do happen, particularly in children of secondary school age. These fractures are usually readily recognized by careful study of the x-ray. The incomplete fracture of the epiphysis may be overlooked and diagnosed as sprain (Figs. 517 to 521). A careful, detailed examination will ordinarily solve this problem since the tenderness and pain will be completely around the epiphyseal plate and strain in any direction will tend to cause pain whereas ligament injury is quite unusual on both sides of the knee at once.

If no displacement is present, *treatment* generally given to injury about the knee will suffice, that is, local measures, compression bandage, ice followed by protection. It should be emphasized that the apparatus applied to protect the knee should result in elimination of pain on stress, otherwise it is not truly protective. When effective it will be adequate for the ordinary incomplete epiphyseal fracture. Any displacement, even of a mild degree, should be corrected (Fig. 522, 523 and 524). Correction becomes increasingly difficult with the passage of time so that in any doubtful situation, x-rays should be made promptly and treatment carried out as soon as possible and under general anesthesia. Epiphyseal fractures do not necessarily affect the growth of the bone and they are much less likely to do so if reduction is anatomical and with a minimum amount of trauma. One should be

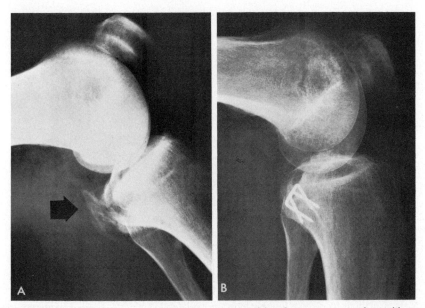

Figure 513.   Avulsion of the posterior cruciate ligament resulting from a motorcycle accident. *A*, X-ray six weeks post-injury. Patient had direct blow to the tibia with the knee flexed, forcing the leg backward. He had four-plus posterior cruciate instability and restriction of extension. Arrow indicates avulsion of the ligament with a fragment off the tibia. *B*, Postoperative film showing removal of some fragments and repair of the posterior cruciate to the back of the tibia with fragmented bone. Nine weeks postoperative the knee would flex to 120 degrees and was stable in this position.

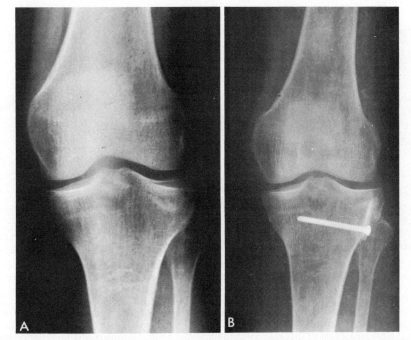

Figure 514.   *A*, Torn medial collateral ligament. Note compression fractures of the lateral tibial plateau. The same force that tears the medial ligament drives the lateral condyle into the tibia. A disappointing result will be obtained if this fragment is not elevated. This is not common in the young athlete.

   B, Postoperative film shows fragment completely elevated and held in place by a strut of bone. Medial collateral ligament was repaired. Good stability.

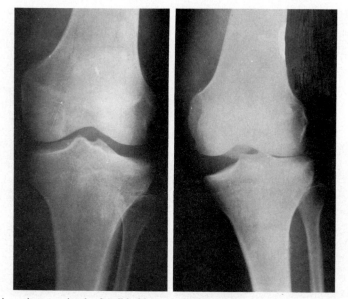

Figure 515.   This patient received a forcible blow on the lateral side of the knee. *A*, Anteroposterior view showing depression of the central portion of the lateral tibial plateau. *B*, The stress picture reveals that his marked instability was due not only to depression of the plateau but to severance of the medial collateral ligament. Note that the femur has moved slightly medially and the edge of the condyle rests on the depression of the tibial plateau. This should be treated by elevation of the plateau but of equal importance is repair of the medial collateral ligament.

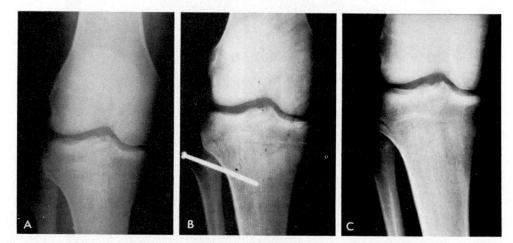

Figure 516.   Gymnast, vaulted over a horse and landed off balance, with his knees stiff, and with considerable force. Left knee snapped and hyperextended. He had severe pain posteriorly and to the outer side of his knee over the head of the fibula. The injury was treated with heat for 10 days and then put in a cast. While in a cast it was still painful. The patient was seen here two weeks post-injury. Examination revealed a very tender, painful fibula which was quite prominent on the left side compared with the right. Flexion of the leg against resistance was painful in this area. X-ray was suggestive but nonconclusive. Surgery revealed that there was a tear of the ligament (proximal tibiofibular ligament) which permitted the fibula to displace away from the tibia. This was held with a transfixion screw and fascia was repaired. The screw was removed three months later. Six months later there was a little prominence of the fibular head. Patient was otherwise asymptomatic. X-ray was negative. *A*, Preoperative x-ray. Note evident widening of fibula from tibia. *B*, Internal fixation. *C*, Six months post-injury, asymptomatic.

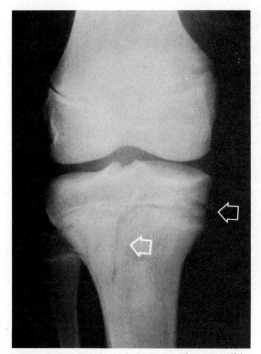

Figure 517. Epiphyseal fracture of upper tibia. Note slight separation of medial half of epiphysis with it split down the shaft. As a result of the injury the fractured part of the epiphysis closed, necessitating surgical closure of lateral tibia and fibula.

able to reduce these fractures by closed manipulation but they may require internal fixation, preferably not crossing the epiphyseal plate, to prevent recurrence of the displacement. If open reduction is decided upon one must be particularly careful in handling the epiphyseal cartilage. Prying against the cartilage or levering the fragments into place with instruments may well do more damage than the injury itself. The epiphyseal cartilage as a rule remains with the epiphysis, the diaphyseal portion of bone being denuded, hence one must be particularly careful in handling the smaller fragment.

Fabella

The fabella (Fig. 434) is a sesamoid bone frequently found in the tendon of

the lateral head of the gastrocnemius muscle as it passes under the femoral condyle. Fracture of the fabella is extremely uncommon but is of quite serious consequence when it occurs. One should be aware of the fabella and not mistake it for a foreign body or a loose fragment in the joint. If it is in two or more pieces the opposite knee should be carefully checked since as a rule the bipartite fabella will be bilateral. The location of the tenderness and pain on function of the gastrocnemius are diagnostic points. The x-ray may be quite deceptive. If the fabella is actually involved, either by a fracture or by osteochondritis or chondromalacia, it should be removed. The approach is a lateral one behind the fibular collateral

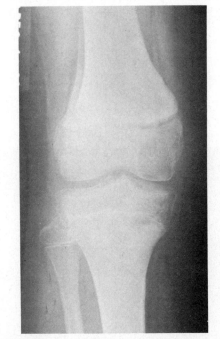

Figure 518. Illustrating a case of slight epiphyseal subluxation of lower femur. Note the callus formation where the periosteum was stripped up laterally. This is the same mechanism as sprain of the medial collateral ligament and in fact was diagnosed as such until careful examination localized the tenderness on both sides of the lower femoral epiphysis and x-ray showed the fracture across the lateral corner of the metaphysis.

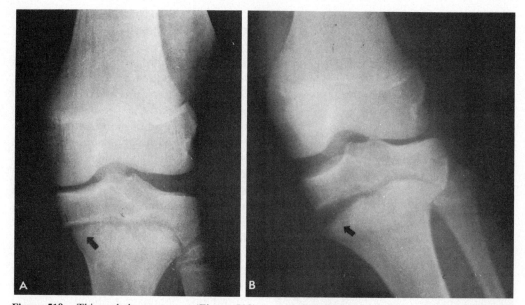

Figure 519. This and the next case (Figure 520) represent a diagnostic problem. Both had what appeared to be medial instability of the knee joint. *A*, The original picture with suggestion of separation of the medial upper tibial epiphysis. *B*, Confirmed by stress x-ray under anesthesia. The apparent widening of the medial joint space is normal for this individual when compared with the opposite knee. This was treated by closed manipulation and repair of the long fibers of the medial collateral ligament. See also Figures 522, 523 and 524.

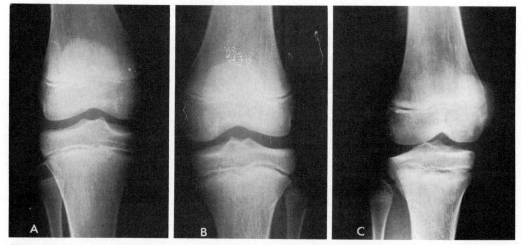

Figure 520. Another medial side injury (see Figure 519) showing apparently normal upper tibial epiphysis but suspicious buckling of the lateral cortex. *A*, The normal side. *B*, The involved side. *C*, Oblique view confirms the true pathology, separation of the medial upper tibial epiphysis with compression of the lateral plateau. Closed manipulation corrected the deformity.

Growth disturbance may become a factor here as well as in the case presented in Figure 519.

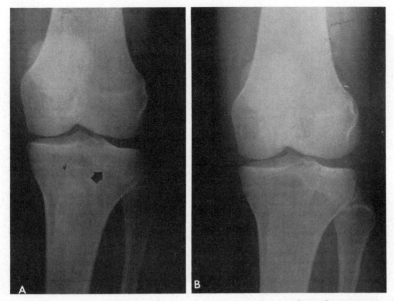

Figure 521. Patient injured by collision with another player. He experienced severe excruciating pain down the lateral side of his leg which was attributable to "nerve." He continued to have trouble and finally developed an effusion in his right knee with ecchymosis in the calf. Careful restudy of his x-rays revealed the fracture line running from across the lateral quadrant of the tibia, beginning just at the head of the fibula and crossing obliquely up through the interspinous area. *A*, Arrow indicates the fracture line at the time of the injury. *B*, Three months later the line of the fracture is still apparent.

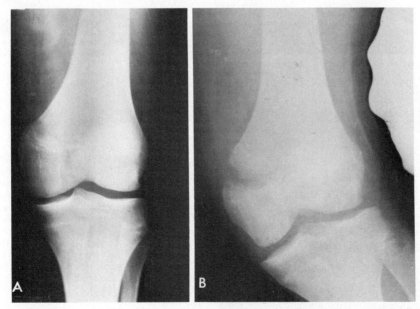

Figure 522. This 17 year old boy was sent in with diagnosis of acute rupture of the medial collateral ligament and instability of the knee. *A*, The picture sent in was interpreted as normal, but note the suspicious vertical line extending upward from the intercondylar notch. *B*, X-ray made with lateral stress under anesthesia revealed the true pathologic condition, an epiphyseal fracture across the medial condyle split down into the intercondylar notch. This was treated by transfixion screw in order to permit more rapid mobilization.

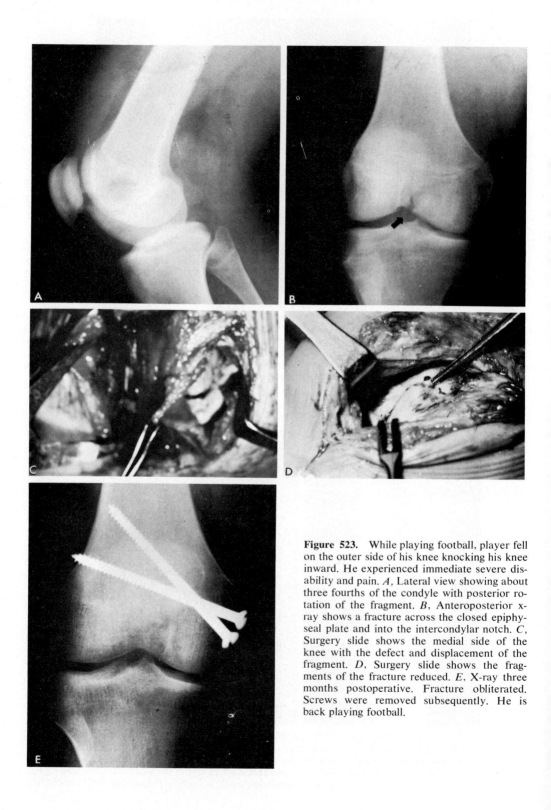

Figure 523. While playing football, player fell on the outer side of his knee knocking his knee inward. He experienced immediate severe disability and pain. *A*, Lateral view showing about three fourths of the condyle with posterior rotation of the fragment. *B*, Anteroposterior x-ray shows a fracture across the closed epiphyseal plate and into the intercondylar notch. *C*, Surgery slide shows the medial side of the knee with the defect and displacement of the fragment. *D*, Surgery slide shows the fragments of the fracture reduced. *E*, X-ray three months postoperative. Fracture obliterated. Screws were removed subsequently. He is back playing football.

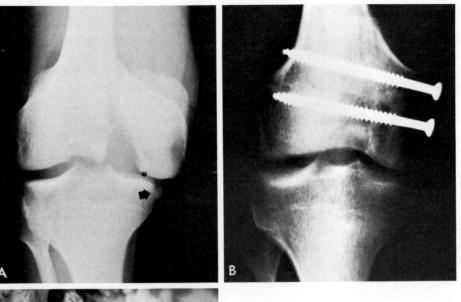

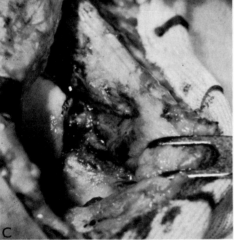

Figure 524. Patient fell about three meters, landing on the flexed knee. He had immediate instability and disability. *A*, X-ray revealed splitting off of the medial femoral condyle and displacement of the patella with the fragment, and avulsion of part of the medial collateral ligament from the tibia. *B*, Twelve weeks post-injury showing repair of the fracture prior to removal of the screws. *C*, Surgical film when screws were removed showing that in spite of the fracture being well healed, there is still a definite fissure in the articular cartilage.

ligament and the iliotibial band—the same approach utilized to expose the posterior horn of the lateral meniscus.

CHRONIC SYNOVITIS WITH EFFUSION
("Water on the Knee")

To be complete, any discussion of injuries to the knee in athletes requires comment on joint effusion. It must be recognized that this is not a specific diagnosis but a finding. In normal cir-cumstances the fluid balance within the knee is finely adjusted with the fluid formed and absorbed in an equal ratio in order to keep the joint lubricated. There are many and varied causes for irritation of the synovia and recurrent effusion. I want to emphasize that there is no such thing as "water on the knee" as a disease or an injury. This excess fluid formation results from a pathologic condition within the knee. To examine the knee and say "He has an effusion" is like examining an abdomen and say-ing "He has rigidity." The effusion must be and ordinarily can be accounted for. If one is unable to explain the cause of the effusion, his management of the case must perforce be extremely inadequate. If the effusion followed an injury one may ordinarily dismiss the systemic and indeed most of the inflammatory causes of effusion. However, a word of caution is necessary since the active young athlete will almost always be able to explain the effusion in the knee on the basis of having injured the knee, since he is bumping his knees constantly. Unless the diagnosis is immediately obvious, measures must be made to rule out in succession the various causes of effusion. Here the routine examination of the knee becomes extremely valuable.

First, the *history*. Is there an immediately determinable cause for the fluid or did it develop insidiously? Has there been a change in the activity habits of the patient? For example, if a boy has run ten miles when he was not accustomed to this degree of activity, this might well account for the irritation and effusion. This cause could easily be overlooked since to him it might not suggest an injury. Inquire as to his general health. Are there signs of a rheumatic disturbance or an infectious process?

On *examination* observe the knee carefully. Is the knee swollen, tense and obviously inflamed, or is the suprapatellar pouch merely filled with fluid? On palpation much can be learned as to the nature of the effusion. The ordinary traumatic effusion, even with hemarthrosis, causes little local heat whereas an inflammatory knee will ordinarily be hot. Careful examination for tenderness around the menisci or over the condyles or around the patella may give a lead. Is there a local area of tenderness?

Careful manipulative examination of the knee will help to determine whether there has been ligament damage or whether there is persistent meniscus reaction. Is motion in the knee painful? After careful evaluation and x-ray study the knee joint should be aspirated and close attention given to the fluid. Cloudy, turgid, viscous fluid is very suggestive of acute inflammatory reaction, and conversely, clear, straw colored, thin fluid will pretty well eliminate this possibility. If there is gross blood one may immediately presume an injury. Careful study of the fluid is necessary to determine whether it is actually blood or bloody fluid or merely blood-tinged fluid. If the fluid is at first clear, then toward the end of the aspiration becomes bloody, one may assume the presence of an inflamed synovium in which the irritation from genupuncture has caused local bleeding at the site of the puncture. Culture of the fluid for the presence of infection is of undeniable importance. Routine microscopic or laboratory examination of knee joint fluid is of some value in diagnosis and may be a useful aid in eliminating systemic causes of effusion. The blood count is important and urinalysis may give a lead. The best single laboratory procedure is the blood sedimentation rate, which should be negative in cases of trauma.

The *treatment* of an effusion in the knee is the treatment of the underlying cause. This predicates accurate diagnosis. If the diagnosis must be deferred or is not possible, certain local measures are of value in the interim. The extent of treatment will vary considerably according to the symptoms. Certainly the joint should not be permitted to remain grossly distended over a long period of time since this very distention of the capsule will often perpetuate an effusion long after the causative lesion has been arrested. In general, then, the treatment should be aspiration, pressure and protection. Aspiration is repeated as often as the fluid recurs even though this may be every few days or, in certain very acute circumstances, daily. Injection of various medicaments into the joint may be indicated. I would not recommend injection of an antibiotic into the knee unless definite infection is demonstrable. In chronic inflammation the corticoid preparations are of value. In my opinion they should not be repeated more than once a week even though aspiration may be needed more frequently. Corticoid should not be injected over a long period of time.

One of the most difficult decisions in the presence of chronic or so-called idiopathic effusion concerns the amount of protection necessary. If the condition seems to be relatively minor and there is no pain or other local symptoms, one may be under considerable pressure to permit unrestricted activity, particularly in the athlete. I believe that under certain circumstances athletic activity may be continued with an effusion in the knee, but I would feel extremely uneasy about permitting it unless I were sure of the underlying pathology. To be more specific, in a patient recovering from a meniscectomy where the rest of the knee appears to be in good condition, one might permit considerable activity in the presence of definite effusion since he can readily account for the symptoms. On the other hand, if the effusion is spontaneous one must be very sure of the nature of the pathology before permitting activity. This can often mean complete immobilization of the joint until either the diagnosis is determined or the effusion has been eliminated. While ordinary wrap-on elastic bandage is of little value in the knee for protection of the ligaments, it is of great importance in the presence of an effusion into the joint. Following aspiration of the fluid, if it is not necessary to immobilize the knee for other reasons a snug pressure bandage should be ap-

plied routinely, since it exerts the same restraining influence on intercapsular bleeding or effusion as does the pressure of a capsule full of fluid. I much prefer the wrap-on to the pull-on bandage since the pull-on bandage inevitably fits very few people. It is either too tight or too loose in its ordinary application. Since the elastic bandage does put pressure on the synovium, pushing the irritated surfaces together, it is not advisable to put on a tight elastic bandage and then encourage activity. In other words, if you are going to permit a player to return to play while he still has effusion, it probably would be better to tape his knee, which does give some restriction of motion but does not put the pressure on the synovium that the elastic bandage does.

Physical therapeutic measures are of considerable value in synovitis, whatever its cause. For this reason we recommend modalities such as diathermy, electric pad, whirlpool, hot packs and analgesic packs. It will be noted that with all of these measures the whole knee is encompassed by the heat. Such modalities as microtherm and infra-red or other rays are so restricted in their application that they tend to get the knee much too hot in one location and not hot enough in another. If only the bulb or infra-red ray is available, it should be used in the form of a baker so that the knee is exposed to the hot air rather than primarily to the ray.

Rehabilitative exercises would seem to be the antithesis of what is beneficial in effusion since effusion is encouraged by irritation of the synovium by motion. Obviously a compromise must be reached in a given case to decide what degree of rehabilitation will be compatible with recovery of the irritation. There are some rehabilitative measures, however, that are perfectly consistent with treatment of synovial irritation in the knee. These are the exercises for the foot, the hip and the rest of the body and also the isometric contractions of the quadriceps and hamstrings that have been shown to be very effective in rehabilitation and yet do not entail any degree of motion of the knee and may be carried out with the knee straight. Since rehabilitation of the quadriceps is extremely important, we routinely encourage straight leg raising with a progressive weight program. This does not cause the synovium to slide and so should not increase irritation. We ask the player to discontinue weight lifting exercises that cause flexion of the knee, such as sitting with the foot hanging down and bringing it up to the horizontal level. They can build the same mass by isometric straight leg raising and by resistive extension exercises. (See Chapter 22.) If effusion persists, synovectomy may occasionally be indicated.

APOPHYSITIS OF THE PATELLAR TUBERCLE
(Osgood-Schlatter "Disease")

Apophysitis of the tibial tubercle is a particular type of involvement that is commonly called Osgood-Schlatter disease. The word "disease" is a misnomer since the condition is not a disease. Actually, three manifestations parade as Osgood-Schlatter disease. One is *bursitis of the infrapatellar tendon bursa* (Fig. 430). This bursa lies between the infrapatellar fat pad and the patellar tendon just proximal to the patellar tubercle of the tibia. The tenderness in this condition is elicited at a point slightly higher than the tubercle. The condition should be treated as a bursitis (see page 548).

The second type of Osgood-Schlatter disease is an *aseptic necrosis of the tip of the epiphysis* for the patellar tubercle of the tibia (Fig. 525). The necrosis occurs in the patellar tendon at-

tachment and is probably traumatic in origin and it is initiated by a fracture or by an avulsion of the tip of the patellar tubercle. Because of poor circulation the fragment fails to heal and the constant irritation or traction of the patellar tendon makes it symptomatic. The mass tends to enlarge with reactive inflammation so that a rather large tumor may result. The tumor is tender to touch and there is pain on active extension of the quadriceps against resistance.

The third type of Osgood-Schlatter disease is a *true epiphysitis involving the whole epiphysis* (Fig. 526). This type is not particularly frequent but generally is more severe than the others when it occurs.

The *symptoms* of the latter two conditions are pain on direct pressure and pain on active use of the quadriceps. Rather sharp limitation of the activity of the patient may result. As is true of epiphysitis in other areas, the reaction itself is self-limited but there may be considerable residue, usually in the form of a large patellar tubercle with separate fragments lying within the patellar tendon attachment (Fig. 527). This may or may not remain symptomatic after the active condition subsides.

Treatment varies with the type of pathology and until recently has usually been nonsurgical, an attempt being made to relieve the tension in the mass by measures reducing the activity of the knee. They may range from cutting down the patient's activity to putting his leg in a cast. However, following arrest of symptoms there is a strong tendency for them to recur, so that until the epiphysis closes it remains a constant source of irritation. Even after the growth period, local symptoms may persist. Surgical treatment will result in much more prompt and complete recovery in Types 2 and 3, once frank involvement has occurred.

At operation the patellar tendon is

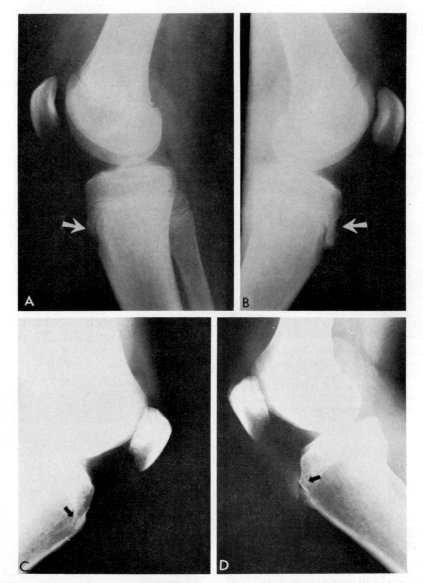

Figure 525. *A*, Normal tibial tubercle epiphysis. *B*, The excavated necrotic area with fragmentation which requires curettement. *C* and *D*, A similar case. Patient had persistent trouble in the knee with a large mass distal to the patella which had bothered him since adolescence and had gradually increased in severity. Surgical excision was essential. This outcome from untreated apophysitis of the patellar tubercle is not unusual although the size of the mass is.

split over the area of the involvement and in the second type the sequestrated fragment is carefully removed and the area thoroughly curetted down to normal bone. The epiphyseal plate between the tubercle and tibia is not disturbed. The split tendon is resutured over the area and the knee protected for about four weeks by a cotton cast. If a large mass of bone and cartilage has developed it should be trimmed down with an osteotome to leave a fairly flat area. Following four weeks of immobilization and a few weeks of rehabilitation, re-

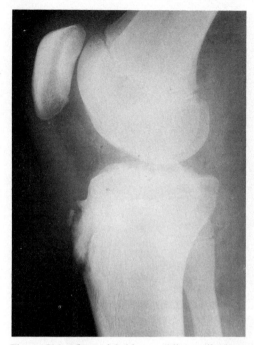

Figure 526. Osgood-Schlatter "disease," showing epiphysitis of the entire epiphysis with irregularity of the epiphyseal line. Since this epiphyseal cartilage is continuous with that of the upper tibia, it should not be disturbed. If surgery is utilized, exposure should be superficial to the epiphyseal cartilage.

OSTEOCHONDRITIS DISSECANS
(Osteochondral Fracture)

Over three-fourths of recognized cases of osteochondritis dissecans occur at the knee, and usually on the lateral margin of the medial condyle. They extend from the articular margin at the notch toward the medial side of the knee, a position coinciding almost exactly with the femoral attachment of the posterior cruciate ligament. The reader is strongly urged to refer to Chapter 4, page 104 for a more complete discussion of this condition.

Etiology. It cannot be doubted that some of these cases are caused by excessive traction on the attachment of the posterior cruciate ligament, resulting in fact in an avulsion or at least a partial

covery should be complete. Great care must be taken in the actively growing person that the epiphysis is not surgically closed. If the epiphysis is continuous with the proximal tibial epiphysis, back knee may develop owing to arrest of growth in front while growth persists in the posterior one-half of the plate. It should be emphasized to the parents that the condition is self-limited and will not develop into a malignant tumor, and if adequately treated it will not limit physical activity. Most parents and patients will accept surgical treatment if the alternatives are carefully explained. The recurrence rate is extremely low after surgical treatment and quite high after nonsurgical treatment. Acute fracture of the patellar tubercle is discussed on page 535.

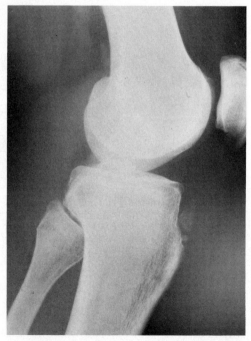

Figure 527. Old apophysitis of the patellar tubercle with fragmentation and painful, unsightly tumor. Treated by excision of the fragments, flattening of the tubercle and reattachment of the patellar tendon which has been split longitudinally and has become partially detached.

avulsion of a fragment of bone by the ligament. I have seen many cases in which the osteochondritic fragment contained a major portion of the attachment of the posterior cruciate ligament (Fig. 528). It is not my contention that all of these cases are caused by trauma but simply that many of them are. Trauma would seem to account more plausibly for the frequent occurrence of the lesion in this location than any of the other stated explanations. The theory of spontaneous ischemia is not wholly tenable. This theory implies that ischemia is more marked in this particular location on the femoral condyle than elsewhere, but actually circulation should be somewhat better here because the posterior cruciate ligament attaches at this point. However, osteochondritis dissecans occurs occasionally in other areas in the knee and also in this same general area without actually including the attachment of the posterior cruciate, so

that avulsion by the posterior cruciate cannot be the universal cause.

The lesion is most common at the extreme distal arch of the condyle, an area that is obviously quite subject to trauma, particularly in a fall on the flexed knee. With the knee flexed the patella rides directly over this area of the femoral condyle and the transmitted force strikes directly here. The principal argument against direct trauma as the occasional cause is that one would expect the lateral condyle to have received at least equal trauma, whereas actually osteochondritis dissecans is quite unusual in the lateral condyle of the femur. The explanation may lie in the fact that the patella is so much thicker in its medial portion and so transmits the trauma more directly.

In summary, the cause of osteochondritis dissecans at the knee may be said to be (1) ischemia with loss of circulation to the bone of the epiphysis,

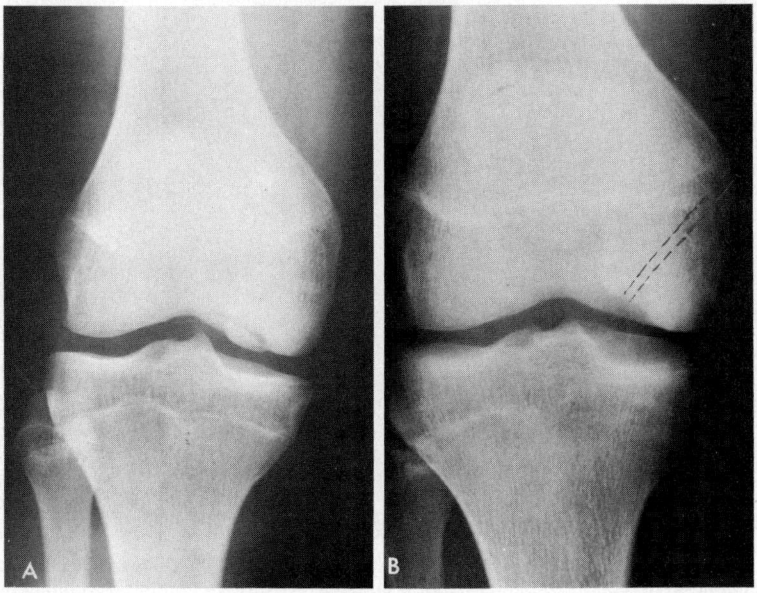

Figure 528. *A*, Osteochondritis dissecans. Actually an osteochondral fracture of the femoral condyle with almost the entire femoral attachment of the posterior cruciate ligament remaining attached to the fragment. *B*, Three months following repair of posterior cruciate to femur. Excellent function. One probably cannot expect complete filling in of this defect at this age.

(2) avulsion of the posterior cruciate ligament attachment, or (3) direct trauma transmitted through the patella directly against the condyle.

Diagnosis. Some cases give no positive clinical findings and are discovered incidentally in an x-ray examination for other conditions (Fig. 511). It should be recognized that the x-ray has been made for *some* reason and most frequently this is a chronic complaint of the joint, nonspecific in character and not suggesting internal derangement, ligament injury or chronic synovitis. In such a case x-ray may show a well defined lesion of the medial femoral condyle on its articular surface and one may presume that the lesion may well be the cause of the slight complaint (Fig. 529). As symptoms develop the condition becomes more acute with chronic synovitis and often mild effusion. Pain occurs after forced exertion.

Examination at this time will reveal no specific findings. Tests for ligament injury are negative. Meniscus tests are negative. Occasionally percussion on the patella with the knee flexed to beyond 90 degrees will elicit discomfort. X-ray examination reveals the lesion. As the condition progresses, the bony sequestrum separates from its bed, the cartilage fissures and the fragment may become detached (Fig. 530). The symptoms then become that of a foreign body in the joint, occasionally a palpable foreign body with locking, increased synovitis, pain and loss of rhythmic motion of the knee (Fig. 531).

Treatment. If osteochondritis dissecans is seen incidentally without preexisting symptoms, the degree of needed protection will depend upon the size of the fragment and the extent of the necrosis. If the fragment is large, involves a considerable portion of the

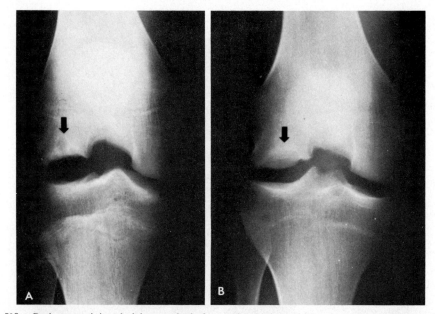

Figure 529. Patient was injured eight months before and experienced lateral meniscus symptoms. X-rays revealed large chondral defect in the lateral femoral condyle. At surgery condyle was filling in, and the lateral meniscus was indeed torn and was removed. Inspection of the condyle revealed (as suggested in x-ray *A*) that the defect was apparently beginning to fill in. Thus it was not disturbed. *B*, Same view three years later. Knee is basically asymptomatic. Note the uniformity of the bone and the normal contour in spite of some marginal irregularity.

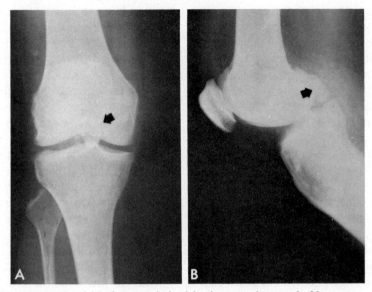

Figure 530. Large osteochondritic fragment lodged in the posterior pouch. No source of the cartilage was demonstrated at surgery.

weight-bearing surface, and necrosis seems quite extensive, the treatment will vary according to the age of the patient. In a patient under 12, prevention

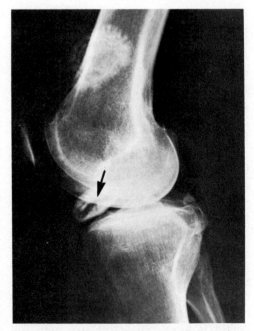

Figure 531. Old neglected case of osteochondritis dissecans with multiple fragments and diffuse arthritis. Note calcareous layers surrounding the original piece.

of weight bearing and immobilization of the knee may well permit spontaneous healing. This will require a period of 8 to 18 months, which becomes quite disheartening to an active youth. In most cases a cast will be necessary with the knee flexed since the youngster can hardly be expected constantly to remember not to bear weight. In an older patient it is quite unlikely that complete resolution will occur. If it does, it will be so slow as to justify operative treatment to expedite recovery, if for no other reason. Surgery under these circumstances begins with arthrotomy of the knee and careful exploration of the area. If the fragment is completely detached it should be removed. If the cartilage appears to be intact without separation or depression one may be justified in drilling multiple 0.3 mm. drill holes through the fragment into its bed in order to increase its circulation and encourage revascularization. It is difficult to assess this method because one can never be certain that healing would not have taken place without operative interference. If there appears to be a defect in the cartilage with any undermining at all, the case should be treated as if the fragment had been completely detached and the fragment should be removed. I have had little experience with replacement of the fragment and fixation by pins or screws. It does not appeal to me unless the fragment is large and vital to joint function.

If the condition is symptomatic, operative treatment is the treatment of choice. The knee is exposed by a medial parapatellar incision with the knee flexed over the end of the table. The medial compartment is carefully explored, special attention being paid to the medial meniscus, to the fat pad and to the cruciate ligaments. Careful scrutiny is given to the femoral attachment of the posterior cruciate ligament. The condyle is then inspected and the defect examined. If the fragment is completely loose the knee should be searched until it is found and removed. At this stage it is important to examine the undersurface of the patella since frequently patellar malacia will be present, particularly if the osteochondritis dissecans has been present for a very long time. Following careful exploration in this position the end of the table is raised again with proper aseptic precautions to a position that directly presents the lesion itself in the wound (30 to 0 degrees). If the fragment is still in place, it is carefully removed by sharp dissection. If it includes the attachment of the posterior cruciate ligament this should be detached from the fragment, care being taken to preserve as much ligament as possible. The posterior cruciate ligament is carefully inspected and this detached portion sutured down to the remaining portion of the ligament. However, if as much as one-half of the attachment is torn it is advisable to make two parallel drill holes from the medial femoral epicondyle into the bed of the defect which is in the intercondy-

lar notch at the articular margin (Fig. 528, *B*). The suture is passed through one of the drill holes, plicated through the loose end of the the torn section of the posterior cruciate and passed out through the other drill hole to emerge on the medial epicondyle. Proper tension will permit close apposition of the cruciate ligament to the bone. Before this fixation, the crater remaining following removal of the fragment is inspected and curetted down to fresh bleeding bone. The surrounding margins of the articular cartilage are trephined so that there is a vertical margin rather than a beveled edge. Great care is taken to remove any cartilage that is undermined. If the bone in the bed of the crater appears to be eburnated, multiple 0.35 mm. drill holes are made through to fresh cancellous bone. The knee is now carefully lavaged by warm saline to wash out any fragments or debris. If the patella has been found to be irregular and malacic the knee is then extended completely, the patella elevated by grasping its margins with tenaculi and a chondroplasty carried out designed to leave firm, smooth cartilage. This is similar to the procedure done in primary patellar malacia (see page 669). The knee is then closed in layers in the usual manner and a cotton cast applied, followed by the usual postoperative care for arthrotomy of the knee.

In postoperative management, active use and active motion should be encouraged. It has been shown conclusively that articular cartilage regenerates better with active use. Hence the belief that trephining, which leaves a smaller defect with vertical margins, is better than shaving, which leaves a larger defect. With a well-defined hole in the cartilage no actual weight will be borne on the regenerating cartilage until the defect is filled. So active use with full weight bearing is recommended as soon as operative reaction has subsided.

With a larger lesion on the femoral condyle I would recommend full activity but not full weight bearing. This may be hard to accomplish in the young active athlete. I would prefer him to have full weight bearing than to immobilize him completely just to prevent weight bearing.

PATELLAR MALACIA

The term "patellar malacia" has been used as a catch-all to include the many processes that involve the undersurface of the patella. Many of these conditions are not particularly pertinent to sports. True malacia is a softening or breaking down of a part or tissue. When chronic synovitis of the knee causes the patellar cartilage to break down and the bed to eburnate so that denuded bone is exposed, the condition is called malacia. So also is fragmentation of the patellar cartilage in the young individual with no signs of arthritis. The previous discussion (page 92) of chondral fractures and their treatment applied particularly to the patella.

Etiologically, patellar malacia falls naturally into three groups.

GROUP I. In the athlete, a relatively young individual, *trauma* may be the cause. This may be a chondral fracture or infraction either by acute trauma or by repeated lesser traumata to the patella. Infraction of the patellar cartilage subsequently causes irritation of the patellar groove on the femur and gradual changes supervene with fissuring, absorption and fragmentation of the cartilage. The findings at operation will depend upon the duration of symptoms. I once operated upon a girl who was injured while riding horseback. The horse got a little eager to turn into the barnyard and made a sharp turn that drove her patella forcibly into the gate post. She had an immediate severe reaction in the knee joint. The x-ray was consistently negative. At operation some four weeks later under diagnosis of chondral fracture of the patella, there was, indeed, a fracture of the cartilage of the patella which was already undergoing degenerative change. It was early enough, however, that there was still injection of cartilage with hemorrhage into the crater of the fragments so that there could be no question as to the etiology. Similar changes were present in the contiguous portion of the patellar groove. Had operation in this case been postponed for several months as in the ordinary case, typical chondromalacia of the patella would have been present. In my opinion trauma accounts for many of the cases of isolated patellar involvement in the young athlete (Fig. 485).

GROUP II. Another etiological factor in involvement of the undersurface of the patella is *disturbance of rhythm of the patellar function.* This is the type of malacia that accompanies intrinsic injury to the knee (Fig. 532). Any condition that causes a disturbance in the rhythm of the knee action frequently results in involvement of the undersurface of the patella. The knee is checked abruptly and motion is reversed. The patella is driven against the femur. In fact, in an analysis of 350 cases* of intrinsic injury to the knee we were able to demonstrate some degree of patellar involvement in 65 per cent of the cases treated by operation, and in 15 per cent of these it was Grade 4. We were able to show a direct relationship between the number of lockings of the knee and the degree of malacia (Fig. 533), and further, that the duration of symptoms and the degree of malacia (Fig. 534) also correlate. These two factors were much more important in indicating the amount of malacia present than was the age of

_____

*Bulletin of Hospital for Joint Diseases, Vol. 17, No. 1, April, 1956.

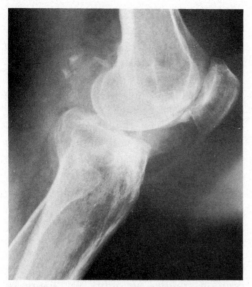

Figure 532. Severe chondromalacia of the patella following neglected ligament injury.

the patient. This seemed so definite that we make a positive recommendation that surgical intervention should be prompt in intrinsic injury of the knee if for no other reason than to prevent damage to the undersurface of the patella. The exact mechanism of this breakdown of the patella has never been wholly explained. This condition also probably occurs as a result of various other causes including direct trauma, synovitis of the joint and general chondrolytic changes. The particular pathologic changes described usually accompany other intrinsic conditions of the knee.

GROUP III. A third classification is *primary malacia of the patella,* usually bilateral without any demonstrable etiological factor. These cases are truly puzzling. One cannot rule out the effect of repeated traumata since the young patients are usually very active physically. They could be expected to traumatize their knee caps repeatedly. However, the simultaneous involvement of both knees with relative lack of involvement of other chondral surfaces

equally susceptible to trauma prompts us to seek a cause other than simple contusion.

Careful evaluation of the anatomical developmental condition of the knee may give a definite lead to the cause of so-called idiopathic malacia. Patellar alta (Fig. 473) is very prone to alter the mechanism of the gliding surface of the patella on the trochlear groove and so contribute to malacia. Lateral subluxation of the patella as the knee comes into complete extension may cause malacia of the patella without actually giving any gross evidence of displacement. This may be documented further by the silhouette view of the patella which shows the patella displaced somewhat laterally (Fig. 535). A negative finding is not very significant, however, because the silhouette view is made with the knee flexed somewhere between 30 and 45 degrees and in this position the patella may well have slipped back into the patellar groove and appear to be entirely normal. A significant examination

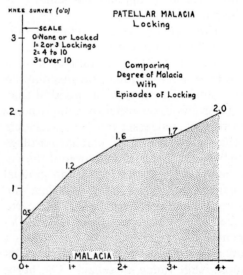

Figure 533. It should be noted in the above graph there is direct correlation in the number of times the knee locked prior to operative treatment and the degree of malacia. The knee which locked as many as ten times (category 2) showed 4+ malacia. (Hosp. for Joint Dis. Bull. *17*:5.)

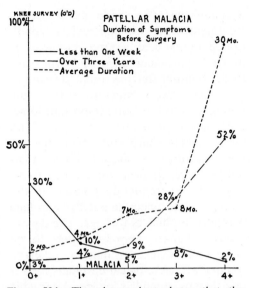

KNEE SURVEY (o'd)

PATELLAR MALACIA
Duration of Symptoms
Before Surgery

———Less than One Week
— —Over Three Years
-----Average Duration

Figure 534. The above chart shows that the great majority with symptoms of less than one week in duration showed no symptoms of patellar malacia; whereas only 2 per cent of those patients with symptoms of less than one week had 4+ malacia, 52 per cent of those with symptoms over three years showed 4+ patellar malacia. (Hosp. for Joint Dis. Bull. *17*:10.)

is made by having the patient sit with the leg hanging pendant off the edge of the table at 90 degrees. As he brings the knee up into extension it will be noticed

that the patella takes a sharp slip laterally in this position and as the knee is bent, it slips back into the groove. In this instance treatment of the malacia will basically be treatment of the subluxing patella. Obviously, the prognosis for patellar malacia is sharply improved if the underlying cause can be well defined.

Diagnosis. Group I caused by a single severe trauma is usually found in the knee that has been seriously contused to the point that a fractured patella is suspected. The findings remain localized about the patella: pain on pressure of the patella into the groove, pain on active extension of the knee particularly against resistance, pain on patellar ballottement. The severity of the symptoms will be increased by continued activity of the individual.

In Group II occurring coincidentally with other intrinsic conditions of the knee, the patellar symptoms may well be completely masked by the other condition so that the patient may present himself with his knee locked and swollen with effusion but with no demonstrable patellar symptoms. At arthrotomy one may be surprised to find

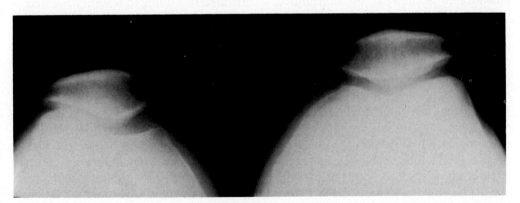

Figure 535. This 35 year old male had a long history (15 years) of trouble with his knees. He has obvious malacia of the patellae with crepitation, pain, and disability. Silhouette view reveals lateral slipping of the patella on the left with definite, rather marked narrowing of the patellofemoral space on the lateral side. At surgery the patella was very seriously involved, the central facet being down to bare bone. There was also a chondromalacic area on the trochlear groove of the femoral condyle opposing the area on the patella which was severe. The patella was removed. (For x-ray positioning of the silhouette view, see Fig. 482.)

extensive involvement of the undersurface of the patella. More frequently, however, careful examination prior to operation will reveal subpatellar crepitation and pain on pressure over the patella provided the condition is fairly severe.

In Group III with spontaneous degenerative changes, the joint is asymptomatic except for the patella. There will have been gradually increasing discomfort and disability in the knee centering around the patella without a history of previous trauma. The signs of involvement of the patella are quite obvious. If the undersurface of the patella is rough and irregular, the patella will not glide smoothly in the patellar groove and gross subpatellar crepitation is usually the first symptom. This is more severe on extension against resistance or on extension of the knee while the patella is held firmly against the patellar groove. There is also pain on going up or down stairs, squatting or anything that forces the patella against the patellar groove. This may become so severe as to become grossly disabling.

Treatment of the knee having these conditions of the patella is surgical. True enough, the symptoms may be ameliorated somewhat by nonsurgical treatment such as aspiration, injection of a corticoid, splinting and prevention of weight bearing but the future is bleak indeed since the defect in the patella remains and the symptoms will promptly recur with resumption of activity. Surgery may be directed primarily toward the patella or may be incidental to other operations. After arthrotomy by median parapatellar incision, the patella is carefully inspected with the examining finger and the extent of the pathologic involvement determined by palpation and observation. If the diagnosis is confirmed, the incision is enlarged sufficiently to permit the patella to be turned up on edge for thorough inspection of the undersurface. At this time a decision must be made on definitive treatment. This decision will be conditioned a great deal by the circumstances in each particular case and will vary from chondral shaving to patellectomy.

CHONDRAL SHAVING. In the young athlete it is quite important to retain the patella if this is possible. With an extremely sharp knife blade the patellar cartilage is shaved down in attempt to reach firm, uninvolved cartilage. This is frequently possible in the young athlete since the patellar cartilage is relatively thick at this age. The degenerative changes may be found to be quite superficial. Care must be taken to remove all pathological cartilage even if this leaves denuded bone. After this step has been completed the patellar groove is carefully inspected and if necessary chondroplasty is done here also to eliminate all abnormal cartilage. At the conclusion of the chondroplasty the patella should slide smoothly in the patellar groove with minimal irregularity either of the patella or of the groove.

At this stage considerable surgical judgment is required to determine whether or not the patella should be retained. If the patient is young and otherwise has an excellent knee, one may be justified in leaving in a somewhat defective patella. On the other hand, if there are degenerative changes throughout the joint with marginal osteophytes and rather poor femoral cartilage, the patella probably should be sacrificed.

TREPHINE AND DRILLING. The cartilage of a young person has a great deal more regenerative power than the cartilage of an older individual and a crater such as is left following removal of an osteochondritis dissecans fragment may readily fill in the former if it is curetted down to raw bone and no degenerated cartilage is left behind. In the older individual with very thin cartilage this regeneration does not occur. Localized lesions in the patella in young people are probably traumatic. It is not advisable to shave all of the patellar cartilage in order to smooth out such a defect. The area should be trephined and all involved cartilage removed down to the underlying bone leaving sharp vertical margins. If sclerotic, the bed should be drilled with a very fine Kirschner wire (0.3 mm.). Sometimes with more extensive involvement of the patellar cartilage a substantial portion of this may be shaved down leaving a smaller area in the center in which the involvement extends to the bone. In this instance preliminary shaving down to the normal cartilage over the major defect may be followed by trephining the small defect in the center of the area for the reasons indicated.

The exact technique of trephine and drilling is quite important. Our major aim here is to retain as much normal cartilage as possible so that the margin of the pathologic cartilage is definitely defined with a degree of conservatism. In other words, if there is any doubt about it, leave it on the first cut. Using a No. 15 blade with a short tip, simply cut around it with the incision in a vertical direction, much as you would take out a defect with a cookie cutter. After this first area has been cut clear around and the center curetted down to subchondral bone, the margins are very carefully inspected to be sure there are no loose fragments or underlying edges left. This margin should be exactly vertical to the underlying bone, if the major part of normal cartilage is to be preserved. If, on the contrary, the margins are beveled off or smoothed off, this simply enlarges the hole and does not add anything. In fact, it detracts because the fibrocartilage or hyaline cartilage, whichever replaces this pathologic cartilage, will appose better to a vertical edge than it will to a sloping one, whether the bone grows up from the bone below or from the periphery. Each process has been described as the way cartilage regenerates. As this hole is rather small, approximately 1 cm. in diameter, the patella will glide perfectly smoothly in the patellar groove (Figs. 536 and 537).

FACETECTOMY. Often the malacia will involve either the medial or lateral facet of the patella, while the rest of the cartilage is relatively normal. In these cases facetectomy is a gratifying procedure. One may safely remove up to one third of the patella either medially or laterally without appreciable dysfunction or noticeable deformity (Fig. 538). I find the indication for this procedure much more frequently now than previously, since it does eliminate all the portion of the patella which is pathologic and yet leaves essentially normal function of the bone. In the course of treating marginal fractures of the patella, it has long been my practice to remove the fragments rather than to repair them. Results have been so gratifying that the same thing has been done in other defects of the articular cartilage with equally good results when the remainder of the patella is normal.

The technique for facetectomy is relatively simple, particularly when it is done in conjunction with exploration of the patella. For such an exploration either a medial or a lateral parapatellar incision is made in order to visualize the involved area. Now if it is decided that the pathology is largely confined to either the medial or lateral facet, a careful dissection is made to detach the tendon covering the damaged portion of the patella as one would do for a patellectomy. This dissection should be carried back as far as it is felt to be necessary in order to remove a sufficient amount of bone to eliminate all of the pathology. Approximately one third of the bone can be removed without any appreciable loss of function. After this tendon, which passes over the patella, is reflected, the facetectomy can be carried out either with an osteotome or with an oscillating saw. I prefer the oscillating

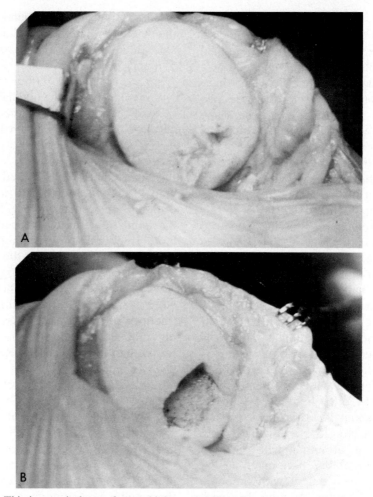

Figure 536.   This is a typical case for trephining and drilling. Notice the localized area of the malacic cartilage with essentially normal cartilage surrounding it. The patient had a history of falling directly on his knee cap a year before with definite symptoms here. Notice the postoperative crater. This is a large defect—larger than is ideal. The drill holes are evenly spaced around the lesion but not enough to destroy the structure of the bone. The shape of the hole is pertinent. It should be shaped exactly to fit the defect rather than square, round or oval. *A,* Preoperative view. *B,* At surgery.

saw. The patella should be carefully immobilized with a forceps and a vertical cut made with the saw extending completely through the bone and cartilage. There seems to be no particular advantage in making this section of the facet exactly vertical as shown in Figure 538. I have more recently been making this at an angle so as to remove less of the anterior surface of the patella and so disturb less of the patellar tendon traversing it. This angle should not be so flat that there is not any possibility of the bony surface articulating with the trochlear groove. The damaged segment is then removed, leaving a clean, smooth cut. This area is carefully smoothed off and covered with a very thin layer of bone wax. Then the retinaculum is closed as it would be had the patellar segment not been removed. In other words, it is not desirable in the ordinary case to tighten the retinaculum by overlapping unless there is some specific reason for doing so, not related to the facetectomy.

The aftercare of this patient is not altered by the facetectomy. If the wound immobilization is to be two weeks, there is no reason to add more time than this because of the procedure described. The follow-up care proceeds as indicated for any other pathology encountered in this particular case. If the facetectomy is the only procedure carried out, it is advisable to immobilize the knee for two weeks during which time the usual patellar setting, straight leg raising, and so forth may be carried out since the major tendinous attachments of the patella have not been disturbed.

PATELLECTOMY. If one decides to remove the patella because of defective

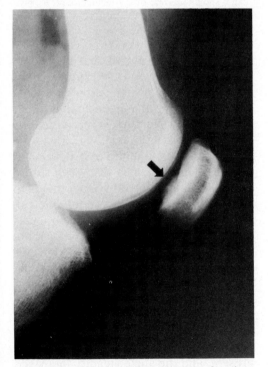

Figure 537. This boy had a history of serious trouble with both knees. The left knee sustained injury when he fell on the flexed knee. He had pain laterally and a cast was applied. One month later an arthrogram showed a torn lateral meniscus. X-ray showed a very localized area of malacia. The patella was treated by trephining and drilling. This particular patient did not do well. The hole actually filled up with bone, as visualized in the lateral view of the patella. The knee was quite symptomatic.

articular cartilage, the technique of removal is extremely important. The patella should be removed by sharp dissection, care being taken to remove all fragments of bone. The knee is then thoroughly lavaged and the quadriceps tendon and patellar tendon are inspected. At this stage it is important to remove with an osteotome the superolateral and superomedial margins of the anterior articular surface of the femur since these margins stand up as a bony prominence upon which, later, the edge of the quadriceps lateralis tendon may catch with a painful snap. This is particularly important on the lateral side since the patellar tendon does tend to slide laterally. After this has been carefully taken off and the raw bone covered with bone wax, the adjacent tendons are inspected for roughness or any undue thickening. If either is present the area is smoothed down. Using No. 1 cotton suture and a relatively long curved needle, sutures are placed beginning at the lateral edge of the quadriceps tendon, going from anteriorly to posteriorly through the edge of the quadriceps tendon to emerge anteriorly through the portion of the tendon which had been lying over the patella about two-thirds of the way toward the patellar tendon. This suture passes back through the portion of the tendon over the patella again to pass through the patellar tendon from back to front. This tends to loop up and invaginate the thin tendon between the patellar tendon and the quadriceps tendon. About eight of these sutures are placed across the knee. As each suture is placed the palpating finger determines that the undersurface is smooth. With this invagination of the thin part of the tendon two things are accomplished: the quadriceps apparatus is shortened by about two-thirds of the length of the patella, and the relatively thicker portion of the tendon occupies the previous position of the patella. The

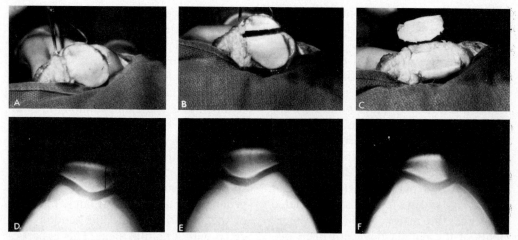

Figure 538.   This 25 year old athlete had internal derangement of the knee for about three years with increasing trouble in the patella. Involvement of the medial facet of the patella was noted when medial meniscectomy was done. *A*, Denuded bone along the medial facet. *B*, The line of the saw cut. *C*, The fragment, showing the square edges. Note the remaining normal looking cartilage of the patella. *D* and *E*, Silhouette views of the right and left patellae. The pencil mark shows the line of the facetectomy. *F*, Five months postoperative. Excellent functional result.

repair is then continued in the retinaculum by direct over and over suture. The previously placed sutures are then tied with the knee in complete extension, closely approximating the quadriceps tendon to the patellar tendon and obliterating entirely the patellar fossa in the tendon. After these sutures are tied, a finger is passed underneath the suture line to make sure that the imbrication is smooth. After all these sutures are tied it should be possible to flex the knee to 90 degrees and determine whether or not the repaired tendon has a smooth gliding surface. By careful attention to this shortening of the quadriceps tendon mechanism, one will avoid the extremely disabling effect of loss of complete active extension of the knee which so frequently follows patellectomy. One can cheerfully sacrifice some degree of flexion in order to obtain complete active extension of the knee. Usually full motion is regained. If the suture line appears to be very secure and there is no undue tension on the sutures, immobilization may be carried out in a cotton cast (Fig. 433) although I really prefer a

little longer dressing so that instead of using the basswood or yucca board splints, we use plaster strips extending from just above the ankle to the upper thigh. Weight bearing is permitted as soon as it is comfortable, which may be the first day postoperative. If your clinical judgment indicates that your suture is secure in good healthy tendon (which is very likely to be the case in athletes), the patient can probably begin motion as early as the second week providing there is no severe reaction within the knee itself. If there is no synovitis with effusion, and if there is no swelling or edema at the end of two weeks a long leg brace may be applied with a caliper heel and a dial knee. The dial knee may be set just beyond the degree of flexion which is present, and the angle steadily increased as range of motion increases. By this mechanism one may permit free weight bearing, utilizing what motion is present in the knee and yet protecting the knee against undue force caused by the patient accidentally stumbling and overflexing the knee. It will require a considerable degree of judgment to decide

KNEE SERIES

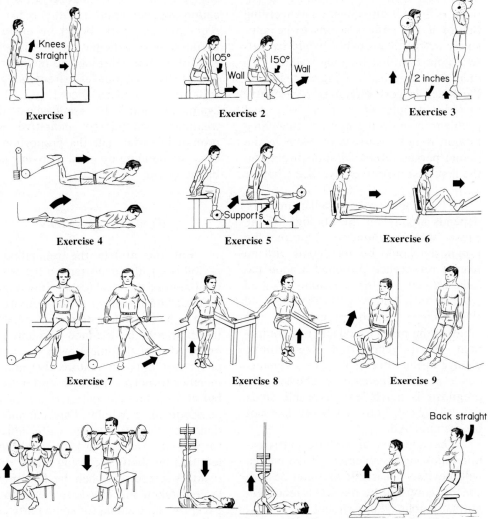

Knee Series. The diagrams above depict the series of exercises utilized by West Point cadets following knee injury or knee surgery. These exercises are instituted following the acute phase of medical care and initial physical therapy. In general they are instituted about the time a patient is ready for brisk walking or light jogging.

Specific notation should be made of the total lower body reconditioning program. All major muscle groups of both thigh and lower leg are challenged. The cadet is started with a low weight, low repetition work-out and is progressed as tolerated until he is ready for competitive athletics.

In conjunction with the above exercises, a program of guided running and jump rope exercise is employed. Running begins with a slow ½ mile and progresses to a 2 mile run in 13 to 16 minutes. Rope jumping begins with jumping on both legs and progresses to three sets of *one* legged jumping (injured extremity) 90 to 120 times in 60 seconds.

It is felt that by employing the above program, re-injury of the involved part or new injury to an adjacent part has been minimized. The above work-out should take at least 30 minutes even if done by the most aggressive athlete. The cadet is returned to full unrestricted activity when lower body performance is approximately symmetrical.

The exercises contained in the diagrams of the West Point knee reconditioning program represent the evolution of rehabilitation spanning many years and many individuals. The West Point Orthopaedic Service, Physical Therapy Department and Office of Physical Education have all contributed to the program now in use.

which patient should be trusted with a brace since it can be taken off by the patient. If there is any question concerning this or if the patient seems to be unusually active, it probably would be better to put him in a long leg walking cylinder or a long leg walking cast. I think the brace is very effective, particularly in older people where there is a real problem in regaining motion. Regaining motion is not a serious problem in the young person. Rehabilitation begins on the first postoperative day. (See Chapter 22.)

The *prognosis* in patellar malacia depends largely on the etiology. If the cause was a chondral fracture, the prognosis should be very good with no fear of recurrence provided a good patella was left. If the condition resulted from intrinsic pathology in the knee and this is corrected, the prognosis is also good. If the patellar malacia is a component of a generalized degenerative change in the knee or if it is a spontaneous type of degenerative change, the prognosis is much less favorable since the etiological factor probably has not been eliminated.

The question of athletic participation following involvement of the patella will inevitably arise. If one can be reasonably sure that he has left a relatively normal patella, there should be no reason to forbid participation. Such would be the case in chondral fracture or malacia following rupture of the medial meniscus, for example. In the more chronic type one would hesitate to permit active competitive sports which cause overuse of the patella. If it is already questionable that the patella will withstand the rigors of ordinary use, one is not justified in encouraging athletic participation, which would only precipitate the trouble. The decision here rests on the same considerations as following any other pathologic condition, and must remain a matter of personal judgment. Particularly to be considered is the im-

portance to the individual of athletic competition. If his livelihood or his education depends upon it, if this is his career, greater effort should be made to permit him to participate. If on the other hand it is a casual thing and his interest can be diverted into less strenuous pursuits, this should be encouraged. Once again, it should be emphasized that treatment should be definitive and prompt in order that the proportion of cases responding by good recovery may be increased.

REHABILITATION

For the athlete the rehabilitative period is equally important to the actual treatment of the local lesion. It is important for him to return to full activity as soon as he can safely do so. So, rehabilitation should be planned and initiated on the day of the injury with particular effort not only to restore the injured member to normal strength and activity but also to prevent deterioration of his physique as a whole. This cannot be done casually. It may be quite difficult to persuade the young high school athlete that he should be doing rather rudimentary exercises when he has pretty largely taken his physique for granted except when training for some particular activity. Dr. Fred Allman, a nationally known authority on the subject of rehabilitation of the athlete, has kindly provided a chapter on this subject for this book. I urge the reader of this material on the knee to carefully study his recommendations in Chapter 22.

The West Point Military Academy also has long had an excellent program of rehabilitation and has given me permission to reproduce the exercise schedule that they use on these rehabilitation procedures on the knee. We gratefully acknowledge their contribution to this problem. These exercises are listed on page 677.

CHAPTER 19

INJURIES OF THE LEG

For the purposes of this discussion the leg will be considered to be the area between the knee and the ankle and not immediately concerned with the two joints themselves.

ANATOMICAL CONSIDERATIONS

The upper portion of the leg receives the muscles from the thigh and involvement of these attachments has been discussed elsewhere (page 535). Likewise, the lower portion of the leg is intimately involved with the function of the ankle joint, which also will be discussed in detail (page 701). The shafts of the tibia and fibula serve for origin of the muscles that move the ankle and foot. The tibia is the only weight-bearing bone since the fibula does not have a weight-bearing component. The fibula situated posterolaterally is not directly involved in the knee joint but forms a vital part of the ankle.

Throughout its length the fibula is bound to the tibia by the interosseous membrane. The interosseous membrane forms a "Y" above to surround the upper tibiofibular joint, the anterior division being called the anterosuperior tibiofibular ligament and the posterior division the posterosuperior tibiofibular ligament. A similar arrangement is formed below, the interosseous membrane thickening and dividing to surround the inferior tibiofibular syndesmosis, the two components being called the anterior and posterior inferior tibiofibular ligaments. Whereas the upper portion of the fibula is largely for muscle attachments and may serve to some extent as a brace, it has no vital function and in fact may be sacrificed without material loss of function provided proper security is made for the structures attaching at the top of the fibula. The lower one-third, as mentioned, is extremely important since it is vital in the formation of the ankle mortice.

The interosseous membrane serves as the floor of the anterior compartment of the leg (Fig. 541). This is a closed space, the boundaries being the anterior fascia of the leg in front, the interosseous membrane behind, the fibula laterally and the tibia medially. This space permits little, if any, expansion of the structures contained within. The posterior compartment on the contrary is a loosely contained space with a relaxed and redundant fascia. This space is not subject to constriction to the same degree as the anterior compartment.

The tibia, the main weight-bearing

679

bone, is roughly triangular in cross section and has muscle attachments at the posterolateral and posterior surfaces. The anterior border, the anteromedial surface and the posteromedial border are all subcutaneous.

CONTUSION

Contusion is extremely common in the lower leg since this part, particularly in athletics, is very much exposed to direct blows. The nature of the contusion will vary according to the location of the blow. If the blow is over the subcutaneous portion of the tibia, the contusion is much more likely to be severe since the integument and periosteum are caught between the external force and extremely hard bone. This may result in a simple bruise with extravasation of blood in a localized area or the periosteal damage may result in severe traumatic periostitis, also usually localized. It is also possible to have contusion over the muscles of the anterior compartment; the resulting swelling within the compartment may be extremely uncomfortable owing to the closed nature of the space. Contusion of the muscles of the calf is also common but circulatory embarrassment is not usual here. An unusual type of contusion is of the peroneal nerve as it winds around the upper portion of the fibula (Fig. 539). This may result in a painful neuritis or even transient paralysis of the peroneals with drop foot which may be very distressing to the athlete.

Contusion and Hematoma

Implicit in the pathology of a contusion is some degree of hematoma. In the lower leg this may be extremely disabling. A severe hematoma in the anterior enclosed space may become a surgical emergency since it may go on to actual ischemia and necrosis of the muscle (see Anterior Compartment Syndrome, page 684). A subperiosteal hematoma complicating contusion of the skin may also be painful and actually disabling if it is severe. Hematoma within the muscle is not as common in the calf as in other areas in the body.

Diagnosis. Following injury of the lower leg, careful analysis should be made of the actual history to determine, if possible, the type of blow and the type of the instrument since a large blunt object such as a player's helmet will usually cause a different type of injury than a relatively sharp one such as a cleat or hard toe of a shoe. The part should be carefully examined to determine the degree of swelling and whether a hematoma is present. Function should be carefully checked since this may well give some indication as to whether the muscle is involved or whether there is involvement of a nerve. The leg should be carefully examined for a possible fracture from a direct blow on the tibia or fibula. The tibia is readily palpable but it may be more difficult to examine the fibula since it is well surrounded by muscle. If there is any question as to the degree of localized injury in either bone, x-ray study should be done.

Treatment. If a diagnosis of contusion or hematoma is made, treatment will depend upon the degree of involvement. If hematoma is present it should be aspirated under aseptic technique and injected with hyaluronidase. These measures should be immediately followed by pressure bandage and cold pack for six to eight hours. Further analysis can then be made as to the severity of the injury. If fluid or blood has recurred it should be re-aspirated. At the end of 24 to 48 hours, depending upon the degree of injury, heat should be substituted for cold. The degree of protection of necessity will depend upon the location of injury. If the injury involves the bone and periosteum and is not severe, treatment should be by protective pad and function need not be interfered with unless it is major injury. If, on the other hand, the blow involves the muscle, the muscle should be kept at rest by proper strapping or splinting until it is determined there is no major bleeding or laceration within the muscle. Protective strapping should be used until such a time as the part is symptom-free.

Contusion of the Peroneal Nerve

As the peroneal nerve continues downward after leaving the popliteal space and passes laterally, it crosses directly behind the neck of the fibula (Fig. 539) and winds around the lateral surface of the fibular neck to pass into the extensor muscles anteriorly. It is extremely vulnerable to injury either posteriorly or laterally since it lies directly between the skin and the bone. An ideal situation is present for contusion of the nerve since the nerve will be caught between the hard contusing object and the un-derlying bone. A relatively minor blow may cause serious nerve injury.

The *pathology* will vary greatly according to the severity of injury since the nerve may be only slightly shocked or may be crushed in two. The usual effects of contusion are congestion and edema with local swelling. Since the nerve is contained within a sheath, this swelling will cause pressure on the nerve fibers with resulting symptoms of pain, numbness and paresthesia. If there is actual hemorrhage into the sheath, the increased tension may proceed to actual paralysis due to intrinsic pressure. Indeed, this may result in necrosis of the nerve fibers with permanent functional loss. As a rule, the congestion diminishes, the swelling subsides and the nerve slowly returns to normal. If there has been actual damage to the nerve fibers themselves, they may be replaced by fibrous scar and greater or lesser loss of function results depending upon how many nerve filaments remain undamaged.

Contusion may cause hemorrhage in the surrounding tissues and this may

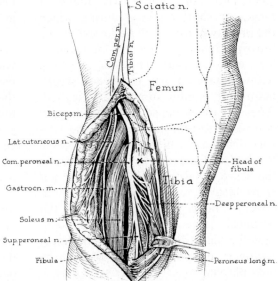

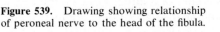

Figure 539. Drawing showing relationship of peroneal nerve to the head of the fibula.

cause secondary pressure on the nerve. This is not likely in this particular area.

The *symptoms* will be those of the local blow plus the effect on the nerve itself. The immediate symptom is almost always a "shocking feeling" with pain shooting throughout the distribution of the nerve to the lateral side of the leg and foot. Acute tingling and numbness remain after pain subsides. These may be transient and may disappear within seconds or minutes if actual damage to the nerve has not resulted. In such a case the patient may completely recover before he is ever examined by the doctor.

If the injury is more severe, a different pattern of symptomatology will emerge. The initial symptoms may be as indicated above but are followed by a completely asymptomatic period to be followed in turn by symptoms of pressure within the nerve. The pain and paresthesia will return and will increase in severity. As the pressure continues, signs of loss of function will develop. This will be evidenced by hypesthesia throughout the distribution and by weakness in dorsal flexion of the foot. This may progress to complete paralysis of the nerve with sensory loss and muscular afunction. There will follow a longer or shorter period during which the only symptoms will be loss of nerve function; namely, sensory and motor loss with no pain. This may develop within days or it may be several weeks before the painful stimuli have ceased. After a variable lapse of time, function will begin to return, usually in the sensory distribution first. One may be able to elicit a Tinel sign by tapping along the nerve distal to the injury and so get some idea as to the progression of recovery. This is rather difficult since the peroneal nerve becomes rather deep-seated a short distance below the knee. Recovery may be complete or may be only partial.

This whole train of symptoms may be interrupted at any time by the recovery process. The earlier the recovery begins, the more rapid and complete it will be. Very careful examination of the leg and foot in a case involving the peroneal nerve will be extremely rewarding since it is quite important to be able to follow accurately the succession of events. If the paralysis is immediate and complete, one may assume a major injury and govern treatment accordingly. Rapidly progressing development of signs of nerve pressure indicate increasing swelling within the sheath. The rate of its development is of considerable importance in determining the proper treatment. One should carefully outline the area of sensory involvement and determine not only touch but sharp and dull and hot and cold sensitivities, although this is not as important here as it is in central nervous system lesions. A good practice is to outline in ink on the skin the area of involvement or to record it faithfully in notes. It is very gratifying to find on re-examination of such a patient that the area of his involvement has lessened and to be able to give him a favorable prognosis. On the contrary, if the area increases one can be prepared to modify his treatment accordingly.

When one is faced with involvement along the peroneal distribution without definite history of an injury, he may be able by careful palpation around the fibular head to locate areas of local tenderness that give some clue as to the possibility of a direct blow on the nerve. In the heat of an athletic contest, such a blow may be readily overlooked and the patient have no knowledge of an injury.

Treatment. The vast majority of these cases will require no specific treatment. If the blow is severe enough that the soft tissue contusion requires care, the customary treatment is in order—ice pack early, local heat later. However, as the nerve symptoms develop and there is motor paralysis or specific weakness, the muscles will require protection. Support of the ankle and foot must be provided by cast, splint or brace. A carefully applied drop-foot brace holding the foot to a right angle by a mechanical spring will permit ambulation without disconcerting drop foot. This will make walking easier and will prevent overstretching of the paralyzed muscles. Some such apparatus is also important in rehabilitation as the muscle strength returns. During the early phase of such a condition, we would recommend wearing the brace and shoe during sleeping hours to prevent contracture of the calf. Once the acute symptoms have subsided there is no particular interdiction to activities. The presence of a drop foot is a real handicap in running, particularly in cutting and turning, and the player's efficiency will be sharply reduced until the drop foot recovers. Overfatigue of any weakened muscle should be avoided and strength should be painstakingly restored by graduated exercises. An example of the type of exercises we use is included at the end of this section (Fig. 540) and also shown in Figure 593.

Should a blow be followed by a quiescent period and then by a rapidly developing paralysis, one is justified in exploring the peroneal nerve and performing neurolysis to be sure that the tight sheath is not constricting the nerve beyond the point of its tolerance. This is not often indicated. Even if the paralysis is immediate and complete, one is justified in a period of watchful waiting to give the nerve a chance to recover spontaneously. If there are no definite signs of recovery within three months I would recommend surgical exploration of the nerve with neurolysis or nerve suture as indicated.

In other instances, the quiescent period may be much longer only to be

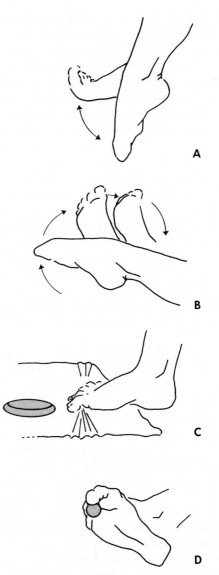

Figure 540. Reconstructive exercises for the foot and leg. See explanation on page 684 of text.

followed by the same pattern of progressively increasing nerve symptoms. This is due to scar formation with gradual constriction of some of the fibers of the nerve by the maturing scar. In such an instance, if the condition is steadily progressive there is no advantage in undue delay and early neurolysis should be done.

Another indication for surgery is

the case in which there is intractable pain along the nerve that persists for several weeks. These cases should be treated by exploration of the nerve. The nerve should be carefully dissected free of all adhesions and appropriate neurolysis carried out, either surgically or by saline injection in order to expand the sheath.

Some typical sets of exercises are shown as follows. (Also, see Fig. 593.)

1. First Stage (Check range of motion):

A. Flexion—flex foot as far as possible (point toes upward) (Fig. 540, A).

B. Extension—extend foot as far as possible (point toes downward) (Fig. 540, A).

C. Inversion—turn soles of feet inward.

D. Eversion—turn soles of feet outward.

2. If the above exercises can be done in full range of motion and without pain, do the following exercises:

A. Foot circles—foot circumscribes a small circle. Ball of foot down first, then in, up and finally out (Fig. 540, B).

B. Alphabet—sitting on table with knee straight and only ankle extended over the end of the table, print in capital letters the entire alphabet with your foot.

3. If the above exercises can be done in full range of motion and without pain, do the following exercises:

A. Towel exercise—sitting on a chair with foot on a towel, pull towel up under foot with toes. After completing the above part successfully, place a weight on the other end of the towel to offer resistance (Fig. 540, C).

B. Pick-up exercise—with the toes pick up marbles or a small piece of sponge rubber. Alternate placing the object in the hand in front of and behind the opposite leg (Fig. 540, D).

C. Toe rises—stand with feet one foot apart and toeing in. Rise on toes as high as possible without pain. Also repeat this exercise with toes pointed straight ahead and pointed out.

STRAIN

Strain of the muscles and tendons about the ankle and foot will be discussed elsewhere (page 750). Here, in addition to the well delineated entities of strain involving the leg proper, some rather unusual conditions will be covered although there may be some argument as to whether strain is actually the cause.

Anterior Compartment Syndrome

It will be recalled that in the anterior compartment of the leg the anterior tibial, the extensor hallucis and the extensor digitorum longus muscles arise from the sides of the tibia, fibula and interosseous membrane, completely filling the anterior compartment. This compartment is tightly roofed by the anterior fascia of the leg (Fig. 541). In the anterior tibial syndrome for various reasons there is a rapid swelling of the muscle within this compartment. This may come on following active exercise alone and in theory is due to the fact that muscles which have not been previously conditioned are overused and respond by swelling and edema. It may also come on following direct injury in which there is excessive swelling and hemorrhage into the space. The condition can also be caused by localized infection within the space. In fact, anything that causes intractable swelling may cause this syndrome.

At onset there is severe pain over the involved area and loss of function so that contraction of the muscles contained in the space rapidly becomes impossible and a drop foot ensues (Fig. 542). Very soon even passive stretching of the muscles becomes quite painful. This is not ordinarily preceded by the symptoms of tenosynovitis however. The skin over the area becomes red,

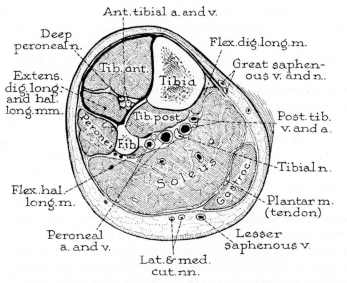

Ant. tibial a. and v.

Deep peroneal n.

Flex. dig. long. m.

Great saphenous v. and n.

Extens. dig. long. and hal. long. mm.

Tib. ant.

Tibia

Post. tib. v. and a.

Tib. post.

Tibial n.

Flex. hal. long. m.

Plantar m. (tendon)

Peroneal a. and v.

Lesser saphenous v.

Lat. & med. cut. nn.

Figure 541. Cross section of leg showing its anterior compartment outlined by heavy line indicating muscles and vascular bundle within the compartment.

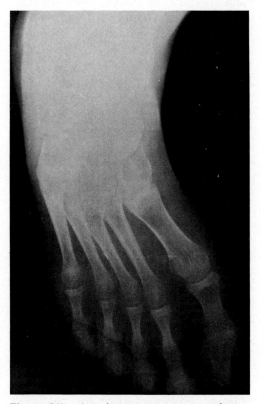

Figure 542. Anterior compartment syndrome, late. This is an intractable deformity of the foot due to pressure of the vessels in the anterior compartment of the leg. Triple arthrodesis was necessary.

glossy, warm and markedly tender with a feeling of woody tension even to the point of real hardness of the fascia over the space. There may occasionally be involvement of the peroneal nerve with sensory loss, but the loss of muscle function is usually not due to nerve involvement but to pathologic change within the muscle itself. The muscles go on to ischemic necrosis, often called "Volkmann's ischemia of the leg," with swelling, edema, extravasation of red blood cells, destruction of blood cells and replacement of muscle tissue by fibrous scar. The result is a firm, inelastic, noncontractile muscle group. This can be extremely disabling and defies reconstructive treatment.

Treatment depends upon the extent of involvement. Any delay is disastrous. Early treatment should be prompt application of ice without pressure dressing. If the symptoms do not respond within a few hours, treatment must be surgical. If the anterior fascia of the leg is promptly sectioned, complete relief is obtained from pain and the other symptoms. If the operation is postponed until necrosis of the muscles has already occurred, fibrous replacement will still leave irreparable scarring.

This condition is not common but when it occurs it is an extreme emergency. The danger lies in the similarity of the early symptoms to so-called cramping, muscle spasm, "shin splints" or contusion. Any of these conditions that do not respond promptly to treatment should be carefully investigated. Of particular importance is the patient's complaint of constant, boring, aching pain made more severe by function but not disappearing under rest. The anterior compartment syndrome may spell the end of athletic competition for the affected individual. Because of the extreme urgency of this situation, any time there is intractable pain in front of the leg accompanied by some loss of function of the toes which is not relieved by ordinary sedation, it must be assumed to be anterior compartment syndrome and preparation must be made for surgical release of the fascia of the leg. If one waits until this is completely defined, necrosis of the muscle has occurred and surgery is of little value. This often results in complete drop foot as well as the symptoms of ischemia of the leg.

Shin Splints

Another condition unique to the leg is so-called "shin splints." As with many names in common use, there is considerable and often raucous argument as to what is actually meant by the term. As is usual in these circumstances the title "shin splints" is a waste basket including many different conditions. The authors of various articles on the subject are inclined to state very definitely that it is caused by one particular thing to the exclusion of all others. This causes great confusion.

Shin splints ordinarily occurs early in the training period, frequently in training on hard floors such as indoor track. It also may occur on the hard ground in the early fall or on the basketball court. One of the conditions sometimes called "shin splints" is irritation of the attachment of the posterior tibial muscle along the posterior face of the tibia with resulting periostitis. Here the tenderness will be along the posterior medial angle of the tibia and pain will be on function of the posterior tibial muscle. Another cause is an actual tearing of the attachment of the posterior tibial muscle along the tibia. "shin splints" may also be caused by irritation at the interosseous membrane, in which case the symptoms are somewhat more posterior and seem to be deeper in the muscles of the calf. An ordinary periostitis along the posteromedial angle of the tibia may also be called "shin splints." Indeed, the involvement of the anterior tibial muscle at the anterior border of the tibia and onto its anterolateral face is by some called "shin splints." The last named condition may go on to serious involvement of the anterior compartment. A stress fracture of the tibia may also be misdiagnosed "shin splints" by the unwary.

Treatment. A condition having so many etiological factors must of necessity require varying types of treatment. However, certain basic measures are of importance regardless of the etiology, the primary ones being rest and local heat. A word of caution is nevertheless needed about use of heat in involvement of the anterior compartment since heat may only aggravate the tension within the space. In the ordinary case of "shin splints" local heat, rest of the part, and strapping to prevent stress of the posterior tibial muscle will give marked improvement. The outcome may be disappointing, however, since the condition has a great tendency to recur and may indeed keep a track man off the boards a whole season. A longer initial period of rest and protection will pay dividends in a more complete recovery. Various measures have been recommended such as binding of the leg with elastic or adhesive over foam rubber or various other types of padding. This has but little effect upon a condition that is basically due to overuse of the muscles. Physical therapeutic measures should be continued until the leg is symptom-free. Resumption of activity should be on a very carefully supervised basis and function should always be kept below the level that causes pain.

There has recently been a great deal in the literature and at various meetings about treatment of shin splints by support under the arch of the foot. I call your attention again to the fact that I think you should really determine the cause of the shin splint. If so, the treatment can be much more intelligent. If the patient has a tendency to pronate the foot, he may well be susceptible to chronic stress of the muscles of the leg. If the deficiency of the arch is corrected by overtension on the posterior tibial, or even occasionally on the anterior tibial muscle, this can cause extreme overfatigue of these muscles with resulting muscle spasm and that condition which we, for lack of a better word, call shin splints. Certainly careful analysis of the arch should be carried out. If there is any tendency toward pronation, appropriate support should be put under the arch of the foot. This is particularly pertinent since most athletic shoes have no support to the arch. Many of them do not even have a heel of any sort. Possibly simply elevating the heel by a $\frac{1}{2}$ inch felt pad inside the shoe and/or the inserting of a cork and leather arch support flexible enough to permit the foot to flex, yet still give some support on the inner arch, may solve what has seemed to be an insolvable problem. Again, the emphasis must be on accurate diagnosis of the actual trouble so that you are not treating "shin splints" but you are treating the cause of the pain and disability in the patient's leg.

Rupture of the Plantaris Muscle

Another condition unique to the leg is rupture of the plantaris muscle. This is a pencil-sized muscle arising from the lateral condyle of the femur, passing beneath the gastrocnemius and soleus muscles to attach to the tendo Achilles or the tubercle of the calcaneus on the medial side. The tendon is no larger than a piece of twine and is easily broken. To the freshman anatomy student it is the "fool's nerve." This muscle itself is sometimes completely ruptured, in which case pain will be deep in the calf and may be quite disabling. Actually function of the muscle is of little importance in the human and there is no necessity for repair. A relatively short period of protection will result in complete recovery.

One must carefully distinguish between the above condition and *rupture of a portion of the calf,* in which case the symptoms will be much more severe and much longer lasting. Because of the extremely explosive action of the calf muscle, a vessel in the muscle or in the subcutaneous or fascial area will not infrequently be ruptured. This also gives a sharp stinging pain without serious disability but with development of ecchymosis which may be disquieting. This ruptured vessel requires no treatment other than symptomatic, but the condition must be distinguished from rupture of the plantaris which may be somewhat more disabling.

Muscular Strain

The muscles of the lower leg are particularly subject to strain and this will be discussed at greater length elsewhere (see Ankle Strain, page 701).

One of the most common locations for strain is at the musculotendinous junction of the calf. Much of the accustomed activity of the athlete involves forcible contraction of the calf so that the whole body weight is abruptly thrown on the calf mechanism. Strain here may be caused either by chronic overuse in the poorly conditioned calf or by a single violent stress. Strain in the calf mechanism may be extremely disabling.

Treatment. Ordinarily strapping or taping is of little benefit except to prevent overstretching of the strained area. The athlete must be withdrawn from competition and instructed to do nothing that causes pain. The condition will frequently progress to chronic strain. Early treatment consists of rest, local heat, immobilization, followed by protective strapping and very gradual return to activity. In the early period the most efficient immobilization is a walk-

ing boot cast that will permit the patient to have fairly good activity and still prevent any strain on the calf. If the strain is less severe, primary elastic adhesive strapping will be adequate. Strapping is also used subsequent to removal of the cast (Fig. 543). This strapping is of the type designed to prevent dorsal flexion of the foot. The foot should be placed in equinus and the major anchor strap should begin above the bulge of the calf and pass directly down the back of the leg, over the heel and along the sole of the foot to the toes. The cross stretch adhesive that stretches laterally rather than longitudinally serves well for this purpose. It has the advantage of rigidity in its long axis while the lateral stretch permits it to be molded well around the ankle and heel without wrinkling (Fig. 543). This can be placed to limit dorsal flexion to any desired degree and the foot may ac-

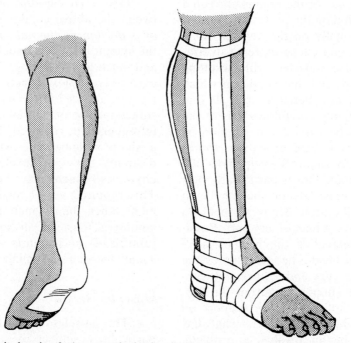

Figure 543. A 3-inch strip of cross-stretch elastic adhesive is run down the back of the calf and over the sole of the foot to the metatarsals. It is anchored in place by a Gibney-type basket weave as shown on the right.

tually be held in plantar flexion. If the foot is held in plantar flexion by the strapping, the shoe heel must be built up a proportionate amount. Even after recovery it is advisable to elevate the heel of the street shoe and put a ½ inch pad in the heel of the athletic shoe to give some degree of relaxation to the calf. Once a strain has occurred it is advisable to strap the foot at each practice session or game so that it cannot be dorsiflexed beyond the point where it becomes painful or sensitive. By this means one may at least prevent the strain from excessive dorsal flexion although he cannot limit the strain caused by violent muscle contraction.

In a similar manner there may be strain to the anteromedial muscles of the foot, most often the anterior tibial, less frequently the posterior tibial except in relation to the muscle origins (see Shin Sp ints, page 686). In these instances the strapping should be so applied as to relieve the tension on the muscle involved. The peroneal group is not frequently involved since athletic activity does not ordinarily subject these muscles to the same tensions received by the posterior and medial groups.

Severe (Third Degree) Rupture

The calf muscle may be ruptured partially or completely any place from its origin on the posterior part of the femoral condyles and back of the tibia to its attachment to the calcaneus. The tear may be in the muscle belly itself: more frequently in the musculotendinous junction between the gastrocnemius and the conjoined tendon with the soleus. The unit may rupture through the tendon itself or at the attachment to the heel, sometimes avulsing a fragment of bone. As in a muscle rupture anywhere, determination of the location and extent of the injury is extremely impor-

tant. The location is usually readily determined when the injury is examined early since the tenderness will be found to be quite localized. After several hours, swelling, edema and inflammation become diffuse and the exact location may be in doubt. Both active contraction of the muscle and passive stretching will cause pain. If there is complete severance of the whole muscle-tendon unit such as (1) the head of the gastrocnemius or (2) the entire gastrocnemius from the conjoined tendon or (3) rupture of the tendon, loss of function will be noted so that the muscle on contraction will bunch up rather than flatten down as it normally does. If the rupture is in the tendon or musculotendinous junction a palpable defect can often be felt. The condition is quite disabling even with a relatively minor degree of tearing. It interdicts running or any activity that causes the athlete to be on his toes. This loss of function may be due to actual loss of continuity of the tendon but it is more frequently due to muscle spasm and pain. If the rupture is complete and seen early, repair is quite feasible even in the muscle belly.

Treatment. Surgical repair of the tendon is mandatory even if the case is seen late (Fig. 544). In the early case incision is made directly over the involved area, the underlying muscles are inspected, the clot is evacuated and the muscle ends are apposed by mattress sutures placed with the knee flexed and the foot in plantar flexion. The extremity must be kept in this position for about four weeks if the repair is in the muscle itself. If the repair is in the tendon or tendon to bone, a much firmer internal fixation may be obtained and the extreme flexion position may not be necessary. In any instance, it is advisable to hold the foot in equinus for a period of time. When a fragment of bone is avulsed, this fragment should be excised unless it is so large as to be vital

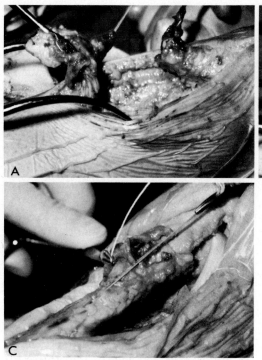

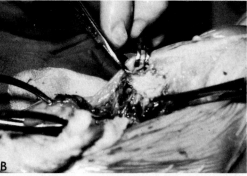

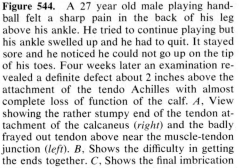

Figure 544. A 27 year old male playing handball felt a sharp pain in the back of his leg above his ankle. He tried to continue playing but his ankle swelled up and he had to quit. It stayed sore and he noticed he could not go up on the tip of his toes. Four weeks later an examination revealed a definite defect about 2 inches above the attachment of the tendo Achilles with almost complete loss of function of the calf. *A*, View showing the rather stumpy end of the tendon attachment of the calcaneus (*right*) and the badly frayed out tendon above near the muscle-tendon junction (*left*). *B*, Shows the difficulty in getting the ends together. *C*, Shows the final imbrication of the stumpy distal end into the more frayed out proximal end with marked plantar flexion of the foot. Result equivocal even though reconstructive support by the peroneus brevis was added.

to calcaneal function. One of the major sources for tension on the suture following repair of any part of the gastrocnemius-soleus complex is a spasm in the calf muscles. If the rupture is actually in the muscle, this is not quite so pertinent since the lesion in the muscle will tend to prevent overcontraction. However, if the lesion is in the tendo Achilles or at its attachment, it is necessary to undertake some measure to prevent overstress of the calf during the convalescent period. For this reason a mattress suture holding the calf muscle down with a pull-out wire to take out the wire suture later is extremely important. Technically, the wire is woven back and forth through the muscle above the level of the lesion, terminating with one wire on either side of the tendon. These wires are led down along the side of the calcaneus and through the sole of the heel where they are tied

over a suitable block or button to securely accept the tension of the calf muscle. The pull-out element is a wire loop passed through the proximal portion of the mattress holding the calf. This exits through the skin on the calf above the level of the wire suture holding the muscle. By such a measure it is not necessary to hold the foot in such extreme equinus for a long period of time which often results in equinus contracture. At eight weeks or so the wire can be cut on the button at the sole of the heel, and, using the pull-out wire, can be pulled out. This aids materially in the general management of rupture of the tendon below the level of the muscle-tendon junction. It is important to be sure that the mattress wire will slide freely through the muscle with no kinks which may make it difficult to remove with the pull-out loop.

Good surgical judgment is required

to determine just how long the foot needs to be kept in equinus after the repair. If it is held too long it may be difficult to get the calf muscle stretched out to its normal length. If the injury is fresh, the tissues strong and the suture material well placed, it may be possible to put the foot at right angles immediately after suture. If the strength of the fixation is questionable because of shredding of the tendon, the equinus position must be maintained longer. It should be borne in mind that at least four weeks are needed for the tendon to start to heal and even then union is quite insecure. In order to minimize morbidity a walking cast may be utilized after a week or ten days so that disability is not unduly prolonged. One should not anticipate return to competition in the same season in which the injury occurs. A little more time spent to get a complete recovery is well rewarded by the completeness of the recovery. A tendon as large as the tendo Achilles could not be expected to resume anything like its normal strength under three or four months although some

function may be permitted as early as eight weeks.

SPRAIN

Sprain occurs in the leg proper only at the upper end of the fibula. The upper end of the fibula does not participate primarily in the knee joint but may be involved in a knee injury. This is especially likely in relation to the fibular collateral ligament attachment (see page 558). There may be damage to the upper tibiofibular ligaments to the extent of an actual dislocation of the upper end of the fibula. The exact mechanism of isolated strain of this area is difficult to determine. It may be that some of the lesser sprains are caused by forcible traction of the biceps tendon with the knee in flexion (Fig. 545). The type of injury that damages the fibular collateral ligament of the knee would not ordinarily damage the tibiofibular ligament since its force tends to pull the fibula toward the tibia. If, however, the distracting force occurs with the knee

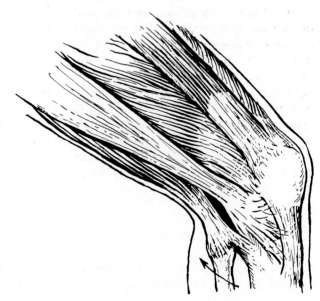

Figure 545. Drawing showing flexed knee, the biceps tendon pulling the fibula back.

flexed, the lateral collateral ligament may possibly pull the fibula backward in relation to the tibia. Certain it is that sprain to the extent of complete dislocation may occur from a direct blow to the upper end of the fibula, driving it away from its tibial attachment.

It may actually be possible manually to subluxate the head of the fibula back and forth or to dislocate it from the tibia if the ligament tear is severe, since the bone is subcutaneous and can be readily manipulated. Distinguishing symptoms are pain and tenderness around the anterior and posterior tibiofibular sulci at the superior end.

Treatment. If the fibula has dislocated and spontaneously replaced, it may be difficult to determine that there has actually been a rupture of the ligaments. Occasionally the dislocation remains unreduced (see Fig. 516, page 654). If it is seen early it may be readily reduced by manipulation. It may be held in place by simple splint fixation protecting the knee. The splint should extend from above the ankle to the groin. One must be extremely wary of trying to hold the fibula to the tibia by a constricting circumferential bandage because of the extreme vulnerability of the peroneal nerve. There may be a chronic dislocation of the upper end of the fibula and in many instances this will not be troublesome. However, the fact that the biceps and fibular collateral ligament attach to the fibula may cause this condition to become symptomatic. If it is symptomatic to the degree that it causes disability, surgical repair should be carried out by screw fixation across the upper end of the fibula into the tibia. This is rarely necessary.

FASCIAL HERNIA

Fascial hernia occurs in various areas of the body. One of the most common hernias of this type and one of the most likely to be symptomatic occurs in the anterior fascia of the leg. This rent usually takes place at the attachment of the anterior fascia to the anterior border of the tibia. The early symptoms will be those ordinarily connected with "shin splints," periostitis, or in fact simple contusion. As acute symptoms subside, the patient will complain of a sharply localized mass that appears just lateral to the tibial crest but is not constant. It may or may not be tender. He may notice aching pain in the leg after continued use but at other times the condition may be almost wholly asymptomatic. Careful examination reveals a palpable defect in the fascia through which bulges a tumor mass particularly noticeable when the muscle is relaxed. When the anterior tibial muscle is contracted the mass will disappear, since on contraction the tension in the muscle prevents it from bulging through the defect. The rim of the defect may readily be palpated.

Treatment. Ordinarily a careful, detailed explanation to the patient of the nature of his defect will suffice to reassure him and permit him to go on without further management. Occasionally, however, the condition is symptomatic enough that it causes disability by pain chronic in character involving the anterior tibial muscle. In these cases the defect is usually relatively small and there may be impingement of a portion of the muscle or soft tissue between the sharp edge of the fascia and edge of the bone. Here surgical interference is justified and consists in suture of the fascia to the tibia. This is successful if the sutured edge of fascial tissue is firm. Frequently, however, the edge of the fascia will be torn and effort to draw it to the tibia simply results in splitting it further. In this instance, extending the rent to a distance of 2 to 3 inches will give symptomatic relief so far as pain is concerned. The bulging will persist but its discrete character has been lost so that it no longer resembles a tumor mass.

EXOSTOSIS

There is no particular propensity toward traumatic exostoses in the leg. Although they frequently occur at the upper and lower ends of the tibia (Fig. 546) they are not frequent in its shaft. If they do occur they are managed as exostosis anywhere except that a much smaller exostosis will be symptomatic in a subcutaneous bone than in one surrounded completely by muscle. If the condition is symptomatic and cannot be handled by a simple protective pad, surgical excision should be entirely successful. Occasionally a small exostosis at the upper end of the tibia will lie directly under the pes anserinus. While a player is running, or more particularly, cutting, one of the tendons of the pes may snap over the exostosis and in fact may even catch on it and simulate lock-

ing or catching of the knee. Careful attention to the location of the tenderness and to the absence of knee symptoms will prevent an embarrassing error in diagnosis. The condition is readily relieved by removing the exostosis surgically.

FRACTURE

It is not our intention to relate in detail the treatment of fracture of the bones of the leg. The tibia and fibula are both very subject to fracture from unusual forces.

Tibial Fracture

Fracture of the tibia is not common as an athletic injury but does occur. A complete fracture of the tibia will be symptomatic enough that x-ray studies will be made and the condition readily determined. Needless to say, treatment should be prompt and definitive. Competition within a season would not be expected following a fracture of the tibia even though it were an incomplete one.

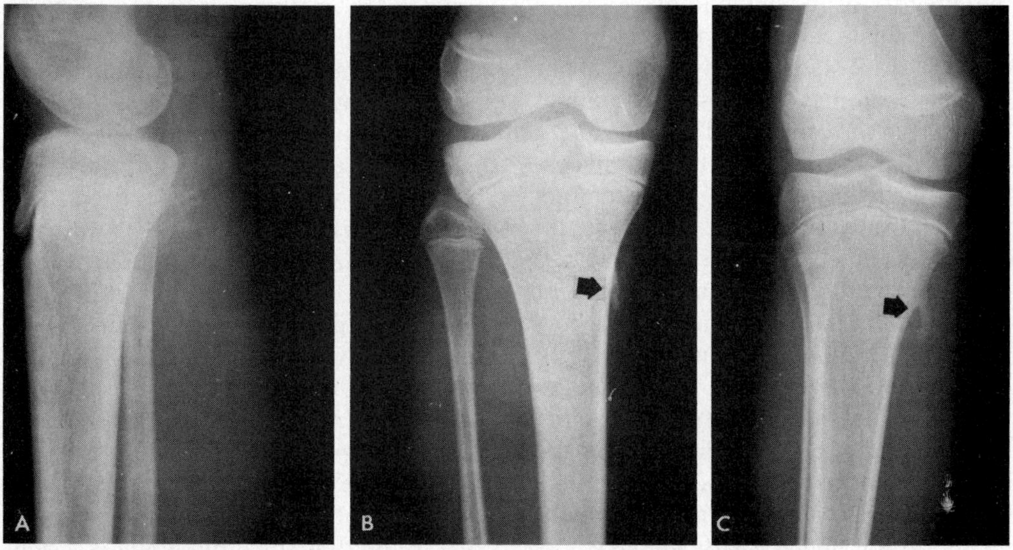

Figure 546. Exostosis of tibia. Note that the lateral view *(A)* is negative. The anteroposterior view *(B)* is inconclusive as to the nature of the mass, whereas the oblique *(C)* reveals the tumor very distinctly.

Fibular Fracture

Whereas fracture of the tibia is relatively infrequent in athletic injury, fracture of the fibula is relatively common. In any fracture of the fibula, one is obligated to rule out associated injury to the ankle joint and I shall categorically state that any time there is a complete fracture of the fibula (see Ankle, page 705) above the level of the lower tibiofibular syndesmosis one is obligated to rule out accompanying complete rupture of the inferior tibiofibular ligaments. This is without doubt the most serious, most important consideration in the fracture of the fibula. The actual fracture of the fibula is usually quite inconsequential except that it does require a certain period of healing, but if the fracture is accompanied by a rupture of the tibiofibular ligament with resulting instability in or separation of the ankle mortice (see Fig. 561), the outcome is a serious permanent disability. The condition is readily handled if it is recognized early and treated promptly. It is very difficult to handle as a reconstructive measure. So the first step in considering the fracture of the fibula is to determine the integrity of the ankle joint.

The fibula is subject to fracture by direct blow. This is usually in the lower one-third and may be caused by contact with a shoe or other hard object. There is immediate severe pain but not necessarily severe disability. Upon examination local tenderness will be present at the site of the injury. There may or may not be local crepitation. There is prompt swelling with localized hematoma formation. The individual can usually walk quite well, in fact, may complete the football game since in a fracture of the fibula by direct blow the integrity of the ankle is not involved and disability is due to contraction of the muscle attachments on the fibular shaft. Diagnosis is confirmed by x-ray study which should always be made in a case of localized tenderness over any bone.

Treatment consists of management of the localized area and protection of the part. If there is definite hematoma with localized swelling, aspiration under surgically aseptic technique and infiltration of hyaluronidase is of some value. These measures are ordinarily not necessary. After a short period of packing in ice or compression bandage the extremity should be placed in a walking boot which should be worn for about three weeks. Union will not then be complete but by this time it is usually possible to so strap the extremity that some degree of function may be resumed. At least activity may be permitted to the point of starting rehabilitation but nonparticipation in contact sports probably is advisable for as long as six to eight weeks. One has a quite effective indicator in the degree of the patient's discomfort.

Stress Fracture (Fatigue Fracture) (See Page 86)

The fibula is particularly prone to stress fracture (Fig. 547), being second only to the metatarsals in this respect. This condition arises early in the training period and appears as aching pain, soreness and some distress on function, usually localized near the neck of the fibula. There is no history of injury. Examination will reveal localized tenderness over the bone. Early x-ray will usually be negative. The patient will be treated for contusion or sprain. The complaint persists and remains quite localized. X-rays after 10 to 14 days will often reveal a transverse crack across the bone. Possibly callus formation will appear with no fracture line visible. The significance of stress fracture of the fibula is not as important as that in the foot since the fibula is a non-weight-bearing bone, but the patient

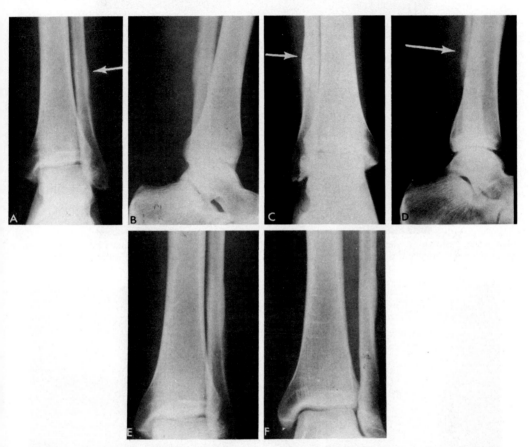

Figure 547. This boy was examined by a physician because of persistent pain in the lower fibula. X-ray was made (*A, B*) and he was advised that he had a malignant tumor and operation was scheduled. On seeing him in consultation a careful history elicited the fact that three weeks before he had sprinted off the curve of the track and up an incline and pulled up lame in his left leg. Two days later he ran in a race and had increased pain, particularly after the race. The pain and tenderness persisted but actually had seemed somewhat less in the past several days. He was advised that he probably had a stress fracture. The subsequent pictures (*C, D*) three weeks later show some increase in the extraperiosteal shadow but also some increased modeling. Meantime, the clinical symptoms had materially improved. Eight months later (*E, F*) the films show almost complete resolution. The patient had long been asymptomatic.

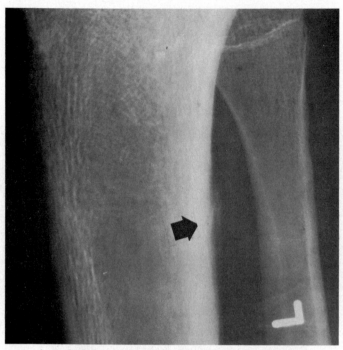

Figure 548.   Blown-up view of "fatigue" fracture of the tibia. Differential diagnosis here was of tumor because of no injury and the presence of severe aching pain. Time gave complete relief.

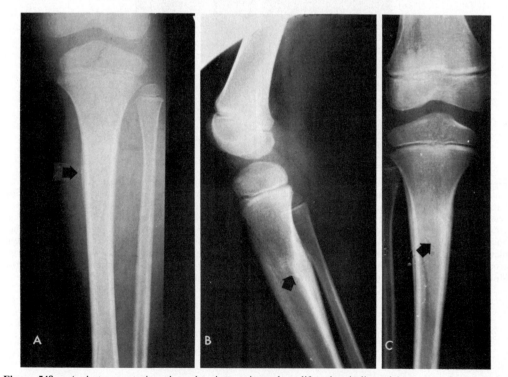

Figure 549.   *A*, Anteroposterior view showing periosteal proliferation indicated by arrow, four months after onset of pain. Patient had no specific injury. *B* and *C*, One month later, anteroposterior and lateral views show definite callus solidification at the fracture line.

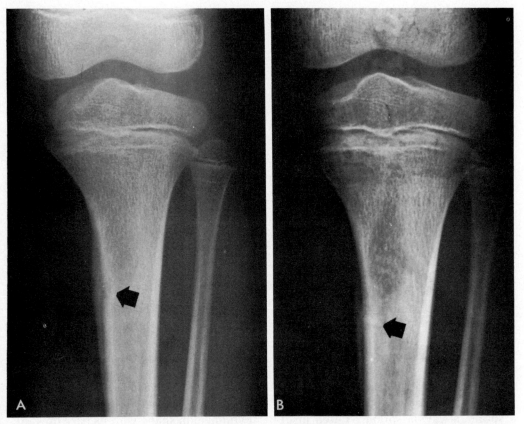

Figure 550. *A*, Four weeks following the onset of pain radiograph shows callus (indicated by arrow) with an indefinite line. *B*, Four weeks later radiograph shows the solidification of callus and obliteration of fracture line. This is a typical stress fracture which should not be confused with a tumor.

should be carefully rehabilitated lest he develop chronic muscular disability in the leg. Frequently by the time the fracture is found the time for immobilization will be past and treatment will be by careful muscular rehabilitation and other physical therapeutic measures such as local heat and muscular massage. Stress fracture of the tibia is not as frequent as of the fibula but it does occur principally in athletes (Figs. 548, 549 and 550). It is of necessity more disabling than in the fibula since the tibia is a weight-bearing bone. When the fracture is recognized a protective cast should be applied until union has progressed to the point of good stability with no pain.

CHAPTER 20

INJURIES OF THE ANKLE

ANATOMICAL CONSIDERATIONS

Injuries to the ankle joint are the most common conditions encountered in the treatment of injuries to the athlete. There is no doubt that many ankle injuries are treated overcasually, which may account for the expression "Once a sprain, always a sprain." Often insufficient consideration has been given to the exact nature of the damage in the individual case. In order to be able to treat intelligently any injury of the ankle joint, a definitive diagnosis must be made. This predicates a working knowledge of the anatomy of the region involved.

Let us consider those anatomic characteristics of the ankle joint that have a direct bearing on the type of injury that occurs in response to various forces applied (Figs. 551, 552 and 553). The ankle joint is functionally a hinge joint having motion in only one plane—flexion and extension. The bony structure is designed as a mortice and tenon with considerable inherent stability (Fig. 551). The mortice is formed by the lateral malleolus, the undersurface of the tibia and the medial malleolus. The tenon is the body of the talus which is shaped to fit snugly into the mortice.

It should be noted that the lateral malleolus is longer than the medial malleolus. Its distal tip extends to the bottom of the talus at the level of the talocalcaneal joint. It is roughly rectangular in outline but actually somewhat narrower at the level of the lower end of the tibia. The medial malleolus, on the other hand, is short and thick, being roughly pyramidal in shape with its base upward.

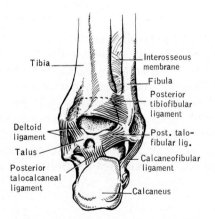

Figure 551. Anatomical drawing of ankle, posterior view, showing the tibiofibular ligament which is heavy distally, thinning out to become the interosseous membrane proximally. The posterior and lateral fasciculi of the lateral collateral ligament and the posterior and medial fasciculi of the medial collateral ligament are shown. Note the different lengths of the two malleoli. The guide line indicates top of dome of talus.

698

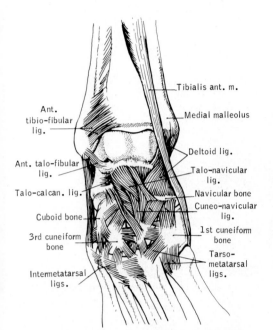

Ant. tibio-fibular lig.

Tibialis ant. m.

Medial malleolus

Deltoid lig.

Ant. talo-fibular lig.

Talo-navicular lig.

Talo-calcan. lig.

Navicular bone

Cuneo-navicular lig.

Cuboid bone

1st cuneiform bone

3rd cuneiform bone

Tarso-metatarsal ligs.

Intermetatarsal ligs.

Figure 552. Anatomical drawing of ankle, anterior view. Note massive deltoid ligament and very weak anterior talofibular ligament. Note no ligament from front of tibia to top of talus. The joint capsule has been removed.

Its distal tip extends only halfway down on the body of the talus.

The distal tibia and fibula are bound together by the anterior and posterior tibiofibular ligaments which are really thickened expansions of the interosseous membrane that fastens the two bones together throughout their length. Although some motion is present in the syndesmosis between the tibia and fibula at the lower end, there is to all practical purposes complete stability between the two bones. Definite motion has been demonstrated in the distal tibiofibular syndesmosis so that a certain amount of disability occurs from ankylosis between the tibia and fibula at the ankle joint. Thus, the ankle joint has stability from two sources: first, the mortice and tenon bony structure, and second, the extensive investiture of ligaments that surround the joint.

The ligaments are thin fore and aft (capsule) to permit flexion and extension of the joint, but on each side the ligaments become heavier and stronger as the tibial and fibular collateral ligaments. The medial collateral, or deltoid, ligament is particularly strong, has a very broad attachment to the internal malleolus and extends downward in many bands to become intimately connected to the ligaments supporting the arch of the foot. In addition to stabilizing the ankle joint on the medial side, it serves to support the arch and hence is a doubly vital structure.

It is possible to dissect the lateral collateral ligament into many separate ligaments but there are three primary fasciculi: (1) one running forward to attach to the talus anteriorly (anterior talofibular), to attach to the lateral margin of the nonarticular portion of the body of the talus just in front of the articular surface; (2) another backward to attach to the posterior portion of the talus (posterior talofibular), again just adjacent to the articular surface on the nonarticular portion near the top of the bone; and (3) one directly downward to attach to the calcaneus (calcaneofibular), bypassing the talus, the second and stronger branch passing from the talus directly to the fibula. These ligaments also blend into the lateral ligaments of the foot, extending forward onto the cuboid and to the base of the fifth metatarsal. Together the medial and lateral ligaments, acting in conjunction with the two malleoli, serve to prevent lateral instability at the ankle joint.

The long lateral malleolus, acting with the medial ligament, prevents excess motion to the outer side. The length of the lateral malleolus firmly holds the body of the talus so that lateral motion in the tarsus is more restricted than is medial motion. A normal range of flexion-extension is permitted with its axis at the tip of the medial malleolus.

The body of the talus is not rectan-

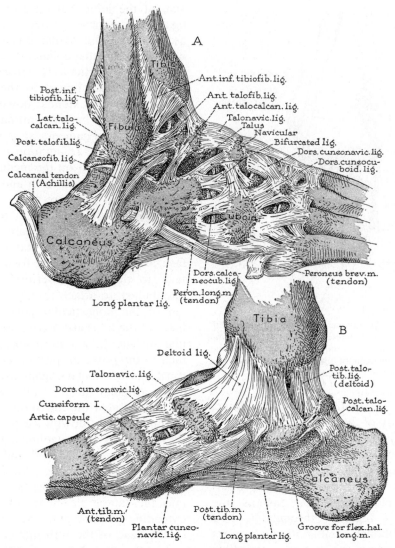

Figure 553. Ligaments of the ankle and foot. *A,* Lateral side. Note very weak lateral ligaments. Distal end of fibula is at level of talocalcaneal joint. *B,* Medial side. Note massive deltoid ligament and short medial malleolus. Deltoid ligament extends down over medial side to support arch. The calcaneal tendon has been removed in *B.* (From Jones and Shepard, A Manual of Surgical Anatomy, p. 116.)

gular in its general shape. The anterior portion of the body is distinctly wider than the posterior portion so that, as the foot goes into dorsiflexion, the wider part of the talus is forced between the two malleoli and the ankle is very stable in this position. As the foot goes into plantar flexion the narrower part of the body of the talus moves into the mortice and some lateral instability results in this position, predisposing to injury. It also adds distinctly to the mobility of the foot so that with the foot in equinus there is definite lateral motion in the ankle joint, whereas with the foot in dorsiflexion there is no lateral motion. On dorsiflexion of the foot the fibula is forced away from the tibia and injury may result. On forcible dorsiflexion of the foot the anterior edge of the tibia nestles into the sulcus between the head and body of the talus. The anterior inferior angle of the tibia inclines slightly backward in order to prevent direct impingement between the talus and the tibia. As the foot dorsiflexes and everts, the talus is driven forcibly against the lateral malleolus. These factors are of considerable importance in the study of injuries to the ankle.

The two malleoli are subcutaneous and as such are subject to direct injury. The posterior tibial and flexor hallucis tendons medially and the peroneal tendons laterally lie in very intimate association with the back of the medial and the lateral malleolus respectively, whereas the dorsiflexors of the foot have a much less intimate relationship to the osseous structures in front of the ankle.

CONTUSION

There is nothing particularly significant in contusion about the ankle. The contusion is usually to one or the other malleolus. The most critical factor is accurate diagnosis of the injury. Once it has been confirmed that a contusion, and not a fracture or a sprain, is present the treatment is simple. A few words of caution: in many sprains the maximum tenderness will be on the malleolus itself. A negative x-ray does not necessarily mean that the injury is a contusion only. An incomplete or fissure type fracture may simulate a contusion and one should be suspicious of the condition that is particularly slow to heal or causes pain on function. In an ordinary contusion of the ankle, ankle function is disturbed very little unless there has been a severe crushing injury of the soft tissues. A blow over the tendo Achilles may lead to tenosynovitis complicating a contusion. A blow over the peroneal tendons may actually dislocate them from the groove—an injury very much

more serious than simple contusion. These facts suggest that a careful examination should be made to eliminate other possible injuries before treatment for contusion is initiated.

Treatment is the same as for contusion elsewhere: aspiration of the hematoma, local injection (hyaluronidase), compression, cold packs to be followed in a few hours by heat. Immobilization and support per se are not necessary. Protective appliances such as sponge rubber or felt doughnuts are useful. Rehabilitation should be rapid and athletic participation is not unduly interfered with.

STRAIN

The area of the ankle joint is subject to strain perhaps more than any other area in the body. This is due to several factors. In the first place the ankle is a weight-bearing joint and in the athlete is subject to very dynamic forces as a result of the explosive character of its motion under certain circumstances. The broad jumper, for example, not only takes off with a terrific drive but on landing forces both feet into extreme dorsiflexion with resultant strain on the tendo Achilles. This strain may occur either at the attachment of the tendon to the calcaneus or frequently at the musculotendinous junction, occasionally along the course of the tendon. It is frequently complicated by tenosynovitis. Another tendon particularly subject to strain is the anterior tibial. A most annoying disability can arise from strain of this tendon at its attachment to the medial side of the foot. The posterior tibial tendon is unusually vulnerable because of its dual role in supporting the arch of the foot and in supplying plantar flexion and inversion. A frequent problem is a tendinitis at its attachment to the tuberosity of the navicular, or under the navicular in the arch of the foot. Switching from street shoes, which have a heel and a firm medial support with a strong counter, to athletic shoes, which, as a rule, have no heels, minimal support and very little counter, can cause a static strain which is very difficult to handle. The tenderness occurs at the medial border of the arch. Pain and aching may spread around under the arch of the foot and back of the medial malleolus. The peroneal tendons are much less frequently strained since the nature of the activity of the ankle does not require such forcible use of the everters as of the other muscles of the ankle. So it can be seen that strain does not involve the ankle joint proper. It involves the many dynamic forces through the muscle tendon units which encompass the lower leg and foot.

Treatment of the acute condition is rest of the muscle involved, local heat, injection with a local anesthetic, and protection against further injury. The proper degree of protection may be very difficult to decide. Since the condition involves the integrity of the muscle it is obvious that the strain cannot be well protected while activity of the muscle is permitted. An attempt to shorten the treatment period often results in prompt recurrence of the disability and the situation may become quite frustrating to the doctor—doubly so to the athlete. Certain protective measures can be used, however, the general rule being that no function should be allowed that causes pain. In sprain of the tendo Achilles, for example, the pain may be caused mainly by overstretching of the tendon and this can be prevented by adequate strapping to prevent hyperdorsiflexion of the foot (Fig. 542). With such protection the athlete may be able to jog or even run at a relatively steady pace but should not be allowed to charge out of the blocks or to jump or to hurdle. In short, he

should do nothing that requires explosive activity of the muscle. Ordinarily the condition will require at least ten days of relative inactivity and sometimes much more than this. Unrestricted activity should be permitted only when it is entirely pain-free. Since pain is a relative thing it may be very difficult in a given case to decide just when unrestricted activity will be safe. If the strain involves the posterior tibial tendon, a well-fitted arch support may be a useful adjunct. After a period of taping (Fig. 554) to slightly invert the foot and support the arch, a flexible arch support should be used the rest of the season, particularly when the athlete is wearing athletic shoes.

TENOSYNOVITIS

Tenosynovitis is quite frequent about the ankle and, as indicated in the above section, frequently follows strain. Tenosynovitis can result from contusion or infection but at the ankle the most common cause is overuse of the tendon. This causes irritation between the tendon and surrounding tissues with resulting loss of the smooth gliding pattern. The significant findings are pain on motion of the tendon particularly under tension, "snowball crepitation" on motion, tenderness along the involved area, local heat and redness and other signs of inflammatory reaction. Differentiation between tenosynovitis and strain may be extremely difficult, but since their treatment is quite similar this is not a vital problem. In fact, the two often coexist. When they do the condition becomes more resistant to treatment.

Treatment should be prompt. Complete rest of the involved tendon together with the use of a long-acting local anesthetic is indicated. Extreme care should be taken that this is injected around the tendon and not into it. If it is impossible to be sure you

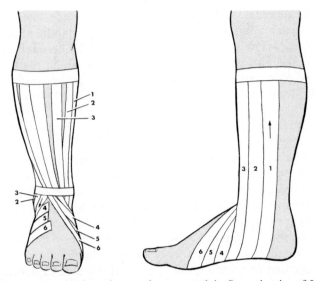

Figure 554. Drawing shows a classic arch strapping on an adult. Several strips of 2.5-cm. adhesive tape will be necessary. Strip 1 starts at just above the lateral malleolus and passes under the heel and up the inner side of the foot to above the bulge of the calf. Strips 2, 3 and 4 pass up the leg in a similar course; the number of strips used depends somewhat on the size of the leg. As the strip reaches the front of the ankle it is then twisted across the front of the leg to the lateral side. Five or six strips are utilized with the arch strapping extending clear up and forward to the base of the head of the metatarsals. Strips are anchored at the calf and above the ankle with one or more circumferential strips. If the injured arch is high, a felt pad should be inserted under the arch and held in place by short strips of tape, particularly if a flat support shoe is worn. This felt pad is probably not necessary in a shoe having a heel and a good support.

are in the tendon sheath, injection should not be carried out. There is a certain resistance given to injection into a tendon which is quite different from that of the sheath, so if you encounter any resistance at all in the injection it should be discontinued. Local injection of anesthetic agents should not lull one into the conclusion that the inflammation has subsided, since return to function under these circumstances will result in prompt exacerbation of the condition. Local injection is of value as a measure of active treatment, not as a means of rehabilitation. Athletic participation is extremely difficult in cases of tenosynovitis of the ankle since the only real way to prevent motion of the tendons of the ankle is to immobilize the ankle and this is not consistent with ordinary athletic endeavor. As rehabilitation progresses, protective measures should be designed to prevent extremes

of motion in the involved tendon. If the heel cord is involved, strapping to prevent dorsiflexion will help (Fig. 542). If the anterior tibial or posterior tibial tendon is involved, strapping in inversion in the early stage (Fig. 554) and later a properly fitted arch support or wedging the shoe on the medial border of the sole and heel will serve to eliminate some of the static stress of this condition.

Tenosynovitis is more likely to be disastrous to a season's play than strain but for the same reason, namely, a marked tendency toward recurrence. The track man who develops a tenosynovitis running on the boards in the winter will frequently have a very ineffectual season since, when he puts out his maximum effort, he is likely to be pulled up short by recurrence of his tenosynovitis. As in so many other instances, early adequate treatment is the very best insurance of success. A period of complete nonparticipation may well be followed by a highly successful season, whereas an attempt to continue athletics in spite of pain and discomfort can result only in continued ineffectual activity.

My best recommendation for treatment in severe acute tenosynovitis in the tendo Achilles or anterior tibial is a period of elevation and hot packs until the acute tenderness has disappeared, followed by application of a walking boot cast to be worn for a period of 10 to 14 days. By this time the symptoms will have largely subsided and adequate strapping can be applied to permit gradual return to function. Protective strapping should be continued for several weeks until one is sure there is no real likelihood of recurrence. The strapping must be specifically designed to protect the tendon involved. Great care must be taken that the adhesive straps do not actually constrict the tendon and so make the condition worse. For anterior or posterior tibial strain the strips should start on the lateral border of the dorsum of the foot, pass under the sole of the foot and swing under the arch and up the medial aspect of the leg (Fig. 554). They are applied with the foot in neutral flexion and slightly inverted.

To support the tendo Achilles the foot should be strapped in plantar flexion (Fig. 542).

DISLOCATION OR SUBLUXATION OF THE PERONEAL TENDONS

A condition unique to the ankle area is dislocation or subluxation of the peroneal tendons. This condition may be acute or chronic.

Acute

In the acute condition the history usually is of a blow back of the lateral malleolus while the peroneal tendons are taut in dorsiflexion and eversion of the foot. The peroneal retinaculum gives way. One or both of the tendons pop out of the groove onto the lateral side of the malleolus. They usually spontaneously reduce. One may confuse this condition with an ankle sprain. Careful history and physical examination will eliminate the confusion, however. Tenderness is directly over the peroneal tendons and it may be confused with tenosynovitis. Indeed, tenosynovitis may be a sequel. In the acute case, it is usually not possible to displace the tendons at examination.

If the diagnosis of an acute dislocation is made, the *treatment* is surgical. Incision posteriorly along the peroneal groove and replacement of the tendons with resuture of the torn or redundant retinaculum may be effective. In many cases there will be a shallow peroneal groove which predisposes to this condition. In this instance, repair should be accompanied by deepening of the groove in order to make the tendons more secure. If the groove is to be deepened, the tendons are displaced forward in order to expose the furrow behind the fibula. With a very sharp osteotome a thin flexible layer of bone is elevated from the posterior fibula beginning on the lateral margin and extending to the medial edge. Care should be taken not to detach the medial margin of the cut. It is important that this thin strip of bone including the fibrocartilage of the peroneal groove should remain attached on the medial side. This may be retracted medially while the furrow is deepened beneath it. This flap includes the smooth membrane which overlies the fibula and forms the floor of the peroneal groove. After this layer is carefully reflected from laterally to medially, the underlying bed is scooped out with a sharp gouge until a smooth deep furrow is formed large enough to contain the tendons. The reflected flap is placed back over the raw bone and sutured down through drill holes in the fibula if necessary to make a smooth bed for the peroneal tendon. The redundant sheath is plicated over the tendons in order to make a strong roof. If the tissue seems too redundant or too inadequate, a strip of periosteum can be resected up from the tibia and pulled back over to help support the roof of the groove. This completes the tunnel. Following surgery, fixation in a stirrup splint for two weeks, then a walking cast for four weeks, will give adequate protection. Active athletics should not be permitted before eight weeks, however.

Chronic

Chronic or recurrent subluxation of the peroneal tendons may be congenital or it may follow an acute episode that was untreated. In the latter instance there will be a history of acute injury with considerable soreness for many weeks, followed by recurrent episodes of feeling something slipping out of place at the back of the ankle, with or without sharp pain. These episodes occur as the athlete everts the foot with tendons tight. They are quite distressing. The tendons slip back into position and all is well until the next episode. Careful history will usually disclose the original accident and the patient can describe the recurrent ones quite graphically. Physical examination will usually demonstrate the shallow groove with thickening of the retinaculum. The tendons often can be slipped completely or partially out of the groove on manual manipulation.

This condition should be treated by surgical reconstruction of the groove and repair of the retinaculum, suitably reinforced by adjacent tissue. The groove should be reconstructed as indicated in the discussion on Acute Dislocation, taking particular care to obtain further soft tissue from the tibial periosteum or even a strip of tendo Achilles in order to

get a very substantial roof over the groove. This is a very successful type of reconstruction. This should give prompt relief but eight weeks of immobilization will be needed to insure stability.

SYNOVIAL HERNIA

Synovial hernia about the ankle will be discussed in the section dealing with the condition in the foot (page 759).

SPRAIN-DISLOCATION-FRACTURE

In injuries to the ankle there is such a close association of these conditions, namely, sprain-dislocation-fracture, that it is unwise to place them in separate categories. This is particularly true in the athlete since the same forces may well cause a combination of injuries. Resultant pathology may be determined more by the strength and duration of the forces causing the injury than by the exact type of stress. In the athlete the injury is usually caused by stress forces which may result in either a sprain, a dislocation, a fracture, or all three at the same time.

MECHANICS OF INJURY

Since the ankle is functionally a hinge joint normally permitting only dorsal and plantar flexion, it follows that injuries to the ankle are primarily due to lateral stresses that force the ankle through an arc of motion which it does not normally possess. Less frequently they are due to hyperflexion or hyperextension. The injuries due to lateral stresses may readily be divided into two categories, namely, inversion injuries and eversion injuries.

Inversion Injury

Inversion injuries to the ankle (Fig. 555) are as a rule not due to pure inver-

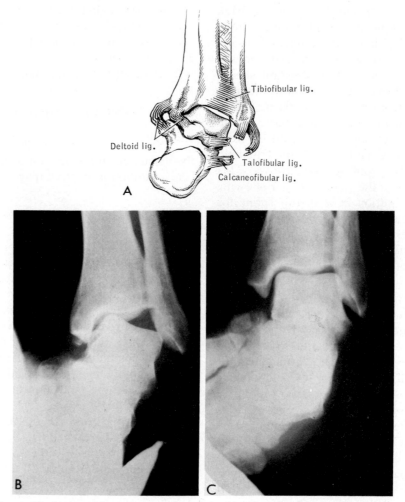

Figure 555. *A*, Mechanics of inversion injury of the ankle. Drawing showing talus rolling over medial malleolus. *B*, Inversion injury showing complete severance of the lateral collateral ligament permitting the talus to roll over the medial malleolus. There is no fracture. The ossicle on the medial side is the os trigonum. *C*, The same stress on a normal ankle.

sion. The force usually consists of inversion, internal rotation and plantar flexion of the foot in relation to the leg so that the foot is inverted and the ankle and leg are thrown to the outer side. It will be noted that the push is against the medial malleolus and that the pull is away from the lateral malleolus. As the foot inverts in relation to the leg, strain is put upon the lateral collateral ligament, which is the ligament primarily constructed to restrict this motion. As a result of this overinversion the ligament will tear slightly, partially or completely according to the severity of the force. If the inverting force continues as the lateral ligament gives way, the ankle "opens up" on the lateral side and the talus is forcibly thrust against the medial malleolus. The medial malleolus, being short and stubby and extending no more than halfway down the vertical height of the body of the talus, will act as a fulcrum with its tip impinging against the central portion of the medial face of the talus. The talus thus rotates over the malleolus rather than pushes it off. In such a case the injury will probably be confined to the lateral side and there will be more or less complete laceration of the lateral collateral ligaments. It is unusual for this type of force to break off the lateral malleolus in the athlete. In the elderly person in whom the bone is brittle and fragile, the lateral malleolus may break rather than the ligament tear. If this same inversion force is continued as the talus is driven against the medial malleolus, the latter may break off. In this instance the fracture line will ordinarily extend more or less vertically up the shaft of the tibia beginning at the lateral margin of the medial malleolus (Fig. 556, A). There is injury on both sides of the ankle. This may be a bimalleolar fracture or perhaps a fracture of the medial malleolus plus an avulsion of the lateral collateral ligament (Fig. 556). If

the x-ray shows a vertical fracture of the medial malleolus as in Figure 556, B, one must presume that the lateral components are torn until proven otherwise. Open repair of the torn lateral ligaments with screw fixation of the medial malleolus is recommended.

Approximately 85 per cent of all injuries to the ankle are inversion injuries and are confined to ligament injury, so-called sprain or "sprain-fracture" of the ankle (Fig. 557). The vast majority of these may be classified as mild (first degree) sprains without any particular loss of function of the ligament. If the force is violent, other fractures may occur such as fracture of the superomedial portion of the talus and fracture of the back of the articular surface of the tibia, but as a rule injury is confined to the ligament injury on the lateral side with occasional instances of avulsion fracture of the tip of the fibula or "push-off" fracture of the medial malleolus.

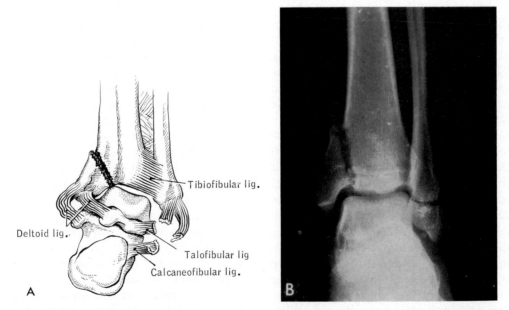

Deltoid lig.

Tibiofibular lig.

Talofibular lig

Calcaneofibular lig.

A

B

Figure 556. Inversion injury of the ankle. *A,* Drawing showing vertical fracture of the medial malleolus, with a split up the shaft and complete tear of the lateral ligament witn no fibular fracture. *B,* Another inversion injury. The talus pushed the medial malleolus off instead of rolling over it and the fibula was fractured. This should be treated by reduction and internal fixation.

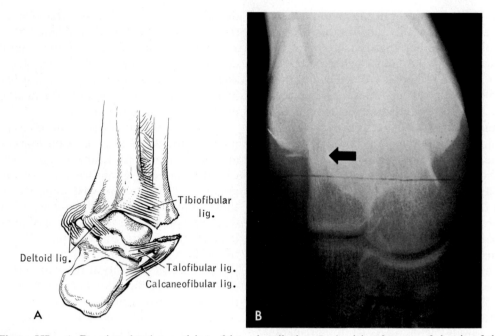

Figure 557. *A,* Drawing showing avulsion of lateral malleolus. *B,* Avulsion fracture of the tip of the lateral malleolus by inversion injury, so-called sprain fracture. The fragment will usually be smaller than is shown in the drawing.

Eversion Injury

If the opposite force is applied and the foot is carried outward in relationship to the leg, the talus is forced laterally and into dorsiflexion (Fig. 558). The anatomic difference between the two malleoli becomes doubly significant here. Whereas on the medial side the malleolus is short and the talus may rotate over it, on the lateral side the malleolus is at least as long as the height of the talus so that it is extremely difficult for the talus to rotate over the lateral malleolus with the malleolar tip as the fulcrum. In eversion force, the push being toward the lateral side, the talus is driven forcibly against the lateral malleolus and severe pressure is applied to the malleolus before overstress of the short medial collateral ligament occurs since it can permit some degree of lateral tilting of the talus. This stress applied to the lateral malleolus may cause one of several types of injuries but all

are due to the same forces. Perhaps the most common injury is fracture of the fibula somewhere below the level of the lower end of the tibia, resulting in a single malleolar fracture (Figs. 559 and 560). This may occur without significant damage to the deltoid ligament but it is more often accompanied by a rupture of this ligament. This same force may actually drive the fibula away from the tibia after rupturing the tibiofibular ligament and so permit separation of the ankle mortice (Fig. 561). In this instance as the force continues, the medial collateral ligament having given way, the tibiofibular ligaments having torn, the fibula is driven further away from the tibia and the fibula may break anywhere along its length. The common location of the break is somewhere in its lower third. If a fibular fracture appears above the level of the ankle joint, one must assume that the tibiofibular ligament has been torn and that the integrity of the ankle mortice has been lost until proven

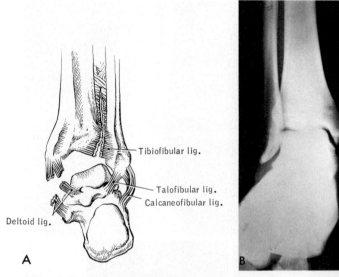

Figure 558. A, Drawing of eversion injury of the ankle. The talus pushes the fibula laterally, rupturing the tibiofibular ligament. The fibula may break at any level above the tibiofibular ligament. The medial collateral ligament is torn. B, X-ray showing normal ankle. C, Eversion injury. Eversion stress would displace the talus further. Severe example of this same injury is shown in Figure 566. There may be no fracture or the fibula may break anywhere in its distal half—usually just above the tibiofibular ligament.

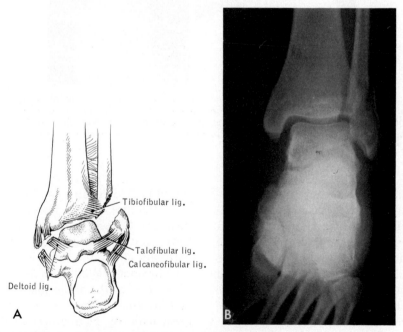

Figure 559. A, Eversion injury, showing fractured fibula without separation of ankle mortice. Note rupture of the deltoid ligament. Tibiofibular ligament is intact. B, X-ray of injury shown in drawing. Note the vertical direction of the fracture line of the fibula, typical of the push-off injury. The deltoid ligament must be repaired and internal fixation of the fibula done. In this instance, with the tibiofibular ligament intact, pin or rod fixation in the fibula will suffice.

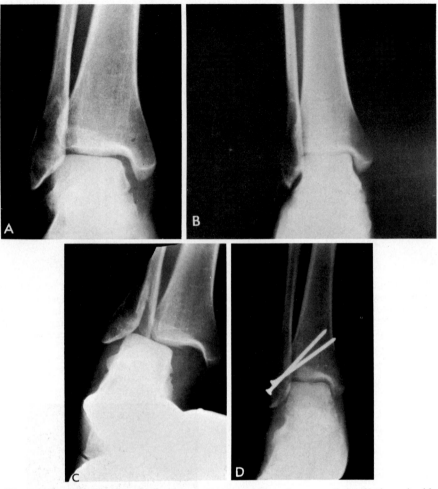

Figure 560. *A,* "As is" picture without stress showing oblique fracture of the fibula and widening of the ankle mortice. *B,* Carefully positioned anteroposterior view shows no pathologic change. *C,* Lateral stress reproducing displacement which occurred at the time of the injury. Note the tibiofibular ligament is intact. *D,* Repair of the deltoid ligament and fixation of the fibula by transfixion screws. Note in this picture the fracture line has again disappeared.

otherwise. This is an extremely important point from the standpoint of treatment. Before this stress laterally is sufficient to push the fibula away from the tibia, something must give way on the medial side of the foot. This may consist in laceration of the medial collateral (deltoid) ligament or an avulsion of the medial malleolus.

Another common injury is the *bimalleolar fracture* (Figs. 562 and 563), namely, fracture of both malleoli at or below the level of the lower end of the tibia. This is also an eversion injury. If a fracture of the lower end of the fibula is observed at the level of the lower end of the tibia, one should very carefully check the integrity of the deltoid ligament. While the great majority of injuries of the ankle joint are sprains and are the result of inversion injury, a great majority of fractures of the ankle are of the lateral malleolus and are caused by lateral angulation, eversion and external rotation.

From the description of the me-

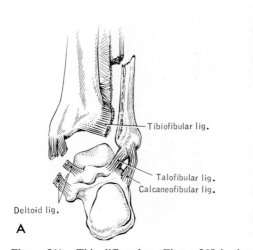

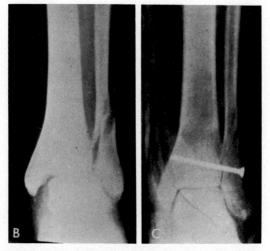

Tibiofibular lig.

Talofibular lig.
Calcaneofibular lig.

Deltoid lig.

A

B

C

Figure 561. This differs from Figure 560 in that the fracture is higher in the fibula and the tibiofibular ligament is ruptured. *A*, Eversion injury. Fracture of fibula in which fibula is actually pushed off with separation of ankle mortice and rupture of the tibiofibular ligament.

B, X-ray of same injury. Rupture of the medial ligament, separation of the tibiofibular ligament, lateral displacement of the talus, fracture of the fibula above the level of the joint. This fracture cannot occur without rupture of the medial ligament and almost always of the tibiofibular ligament.

C, After repair of the medial ligament and fixation of the fibula to the tibia.

chanics of injury it becomes quite apparent that it is of great importance in any individual case to determine if possible the type of forces involved and so be able to forecast to some extent the area upon which the strain is to be expected.

Dorsiflexion Injury

Characteristically, the eversion injury is some combination of eversion, external rotation and dorsiflexion. Thus, strictly speaking, the dorsiflexion injury is a type of eversion injury, but it is so frequent that it merits individual description. As was indicated in the description of the anatomy of the ankle, the talus is broad in front and narrow behind. As the foot is pushed into dorsiflexion, the broad part of the talus seats firmly between the two malleoli and this stress is readily supported by the distal tibiofibular ligament. If the force continues or if some eversion

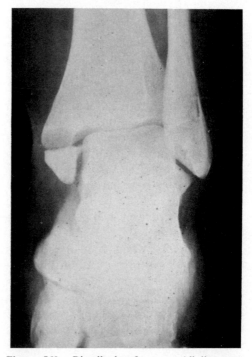

Figure 562. Bimalleolar fracture. All ligaments intact. This should be treated by replacement of the medial malleolus and internal fixation. In this case no treatment was necessary on the lateral side of the ankle, since the fibula is relatively stable by virtue of its intact periosteum. In many cases fibular fixation is advisable (see Fig. 572).

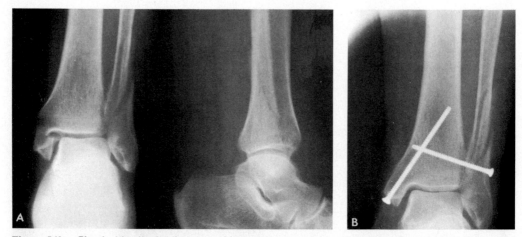

Figure 563. Classic bimalleolar fracture with eversion type injury. Note *(A)* the complete fracture of the medial malleolus which is displaced laterally. Note the oblique fracture of the lateral malleolus, a little higher than usual but still quite typical. Note also that the tibiofibular ligament, although partially torn where it attaches to the distal fragment of the fibula, has remained intact to the proximal fragment of the fibula and the interosseous membrane so that there is complete stability of the fibula. This is properly treated as a bimalleolar fracture *(B)* by reduction of the malleolar fracture, by internal malleolar fracture fixation with a long screw, and by immobilization of the distal fragment of the fibula by transfixion screw through the tibia. It is better for each of these screws to transverse the opposite cortex. View *B* was made the day after the injury. Note the complete disappearance of the fracture line because of the obliquity of the fracture of the tibia.

component thrusts the talus more forcibly against the fibula, the result is unusual strain against this ligament, which binds the two bones together. This same force puts tension against the musculotendinous unit of the calf and may result in strain or actual rupture of this mechanism. Far more frequently the dorsiflexion simply springs the tibia and fibula apart, the force is resolved, the two bones fall back together and the disability does not seem to be severe. Simple dorsiflexion probably will not avulse the ligament completely.

Symptoms. The patient presents himself with a rather indefinite history. He may be able to say that his foot was pushed too far in dorsiflexion. Usually, he cannot be sure. He noticed that he experienced pain at the ankle and this subsided as the foot came down into the normal position. Contrary to the ordinary sprain of the ankle, local swelling is not manifested because the hemorrhage occurs deep in the leg and is not readily detectable under the skin. This is the patient who continues to play, tries to run, who has increasing pain and discomfort as he increases his activities. He may be able to run well at a normal pace but if he puts the pressure on, he will notice pain in the ankle. He will often be able to associate this pain with dorsiflexion of the foot.

Examination reveals a moderate degree of swelling with some fullness in the area back of the lateral malleolus, between it and the tendo Achilles. Palpation directly along the sulcus between the tibia and fibula will demonstrate tenderness posteriorly and anteriorly. The findings at this stage are ordinarily not marked, however, unless the injury has been a severe one. On manipulation of the foot ordinary motion is free and pain-free. Inversion and eversion do not cause pain. Pain will be elicited on complete dorsiflexion of the foot, particularly with the knee flexed to relax the calf. These symptoms are very similar to those of talotibial exostosis, the distinction being that, in the sprain, pain is usually tibiofibular while in the exostosis it is ordinarily in front of the ankle. The two conditions may coexist. If the injury seems severe an x-ray should be taken with the foot sharply dorsiflexed and slightly everted. If this now shows any tibiofibular displacement, as compared with a similar view of the opposite ankle, it indicates that there has been a complete tear of the tibiofibular ligament.

Treatment. Early attention to this injury will result in prompt recovery in the moderate (first or second degree) sprain since it is relatively easy to protect the injured part and even permit a fairly high degree of activity. Measures designed to prevent dorsiflexion, such as strapping of the foot (Fig. 542) and the use of an elevated heel on the shoe, will be effective. The foot should be strapped so that dorsiflexion cannot take place even under very severe stress. In too many instances the condition is minimized by both player and physician and only after weeks of frustration is the true nature of the injury recognized.

If the injury is third degree (severe), treatment must be much more comprehensive. In this case if an anteroposterior view of the ankle, made when the patient is standing, does not show separation at the tibiofibular synchondrosis, as compared to the opposite side, one may treat this condition by plaster immobilization. Posterior and lateral boot stirrup splints should be used with no weight bearing until the swelling is well controlled. Then a boot cast with a walking heel should be worn for at least four weeks post-injury. At this time if the symptoms seem to be minimal, a very adequate strapping may be substituted. This must be continued for at least another four weeks, and longer if active participation of athletics is initiated at that time.

If there is any question about the separation, an oblique view should be made of each ankle in addition to views made in sharp dorsiflexion. If any of these views show a separation between the tibia and fibula, surgical treatment will be much more effective. It is relatively simple to place a transfixion screw through the fibula and across both cortices of the tibia just above the level of the tibiofibular joint through a small lateral incision over the shaft of the fibula. This will maintain continuity of the ankle mortice and so prevent instability of this joint. It goes without saying that the reduction must be complete at the time the screw is placed. This screw should be removed later (eight weeks) in order to permit motion in the tibiofibular joint.

If reduction cannot be carried out under anesthesia, an incision must be made in order to free the space between the tibia and fibula before the fixation is inserted. Although the fibula is situated somewhat posteriorly, visualization is more easily and completely obtained by an anterior approach since this will not disturb the peroneal tendons. A vertical incision, right over the syndesmosis, just lateral to the peroneus tertius tendon, permits ready access to the area with no vital structure involved. It is extremely important that all of the soft tissue debris be trimmed away with minimum disturbance of the bone since a fusion across this syndesmosis is not desirable.

The dorsiflexion injury accounts for the relatively high incidence of ossification noted between the tibia and fibula in x-rays of the ankle, since ossification is prone to occur where chronic irritation takes place (Figs. 564 and 565). The late manifestation of this chronic condition may be quite discouraging. I do not believe there is real justification for removing the ossification unless there is separation between the tibia and fibula or intractable pain on function making it advisable to restore the ankle

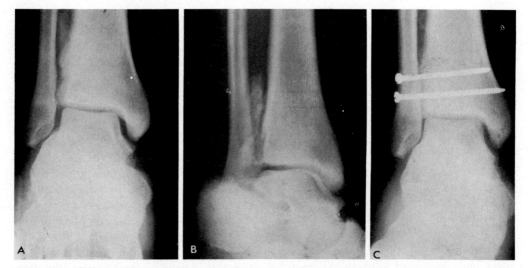

Figure 564. College athlete who had a dorsiflexion injury apparently resulting in a mild sprain. Inadequate treatment which did not prevent dorsiflexion resulted in persistent pain and repeated, unsatisfactory efforts to return to football. The player could not run all out. At the season's end, more thorough study revealed the true nature of the condition with ossification of the tibiofibular ligament over a considerable space. There was mild diastasis. Removal of the bone and screw fixation for eight weeks resulted in improvement but some symptoms persisted.

    A, Anteroposterior view showing slight tibiofibular diastasis with ossification.

    B, Oblique view revealing the extent of the bone deposit and diastasis.

    C, Postoperative view showing reduction of the diastasis and fixation.

mortice. Probably conservative treatment is better in the ordinary case of ossification. The foot should be carefully strapped to prevent the motion causing the pain.

DIAGNOSIS

History. Since the forces that cause ankle injuries are of such significance in the resulting damage, one must determine, if possible, the exact mechanics of the injury. Was the foot inverted or everted? How did the accident occur? Was disability immediate? Is disability the result of swelling and edema? Was there a primary deformity which was corrected by the patient, a friend or the x-ray technician before making the picture? How long ago did the injury occur? What was the treatment? Has heat or cold been applied? All these factors give important leads, not only as to

the type and location of injury but as to its severity. They may be invaluable guides to the treatment indicated.

Examination. Examination of the injured ankle should be preceded by careful examination of the opposite leg in order that a normal may be obtained for comparison. One then proceeds with a meticulous but extremely gentle examination of the involved extremity. If one begins by simple observation, he can obtain the confidence of the apprehensive patient and with it more detailed information. Observation will reveal deformity, the location and amount of swelling, the degree of tension in the skin, and the extent of circulatory impairment. Following observation, by careful palpation one can determine the tension and the degree of swelling. There may be obvious bony crepitation on careful palpation through the skin. Then, by gentle manipulation the pain-

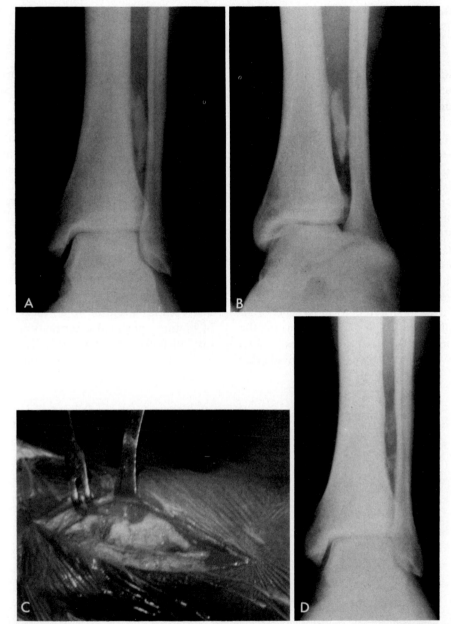

Figure 565. The findings at the time this 20 year old male was first seen were rather nonspecific except for some swelling of the ankle. The lateral ligament seemed to be entirely intact. He continued to play the rest of the season although he could not cut well. X-rays were negative. Three months later, *A*, x-ray revealed ossification between the tibia and fibula. Relatively immature at this time. He was advised to leave it alone until this became more mature. Examination six months post-injury revealed pain on forced motion such as sprinting; tenderness along the front of the fibula from about 5 cm. above the ankle upward for about 8 cm. There seemed to be a hard, firm, bony mass here. *B,* X-ray at this time showed ossification very much more mature, the bone uniting the tibia and the fibula. *C,* At surgery, revealing the plowshare-shaped mass of bone extending directly forward from the fibula and fastening over to the tibia. Note there is synostosis between the two bones. This mass was completely excised. *D,* Although four months later he had some x-ray evidence of recurrence of ossification, he was asymptomatic. Since that time he has gone on with good function and is able to play football. It should be pointed out that these exogenous bony masses should be left alone until they mature. If they are, there is a good chance that significant recurrence will not take place.

free range of motion is determined and a test is made for increased lateral motion. If abnormal lateral motion is elicited, note is made as to whether there is pain on attempting to force lateral motion or dorsiflexion. Any abnormal motion indicates serious ligament or bone injury.

X-ray Examination. Examination of x-rays should be done only after careful clinical examination by the surgeon. If possible, he should examine the foot before the x-ray is made. X-ray technicians are trained to position extremities in certain standard ways and often manipulation of the part to get proper x-ray position will reduce deformities or screen injuries that might otherwise be obvious. The x-ray technician should be instructed to make the original picture without correction of the position of the foot, the "as is" view, since this may provide an invaluable

guide to the degree of injury (Fig. 566). Following this original picture, proper positioning can be made to obtain the standard views. At least three views should be made: an anteroposterior of the foot, an anteroposterior of the ankle, and a lateral of the ankle and foot. Oblique views are invaluable and may reveal fractures not seen in conventional views (Fig. 567). If abnormal motion can be elicited, an x-ray made in the abnormal position is of considerable value. If the x-ray examination does not appear to be consistent with the clinical findings, a careful review of all findings must be made. Further x-ray views may be needed to clarify the situation, such as an anteroposterior view in forced dorsiflexion.

Careful attention to all these details of history, physical examination and x-ray visualization will usually permit early diagnosis of a serious injury. De-

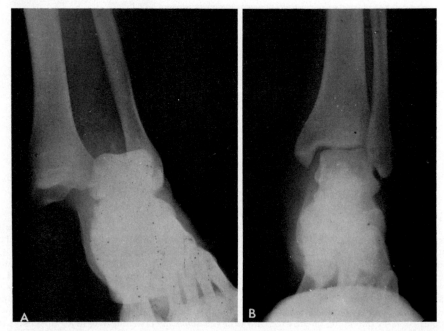

Figure 566. *A*, The "as is" view. Original film of severe sprain, which illustrates dramatically the nature of this injury, namely ruptured medial collateral ligament and ruptured tibiofibular ligament. Repair of medial ligament and fixation of fibula to tibia by long screw resulted in normal ankle. *B*, After reduction the positioned anteroposterior view showed no pathologic changes.

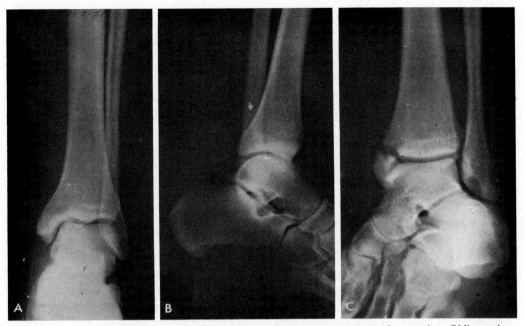

Figure 567. Routine anteroposterior *(A)* and lateral *(B)* x-rays are apparently negative. Oblique view *(C)* reveals true condition, namely fracture of medial malleolus and rupture of tibiofibular ligament. In this instance the x-ray examination did not agree with the clinical findings so further x-ray study was made. This should be treated by reduction and fixation of the fibula to the tibia with a screw. Exact reduction and fixation of the medial malleolus by a screw is vital in this injury.

finitive treatment may then be carried out promptly rather than after a period of time pending determination that the injury is more serious than it was first considered to be. Although the majority of injuries to the ankle will be sprains without bone involvement, it is extremely embarrassing to discover after several weeks that treatment was woefully inadequate because of more extensive damage than was recognized at the time treatment was begun.

Here is a useful checklist indicating the common association of injuries. Given certain x-ray findings as indicated, one might expect the corresponding injury to be as follows:

I. Fracture of the fibula above the tibio-fibular joint
   A. Lateral side
      1. Ruptured tibiofibular ligament.
   B. Medial side
      1. Ruptured medial collateral ligament or
      2. Fractured medial malleolus.
II. Fracture of the fibula below the joint line
   A. Lateral side
      1. Fractured lateral malleolus.
   B. Medial side
      1. Fractured medial malleolus or
      2. Ruptured deltoid ligament.
III. Fractured medial malleolus
   A. Lateral side
      1. Ruptured lateral collateral ligament or
      2. Fractured lateral malleolus.
      3. Ruptured tibiofibular ligament.
         a. Separation between tibia and fibula.
         b. Fractured fibula above the joint line.
IV. Separation between tibia and fibula
   A. Lateral side
      1. Ruptured tibiofibular ligament.

2. Fractured fibula above tibiofibular syndesmosis.
B. Medial side
1. Ruptured deltoid ligament or
2. Fractured medial malleolus.
V. Negative x-ray may not indicate serious pathology but there may be:
A. Lateral side
1. Ruptured lateral collateral ligaments.
2. Ruptured tibiofibular ligament.
B. Medial side
1. Ruptured deltoid ligament.

TREATMENT

Before treatment can be properly initiated in any individual case, it is important to classify the injury not only as to type and to structures damaged but also as to severity. It is axiomatic that the closer an injury approaches the joint the more necessary it is to get completely accurate repositioning of the injured structures. One must not be satisfied with incomplete reduction or partial replacement of fractures or dislocations about the ankle any more than about any other joint. Indeed, it is more important to get accurate repositioning in a weight-bearing joint than in the non-weight-bearing joints in the upper extremity.

Complete reduction must be accomplished by the method that will insure the best result, not by the method that at the time seems the most convenient. A little extra care at the time of injury will save a great deal of time and trouble at a later date. It is well known that surgery will be required in a certain percentage of injuries about the ankle joint. Recognizing this fact, it is extremely important that surgery be considered as a method of treatment per primam. If it is going to be necessary for best results, it should be carried out promptly at the time of injury, rather than backed into after nonsurgical treatment has failed.

Sprains

Sprains, which comprise the majority of injuries about the ankle, can conveniently be classified into three groups—mild (first degree), moderate (second degree) and severe (third degree). This arbitrary division is subject to a good deal of variation according to the views of the individual physician. The groups will, of necessity, overlap.

Mild (First Degree) Sprain. There is no functional loss and treatment is symptomatic. A mild sprain (Fig. 568, *A*) is one in which there has been a partial tear of elements of one of the ligaments at the ankle joint but without any actual functional weakening of the ligament as a whole. In such a case, one would expect to find minimal symptoms: local tenderness, local swelling and mild disability. Indeed, the disability may be so mild that the patient does not even seek advice from a physician.

Examination will reveal no pain on normal motion, no abnormal motion and only a moderate degree of pain on applying the stress that caused the original injury. X-ray examination is negative. This case requires no extensive treatment. This is the type of case that responds dramatically to the local treatment that was so popular a few years ago. Unfortunately, these local methods have been applied in many cases in which they were woefully inadequate.

Local application of ethyl chloride spray tends to break down the cycle of vessel spasm and reduce the local swelling and edema. It can have no effect on the strength of the ligament itself or on its healing. This should be kept in mind since, although it does tend to relieve the symptoms, it does not protect the joint against further damage. However, in the mild case, local injection of procaine and hyaluronidase will tend to permit more rapid absorption of the hematoma and to reduce pain. In this sense it is valuable in treatment.

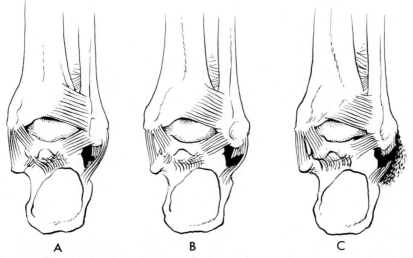

A   B   C

Figure 568. Drawings showing *A*, partial tear of ligament, mild (first degree) sprain; *B*, moderate (second degree) sprain, with more complete tear but still integrity of ligament; *C*, severe sprain with (third degree) tear and loss of integrity.

In this group ideal treatment would be rest with application of ice followed by heat. However, in a mild (first degree) sprain this is usually not necessary. It is not justified if it interferes unnecessarily with the patient's occupation. Local injection followed by adequate strapping (Fig. 569) and a well fitted shoe is all the treatment that is necessary since there is no actual weakness of the ankle joint. It should be pointed out again, however, that if one is to permit activity, one must be extremely sure of the diagnosis. It is unwise in any case to use local treatment that relieves the symptoms and then permit the injured person to participate in active sports immediately. The lapse of several hours will determine more accurately the extent of injury.

Moderate (Second Degree) Sprain. There is definite loss of strength and treatment is protective. A moderate sprain consists of one in which there has been an actual tear of a portion of the ligament but in which the integrity of the ligament has not been entirely lost (Fig. 568, *B*). There is some weakness of the ligament but no abnormal motion is elicited. Ordinarily, the history is of

sharp inversion of the foot followed by a fall with immediate severe pain. The patient is not necessarily wholly incapacitated for walking since direct weight bearing does not put strain on the injured ligament.

Symptoms are usually so severe that medical aid is sought. On examination there is severe pain in the ankle, diffuse swelling through the ankle and foot and tenderness over the lateral side of the foot and ankle, usually sharply increased at the area of the damaged ligament. This may be at the attachment of the ligament to the foot, or at the malleolus, or it may be in the substance of the ligament. The patient may tend to hold the foot in an everted position and any attempt to invert the foot beyond this point will cause severe pain. Even normal motion may be painful. An attempt to reproduce the forces that caused the injury will produce severe pain. However, there will be no abnormal motion since some portion of the ligament is still intact. X-ray is negative except as it may show a sprain-fracture at one or the other attachments of the ligament (Fig. 557).

In choosing treatment it should be

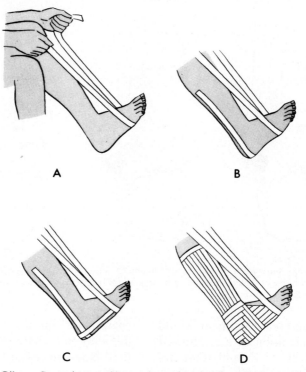

A   B

C   D

Figure 569. Typical Gibney Strapping. *A,* Shows the patient holding the foot with a loop of muslin to keep it at the right angle and inverted or everted as the case may be, depending on the location of the sprain. *B,* Shows the first strip of 1-inch adhesive tape which begins well back on the calf, at the bulge of the calf, extending down under the heel and up the opposite side. If the sprain is a lateral sprain the strip should start on the medial side and come to the lateral side. *C,* Shows the other portion of the weave, a strip running from the base of the first toe around the ankle and back to the base of the fifth toe. *D,* Shows application of successive strips, as many as necessary to reach the front of the foot. In the acute case these transverse strips should not overlap in front because of danger of impairment of circulation. If the strapping is for a chronic case where swelling is not a factor, it would be more secure to overlap the strips in front. The whole is secured by a circumferential strip around the top of the dressing and then further secured by gauze bandage. It should be emphasized again that in an acute case there should be no circumferential wrapping overlapping on the front of the foot or on the front of the ankle. NOTE: The foot is held at a right angle to the leg and inverted or everted, depending upon the location of the sprain.

borne in mind that whereas in the mild sprain there is no weakness and protection is not vital, in the moderate sprain there is definite weakness of the ligament and treatment should be protective. The first aim of treatment is to protect the ankle against further injury until healing occurs, the second to promote repair of the damage already present. Rather mild stresses superimposed over the already weakened ligament may cause complete avulsion.

Treatment consists in local injection of the area with hyaluronidase and procaine, followed by compression bandage and ice pack for several hours. Relief of symptoms by local injection should not permit early ambulation or early function of the part since this will have a detrimental effect upon healing. The patient should be put to bed with a pressure bandage and an ice pack for 10 to 24 hours. At the end of this time, further analysis should be made as to extent of the injury.

Following the period of ice packing, a posterior and a lateral stirrup boot splint is applied from below the knee to the toes in order to maintain the part in the normal weight-bearing position. The patient is then allowed to get up on crutches but should be advised not to bear weight on the extremity. Several days later, after the swelling subsides, this splint should be replaced by a walking boot cast which may be worn for ten days to three weeks depending upon the extent of the damage. Active weight bearing is encouraged as soon as this cast has dried.

It may be argued that a cast handicaps the patient needlessly. Usually, it will be found that, in a ligament injury of this degree, the patient will be substantially disabled in any event. He will actually get around more efficiently and with less pain in the walking cast than he will with ordinary wrapping or strapping. Some liberties with this regimen may be permitted in a well-organized training program. For instance, during the early period of protective splinting, the splints may be removed daily for utilization of physical therapy. Whirlpool is not indicated under these circumstances because it allows the foot to be pendant and so may increase the local swelling. It is not very feasible to remove the walking cast daily since it is difficult to replace it with sufficient security to permit pain-free weight bearing. Sometimes in the exceptional case under ideally controlled circumstances a very thorough strapping is utilized in place of a walking cast and this is removed each day for physical therapy and conscientiously replaced when treatment is finished. This should not be accepted for routine treatment. It should be emphasized again that in the ordinary practice it is not feasible to remove the splints and cast daily for exercise. Certainly this is not acceptable in the high school program. In those cases the cast should be left intact. There will be no particular trouble with limitation of motion in the high school

person. It is unwise to assume that the motion of the ankle will be confined to normal motion unless it is in a very well-controlled, adequately supervised training program which is available in very few high schools.

Following removal of the cast after 10 to 20 days, it is advisable to apply well-fitted adhesive strapping of the Gibney type (Fig. 569) to protect the ligament against further injury. This strapping should be worn until symptoms are minimal, ordinarily at least six weeks from the time of injury. If the original injury is treated adequately in this manner, there is little reason to expect recurrent injuries since the ligament will heal at its normal length and strength. I would like to emphasize again that the ligament injury will heal completely if given adequate opportunity. It takes as long for a ligament to heal as it does a bone. If this is borne in mind and protection carried out for an adequate period, the ligament injury should heal completely and leave no permanent disability.

Severe (Third Degree) Sprain. In a severe, or third degree, sprain there has been a complete rupture of one or more of the ligaments of the ankle so that its function has been completely lost (Fig. 568, C). Treatment here must be restorative to restore the integrity of the ligament and permit it to heal. Either the ligament is torn completely or one or the other of its attachments has pulled loose from the bone. History will be essentially the same as for moderate sprain but all complaints will be more severe. The patient will frequently volunteer the information that the foot had been out of place but had been reduced by manipulation and that pain was relieved by the reduction.

Examination will reveal more serious and extensive findings than in the other groups. The swelling is more extreme. The pain is more severe. The patient resists any attempt to move the foot and is extremely apprehensive. If the foot is examined very early, abnormal motion may be elicited without undue pain. It is justifiable, in certain cases, to inject procaine into the painful area or even to induce short general anesthesia in order to determine whether or not there is complete disruption of one of the ligaments of the ankle joint. An x-ray should be made in the abnormal position if possible (Fig. 566, *A*). These cases are relatively infrequent but when they occur the consequences may be extremely disastrous if the true condition is not recognized and appropriate treatment instituted. Many of the most disabling injuries reveal no demonstrable fracture but are caused by dislocation. Ligament injury may be extremely severe.

An example of these serious injuries to the ankle is disruption of the medial collateral and tibiofibular ligaments, in which case the x-ray findings may be completely negative (Fig. 566, *B*). Also the external collateral ligament may be completely torn and a normal x-ray picture seen. One must recognize the exact condition present in order to plan the best treatment, which obviously must be far more comprehensive than that for an ordinary sprain of the ankle. For this reason the diagnosis must be made at the earliest possible moment. If surgical repair of the ligament is to be carried out, it must be done promptly in order to secure the best results. If there is a complete severance of the medial collateral or tibiofibular ligament, or both, surgical treatment is certainly the treatment of choice.

Complete avulsion of the external collateral ligament has customarily been treated by simple immobilization since it is relatively easy to protect the foot against inversion by splints in an everted position. However, there is no more reason to expect these ligament ends which have been completely torn to fall together on the lateral side of the foot than there is elsewhere. This is the typical patient in whom the injury is treated nonsurgically and who goes on to have repeated sprains due to the overlength of the ligament. True enough, he can tolerate it to some extent since this ligament does not support the weight of the body, but it is extremely distressing to someone who wants to play tennis, hand ball or any other active sport to have recurrent, relatively minor injuries. If it can be determined that a complete tear of this ligament is present, surgical repair will not only speed recovery but will improve the probability of obtaining a perfect functional result.

The warning is explicit that in these serious injuries one must not temporize but must make up his mind whether or not surgery is indicated. The time to carry out an operation is at the earliest possible moment after the need for one is determined. While late surgery is not nearly as favorable as is early operation, it should not be refused simply because the diagnosis was not made at time of the injury (Fig. 570). "Better late than never." However, we have found that if surgery is postponed, after two or three weeks it is impossible to define the ligament ends and under these circumstances reconstruction is necessary to obtain support for the collateral ligaments from some other source. Late repair is usually not successful, but reconstruction may be (Fig. 571).

If nonsurgical treatment is chosen, then the same treatment is indicated as for a moderate sprain, namely local injection, compression, ice packs, splints, walking cast and adhesive strapping. All of these treatment phases must be somewhat more extensive and protection must be carried out for eight to ten weeks since there is marked functional loss in the ligament. If such a long

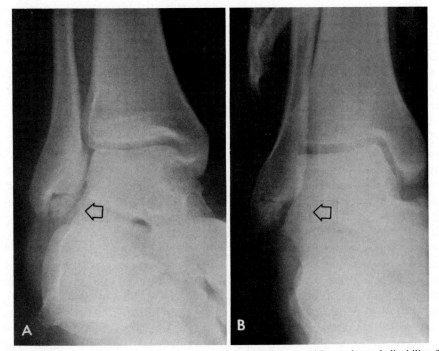

Figure 570. Fracture of tip of lateral malleolus with nonunion, resulting pain and disability from involvement of peroneal tendons as well as lateral collateral ligament. This patient was treated without immobilization. This is in reality a sprain-fracture, the tip having been avulsed by the lateral collateral ligament. Surgical removal of the fragment resulted in marked improvement. Early surgery should have given complete recovery. *A*, Illustrating value of oblique view. *B*, Stress film demonstrating no instability.

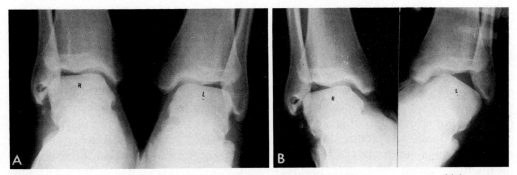

Figure 571. This 19 year old boy received an injury to his right ankle two years ago which was seen here four months post-injury with complete instability of the lateral collateral ligament. A Watson-Jones reconstruction was done four months after the injury, resulting in good stability. The opposite (left) ankle then had an identical situation. He hurt his left ankle one year ago and received the same casual treatment which he received on the first injury and again had complete loss of the lateral collateral ligament.

A, Anteroposterior view of both ankles. Note hole for the reconstruction in right fibula.

B, Stress film on both sides. Right shows good stability with tilt within the acceptable range. Left shows complete dislocation of the talus out of the mortice. The stress film on the right originally looked exactly like the present film on the left. More thorough treatment of the original injury might have prevented this chronic instability. The left ankle has now received a similar type reconstruction of the lateral collateral ligaments with good stability.

period of immobilization is required, formal rehabilitation becomes necessary. Usually rehabilitation is required in direct proportion to the length of time it was necessary to immobilize the joint.

Following operative repair, posterior and lateral below-knee stirrup splints are applied for about two weeks. Then stitches are removed and a walking boot cast is applied which the patient will wear for an additional four weeks. Even six weeks is an inadequate time for healing to occur, but after six weeks careful adhesive strapping should give enough support that rehabilitation can commence. Actually, rehabilitation will be much less necessary if a walking cast has been used, since the muscles in the extremity that are not immobilized by the cast will be in good condition. I do not believe the oft-repeated statement that "ligament injuries are worse than fractures." This aphorism has arisen from the fact that serious ligament injuries have been undertreated and so the consequences have been more severe than those from an adequately treated fracture. Careful investigation of the patient having painful recurrent sprains of the ankle will probably uncover an initial injury that was treated inadequately (Fig. 571).

Fractures

I have noted above that while the most common injury to the ankle is sprain and is an inversion injury, the most common eversion injury to the ankle is actually a fracture. The two most important factors in the treatment of fractures about the ankle are: (1) maintenance of the integrity of the ankle mortice, and (2) complete re-establishment of the weight-bearing surfaces of the talus and tibia.

Uncorrected separation between the tibia and fibula with corresponding widening of the ankle mortice is not compatible with normal ankle function. While irregularity of the weight-bearing surface is usually quite obvious on x-ray examination, separation of the ankle mortice may not be so readily apparent. It is extremely important that one carefully analyze the relationship between the tibia and fibula in order to determine whether there is separation between the two with widening of the mortice. Actually, the vast majority of fractures around the ankle are malleolar fractures. If they are complete, they have been accompanied by some dislocation of the ankle.

If there is a fracture of the lateral malleolus with displacement and with no fracture of the medial malleolus, there is usually avulsion of the medial collateral ligament. If there is a fracture of the medial malleolus by an inversion force, an avulsion of the lateral ligament must be present. If there has been a fracture of the medial malleolus because of an eversion force, either the lateral malleolus must be broken, or the tibiofibular ligament ruptured. The same force that causes a bimalleolar fracture may cause fracture of the medial malleolus with ruptured tibiofibular ligament or it may cause rupture of the medial ligament and rupture of the tibiofibular ligament with no fracture at all (Fig. 572, A). Thus, it can be seen that the treatment of ligament injuries and fractures of the ankle cannot be separated. If the two basic goals are borne in mind, namely, the integrity of the ankle mortice and the restoration of normal weight-bearing surfaces, the type of treatment indicated is clear. Actually, it is not common for the weight-bearing surfaces to be involved. Ordinarily the lower end of the tibia and the upper surface of the talus are not fractured in ankle injuries so that the fracture that is actually being discussed here is the malleolar fracture. This is caused by the same forces that cause sprains.

In bimalleolar fractures, it is virtually impossible to obtain and maintain accurate reposition of both malleoli without internal fixation at least in one of them. In these cases, internal fixation has long been the rule. The excellent results obtained by this method have encouraged me to apply it to injuries apparently less severe. With fracture of the medial malleolus accompanied by a tibiofibular separation, I feel that open reduction should be carried out, and the internal malleolus accurately replaced and held by screw or some other method of fixation (Fig. 572, B). At the same time, the tibia and fibula should be held together by a long metal screw transfixing the lower fibula and crossing both cortices of the tibia. Since it has been demonstrated that under normal usage there is definite motion in the distal tibiofibular joint, I consider it advisable to remove the screw that holds the tibia and fibula together after a suitable interval for healing of the tibiofibular ligament. This period is usually between 8 and 12 weeks. It is not unusual for the screw to break in the interval between the two bones when normal activity is resumed earlier. If this happens it is extremely difficult to remove the tibial section of the screw (Fig. 573). This is of little consequence unless the metal is reactive, since once the screw breaks normal motion is permitted and it is usually not necessary to remove either part of the broken screw. If the injury is a fracture of both malleoli, it is better to use internal fixation on both sides.

Surgical treatment should be carried out only by one well versed in the anatomy of the ankle. The proper surgical environment is a *sine qua non* to success. Although the techniques of these various surgical procedures are available elsewhere, a brief description of the technique may be useful in order to emphasize some of the vital factors involved in the different situations.

Medial Side. If the injury is a fracture of the medial malleolus, I prefer to make a linear incision beginning 2 inches above the tip of the medial malleolus, extending downward along the posterior medial border of the tibia to the tip of the medial malleolus. The incision then should swing forward and downward directly along the line of the posterior tibial tendon as far as the tubercle of the navicular. Reflecting this flap forward, with care being taken to include all of the subcutaneous tissue in the flap, will expose the whole malleolus. One must not bring the incision forward beneath the medial malleolus but should extend it downward parallel to the posterior tibial tendon toward the navicular tubercle. Otherwise, great difficulty may be encountered in exposing enough of the area below the malleolus to permit the insertion of the internal fixation. It is necessary to sacrifice the posterior branch of the saphenous vein in this incision.

After the flap is reflected the fracture is defined and the fracture line exposed. Great care must be taken to remove all soft tissue which is frequently found interposed into the fracture site. By displacing the malleolar fragment it is possible to visualize the medial portion of the talus, including its neck. By retracting the capsular incision forward it is possible to expose a good portion of the dome of the talus, and by plantar flexing the foot one can make an even more extensive examination. One may also inspect the leading edge of the distal end of the tibia. Careful search here may well reveal osteochondral fractures of the talus or of the tibia which are not demonstrated in the x-ray.

When one is satisfied that the joint does not contain any foreign bodies or any other fracture line, the wound should be copiously lavaged with saline. The malleolus then should be fitted me-

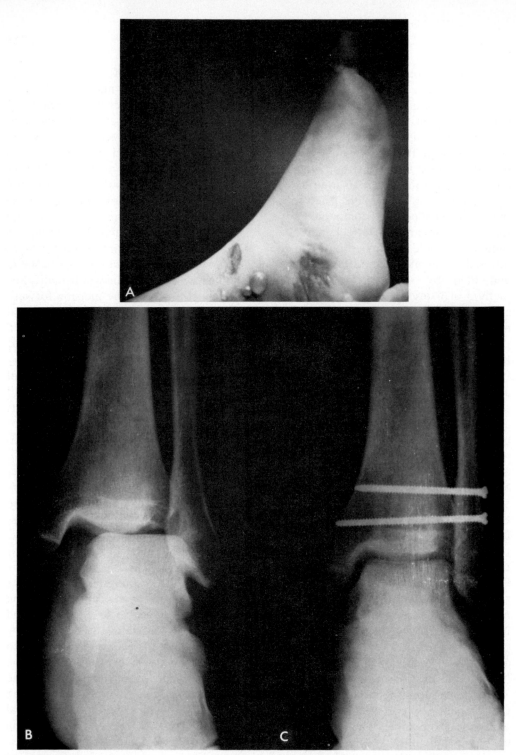

Figure 572, Case A. This 20 year old male received an injury playing football when his foot was forced out and his leg forced in. He had immediate swelling, diagnosed as sprain. *A*, Eight hours after the injury he had tremendous swelling of the calf, foot and thigh with definite lateral instability of the ankle. *B*, X-ray shows lateral displacement of the talus on the tibia with separation of the distal tibiofibular ligaments and ruptured deltoid ligament. At surgery the posterior tibial tendon was lying between the talus and the malleolus, preventing reduction. The deltoid ligament was completely torn and was treated by direct suture. *C*, Since it was completely dislocated, I thought it would be more secure to have two screws across the tibia and fibula rather than the ordinary one screw fixation. His postoperative course was satisfactory. Three months postoperative he had no complaint except soreness over the end of the screws. The screws were removed five months postoperative. He returned to full activity, including football.

726

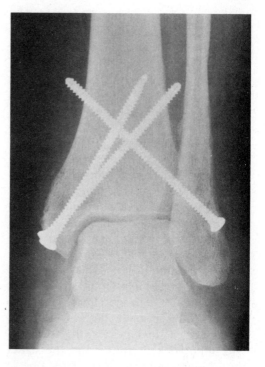

Figure 572, Case B. Bimalleolar fracture with adequate internal fixation. In this instance the lateral screw transfixes the fibular fracture site and enters the tibia, coming through medially far enough that it can be removed from the opposite side if it breaks. In other instances an intramedullary pin may be placed in the fibula if the tibiofibular ligament is intact.

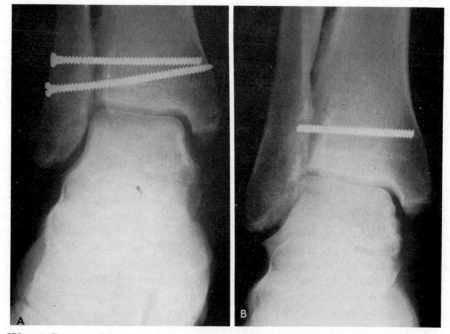

Figure 573. *A*, Fracture-dislocation of the ankle, treated by two transfixion screws. Note that the upper screw is broken whereas the one which is slightly bent is intact. *B*. The screws were later removed but the broken screw was inaccessible. Note that it has freed itself from the fibula by forming a cul-de-sac in the bone around the screw, thus permitting normal tibiofibular motion. (This was visualized even better in the lateral view.)

ticulously into position. This must be done with hairline accuracy. The articular cartilage extending from the malleolus onto the tibia should be exposed to be sure that it is in direct continuity. The fragment may then be held in this position with a Bishop clamp or some similar type of tenaculum; it is very difficult to hold manually. Fixation is then inserted.

If the fragment permits, it is desirable to use two screws at slightly divergent angles. Each must pass through the medial malleolus, across the fracture line, traverse the tibia and penetrate its opposite cortex (Fig. 572, Case B). This requires a relatively long screw but does give much better fixation, particularly in older people where the cancellous bone may seem quite inadequate for fixation. If one uses a single screw, the fragment will often rock or rotate and the exact repositioning may be lost. After one is certain that the fragment is securely held in position and will stand a considerable degree of manipulation of the foot, the wound is closed in layers. It is possible to use various other appliances to fix the medial malleolus, but I prefer the long screw. On occasion the malleolus fragment may be very small and include the articular portion only. This makes it very difficult to screw from below. In this instance retrograde screws can be placed from the tibia into the fragment with less disruption of the fragment and the deltoid ligament.

Medial Approach—Repair of the Deltoid Ligament. This incision is similar to that for the medial malleolus except that it is carried somewhat more distally before it is brought forward across to the tubercle of the navicular. If the incision is extended a little bit further distally before it is extended forward, the deltoid ligament is more readily available particularly if it happens to be torn beneath and behind the tendons. The pathology is carefully defined by metic-

ulous dissection with minimal damage to any of the ligament fibers. If the ligament is pulled off the malleolus, as it frequently is, it is best replaced by mattress sutures, imbricated through the ligament so as to get firm security, and is then passed through multiple drill holes placed in the blunt end of the medial malleolus. My preference here is to use No. 0 cotton and to have at least three and possibly four mattress loops. If the deepest, most lateral portion of the ligament is damaged beneath the tendon bed, this should be carefully sutured by inverted sutures, leaving the knot buried in the ligament. When all the sutures are placed the tendon sheath is closed. It is extremely important that all the components of the ligament be repaired so that the edges accurately appose. Occasionally the fracture in the medial malleolus may be such that it is difficult or impossible to get fixation screws from the malleolus upward into the tibia.

Lateral Approach. The preferable incision for exposing the lateral malleolus and the lateral collateral ligament parallels the posterior border of the fibula and extends down across the tip of the fibula to swing along the line of the peroneal tendons toward the base of the fifth metatarsal bone. Reflecting this flap forward, together with all the subcutaneous tissue, exposes the various components of the fibular collateral ligament. The ligament then should be carefully defined and replaced with as many stitches as are necessary to appose the various fibers. Actually, the ligament is such that No. 0 cotton is probably adequate. Stronger suture tends to necrose the ligament if it is tied too tightly. After all the components are carefully sutured, the wound is closed in the usual manner.

Lateral Malleolar Fracture. The same incision may be used for fixation of the lateral malleolus. It may need to be extended proximally if the fracture is higher up the shaft. It may not be necessary to use the distal curved portion in this instance. There are various ways to fix the fracture of the malleolus. These vary according to circumstances. If the fracture is transverse at the level of the line of the joint, some sort of intramedullary fixation is preferable, either with a long screw, a threaded pin or even a smooth type Steinman pin drilled up the fibula from the distal end. In this instance the tibiofibular ligament is not involved and good stability can be obtained in the malleolar fragment by intramedullary fixation.

If the fracture is oblique and through the tibiofibular joint, as it often is, with the fracture line oblique from above downward and inward, it is probably better fixed by a long screw through the distal fragment crossing the tibiofibular synchondrosis and tibia to engage the opposite cortex of the tibia (Fig. 572, Case B).

If the fracture is above the tibiofibular joint and there is tibiofibular separation, it is not adequate to use simple intramedullary fixation. In this case, the most important consideration is to get fixation between the tibia and the fibula. This is best obtained by a long screw just above this synchondrosis. It should traverse the fibula and both cortices of the tibia, care being taken not to overcorrect the fibula at this level (Fig. 573). If the screw happens to be a little high, it may pull the fibula too close to the tibia and so tilt the tip of the malleolus outward and defeat the purpose of making a stable mortice.

If it is a gross fracture-dislocation with major instability, it may be advisable to put a plate on the fibular fracture above to obtain stability of the fibula. This is not often the case in athletic injuries.

The prime importance in open reduction for a fractured fibula with separation between the tibia and fibula is to be sure that there is no foreign material between the two bones. If the two bones do not completely appose, as checked by x-ray on the operating table, the fracture line and the syndesmosis should be explored and all intervening tissue removed. As indicated on the medial side, if the joint is involved it should be inspected as far as possible by displacing the fragment and determining whether or not there is damage to the articular cartilage of the talus, lateral tibia or lateral malleolus.

Following surgical repair, postoperative fixation should be by posterior and lateral stirrup splints (Fig. 444). Under ordinary circumstances it is better to extend these splints above the knee for at least two weeks while the wound is healing. At the end of that time a cast is applied. A decision must be made whether or not to put on a walking heel and whether or not it needs to extend above the knee (Fig. 446). This depends on the stability of the internal fixation. If there is any danger of displacement of any of the fragments or stress on any of the repaired ligaments by rotation of the foot and leg at the knee, the cast fixation must extend above the knee. For example, an injury involving a ruptured deltoid ligament and tibiofibular ligament should not be subjected to weight bearing this soon. Weight bearing in a walking cast should not be permitted if any weight-bearing bone is involved. Some judgment is required in the utilization of a walking cast to be sure that the cast gives proper fixation. This is much more easily done with a patient who is long legged and slender than it is with one who is short and fat. It is always better to err on the side of adequate protection if there is any question about whether or not protection should be extended above the knee. If you bear in mind that it requires 10 to 12 weeks for a ligament to heal, even with partial strength, and that simple subsidence of symptoms is not an indication that healing is complete, the importance of adequate protection is clear. We have a guide for healing in fractures and these should be carefully checked by x-ray for degree of union. Following removal of the plaster fixation the ankle must be protected against unusual stress by either taping, elastic bandaging or wrapping.

Since in many instances open surgery may be simpler to carry out and easier to manage postoperatively than manipulative treatment, it follows that adequate training is essential before any physician should attempt to manage a serious fracture or dislocation about a joint.

Only by extreme care in examination, conscientious selection of the best method of treatment and thorough preparation in technique can one expect to obtain optimum results in treatment of injuries about the ankle.

EXOSTOSES

This condition in its various manifestations appears quite frequently about the ankle and foot, in fact, so frequently on the top of the talus and the front of the tibia that it has been described as a separate entity, namely, *talotibial exostoses*. An exostosis should be distinguished from a marginal osteophyte. An exostosis is an actual piling up of bone at the site of the irritative lesion, whereas the marginal osteophyte is an osteochondral ridge developing at the joint margin as a result of a chronic synovitis or chronic arthritic change. An exostosis will characteristically develop as a response to direct trauma so that it may be seen on the back or front of the lower margin of the tibia, less frequently in front of the medial malleolus or of the lateral malleolus

due to impingement of the talus. On the talus the exostosis forms just back of the head superiorly (Fig. 576). Here the trauma results from repeated overflexion or overextension, overinversion or overeversion of the ankle joint beyond its ordinary range. For example, with the foot driven into dorsiflexion, the leading edge of the tibia impinges against the concavity of the neck of the talus. The resulting irritation causes a piling up of bone that simply serves to aggravate the condition.

It will be recalled that, in extreme dorsiflexion of the foot, the anterior lip of the tibia nestles into the sulcus which is located on top of the talus between its body and head. It should be noted that the leading edge of the lower end of the tibia normally inclines backward in order to prevent impingement against the talus during dorsiflexion (Fig. 574). There actually is no true ligamentous attachment at either of these locations. The anterior capsule of the joint attaches slightly higher on the tibia and runs forward to the navicular with little attachment to the superior surface of the neck of the talus. Spur formation in this region is the result of direct trauma during forcible dorsiflexion of the foot on the leg. It is not the late result of a ligament injury caused by extreme plantar flexion at the ankle, so-called traction sprain. The injury occurs, not during ordinary running, but during the "drive" of the athlete when his cleats are fixed to the ground with the foot forcibly dorsiflexed and the neck of the talus in direct apposition to the tibia (Fig. 575).

In many instances, much more often than is usually noted, the reaction to direct trauma during such "driving" running is the formation of bone at the area of impingement. This reaction apparently is similar to the formation of calluses on the skin. This mass has an adverse rather than a protective effect, however, for the more bone that is piled

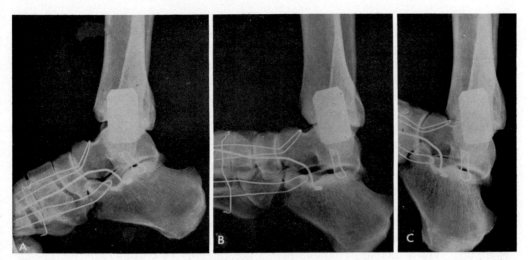

Figure 574. Roentgenograms showing the area of opposition between the tibia and talus. *A*, The foot in a neutral position. *B*, The foot in dorsiflexion. *C*, The foot in hyperdorsiflexion.

up, the more easily the impingement occurs, and so a vicious cycle is formed resulting in gradually increasing disability.

Characteristically, the player loses his "drive." As a rule, he has rather vague complaints which do not seem sufficient to account for his disability. Ordinary examination reveals little; there is no swelling, no pain on inver-

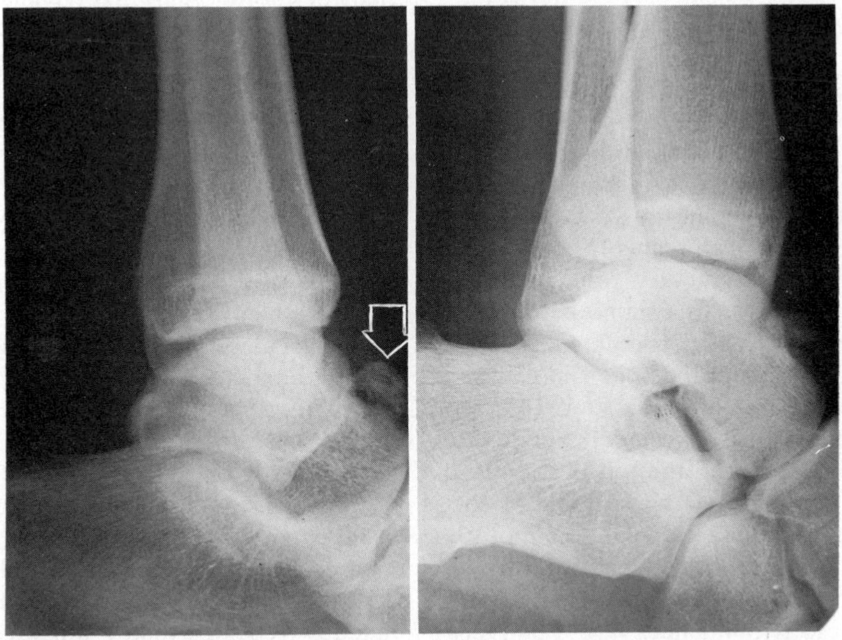

Figure 575. Avulsion of the capsular attachment on top of the talus, together with fragment of bone 18 months after injury. This probably was a relatively big fragment to start with. The patient's complaint now is on forceful running which impinges the fragment against the lower end of the tibia, similar to a talotibial spur.

sion or eversion, and no tenderness around the malleoli. The impression grows among teammates and coaches that the player is "dogging it." This is especially likely since he can often run, cut and jump without pain so long as he does not go at full speed. The result may well be disappointment of the coaches, disheartenment of the player, and the ultimate blighting of an otherwise promising athletic career.

Such a patient presents himself with a history of aching pain in the ankle sharply increased by "driving," often to the point that he feels he cannot "go all out." He is unable to explain his failure to get that extra push that differentiates the star from the ordinary athlete. He simply realizes that his previous speed and force have been unaccountably diminished.

Examination will almost uniformly elicit particular findings. One is pain on forcible dorsiflexion of the foot—an impingement type of pain located at the anterior talotibial sulcus. Another is pinpoint tenderness directly over the spur on the talus or tibia. Roentgenographic examination will reveal that the anterior margin of the lower end of the tibia has lost its slanted character and that the edge is sharp, often with an identifiable exostosis extending forward over the articular surface of the talus (Fig. 576, A). The condition may vary from a simple change in contour to a spur a centimeter or more long. This spur extends along the whole width of the bone and is in reality a ledge rather than a spur. In addition, an exostosis of a greater or lesser size may appear on the top of the neck of the talus. Upon dorsiflexion of the foot, the two will be seen to impinge (Fig. 576, B). Either one or both of these exostoses may be present.

These prominences are relatively small in the early stages but may be tremendous in the later stages, at which time the diagnosis becomes obvious.

The condition may extend onto the front of the medial malleolus and, rarely, to the anterior edge of the fibula; in severe cases it may also occur in other areas of the foot in which there are impinging bones, such as the posterior part of the ankle. These exostoses appear to be similar to but are not etiologically the same as the spurring that is found on adjacent articular surfaces, such as the metatarsal-cuneiform joints. The latter condition is almost always accompanied by degenerative change in the articular cartilage and an actual narrowing of the joint space and falls into the category of chronic arthritic change or so-called marginal osteophytes. This is not the condition to which we are referring when we speak of impingement exostoses of the talus and tibia. The typical impingement exostosis is most common at the anterior edge of the tibia and neck of the talus and is not accompanied by marginal osteophytes, degenerative changes (Fig. 577), or other signs of chronic joint involvement. This is reflected in the prognosis since the result, from an athletic viewpoint, can hardly be classed as excellent if degenerative changes in the foot and ankle or, in fact, any other changes persist. The conditions may coexist, but one is not necessarily the forerunner of the other. When severe, the impingement exostosis may be extremely disabling, precluding athletics or any real activity. In some instances the spur is broken off and is found as a loose body lying on top of the talar neck or elsewhere. As such, it may cause acute disability in an ankle already chronically impaired.

It seems doubtful that the condition is initiated by repeated mild sprain of the very weak anterior capsule. Rather, it would appear that the reaction is initiated by repeated mild traumata caused by direct impingement and is often made severe by acute injury. There seems no question but that repeated in-

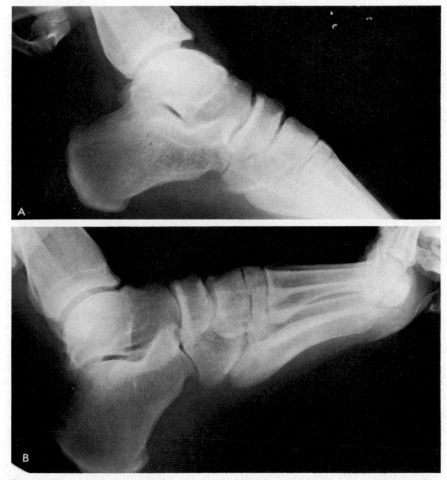

Figure 576. *A*, X-rays showing talotibial spurs, 3 plus. *B*, Showing impingement occurring when the foot is dorsiflexed.

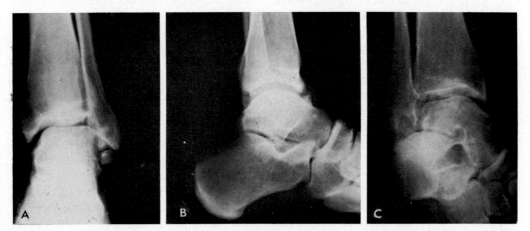

Figure 577. Advanced tibiotalar exostoses. Note fragmentation between talus and fibula. The tarsal joints are not degenerative. This is not degenerative arthritis.

Table 20–1. Roentgenographic Findings in a Survey of the Ankles
of 120 Athletes and Non-Athletes

ATHLETES		NON-ATHLETES	
No exostosis	66 (55%)	No exostosis	101 (84.2%)
Exostoses in only one bone		Exostoses in only one bone	
Talar		Talar	
Grade 1 14		Grade 1 8	
Grade 2 3		Grade 2 1	
17 (14.2%)		9 (7.5%)	
Tibial		Tibial	
Grade 1 4 (3.3%)		Grade 1 6 (5%)	
	21 (17.5%)		15 (12.5%)
Exostoses in both bones		Exostoses in both bones	
Grade 1 22		Grade 1 2	
Grade 2 7		Grade 2 2	
Grade 3 4			
	33 (27.5%)		4 (3.3%)
Total	120 (100%)	Total	120 (100%)

(From the Journal of Bone and Joint Surgery, Vol. 39A, p. 851.)

sult is the definitive factor in this progressive syndrome.

In order to determine its frequency we checked a long series of students of the same age group and of the same general characteristics. One-half of them were scholarship athletes and one-half were nonathletes. We found that the presence of talotibial spurring was much more frequent in the athletes (Table 20–1), 45 per cent of them having some degree of spurring while only 15 per cent of the nonathletes did. It should be understood these were all nonsymptomatic cases.

The mere presence of a spur is not justification for *treatment* since the great majority of them are completely nonsymptomatic. Surgical treatment is highly successful in young, healthy adult males provided the proper indications for it are present. The athlete is, of course, the one to whom surgical correction has the most appeal since if he has to restrict his activity he is no longer an athlete. On the other hand, the casual player may well prefer to give up his athletic activities rather than to submit to surgical correction.

Surgical Treatment

In the ordinary case, an anterolateral approach will suffice to remove both talar and tibial exostoses (Fig. 578). However, in some cases it will be necessary to make both medial and lateral incisions, and occasionally a posterior exposure will be necessary.

Anterolateral Approach. After the usual preparation and the application of a tourniquet, a skin incision is made just lateral and parallel to the peroneus tertius tendon, beginning about 4 cm. proximal to the lower articular surface of the tibia and extending distally for approximately 7.5 cm. (Fig. 578, *A*). The extensor tendons are retracted medially (Fig. 578, *B*), and the incision is carried through the very weak anterior capsule of the ankle joint, including the anterior fasciculus of the talofibular ligament. It is not ordinarily necessary to disturb the short extensor muscles, nor is it necessary to clean out the sinus tarsi. After the capsule has been opened, the anterior articular lip of the tibia is readily apparent, and by firm retraction the neck of the talus may be exposed (Fig. 578, *C*). By means of a sharp osteotome, the exostosis along the lower portion of the tibia is carefully removed and the posterior inclination of the surface restored. The front edge of the lateral malleolus is visualized, and any spurring found is removed. The exostosis on the neck of the talus is best removed by means of a gouge which is shaped to conform to the concavity of the neck; a small osteotome is also useful. The roughened bone is very carefully smoothed and all fragments removed. The area is then thoroughly lavaged and the raw bone surfaces are sealed with bone wax. Following this, the wound, including the divided ligament, is closed in layers.

Medial Approach. The incision on the medial side begins 2.5 cm. above the lower end of the tibia, just medial and parallel to the anterior tibial tendon. The incision extends distally to the posterior edge of the navicular. The saphenous vein may be retracted by cut-

ting either its anterior or posterior branch, and ready access may be had to the front of the ankle by opening the capsule. The procedures described in the previous section for the removal of the exostoses are then carried out.

The medial malleolus and the medial border of the talus are examined by digital palpation. If spurring is found, a portion of the deltoid ligament may be divided in order to obtain better access to the area involved. The same method of closure is used as is used on the opposite side.

Following these procedures, posterior and lateral stirrup splints are applied from below the knee to the toes, with the foot in neutral lateral position and in 90 degrees of dorsiflexion. After ten days the stitches are removed and a walking cast is applied, to be worn for another ten days. Following removal of this cast, three weeks after the operation, further support is used only as indicated. An elastic bandage may be useful if swelling persists, but it is urged that active use, in fact, unlimited activity, be begun as quickly as possible.

It should be re-emphasized that the condition we are calling talotibial exos-

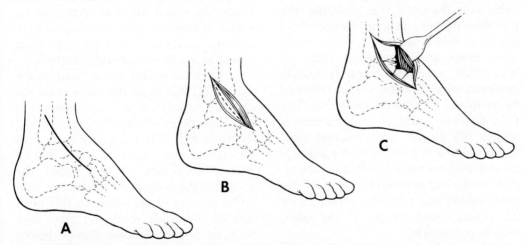

Figure 578. Anterolateral approach: *A*, The skin incision. *B*, The skin has been separated, exposing the lateral edge of the extensor tendons. *C*, The tendon and muscles have been retracted and the capsule has been opened, exposing the spurs.

tosis is not accompanied by degenerative change in the joint. Frequently, as mentioned previously, the ankle joint will be surrounded by marginal osteophytes resulting from chronic degenerative changes in the articular cartilage. These are characterized by roughened joint space, eburnated articular cartilage, chronic pain in the joint and an altogether different picture than that of exostosis. Prognostically there is vast difference since cleaning up of the marginal osteophytes has little effect upon the chronic arthritis that is present, and will as a rule prove disappointing. It may be necessary in case the osteophyte is large or fragmented, but one should not be misled into believing that the ankle will be wholly cured by removing the loose fragment from a degenerative joint. This condition (marginal osteophytes) is also quite frequent in the joints of the foot and will be discussed in that section.

CHONDRAL FRACTURE (OSTEOCHONDRITIS DISSECANS)

Osteochondral fractures have not been recognized as frequently in the ankle as in the knee. It is probably true that they do not occur as frequently. I am sure, however, that a great many more cases are overlooked than are recognized since the lesion is readily confused with an ankle sprain followed by traumatic arthritis in the ankle. The most common cause of the condition is trauma. By far the most frequent location for chondral fracture of the ankle is the dome of the talus where it occurs either on the superolateral margin of the talus, usually in a central location, or on the superomedial margin of the talus, usually posteriorly.

The mechanism of the injury has been described by many authors. It is an inversion type of injury (Fig. 579). Dorsiflexion of the foot forces the broader anterior part of the body of the talus deeper into the tibiofibular mortice so that there is snug contact between the long lateral malleolus and the lateral surface of the talus. If sharp inversion occurs in this position, the superior margin of the talus impinges forcibly against the side of the fibula. The resulting lesion is a snubbing type of fracture in which the cartilage of the superior surface of the talus is "peeled off" the subchondral bone, usually taking a greater or lesser fragment of bone with it. The resulting lesion is a flap of cartilage similar to a piece of linoleum being peeled off the floor. The force may be enough to actually dislodge the whole fragment or may simply hinge it upward, leaving the medial portion of the cartilage flap intact (Fig. 580).

This same inversion force as it drives the talus against the side of the fibula may cause chondral damage to the medial side of the lateral malleolus. The fibular cartilage may be damaged (Fig. 581) but is much less likely to be since there is no margin or edge to be peeled away. I recall one case of an extremely resistant ankle injury with symptoms along the anterior talofibular fissure in which surgical exposure revealed a completely loose fragment of articular cartilage with a corresponding defect in the fibular articular surface.

When the lesion of the dome of the talus (Fig. 582) is on the medial side the cause, strangely enough, also appears to be an inversion injury. Since it occurs at the back end of the superior surface of the talus, one must assume that it occurs in plantar flexion when the weight of the body is on the narrow posterior portion of the talus. In this position of the ankle joint, the talus may rock to a considerable degree before any tension is placed on the collateral ligaments since the narrow posterior

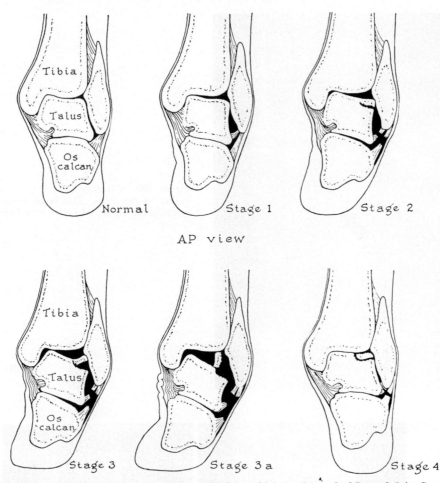

Figure 579. Osteochondritis dissecans showing mechanisms of injury. (Journal of Bone & Joint Surgery, Vol. 41-A, 1959; A. L. Berndt and Michael Hardy.)

width of the talus does not provide good bony stability in the too-wide mortice. Landing from a jump may cause direct trauma to a relatively small area, the typical instance being the basketball player who leaps in the air and lands on his toes with his foot slightly inverted. The mechanism in this instance is a compression type which dislodges the talar cartilage, together with some subchondral bone, quite similar to that which we visualize as happening at the knee in a direct blow on the patella with the knee flexed. These osteochondral fractures may occur at other places in the ankle or foot (Fig. 583). I do not

recall having seen a case involving the head of the talus unless there was an actual fracture of the talar head in which a relatively larger fragment of cartilage and bone was broken off.

Osteochondral fracture occasionally occurs at the superior margin of the posterior articular surface of the navicular with characteristic x-ray appearance of the small fragment with a translucent area between it and the parent bone, giving a scooped-out appearance at the cartilage surface (Fig. 584). One must presume that these same fractures occur on the inferior surface of the talus and on the superior surface of the calcaneus,

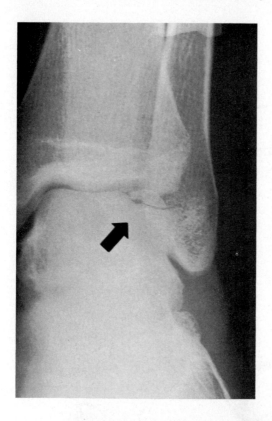

Figure 580. Chondral fracture of superolateral border of the talus. This is an inversion injury catching the corner of the talus against the fibula.

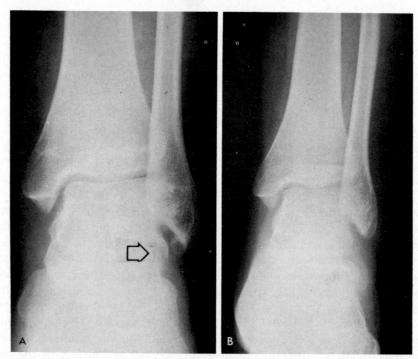

Figure 581. Osteochondral fracture of the articular cartilage of the fibula, old. *A*, The fragment is rounded off and displaced downward. *B*, Following removal.

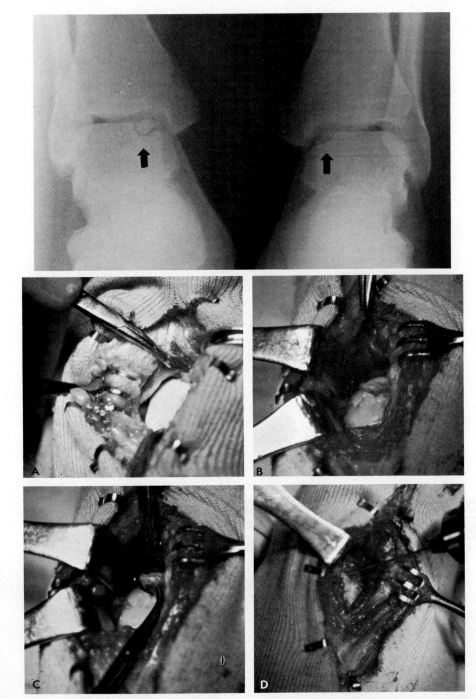

Figure 582. An 18 year old baseball pitcher with persistent "sprain" of both ankles. He had had extensive treatment for sprain with prompt recurrence of symptoms on resumption of activity. Examination revealed none of the classic symptoms of sprain. In fact, interim examination was essentially negative, except for some discomfort on forced inversion. X-ray revealed chondral fractures of the superomedial angle of the talus of each ankle. Surgery through *A*, an anteromedial incision parallel to the anterior tibial tendon, exposed a normal talar cartilage. *B*, Plantar flexion of the foot revealed a chondral fracture with nonunion. *C*, This was a large fragment with only a very small segment of bone attached. It was removed, leaving a wide gap. *D*, The sclerotic bed after curettement, being drilled with multiple drill holes with a K wire. This patient resumed baseball pitching after a few months without symptoms. Earlier diagnosis might have saved many disheartening months.

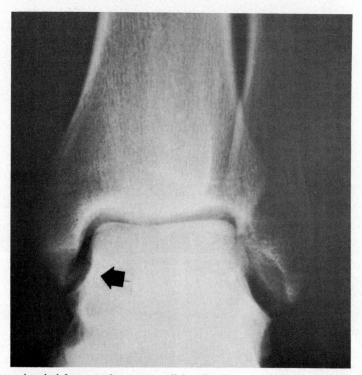

Figure 583. Osteochondral fragment between medial malleolus and talus. This is not in the deltoid ligament. There is also a fragment lying between the fibula and the talus. Removal of these fragments gave substantial relief.

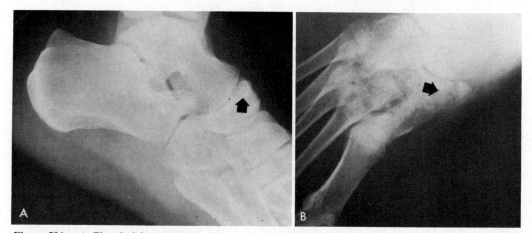

Figure 584. *A*, Chondral fracture of navicular. *B*, Patient treated for sprain of the foot for many months primarily by manipulation and physical therapy. Note fracture through the tubercle of the navicular, unrecognized. Also note extreme atrophy in spite of misguided efforts at making him exercise. Removal of the fragment resulted in gradual improvement. Apparently both of these conditions were from the same injury. The talar tubercle fracture is not an accessory navicular bone.

but if so they are difficult to recognize and must be rare.

The most important single factor in diagnosis of these injuries is an acute awareness that they occur. It is recommended that in any injury to the ankle, x-ray study should be made even though the injury does not appear to be severe. I know of no way to diagnose these conditions in the acute stage except by x-ray examination. We have for many years insisted that x-rays be made. Perhaps too little time has been spent in emphasizing that the films should be adequately studied after they are made. When these injuries occur they are often seen as emergencies. The pictures are frequently taken by a substitute technician. These films may be examined briefly without detailed study for chondral damage. Such casual study will not reveal these lesions. Injuries to the ankle and foot should be x-rayed in at least three positions, namely, an anteroposterior view of the ankle, an anteroposterior view of the foot and a lateral view showing foot and ankle. If there is the slightest doubt about complete visualization, oblique views should be made. In studying the film one should carefully outline each involved bone as a separate entity. In his mind's eye or actually with a pencil he should follow along the line of the superior dome of the talus, being particularly careful where it superimposes over the tibia. The appearance of a cloudy shadow, any type of irregularity or any extra fissure line demands further study from different angles.

Many of these cases are not suspected until the so-called sprain has not responded well to treatment. Indeed, the majority of them will not be examined by a doctor in the early stages since the sprain itself may be relatively minor. These fractures, particularly those of the medial surface of the talus, may occur without any actual tearing of the ligaments of the ankle. The usual history is for the patient to present himself with a painful ankle which has resisted all the usual modalities of treatment. Sometimes the treatment for the original injury was quite inadequate (Fig. 585). At other times completely adequate treatment for a sprain has been carried out. In spite of the measures used, the symptoms persist much longer than they should in a sprain. Careful examination at this time will soon determine that one is not dealing with a "chronic sprain" of the ankle. There is no tenderness along the lateral collateral ligaments. There are no symptoms involving the tip of the lateral malleolus or along the cuboid or superolateral surface of the foot. The local symptoms, if any, will be actually in the ankle joint, either at the anterolateral confluence of the talus, tibia and fibula or along a similar area on the posteromedial side of the joint. Such a case presenting with chronic symptoms that are aggravated by activity and that subside almost completely with rest is very frequently an osteochondral fracture. By that time the condition which we identify as osteochondritis dissecans (although it is neither dissecting nor is it an osteochondritis) may be present. Careful x-ray study will reveal the typical appearance with a crater in the articular surface usually occupied by a line of opacity surrounded by an area of radiolucency (Fig. 586). In many instances only the crater appears since the fragment may be dislodged from the bone or may not throw enough shadow to show in the film. This is particularly true in older cases. One should not withhold treatment simply because the opacity is not present.

Treatment. It is my opinion that, in the vast majority of cases, treatment is surgical. True enough, we have learned (particularly at the knee and

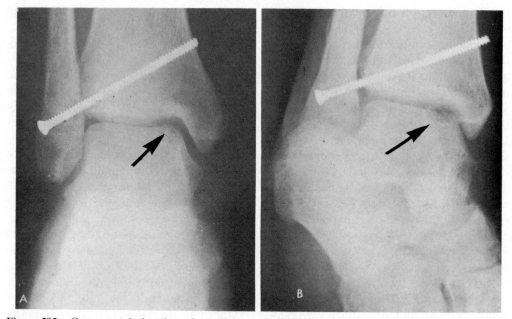

Figure 585. Case treated elsewhere for rupture of deltoid and tibiofibular ligament. Patient remained symptomatic. Examination of x-rays revealed chondral fracture of the superomedial surface of the talus. The patient improved after removal of this fragment and removal of the screw. Note incomplete reduction of tibiofibular diastasis.

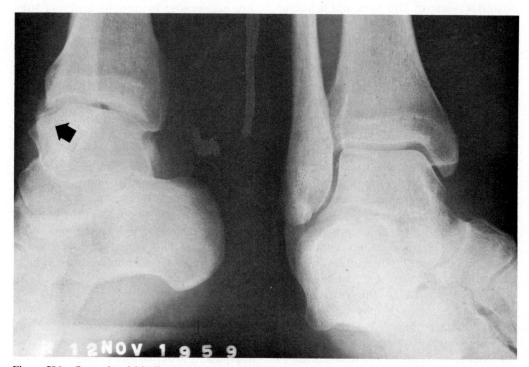

Figure 586. Osteochondritis dissecans of superolateral portion of the talus. *Left,* Arrow shows fragment in oblique view. *Right,* Anteroposterior view was negative.

also at some non-weight-bearing joints) that a prolonged period of protection against weight bearing may permit these conditions to heal, particularly in the young individual. It has been suggested by some that this period should be at least six months and by others as long as a year. In my experience, the success of conservative treatment has not been great enough to justify denying weight bearing to an active young athlete for a period of a year. On the other hand, surgical treatment has been almost uniformly successful in those cases in which a pure lesion was involved. This qualification is made because a long-standing osteochondritis dissecans may cause irreversible chronic arthritic changes in the joint cartilage and in the capsular structures. In such an instance simple elimination of the primary lesion will not cure the condition even though it may result in marked improvement. It is my belief, therefore, that early operation is desirable.

In the unusual instance in which the injury is recognized at once, there may seem to be some justification for conservative treatment. One should bear in mind, however, that no weight bearing can be permitted. Elimination of weight bearing is not accomplished in the walking cast. In fact, the only way I know for one to be relatively certain of no weight bearing is to use a long leg cast with the knee flexed to 90 degrees. Since all admit that many months of casting is necessary, this treatment is not without its hazards and is, to say the least, very onerous to the young and active athlete. It would not be tolerable in an adult. It might conceivably be tolerated by a youngster under 12. The only justification for such nonsurgical treatment would be the risk of surgery and the belief that surgery is not highly successful. Neither of these is a tenable presumption. Treatment, therefore, of these fractures is surgical at whatever stage they are seen.

In the lateral lesion the area may be approached by an extremely atraumatic incision over the anterolateral ankle parallel to and just lateral to the peroneus tertius tendon (Fig. 578). The dorsal retinaculum is divided, the anterior fasciculus of the lateral collateral ligament is sectioned transversely and the capsule is exposed. (See page 734, operation for spurs.) Similarly, the medial side may be exposed by an incision medial to and paralleling the anterior tibial tendon. It is necessary to tie off the anterior division of the saphenous vein below the ankle. Both incisions may be made and the whole mass of tendons, vessels and nerves may be elevated forward out of harm's way. These approaches seem much better than the single incision directly anterior which involves the vascular bundle and the tendons.

In the early case, the capsule will be distended with blood. If the case is of longer duration, a diffuse synovitis will thicken the capsule. (The author recently operated on a patient in whom there was tremendously thickened synovium, at least $3/8$ inch [1 cm.] thick, which presented all the gross characteristics of a xanthomatous synovitis. A classic superolateral talar lesion was found and the other joint changes appeared to be confined to synovitis.) On dividing the capsule along the line of the incision, the anterior margin of the lateral malleolus, the leading edge of the lower end of the tibia and the dome of the talus are exposed. On initial examination all of the cartilage appears to be intact and without any apparent defect, but as the foot is plantar flexed to expose the central portion of the talus, the defect comes into view. In the majority of instances the defect can readily be seen as a separate piece of cartilage, a depressed area with a cartilaginous wrinkle, or a fissure in the cartilage of the superior surface of the talus. In these cases the fragment can be readily lifted up and removed, using a small, curved hemostat or similar instrument. Since the fragment may be as long as 2 cm. or more, it is frequently necessary to go back under the tibia to complete the removal. This can be more easily accomplished if its anterior portion is removed first since this allows ample room to explore the area completely. The chondral margin of the defect should be palpated carefully and any loose or undermined cartilage removed. The crater will present itself as an area lined with chronic granulation tissue which can be scraped away with a curette. The underlying bone is extremely sclerotic. The older the lesion, the more sclerotic the bed will be.

At the conclusion of this procedure there is a dished-out oval of bone including the superior lateral margin of the talus for a major portion of its middle one-third. This crater may be as large as 1 cm. wide, 1 cm. deep and 2 to 3 cm. long, but as a rule it is smaller and is quite avascular even after brisk curetting. If this bed is sclerotic and avascular, it should be drilled (Fig. 582). Using a small size Kirschner wire and a hand drill, my own practice is to drill 8 to 12 holes in the bed deep enough to permit exudation of blood as the wire is removed. Several fresh drill points may be needed if the bone is extremely sclerotic. The area is not plugged with bone wax as in removal of marginal spurs since in this instance we want to encourage exudation of blood and formation of vascular buds at each of these drill holes. The wound is then closed in layers after thorough inspection and copious lavage of the whole operative area. One will be surprised to discover a considerable amount of debris in the basin after lavaging a joint which to the eye appeared quite clean. The lateral collateral ligament and the extensor retinaculum are carefully repaired. Posterior and lateral stirrup splints are applied to below the knee. At the end of 12 to 14 days the stirrup splints are removed, the stitches are removed and the walking cast is applied. This is worn for an additional two weeks depending to some extent upon the attendant joint changes since the ankle joint should be protected longer if there has been long-standing chronic synovitis.

I am convinced that early weight bearing and active use are better than prolonged protection if the defect in the talus is to become filled. Cartilage replaces much better with active use than with immobilization. If the fragment is left in place, prolonged protection is needed to permit it to unite to the talus; on the other hand, after its removal and curettement of the bed, active use will stimulate formation of granulation tissue followed by scar and in many cases by metamorphosis of the scar into fibrocartilage. So, as soon as the operative reaction and attendant arthritic changes have subsided, activity is encouraged. Nor do I see any reason to limit the patient's physical activity provided the ankle remains relatively symptom-free. However, in contact sports I think the ankle should be carefully strapped to prevent recurrence of the type of injury that caused the condition in the first place. The prognosis is extremely favorable in the young and in those cases which have not already progressed to chronic joint changes. Similar lesions occurring elsewhere in the ankle and foot should be treated in a similar fashion.

Some surgeons have recommended that the osteochondral fragment be removed, the bed freshened up and the fragment replaced and pinned to its bed. This seems to me quite unsuitable in the talus. In the first place the lesion is not usually recognized early when the fracture is fresh and union could be expected to occur. In the second place, a major portion of the lesion is pretty well covered by the lower end of the tibia and, while it is available for removal and the bed may be reached for curetting and for drilling, it would be extremely difficult to replace the fragment and pin it adequately without more exposure than seems justified. Exposure can be obtained laterally by transection of the lateral malleolus and medially by transection of the medial malleolus. However, these measures are not without danger of complications and at the very best needlessly prolong convalescence. The success of re-pinning the fragment would seem to depend upon early recognition and treatment. These are the very cases in which removal of the fragment also gives very good results. Following pinning of the fragment, a prolonged period of non-weight-bearing is desirable. As pointed out above, this presents difficulties and is not acceptable to many young patients, so that their cooperation is likely to be poor. For these reasons I do not recommend replacement and internal fixation of the fragment.

SYNOVITIS OF THE ANKLE

Although synovitis is much less of a problem at the ankle than at the knee, some degree of synovitis will occur with any injury involving the capsule of the ankle joint. The manifestations of synovitis at the ankle are quite different from those at the knee. The very nature of the ankle joint is not consistent with extensive effusion. There is relatively little synovium in the ankle, the joint space is snug and tight and there is actually no area of the ankle joint where the synovial surfaces are in contact with each other, as they are for example in the suprapatellar pouch. Therefore, one can infrequently make a diagnosis of synovitis with effusion per se although effusion will occur with injury or with

disease. There is no such evident collection of fluid. The condition appears simply as diffuse swelling of the ankle.

As in other joints, it is extremely important to make a definitive diagnosis if at all possible. In the acute synovitis which may follow an injury or an infection or a metabolic disturbance such as gout, the ankle is painful, swollen, hot and has all the appearance of an acute inflammatory reaction. Aspiration ordinarily will not recover much, if any, fluid. The treatment of such an acute condition is systemic and local. Systemic treatment is treatment of the underlying condition: antibiotics if it is an infection and correction of whatever general condition may be present. Local treatment is rest, elevation, support and local heat. Although it is difficult to aspirate the fluid from the ankle, the ankle may be readily injected. This is not indicated usually in the acute condition. As the acute symptoms subside, it is important to protect the ankle against stress and strain until healing is complete since synovitis will have a great tendency to recur.

Chronic Synovitis

A much more distressing condition is a chronic synovitis of the ankle. As previously indicated in this chapter, there are many conditions about the ankle which are difficult to diagnose. There is mild tibiofibular separation, osteochondral fracture of the talus and instability of the lateral collateral ligaments. All of these will cause the symptoms of a chronic synovitis, namely, swelling, pain and disability, yet the synovitis is simply secondary to a primary condition which may well be amenable to treatment. If careful search does not reveal any particular etiology, treatment must be local. Of prime importance is a period of rest for the ankle. Since this is difficult to obtain in the athlete, rest should be carried out by plaster fixation. Stirrup splints should be used if swelling is marked. As swelling subsides a walking boot cast may be substituted. It will take several weeks of adequate protection followed by a period of strapping and wrapping in order to permit the condition to heal and athletic endeavor to resume. One of the most distressing situations is to relieve the synovitis only to have it recur because the underlying pathology has not been eradicated. A chronic synovitis is not consistent with athletics.

CHAPTER 21

INJURIES OF THE FOOT

ANATOMICAL CONSIDERATIONS

The foot is an extremely ingenious mechanism designed to transfer the body weight from the leg to the ground. The arch of the foot provides an elastic, springy connection so that the jar of weight bearing is dissipated to a large extent before it reaches the long bones of the leg and thigh. The arch also has the function of improving locomotion by adding speed and agility to the gait. Additionally the foot is capable of rolling from side to side when contacting surface imperfections, so permitting the leg to remain vertical while the foot rolls into inversion or eversion.

The leg contacts the foot, in its posterior one-third, so that the longer lever arm from the heads of the metatarsals to the ankle has a marked advantage over the shorter lever arm from the ankle to the back of the calcaneus. Space does not permit a full description of all the many joints of the foot or of its multiplicity of ligaments and tendons, each designed to improve function. A careful study of the anatomy of the foot is extremely interesting and quite rewarding to the surgeon who has to treat injuries to this area.

Basically, the foot is divided into three divisions: the posterior part, consisting of the talus and calcaneus; the central part consisting of the navicular, cuboid and the three cuneiforms; and the anterior part consisting of the metatarsals and the phalanges (Figs. 587, 588 and 589). Each of these areas has characteristics that account for distinctive types of injuries. Thus, injuries to the posterior division are usually of the compression type as the forceful drive of the leg into the foot collapses the

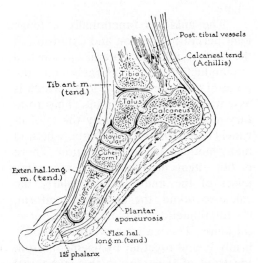

Figure 587. Sagittal section of right foot and ankle, showing bony structure and superficial muscles. (From Jones and Shepard, Manual of Surgical Anatomy.)

747

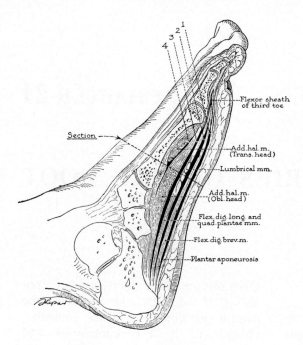

Flexor sheath of third toe

Section

Add.hal.m. (Trans.head)

Lumbrical mm.

Add.hal.m. (Obl.head)

Flex.dig.long. and quad.plantae mm.

Flex.dig.brev.m.

Plantar aponeurosis

Figure 588. Sagittal section through plantar spaces *(1, 2, 3, 4)* of right foot. (From Jones and Shepard, Manual of Surgical Anatomy.)

bone. In the central portion of the foot, the injury is usually an avulsion type as the foot is forced through a range of motion beyond its capacity and either the ligament tears, the bone fractures, or both. In the anterior part, the injury is like that occurring in long bones anywhere.

The ankle is functionally a hinge joint permitting flexion and extension of the foot on the leg. Lateral motion and circumduction occur largely on the pivot of the talonavicular joint, which is essentially a universal joint. This rotatory motion is permitted by the talocalcaneal and talonavicular joints, which in many motions act as a single unit. There is but slight motion in the remaining joints of the midfoot, particularly the calcaneocuboid, the naviculocuneiform, the intercuneiform and the tarsometatarsal joints. This entire area of the foot is firmly bound together by ligaments from the front of the talus to the metatarsal heads. In dissection of the foot it is difficult to delineate the actual joint lines in

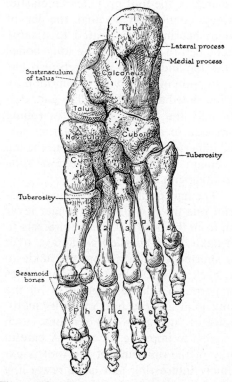

Tuber

Lateral process

Medial process

Sustenaculum of talus

Calcaneus

Talus

Navicula

Cuboid

Cuneif.

Tuberosity

Tuberosity

Metatarsals

Sesamoid bones

Phalanges

Figure 589. The bones of the right foot, viewed from below. (From Jones and Shepard, Manual of Surgical Anatomy.)

the cuneiform-metatarsal areas, so close is the fit. Since there is such intricate apposition of the many bones of the foot, it is very important that the joint surfaces be maintained in the proper position and without undue irregularity. Failures in these respects account for the severity of the disability following what appears to be a relatively minor injury.

The general contour of the foot is a longitudinal arch resting posteriorly on the bottom of the calcaneus and anteriorly on the metatarsal heads. This arch is supported by the plantar ligament arising from the calcaneus and extending forward to attach near the metatarsal heads. In the normal foot the lateral portion of this arch rests on the ground, giving additional support to the foot. The plantar ligament is reinforced by the short flexors and other intrinsic muscles and by the ligaments of the foot. Thus, the integrity of the longitudinal arch is preserved by bony architecture, by strong ligaments and by active muscle.

The undersurface of the foot is covered with unusually heavy skin. The underlying fat pad is compartmented by dense, fibrous bands so that the skin makes a very adherent contact with the deep fascia. The skin of the sole does not slide back and forth as does the skin on top of the foot.

Muscle attachments are arranged to move the foot through its various ranges of active motion and still give static support. The synchronous action of the muscles of the foot is not dissimilar to that of the hand and wrist. The muscle assumes a different function depending upon the starting position of the foot and the motion involved. So also there are different functions of the muscles and varying tensions on the joints depending upon the position of the foot — in equinus, calcaneus, inversion or eversion. The rapidly reversing mo-tions by the athlete cause excessive strain on the various components of the foot.

CONTUSION

Contusion of the foot is a frequent occurrence and may be caused by any sort of direct trauma as by a dropped weight or trampling or striking by another player. Contusion of the dorsum of the foot may be quite distressing because of the extremely sensitive nature of this area. Thin integument overlies the tendons, blood vessels and nerves so that they are caught between the underlying bone and the striking object over thin skin.

The complications of contusion may be more important than the contusion itself. The blow may cause damage to a nerve causing intractable pain over the dorsum of the foot, damage to the blood vessels with phlebitis or hemorrhage, damage to the tendons with resulting tenosynovitis, damage to the periosteum or to the joints. Each of these conditions should be treated appropriately, the important element being recognition of the complication so that one will not continue to reassure the patient that he has a minor condition that will promptly recover when the patient is convinced that he has a rather severe condition that definitely is not recovering. This is particularly true of tenosynovitis which has the same tendency to recur here as elsewhere.

The necessity for weight bearing adds to the seriousness of contusions to the undersurface of the foot. These frequently are caused by a faultily placed spike, a loose cleat, or even a wrinkle in the sock so that the subcutaneous tissue lying between the thick plantar skin and underlying bone and muscle becomes ecchymotic and reacts by inflammation, forming the characteristic "stone bruise." Under the heel or under the metatarsal heads this may be very persistent.

The anatomical characteristics of a particular foot have a great deal to do with this type of injury. The extremely high-arched foot with a tight heel cord puts unusual stress on the metatarsal heads as they strike the floor or track. The tightness of the calf does not permit the ankle to dorsiflex and a good deal of the elasticity of the forefoot is lost. To this is added the fact that the weight is borne on the metatarsal heads and on the heel rather than along the lateral margin of the foot. Thus a contusion to the heel or to the metatarsal heads may result because of the excess pressure of weight bearing. This is particularly pertinent under the first metatarsal head where the equinus of the forefoot throws excess stress against the two sesamoids lying under the first metatarsal head, possibly resulting in severe contusion of these bones. This same type of foot, with a high arch, often has marginal osteophytes at the junction of the metatarsal bases and the cuneiform bones so that the bone is quite prominent under the skin and thus much more subject to damage. Under the heel the relatively vertical position of the calcaneus may cause repetitive bruising in the running gait so that a deep-seated hematoma may form and may develop into an adventitious bursa, thus complicating recovery. The remedy is to relieve weight bearing until the condition has become arrested. This is frequently incompatible with athletic participation. It is particularly distressing to the track man or basketball player since it seems to him to be a minor condition yet it interferes with his effective competition. Early local injection with a long-acting anesthetic agent followed by one of the corticoid preparations is a valuable adjunct in the treatment. Certain ingenuity can be utilized to prevent weight bearing on the tender part and so permit running. Various types of felt pads combined with strapping of the foot may give substantial relief. In this instance it is not the pull of the muscle or the motion itself which causes the distress; it is the blow against the hard surface. In some instances foam padding will give a good deal of relief. This is a good deal more feasible in football shoes than it is in track or basketball shoes. The usual physical therapeutic measures are of some value in expediting recovery since they serve to improve the local circulation, relieve congestion and promote absorption.

STRAIN

Strain is particularly common in the foot. The complex of intrinsic muscles making up the foot is extremely extensive and is subjected to great forces by athletic activity. Some areas are much more frequently involved than others, one of the most common being the insertion of the TENDO ACHILLES to the calcaneus. Strain here may be severely incapacitating since, each time the calf is contracted in walking or running, severe pain occurs at the attachment of the tendon to the heel. Occasionally, chronic strain in the tendo Achilles may result in calcification in the tendon, with distressing recurring pain on function (see Fig. 590). Another common location is at the attachment of the ANTERIOR TIBIAL tendon on the medial side of the foot. Strain is particularly likely to occur here if there is a tendency for the athlete to pronate the heel so that the talus tends to rotate downward and inward in relation to the foot. The anterior tibial is the most active muscle in dorsiflexing the foot and is the opponent of the tendo Achilles. Early in the season, running will frequently cause irritation at either site. Less frequently there will be strain at the attach-

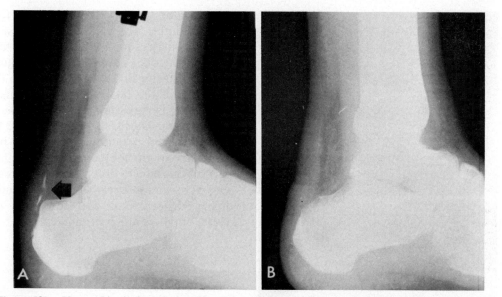

Figure 590. Young skier had persistent pain at the attachment of the tendo Achilles to the calcaneus. *A,* Note calcification in tendon. Pain had become so severe that skiing was impossible. Removal of calcification and scarification of the attachment plus immobilization resulted in complete recovery. *B,* One year postoperative. In this case the prominent superior tubercle at the back of the calcaneus was excised.

ment of the PERONEALS or of the POSTERIOR TIBIAL or of the FLEXORS OF THE TOES (see page 701).

Treatment of strain has been detailed elsewhere (page 62). Elimination of stress is of prime importance. In the heel, strapping to prevent dorsiflexion of the foot and elevation of the heel by a pad in the shoe or an extra rubber heel will serve to relieve the condition provided violent activity is prevented. Physical therapy, especially local heat, is of value but protection is the true remedy for the condition. A longer period of complete disability will be rewarded by complete recovery, whereas temporizing measures often will result in repeated recurrence. If the patient has had a strain of the attachment of the tendo Achilles he probably should keep the foot strapped throughout the remainder of the season to prevent forcible dorsiflexion. True enough, this will not prevent active traction by the calf muscles. It will reduce passive stretching which may be an important

factor, particularly in contact sports. On the other hand, if the anterior tibial is injured the foot should be strapped to prevent extreme plantar flexion. The shoe should be wedged on the inner side of the heel to throw the weight toward the outer side of the foot (page 688). An arch support may be helpful.

While discussing strain of the tendo Achilles attachment, one should mention APOPHYSITIS OF THE CALCANEUS (Fig. 591). This is another of the group of aseptic necroses which occur at various places in the epiphyses of the young athlete. At the calcaneus it is not ordinarily as disabling as at the hip or knee. The calcaneal epiphysis has a wide attachment to the calcaneus and therefore is not particularly subject to extensive irreversible necrosis. Faulty circulation is manifested by sclerosis of the apophysis, frequently accompanied by fragmentation, but the condition is self-limited and usually does not demand drastic treatment. Symptomatically there is pain at the posterior point

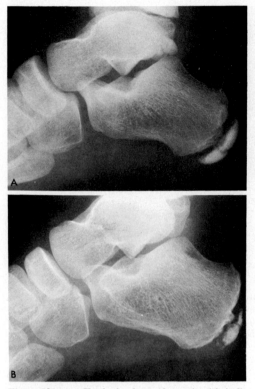

Figure 591. *A*, Typical calcaneal apophysitis indicated by sclerosis and fragmentation. *B*, Another manifestation of calcaneal apophysitis with irregular and delayed epiphyseal formation.

of the heel, usually somewhat below the actual attachment of the tendo Achilles. Pain is elicited by forcible activity so that the adolescent can usually go about his regular activity without trouble only to have recurrence of pain if he starts to run or jump, or violently exercises his foot.

Unlike strain of the tendo Achilles, this condition can usually be completely relieved by restricting dorsiflexion of the foot so that adequate strapping down the back of the leg and over the sole of the foot anchored properly around the ankle, combined with elevation of the shoe heel, is usually all the treatment that is necessary. In my experience a few weeks' reduction of activity will usually result in complete relief from symptoms although the x-ray

evidence of apophysitis will persist for many months. The very acute or resistant case may require a walking cast for six to eight weeks. There is no residual except occasionally some prominence of the back of the heel which may cause symptoms by pressure against the heel of the shoe. During the acute stage, if the tenderness is quite acute, it may be necessary to cut the counter out of the back of the shoe in order to relieve pressure here, and to apply suitable felt padding. Obviously, if the condition is acute, athletics are contraindicated.

SPRAIN

We have defined sprain as a ligament injury and have discussed it particularly from the standpoint of the acute sprain. However, in the foot one must definitely distinguish between static sprain and the acute traumatic sprain.

Traumatic Sprain

Traumatic sprain of the foot is similar to sprain elsewhere and may be acute or chronic. It is caused by violent overstretching of a ligament or ligaments by forcing the involved joint through a wider range of motion than the ligaments will normally permit. The same force applied repeatedly may result in a chronic irritative lesion in the ligament itself. It is basically due to abnormal motion.

Treatment is similar to that of sprain anywhere. In the early stage local injection into the hematoma, compression, ice, followed by adequate support and local heat, is the treatment of choice. Usually support can be accomplished by adequate strapping and elimination of weight bearing, the exact type of support depending upon the ligament involved. Thus, if the sprain involves the calcaneocuboid ligament, it will be treated much like sprain of the ankle. In the plantar ligament it will be treated by support under the arch to prevent distraction between the heads of the metatarsals and the calcaneus. Acute sprain should be evaluated as to its severity since this will to a considerable extent determine the degree of immobilization and its duration (see Fig. 592). If the sprain has been due to inversion or eversion of the foot, suitable strapping of the ankle type (Fig. 569) is advisable since it is difficult to immobilize the foot properly without including the lower leg. This is particularly true of sprain of the arch where it is important to keep the foot inverted (Fig. 554). Additional support can be given by a wedge on the shoe heel so that, if an arch sprain is present, a medial heel wedge to invert the foot will relieve tension. If the sprain is in the lateral ligaments of the foot a lateral wedge on the heel or on the sole worn on a temporary basis for a matter of a few weeks will be of considerable value in relieving the stress until healing is complete.

If the injury appears to be quite severe at the time of the initial examination, careful x-ray study must be made to rule out any fracture or dislocation. The proper local treatment should then be instituted followed by elevation of the foot, compression bandage and ice pack overnight. Evaluation the next day will permit one to determine somewhat better the extent of injury. In some instances it may be necessary to continue elevation and cold followed by heat until swelling subsides sufficiently to permit application of plaster splint for a few days, followed by a plaster boot. This boot should be worn for ten days and followed by adequate strapping, arch support and wedge on the shoe heel until the foot is symptom-free.

The acute sprain may involve the intermetatarsal ligaments at the distal end of the metatarsal. It is particularly likely to occur in the track man who runs in a very light shoe or may run barefooted and receive an injury to his anterior ligaments. This should be treated in the usual manner but the strapping in this

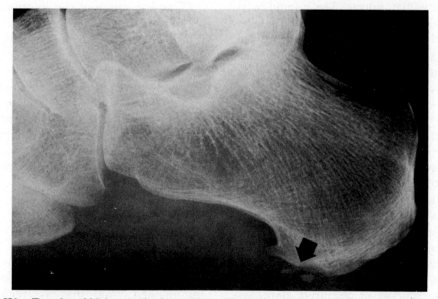

Figure 592. Two day old injury to the foot with swelling and exquisite tenderness under the heel. Note avulsion of plantar ligament with fragment of bone, so-called sprain fracture. No relationship to calcaneal spur.

case should be circumferential around the forefoot. This must not be confused with chronic sprain of the intermetatarsal ligaments, which may be extremely resistant to treatment. Once the acute sprain occurs, the forefoot should be strapped for the remainder of the season (see page 720).

Static Sprain

Static conditions of the foot can be a very complicated and serious problem but will not be dwelt upon at length here. However, one will be called upon frequently to distinguish between a chronic sprain of the foot and a static sprain of the arch. Whereas the chronic sprain is due to repeated episodes of overmotion, the static sprain is due to the constant stress of superimposed weight on the arch of the foot. This is most frequently manifested by pain along the plantar ligament from the attachment of the calcaneus to its attachment near the metatarsal heads. It is promptly relieved by elimination of weight bearing. There is no history of any particular injury. The condition is more likely to occur early in the season when the patient abruptly changes from his regular shoes which have considerable support in the arch to the flat shoes of athletic equipment. This plus the superimposed weight of his equipment and more violent exercise plus long hours on his feet may combine to cause a sprain of the arch. The diagnosis is often suggested by the fact that the player has had foot trouble before and frequently is wearing arch support shoes or arch supports in his street shoes.

Treatment. Static sprain of this type will not respond well to treatment indicated for acute sprains but should receive the treatment given for flatfoot, namely, support of the arch, improvement of the posture of the foot and reconstructive exercises (Fig. 593) to improve the muscle tone of the foot. When one recalls that the muscles of the foot are very similar to those of the hand, he will recognize the importance of proper specific exercises for the so-called weak foot or chronic sprain. Participation in sports cannot be permitted without adequate support by means of either arch supports or adequate strapping since every recurrence of symptoms simply makes it more difficult to effect a complete recovery. This type of condition is not at all limited to "flatfoot." In fact, some of the most painful arches are the very high ones in which case most of the body weight is carried on the metatarsal heads and on the heel. This subjects the plantar ligament and other inferior ligaments of the foot to considerable stress on weight bearing. A carefully outlined program meticulously followed by the patient will give gratifying results. It should be emphasized again that during the violent exercise of athletics the arch should be protected by flexible cork and leather arch supports once it has been subject to chronic sprain.

Chronic sprain of the intermetatarsal ligaments is evidenced by pain in the area of the metatarsal heads. This may be a sequel of acute sprain or may be due to static stretching of the ligaments. It must be treated by circumferential strapping, metatarsal pad and anterior heel, but here again the treatment will likely be incompatible with athletic activity. Chronic sprain may be accompanied by or confused with plantar neuroma.

PLANTAR NEUROMA
(MORTON'S TOE)

Plantar neuroma is a static condition of the foot that is relatively frequent in athletes (Fig. 594). The player usually complains of a "sprain"

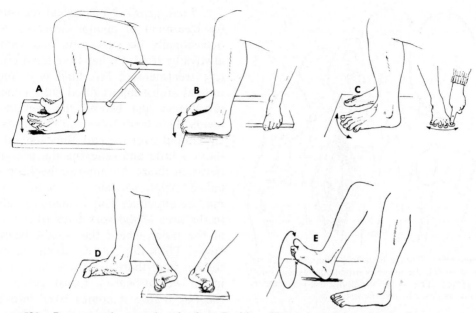

Figure 593. Reconstructive exercises for foot. Position: The patient sitting with the feet on a smooth, flat surface. These exercises should be done slowly and forcibly with maximum effort maintained for three seconds, 1–2–3.

A, Actively lift the toes, keeping the ball of the foot on the floor. This should be done 30 times.

B, Slide the foot forward so that the toes protrude beyond the edge. Flex toes downward 30 times.

C, Spread the toes widely 30 times. At first it may be necessary to assist this movement with the hands.

D, Raise the inner margin of the foot with the weight thrown on the outer margin. Curl the toes downward and backward in attempt to "make a fist."

E, Holding one foot firmly on the floor, place the other foot forward until it rests on the heel. In this position, rotate the anterior part of the foot from the outside inward, so the tip of the right big toe makes a complete circle in a clockwise direction. Definite effort must be made to force this motion to the extreme. The left should turn counterclockwise.

These exercises must be done slowly to the count of 1–2–3 seconds, with a similar period between each movement. Distinct effort must be made to get the most possible motion, and if this is done a definite strain will be felt upon the involved muscles. Exercises should be begun at about ten times apiece, gradually increasing it to 30 times apiece. They should be done twice daily.

You must not hurry through these exercises.

of the anterior arch. The symptom that distinguishes it from sprain is intermittent, excruciating pain in the lateral part of the forefoot usually running into the adjacent sides of the third and fourth toes and occasionally up the dorsum of the foot toward the ankle. There is often a feeling of an electric shock running out into one or both of the toes. Numbness of the adjacent sides of these two toes may be frequently present but it is not as common as the tingling sensation or shock feeling which runs down into the toes. The condition is not ordinarily brought on by any specific motion or any specific sprain. It comes on spontaneously when least expected. The patient is usually much more comfortable barefooted, whereas in sprain of the arch the foot is not comfortable without the support of shoes. On examination tenderness will be found between the third and fourth metatarsal heads, and it will be exquisite on localized pressure in the plantar surface of the web between the third and fourth toes when pressure is directed back toward the third and fourth heads. This finding is best elicited by pressure of the rubber end of a pencil. Compression of the metatarsal

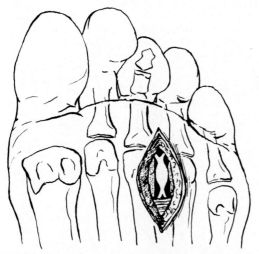

Figure 594. Plantar neuroma. Plantar aspect. In this approach the nerve is subcutaneous and readily treated. The more commonly used incision is dorsal, as described in the text.

heads, particularly by rolling the heads across each other by lateral pressure, will often elicit a definite click accompanied by pain, usually referred to the third and fourth toes. An almost diagnostic description by the patient is that while he is walking or dancing or running he suddenly gets a severe pain in the forefoot; he snatches off his shoe and massages his foot with almost immediate relief.

The cause of this condition is a thickening of the plantar nerve at the point where the medial and lateral branches join and then separate to pass to the adjacent sides of the third and fourth toes. The thickened area where the "x" is formed is subject to trauma when caught between the metatarsal heads. A predisposing factor is relaxation of the intermetatarsal ligaments which permits splaying of the forefoot. As a result of this irritative pressure an extremely large mass of nerve and fibrous tissue may gradually be formed. The larger the mass the more frequently it is caught between the metatarsal heads and the more severe the symptoms.

Treatment. Nonsurgical measures for treatment of plantar neuroma may occasionally be successful and should always be tried. Perhaps the most effective treatment of this kind is a longitudinal arch support fitted with a metatarsal pad just behind the metatarsal heads. This tends to permit the heads to spread out over the pad, thus separating them a little and relieving the pressure between them. An anterior heel, or so-called metatarsal bar put on the shoe, may be effective. This is made by filling in the area at the very back of the sole at the point where the weight bearing stops. Thus the sole is about 1/8 inch thicker here than elsewhere so that the initial weight-bearing thrust comes on the bar before it comes over into the sole of the shoe. Since the pinching is usually quite transient, measures such as heat, massage and elevation usually are not effective. *Surgical treatment* usually is extremely effective if properly carried out. It is extremely important to resect the mass completely. While this may be done through the sole of the foot the general distaste for leaving an open sore on the plantar surface of the foot has made the dorsal incision much more popular although it is considerably more complicated.

It should be recalled that the medial plantar nerve ordinarily supplies three and a half toes and the lateral plantar nerve, one and a half. As a rule, the lateral plantar nerve sends a communicating branch over to the most lateral component of the medial plantar nerve and they join just proximal to the heads of the third and fourth metatarsals. As they pass distally, they divide to form the lateral digital nerve to the third toe and the medial digital nerve to the fourth toe. The resulting thickening makes the nerve particularly susceptible to pressure between the adjacent metatarsal heads. The nerve courses in the plantar surface of the foot beneath the intermetatarsal ligaments but superior to the plantar aponeurosis, lying in the interval between the long flexor tendons.

Approach then is as follows: A linear incision is made, beginning at the web between the third and fourth toes and extending parallel to these two metatarsals and between their extensor tendons. The skin is divided and the extensor tendons are retracted, exposing the dorsal interossei tendons adjacent to each metatarsal. These are retracted, exposing the ligament extending between the two metatarsal heads. This is divided transversely, and the two metatarsal heads are retracted, permitting access to the space just superficial to the plantar subcutaneous tissue. The digital nerves should be defined and cut distally. They are then reflected back freeing the tumor mass which can be pushed up by pressure under the sole of the foot. The mass is carefully elevated out of the intermetatarsal space, and dissection is carried proximally until the normal nerve trunk is identified. Ordinarily there will be a medial and a lateral trunk.

Dissection of the nerves should continue as far as the middle of the metatarsal shaft before they are divided. This should prevent recurrence of pain by constriction of the nerve in the scar. Usually there will be a discrete mass of fatty, fibrous and nerve tissues with two digital nerves which appear relatively normal and two proximal nerves which appear relatively normal. We recently have reoperated on a patient who had intractable pain following excision of a plantar neuroma. We found an extremely large edematous nerve extending right into the masses of scar and very adherent to it. It did not have a neuroma on the end but its adherence to the scar between the two metatarsal heads caused the pain which was promptly relieved by resection of the nerve back up under the metatarsals. In the repair, care should be taken to approximate the divided intermetatarsal ligament, and in the aftercare, the metatarsal heads must be supported by a snug bandage in order to prevent further separation between these two heads.

TENOSYNOVITIS

The foot is quite subject to tenosynovitis since its tendons are charged with the responsibility not only of motion but also of supporting considerable weight. The cause of tenosynovitis here is the same as in other locations, namely, a direct blow or chronic overuse. The latter is more important in the athlete. Frequently tenosynovitis is combined with other conditions such as strain of the tendon attachment. The resultant irritation causes friction between the tendon and its surrounding sheath with edema, inflammation and adhesions, all of which cause pain on active function. Characteristic findings are pain on passive stretching of the involved tendon, pain on active motion of the involved tendon, and tenderness over the tendon at the point of the irritation. Careful palpation over the tendon while active motion is carried out will often elicit "snowball" crepitation, which is diagnostic of tenosynovitis. The tendon sheath does not usually distend with excess fluid as does the joint with synovitis. Tenosynovitis is particularly prone to occur in the early phases of training, being especially frequent in track men particularly when they are training on the boards.

Treatment. Tenosynovitis is another of those conditions which can be treated well only by elimination of the stress involved. This of necessity means elimination of competitive athletics. Other measures of importance in expediting the cure are local injection, local physical therapy and protection. In the foot it is difficult to prevent stress on the tendon without giving support to the arch. These cases frequently should be treated by a splint to prevent motion altogether, followed later by adequate strapping and wrapping to prevent excess motion. At the same time the splint and the strapping should support the arch of the foot. Caution should be used in application of the strapping so that it does not compress the tendon between the strapping and the underlying bone since this may increase the irritation rather than diminish it.

Tenosynovitis involving the dorsiflexors, namely, the anterior tibial, peroneus tertius and toe extensors, should be treated by strapping the foot to prevent plantar flexion (see Fig. 14). Tenosynovitis of the posterior structures such as the calf, peroneals and posterior tibial should be strapped so that the foot will not dorsiflex beyond neutral and also to give lateral support (see Fig. 542). All too often, however, the irritating factor is function of the muscle rather than passive stretching of the tendon and continued forcible motion is incompatible with prompt recovery. Once recovery is complete, strapping is of great importance in preventing recurrence. If strapping does not give complete relief, a time period of about 10 to 14 days should be spent in a walking cast before the strapping. This will expedite recovery.

BURSITIS

Bursitis is not a common problem in injury to the foot although it is well to bear in mind that it may occur. A particularly distressing type of bursitis is that of the bursa between the calcaneus and skin on the plantar surface of the heel. This can be readily mistaken for strain of the attachment of the plantar ligament, particularly if spurs happen to be demonstrable at this attachment. It can usually be distinguished by the fact that tenderness is considerably further posterior on the heel than is usually the case in involvement of the plantar ligament. *Treatment* is by local injection, local application of heat, protective sponge rubber in the shoes and in severe cases by excision of the bursa. There may be a bursitis of the bunion joint but this is not frequent in athletes and requires no discussion here.

Another bursa frequently involved in the foot is that between the tendo Achilles and the back of the calcaneus. The symptoms here may be readily confused with those of strain of the attachment of the tendo Achilles. However, active contraction of the calf should not cause increase of symptoms in bursitis although local pressure does. Careful examination will usually distinguish the condition, the pain being just proximal to the attachment of the tendon to the calcaneus and anterior to the tendon. Tenderness may also be elicited by pressure in the space anterior to the tendo Achilles. Rarely does the bursa enlarge enough to permit the fluid to be palpated or aspirated. *Treatment* consists of local injection and protection against pressure. In the acute phase, dorsiflexion of the foot should be prevented by strapping. This bursitis is not usually as resistant as apophysitis and not as recurrent as strain of the tendo Achilles attachment.

Another common bursitis which particularly frustrates the athlete, especially a track man, involves the bursa lying under the first metatarsal head between the skin and the medial sesamoid. A callus often develops in this area and the skin becomes quite firm and hard. This is apposed to the tendon aponeurosis containing the medial and lateral sesamoids, and the increased weight bearing on these two hard surfaces encourages the development of bursa between them. While this bursa may be protective, permitting the surfaces to slide more freely over each other, it often becomes inflamed and causes severe pain on weight bearing, particularly on running. This requires the treatment given for all bursitis conditions; that is, protection against irritation, aspiration and injection if indicated. The condition may be extremely distressing to the athlete since any attempt to resume his athletic endeavors before the bursa is entirely healed will simply result in aggravation of the bursitis. This should not be confused with involvement of the articular cartilage on the sesamoid itself, although the subjective symptoms may be quite similar. If the bursa becomes chronic, with thickened walls, it may be necessary to excise it surgically.

SYNOVIAL HERNIA (GANGLION)

Whereas synovial hernia is not particularly common in the ankle, it is frequent in the foot. This is explained by the multiplicity of joints and tendons in the foot, making legion the areas where chronic sprain followed by weakness of the capsule and herniation of the synovium may occur. It is not necessary to discuss these in detail in their various locations, but one or two deserve special mention here. One frequent area is near the peroneal tendon distal to the lateral malleolus. In this instance the herniation may be of extremely large size as in the case recently operated upon in which the mass was about the size and shape of one's long finger but came down to a single defect in the tendon sheath no larger than the point of a lead pencil (Fig. 595). Another frequent area of involvement is the dorsum of the foot in the long extensor tendons where it may come off the tendon sheath or from the tarsal joints.

The *treatment* is the same as treatment of synovial hernia elsewhere (page 85). It cannot be overemphasized that if surgical treatment is undertaken it should be done as a major procedure under general anesthesia so that the sac can be meticulously dissected out. If at all possible the defect in the sheath or capsule should be repaired. Chopping off the top of the mass through a $1/2$ inch "medical" incision only results in scarring which makes a later surgical procedure extremely difficult. Surgical excision should be followed by complete immobilization for at least the three weeks needed for ligament or capsule to begin to heal. Resulting stiffness is not as common in the foot as it is in the wrist. No particular rehabilitation is necessary other than for the muscles which have been immobilized.

One can only condemn the treatment of these lesions by violent direct trauma, such as a sharp blow. Aspiration of the mass followed by pressure dressing can be readily done in the foot and is an acceptable measure. Some have reported unbelievably good results from injection of steroids but in my experience this has rarely had any more effect than simple aspiration of the lesion. Repeated aspiration particularly in the foot entails the hazard of ultimate infection and is probably not justified by the results. In several cases in which surgery has followed corticoid injections we have seen plaques of calcific-like material within the sac or in the adjacent tissues. These have been ascribed to irritation from the injection but the matter will require further investigation.

A synovial hernia of moderate size is not incompatible with athletic activity. There is really no objection to permitting athletic competition and postponing removal of the hernia to a later time, provided adequate strapping is utilized and symptoms are not severe enough to interdict active use.

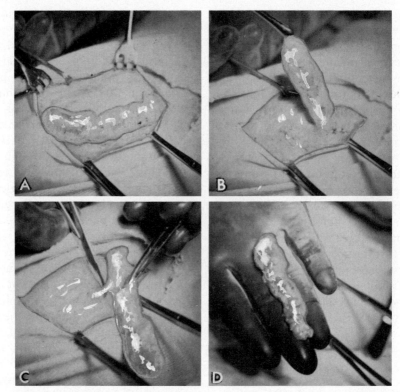

Figure 595. Lateral side injury of the peroneal tendons with resulting painful tumor alongside peroneal tendons. Section proved it to be a synovial hernia off the tendon sheath. *A*, The exposed mass. *B*, The dissection. *C*, Down to match-stem pedicle. *D*, The intact mass removed.

DISLOCATION

Dislocation of the foot is not frequent in athletics. It is much more infrequent than ankle dislocation for obvious reasons. The foot is protected by the shoe and frequently by wrapping and is not subject to the violent disruption stresses that may dislocate the ankle or knee. When a severe injury to the foot occurs, careful study of the x-rays should be carried out, comparing them with films of the opposite foot. Particularly to be looked for is a possible separation of the tarsal joints. A common type of dislocation is one extending along the foot between the first and second metatarsal bases, between the internal and middle cuneiforms, and across the foot laterally at the level of the metatarsal cuboid joints (Figs. 596 and 597). This may be suspected from a tendency of the foot to be broader in this area with characteristic widening of the joint space, the wider space angulating across the foot. The base of the fifth metatarsal is more prominent than normal and pressure here is quite painful. The tip of the base of the metatarsal may be broken off so that the shaft is actually lateral to the proximal tip. This represents a serious disruption of the ligaments of the foot and should be treated by complete reduction and internal fixation. If it is not treated or is treated overcasually, the result is broadening of the forefoot, chronic strain of the tarsal joints and marked incapacity which is extremely difficult to treat at a later stage (Fig. 598). In such obviously severe injuries of the forefoot a particular effort must be made to be sure that

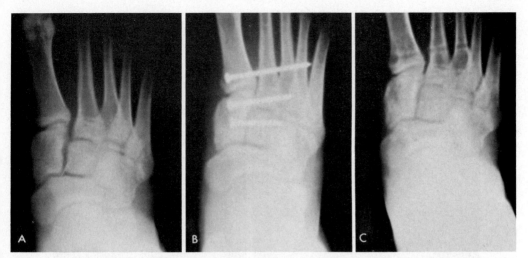

Figure 596. *A*, Dislocation between the first and second metatarsals, the inner and middle cuneiforms, the middle cuneiform and navicular, and the navicular and cuboid. Note definite increase in space between middle and medial cuneiform and the medial cuneiform and distal side of the navicular. *B*, Early, very firm fixation with three screws was done. Immobilization in a walking cast for four weeks was followed by weight-bearing in a stout boot for four weeks. *C*, Twelve weeks postoperative: the screws were removed and arch support recommended for one year with no athletic activity permitted. Good recovery.

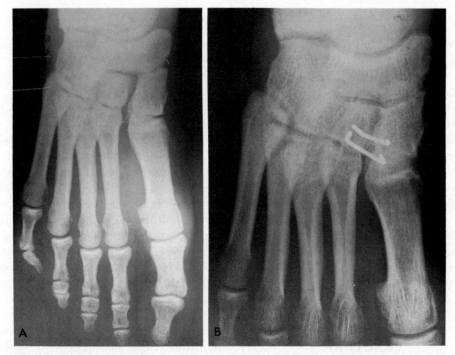

Figure 597. Overlooked dislocation. It was necessary to fuse the two middle and medial cuneiforms. There was some resultant disability. This dislocation is between the first and second metatarsals, medial and middle cuneiforms. The joint between the proximal end of the medial cuneiform and the navicular was not seriously damaged.

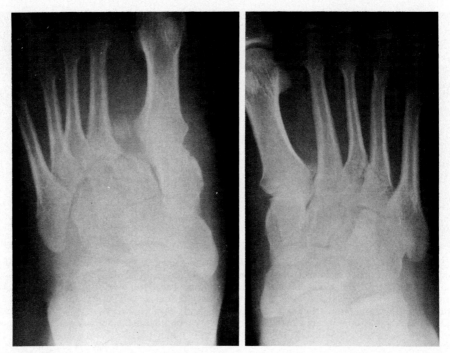

Figure 598. Result of unreduced dislocation similar to that in Figure 596 with gross disability. Note the displacement between the first and second metatarsals extending along the metatarsal cuneiform and cuboid joints with lateral displacement. Note base of M-5 displaced proximally and laterally. *Right,* The normal foot for comparison.

the swelling, pain and disability are not actually due to a persistent displacement or to a spontaneously reduced dislocation.

Other examples of dislocation are illustrated in Figures 599, 600 and 601.

Dislocations of the toes are not frequent but should be promptly recognized and completely reduced. Adequate support is usually provided by strapping the injured toe to the adjacent toes, which are used as splints. With well-fitted shoes and firm soles, continued activity is justifiable. The habit of playing competitive sports in sock feet is to be deplored since the shoe is an excellent protection for the foot.

FRACTURE

The anatomical division of the foot into posterior, middle and anterior por-

tions has definite clinical value in consideration of fractures.

Fracture of the Posterior Portion of the Foot

This section of the foot, including as it does the talus and calcaneus, is rarely fractured in athletics if sprain-fractures are excluded. The ordinary fracture here is by direct compression as in a fall from a height or from driving the foot into the floor board of a car (Figs. 602, 603 and 604). Fortunately, neither of these causes is common in athletics. Certain fractures do occur in special situations such as have been described in the section on the ankle. Abnormal forceful motion may cause avulsion (Figs. 605, 606 and 607) or snubbing fractures of the talus (Fig. 608). So also the sustentaculum tali may be broken by forceful eversion of the

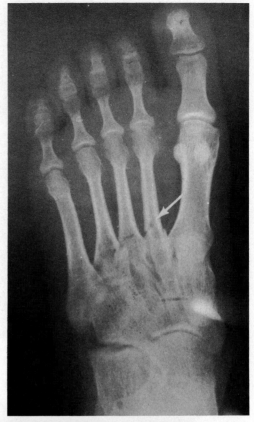

Figure 599. Fracture-dislocation of the foot. Note fracture extending across the bases of metatarsals 2–3–4 with lateral dislocation of the base of M-5. The whole unit is displaced laterally. This is a disabling type injury if not reduced by approximating the shaft of M-2 to M-1. This is similar to the injury in Figure 596.

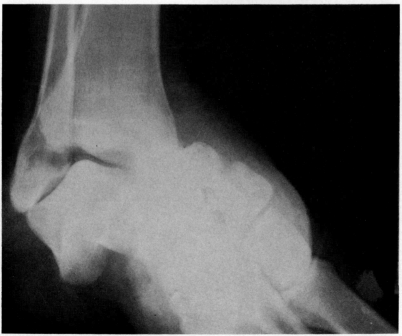

Figure 600. Unusual case of compound dislocation of ankle and foot. Note that the talus is tipped out of the ankle mortice but the deltoid ligament is apparently intact. Talus is also dislocated on the tarsus.

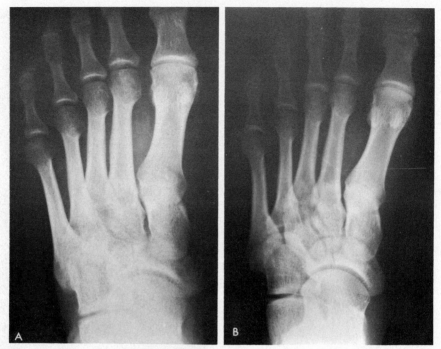

Figure 601. *A,* Fracture-dislocation in tarsal-metatarsal region. This is similar to that of Figure 596 except that the defect continued back through the navicular by breaking its middle third. *B,* The follow-up shows good healing of the navicular but widening of the space between the first and second rays. This probably could have been prevented by early open reduction and internal fixation.

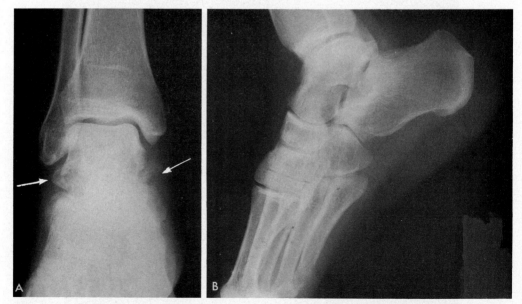

Figure 602. Compression fracture of the calcaneus as the pole vaulter landed on the edge of the pit. *A,* Showing medial and lateral expansion of the calcaneus with fracture through the sustentaculum tali. This could easily be overlooked. *B,* Lateral view is not definitive.

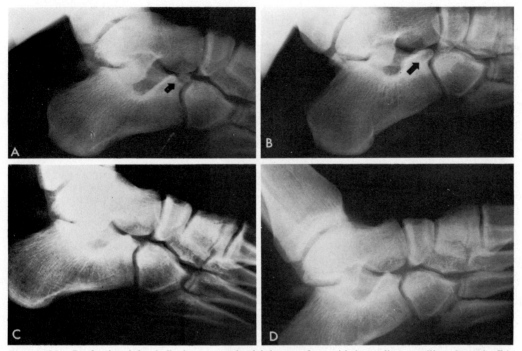

Figure 603. Professional football player sustained injury to foot with immediate swelling. Stayed off it for four weeks then continued playing, but with increased trouble. *A*, X-ray six months post-injury revealed fracture of anterior process of the calcaneus. At removal, the fragment was found to be one inch long, extending right into the talocalcaneal joint. *B*, There was a normal anterior process on the opposite foot. *C*, One month postoperative. *D*, Two months postoperative.

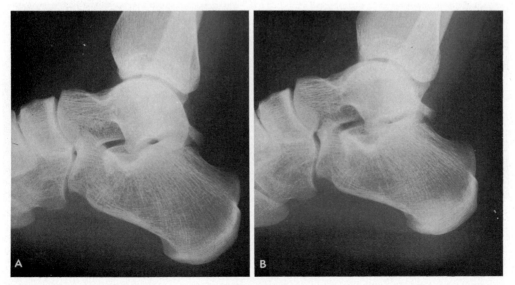

Figure 604. Persistently painful heel after sharply striking the ground. *A*, The negative lateral film. *B*, Two weeks later showing condensation at the ball of the calcaneus, indicating a compression fracture.

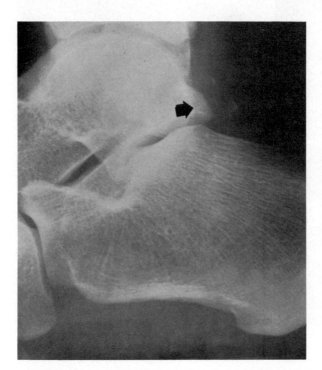

Figure 605. Avulsion of the posterior portion of the talus three weeks old. Note the shape of the avulsed fragment which would fit right on the posterior end of the talus. This is not an os trigonum. This is the result of a dorsiflexion injury, the same forces that cause tibiofibular separation.

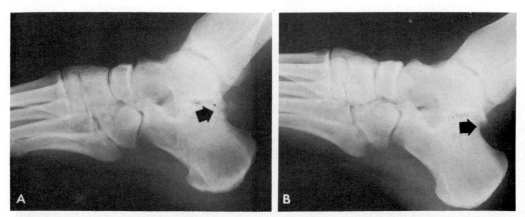

Figure 606. *A,* A forcible dorsiflexion injury. Note the separate fragment at the back of the talus. This is an actual fracture of the posterior process of the talus, not os trigonum. Note normal foot *(B)* showing unusually long posterior process. The mechanism here is probably snapping off of this posterior process as the back of the talus comes forcibly against the top of the calcaneus. This patient had been treated for a "minor strain" and was still very symptomatic three months later. Removal of the fragment relieved the symptoms.

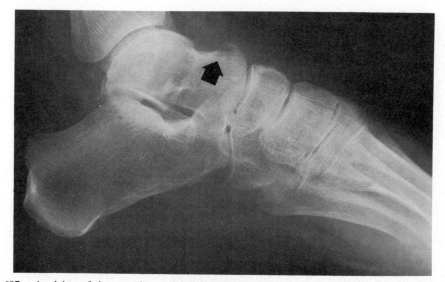

Figure 607. Avulsion of the superior margin of the head of the talus. Detachment of the anterior capsule. This should be treated by excision of the fragment and repair of the capsule.

foot (Fig. 602). It is extremely important to restore the contour of the calcaneus and particularly the integrity of the talocalcaneal joint. Adduction or abduction of the foot may cause a snubbing or avulsion fracture of the superior portion of the calcaneus at the calcaneocuboid joint. If the fragment is large and displaced it should be replaced surgically if necessary. The smaller fragment may be treated as a sprain and recovery will be good (Fig. 609).

Fracture of the Central Portion of the Foot

This portion of the foot includes the navicular, cuboid, and first, second and third cuneiforms. This section is extremely well bound together by the various ligaments and moves almost as a unit. Compression fractures may occur in these bones but they are usually not recognized as such unless there has been a major injury to the foot. A much

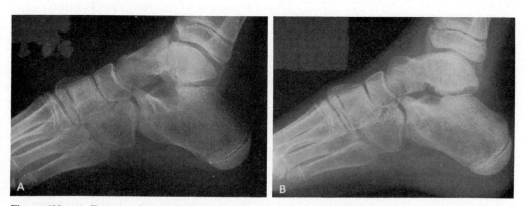

Figure 608. *A*, Fracture through anterior portion of the body of the talus, result of forcible plantar flexion injury. *B*, Result nine months after open reduction and internal fixation.

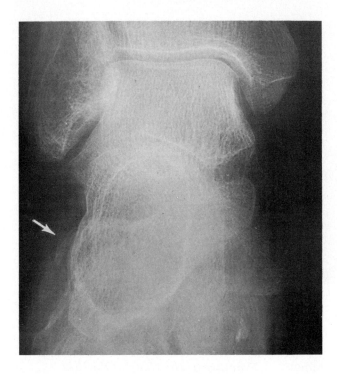

Figure 609. Sprain-fracture of lateral margin of calcaneus, an inversion injury.

more common fracture in athletics is avulsion of an adjacent fragment of bone by the ligament at the time of dislocation or subluxation of the joint. This may be between the cuneiforms or between the cuneiforms and the cuboid or navicular. In the dislocation between the first and second metatarsals, then between the first and second cuneiforms and then across between the navicular and cuboid, there may be one or more areas of fracture (Fig. 601). That is, the injury may split the middle cuneiform rather than cause dislocation between the first and second; the posterior portion of the cuboid may fracture rather than dislocate between the cuboid and navicular. These are modifications of the same injury and require the same treatment, namely, firm fixation in perfect position until union occurs. Surgery may be necessary to accomplish this end. Bony fusion of the joint is considerably more functional than hypermobility or painful motion and results in little handicap. Several weeks will be needed for

union and during this period the foot should be carefully immobilized in a cast that molds the arch into perfect position. A walking cast is not advisable. When the cast is removed and tape applied, protection should be supplied by a molded arch support for many months since chronic disability of the foot is frequent following fractures in this area.

Fracture of the Anterior Portion of the Foot

By far the most common area for fracture is the anterior portion of the foot which consists of the long bones of the metatarsals and phalanges.

Fracture of the Metatarsals. The five metatarsals are long bones that are firmly bound together by overlapping layers of ligament at their bases, held together in the midshaft by the interosseous membrane and at the distal ends by the plantar and dorsal divisions of the distal intermetatarsal ligament.

Fracture of the Base of the Metatarsal. The most frequent fracture is at the base of the fifth metatarsal (Fig. 610). This conical base with its tip posterior is considerably weaker than the quadrilateral bases of the other metatarsals (Fig. 611). The strong attachment of the peroneus brevis plus the massive lateral ligament attachments tend to fix the base of this metatarsal as the forefoot is sharply inverted and adducted and a greater or lesser fragment of the base of this bone may be pulled away. This is essentially a sprain-fracture and may be treated as such. Nonunion of the fragment is not unusual, and while not necessarily disabling, it may be quite painful. Immobilization in plaster splints followed by a walking cast for a total of four weeks will usually give firm enough fixation that taping and a good stout shoe may then be used for support. If painful nonunion persists, the fragment, if small, may be removed and the attachments replaced to the metatarsal. If the fragment is large, internal fixation may be necessary.

On the medial side of the foot the base of the first metatarsal is not often the site of fracture, owing not only to its sturdy structure but to the fact that the stresses applied to this side are not as great as those on the lateral side.

The metatarsal bases may be involved in fracture-dislocation in which a portion of the base is snubbed off as the shaft is forced away from its normal position (Fig. 599). These fractures are usually caused by sharp dorsiflexion or forcible plantar flexion of the foot. The result may be extremely distressing, particularly if the lesion is not recognized. Careful x-ray study will usually reveal the fracture, particularly when one's attention is called to it by sharply localized tenderness. It is important that the integrity of the joint surfaces be restored as fully as possible, particularly if there is tendency for a portion of the bone to subluxate. In these cases reduction should be followed by fixation with a transfixion Kirschner wire, the wire being passed across the bases of the intact bones and through the involved bone after complete reduction.

Fracture of the Shaft of the Metatarsal. Metatarsal shaft fractures are similar to those of long bones elsewhere. The presence of five bones in the same plane allows each one to protect the other to some extent. The cause may be a crushing force applied over

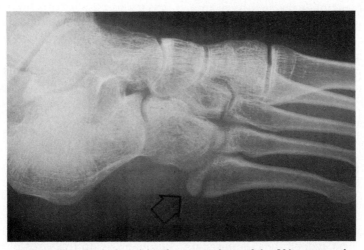

Figure 610. Typical avulsion fracture at base of the fifth metatarsal.

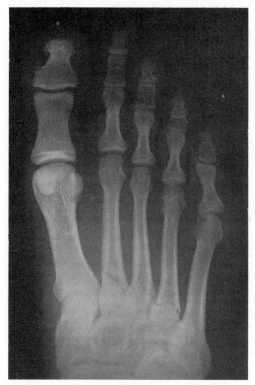

Figure 611. Fracture of the bases of the second, third and fourth metatarsals caused by a sharp hyperflexion injury as the player was hit on the leg from behind. This is one of the hazards of "clipping."

the dorsum of the foot as it is resting on the ground, or forcible torsion of the forefoot on the tarsus. Examination reveals tenderness over the involved area with swelling and hematoma formation. Diagnosis can be confirmed by x-ray study. If there is gross displacement, the fracture should be reduced and held in good position. This may require open reduction. Frequently if only one shaft is involved it may hold well without internal fixation (Figs. 612 and 613). In a comminuted, oblique or spiral fracture of several shafts, skeletal traction may be needed through the toes to secure proper alignment of the bones (Figs. 614 and 615). Particular attention should be paid to the space between the metatarsals, best judged by comparison

with the opposite foot. If the bases of these bones tend to separate, they can frequently be held in good position by threaded Kirschner wires transfixed through several metatarsals after the bones have been placed in normal position. Fracture of the metatarsals is an extremely disabling injury to an athlete and complete healing must be secured before competition is permitted. An arch support should be worn, particularly in athletic shoes.

Isolated fatigue fracture of the metatarsal shaft may occur from strain (pages 86 and 778). Indeed, excessive strain may cause complete fracture with displacement as the leverage is applied to the metatarsal heads with the foot in equinus.

Fracture of the Head and Neck of the Metatarsals. Fracture through this area in the foot is not nearly so frequent as in the hand. Ordinarily there is little displacement and simple fixation and protection from weight bearing will suffice (Fig. 616). However, if the fracture is unrecognized and malunion or nonunion occurs, the metatarsal head may be removed. However, this may be quite disabling. This is not to be recommended for an acute injury since union can usually be obtained without it if good fixation is secured. It may be necessary to pass a Kirschner wire through the head of the metatarsal and down into the shaft in order to hold the head in proper position.

Fracture of the articular cartilage of the metatarsal head is infrequent in athletics and does not constitute a serious hazard. If a portion of the head is broken off in any way and heals in an irregular manner, that head may be removed. It is not advisable to remove more than one head or to remove the first or fifth in an athlete.

Fracture of the Toes. Fractures of the toes do not present as serious a problem as do fractures of the fingers in spite of the fact that similar anatomical structures are involved. While fracture of the toe seems to arouse a sardonic amusement in the minds of everyone but the victim, to the athlete the fractured toe may be extremely disturbing, even to the point of missing a season's play. While it is usually not necessary to carry out the methods for fixation in the toes that are used in the fingers, one should at least take pains enough in the treatment of these conditions to be sure that the end result will be compatible with normal and not unduly delayed function. Many of these accidents occur in the dressing room rather than on the playing field, as by slipping on the wet floor or stubbing the toes against articles of furniture. The tendency for a certain amount of horseplay to work off excess exuberance makes this more probable. Direct forces, as when a bench tips over

on the bare toes, may also result in painful injuries. While the ordinary person may get by pretty well simply wearing a heavy shoe, the athlete with his extremely flexible shoes and with the ever present necessity for forcible flexion and extension of the toes presents a wholly different problem.

Fracture of the First Toe. The first toe should be considered separately since it is much more vital in the mechanics of the foot than the smaller toes. In normal stride, considerable stress is applied to the first toe and after the strike phase when the first toe reaches the ground, it is forcibly flexed to assist in the walkover from heel to toe. As the opposite leg is moved forward, the big toe of the hind foot is kept on the ground in a marked degree of dorsiflexion; and as the toe leaves the ground to swing the leg forward again, sharp flex-

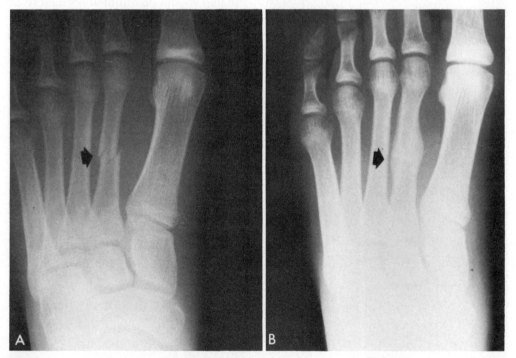

Figure 612. This 15 year old male fumbled a hand-off, and he and another player jumped on the ball. He had pain in his foot and pain on walking. Examination revealed very marked tenderness over the shaft of the second metatarsal. *A,* This fracture through the middle of the shaft with intact bones on either side will heal without any significant displacement, as shown in *B.*

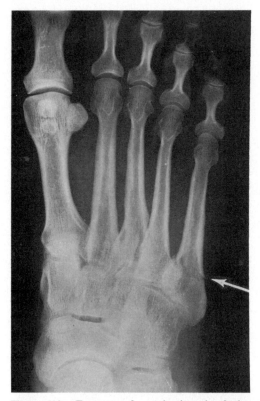

Figure 613. Fracture of proximal end of the shaft of the fifth metatarsal. Note bipartite medial sesamoid to first toe. This may be mistaken for a fracture.

ion of the toe aids in propulsion. A stiff or painful metatarsophalangeal or interphalangeal joint in the first toe that is disabling for ordinary walking is usually remedied by a stiff sole or an anterior heel, but this is not compatible with athletics.

The first toe may be injured by direct force as when the locker room bench falls on it. This results in a more severe contusion with or without comminuted fracture of the distal or proximal phalanx. This is a painful injury with blood extravasation into the tissues, swelling, throbbing and severe discomfort. Careful x-ray study is demanded to determine whether there is fracture involving the joint since this has much more serious implications than fracture of the tuft or shaft (Fig. 617). If the x-ray is negative, careful study of the toe itself will reveal the extent of the hematoma. Any blood under the nail should be drained, preferably by drilling through the nail rather than lifting the nail further away from the nail bed unless avulsion has already taken

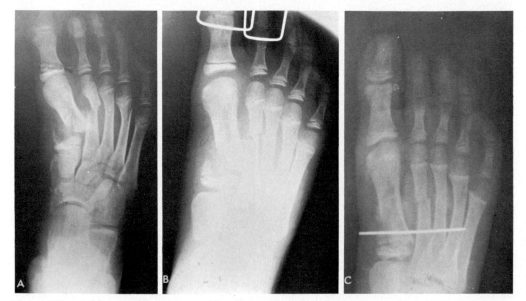

Figure 614. *A,* Metatarsal fractures resulting from a fall from a horse when the foot caught between the horse and road. *B,* Skeletal traction was ineffectual. *C,* Open reduction with transfixion pin and threaded wire resulted in a normal foot. There is no epiphyseal disturbance of the metatarsals.

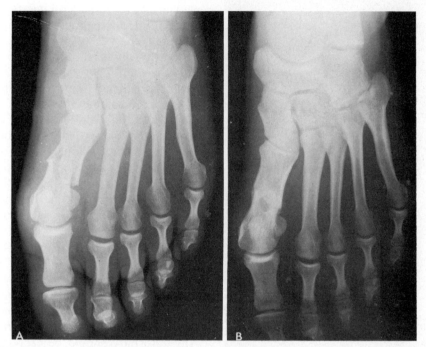

Figure 615. *A*, Fracture of shaft of first metatarsal, treated by skeletal traction. *B*, Six months postreduction.

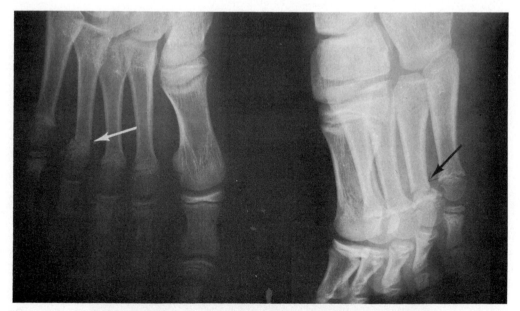

Figure 616. Typical fracture of the neck of the fourth metatarsal. This view shows a little plantar rotation of the head of the metatarsal and clinically the head was quite prominent in the sole of the foot. This deformity should be corrected to prevent painful metatarsal head. There is an incomplete fracture of M-3.

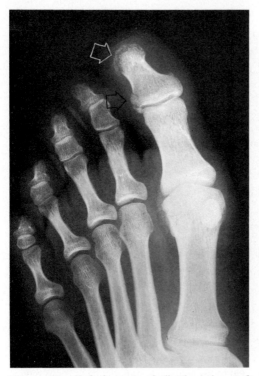

Figure 617. Tuft fracture of distal phalanx of first toe. Note also avulsion fracture of lateral margin of the articular surface of the distal phalanx.

place. The foot should be elevated and packed in ice and walking forbidden. Concentrated treatment the first few hours or days may well save a long period of disability.

A *Fracture of the Distal Phalanx* probably will not require manipulation or even rigid immobilization. If it is at the base of the distal phalanx (Fig. 618) particularly if it extends into the joint, careful reduction should be carried out and a toe spica cast applied. If the fracture is of the articular surface, the fragment may require pinning in place with a small wire. The same rules for treatment of fracture about the joint applies to the first toe as to weight-bearing joints anywhere.

Fracture of the Proximal Phalanx is much more serious than of the distal. The fracture may be of the head, the neck (Fig. 619), the shaft or the base. Any deformity should be corrected and may be held with intramedullary fixation by a Kirschner wire. This is a satisfactory method and obviates the neces-

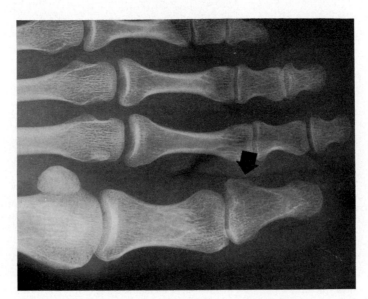

Figure 618. Avulsion fracture of the lateral margin of the proximal end of the distal phalanx of the first toe caused by forcing the distal phalanx inward.

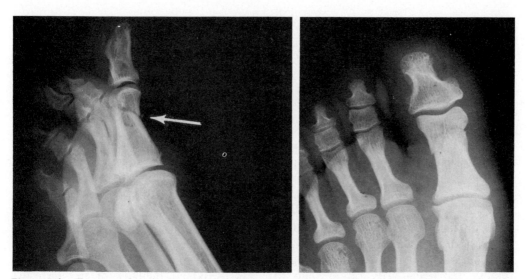

Figure 619. Fracture of neck of proximal phalanx of first toe, treated by plaster cast and later by shoe with a metal plate. The stability of the fracture permitted it to be held without internal fixation.

sity for long periods in plaster. Athletic competition cannot be permitted in these injuries as long as there is a danger of stress causing recurrence of the deformity.

An extremely painful fracture of the first toe comes as the result of a forceful kick that drives the base of either the distal (Fig. 620) or proximal phalanx into the opposing head. This results in osteochondral damage and occasionally comminution of the base of

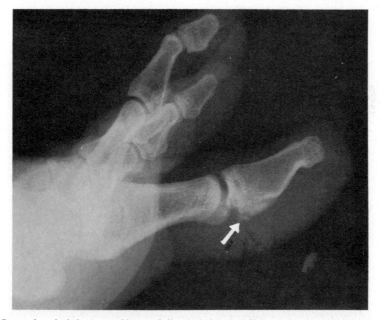

Figure 620. Osteochondral damage of base of distal phalanx of first toe from soccer kicking. This injury may occur from forcing the toe into the end of the shoe as the shoe sticks to the turf.

the bone. In some cases the displacement from a comminuted fracture of the proximal phalanx will be enough to require traction with a wire through the distal phalanx and on an outrigger.

Should a painful traumatic arthritis of the interphalangeal joint occur, it can be best treated by removal of the articular surface and fusion of the joint in the straight position. This results in little disability.

Involvement of the *metatarsophalangeal joint* is much more serious since fusion of this joint is not compatible with the best function of the foot. In this joint one is justified in attempting to remove the irregularity rather than to fuse the joint. Occasionally from sprain or sprain-fracture an irregularity forms around the bases of the bones. Spurs may arise which seriously interfere with dorsiflexion (Fig. 621). Good function may be expected following resection of these spurs provided they are not manifestations of chronic degenerative arthritis involving the articular cartilage.

With the advent of artificial turf there seems to be a sharp increase in snubbing type injuries to the first toe. As the shoe holds in the turf, the foot slides forward within the shoe and forces the distal phalanx into the end of the shoe. The result may be injury to the nail with avulsion. It may be to the interphalangeal joint or to the metatarsophalangeal joint. These injuries may be quite disabling and require careful consideration as to protection of the injury.

Fractures of the Smaller Toes. While fractures of the smaller toes are much less disabling than those of the first toe, they can be extremely exasperating. The most common is fracture of the proximal phalanx of the fifth toe from a nighttime attempt to move the furniture with the toe (Fig. 622). This causes sharp abduction of the toe resulting in a spiral, oblique fracture. In the second, third and fourth toes the fracture is usually from overflexion or overextension and is usually a transverse fracture, often near the joint (Fig. 623). Avulsion of a portion of the articular surface frequently occurs. These fractures have a tendency to heal with

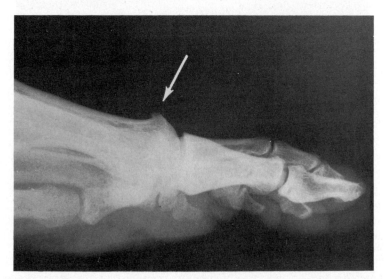

Figure 621.   Spur over the dorsum of the distal end of the first metatarsal, apparently the result of kicking. The opposite foot and the rest of the joints are normal. Complete relief followed excision. The same injury may occur from forcing the toe into the end of the shoe.

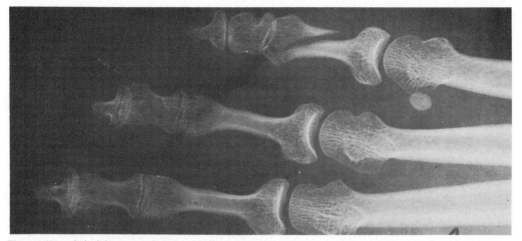

Figure 622. Spiral fracture of shaft of little toe involving the interphalangeal joint. In this toe this fracture can be treated by simple coaptation dressing.

the toe in flexion so that a painful hammer toe may result which will require definitive treatment. X-ray study will reveal the fracture.

An effort should be made to realign the toe. In the fifth toe, abduction deformity usually persists. This can be corrected without anesthesia by inserting a pencil or pen shaft between the fourth and fifth toes at the base and exerting quick, firm pressure outward on the pencil and inward on the head of the first phalanx. Perfect position, while not necessary, is desirable. Following reduction, the toe should be strapped to its fellow if it is the fifth toe or to the toe on either side if it is one of the others. Because of swelling extending back into the forefoot and difficulty in gait, it is also advisable to extend the strapping backward and circumferentially to include the forefoot (Fig. 624). This will result in less

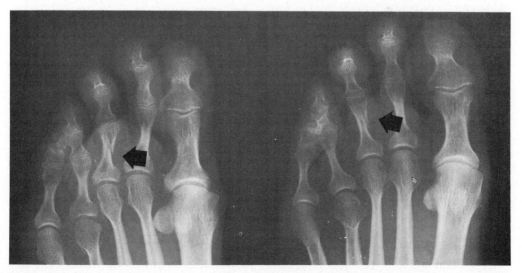

Figure 623. Spiral fracture of proximal phalanx of third toe. Treated by strapping of the second, third and fourth toes together. The forefoot should also be strapped and a hard-soled shoe worn.

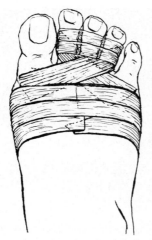

Figure 624. Strapping for fractured third toe. Note that the adjacent toes are strapped to the broken one. The whole is strapped to the forefoot.

disability in the toe and a great deal more comfort on weight bearing. The patient should be able to walk in a shoe that has been cut out to relieve the pressure at the tender area. The decision as to athletic competition may be a difficult one since the player may feel very good as he walks or even runs. To his dismay, he may find as he goes full speed or cuts sharply, throwing the foot into varus or valgus, that he will experience sharp pain which may cause him to fall or lose stride and so cost him a great deal of his effectiveness. A period of rest is probably well worthwhile. In such an injury, packing in ice overnight may mean the difference between rapid, uneventful healing and tedious convalescence since, once the toe becomes badly swollen and edematous, the restoration of pain-free function becomes increasingly difficult.

Avulsion fractures of the toes (Fig. 618) are, strictly speaking, muscle tendon or ligament injuries, and here again there is a tendency for hammer toe deformity to occur. A common avulsion is that of the extensor aponeurosis by sharp plantar flexion. The toe is flexed and painful. At the time of the initial in-

jury, the toe should be strapped straight if the condition is recognized. Usually this condition is not seen by the doctor until persistence of pain brings the patient in weeks later. At this time fusion of the involved joint is the best treatment.

Stress Fracture (Fatigue Fracture)

It was in the foot that the fatigue fracture was first described. This so-called march fracture was reported following mobilization for World War II when many young males who were unaccustomed to being on their feet were equipped with a pack and asked to walk long distances in heavy shoes. The resulting stresses on bones not used to this degree of activity caused a great deal of strain, particularly in the area of the metatarsal necks. The patient develops symptoms similar to those of an arch strain with pain along the forepart of the arch, increased on weight bearing or other activity and relieved by rest. Examination reveals local tenderness over the metatarsals with pain on stretching of the plantar arch but usually none on other motions of the foot. X-ray examination made in an early stage is usually negative. The patient is treated for arch sprain with pads and heat but the condition persists with local tenderness and increasing disability. Subsequent x-rays made after a few weeks will show callus formation around the metatarsal shaft (Figs. 625, 626 and 627). This is sometimes accompanied by evidence of a crack across the shaft but there may be absolutely no indication of a break in the continuity of the bone. This condition has frequently been confused with bone tumor and instances have been reported in which amputation had been recommended under the diagnosis of osteogenic sarcoma with periosteal reaction. A little

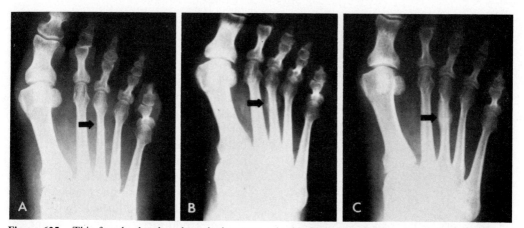

Figure 625. This female developed gradual soreness in forefoot noticed when running up and down stairs. *A,* Negative film, diagnosed a stress fracture. *B,* One month later. Note light abundant callus. *C,* Two months later. Note indefinite, healing fracture line.

patience will usually answer the question since in march fracture callus rapidly consolidates, becomes harder and smaller and ultimately disappears.

This condition is incompatible with active competitive sports during the acute stage and competition should be permitted only after consolidation of the mass of callus is complete. If the lesion is recognized early, the best treatment is with a plaster boot for two to three weeks followed by adequate strapping for a week or ten days, then the use of an arch support and a firm shoe. This type of condition illustrates graphically the value of re-examination by x-ray. If the initial x-rays have been negative but the symptoms persist, careful follow-up films will often reveal the pathologic changes. It should be emphasized again that x-ray is simply an adjunct to the diagnosis and a negative x-ray by no means rules out a bone lesion.

OTHER CONDITIONS OF THE FOOT

Hammer Toe

There is no necessity to detail the treatment of hammer toe. This condition results from a combination of contracture of the flexor and extensor tendons so that one or more joints is in flexion and another in extension (Fig. 628). A frequent combination is for the interphalangeal joints to be in flexion and the metatarsophalangeal joint in extension. This causes pressure on the tip of the distal phalanx and on the dorsum of the

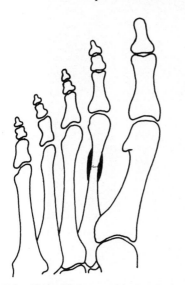

Figure 626. "March" fracture. A sketch showing a classic "march" fracture through the neck of the second metatarsal. This fracture usually occurs through the metatarsal shaft, the callus appearing before the fracture itself is evident.

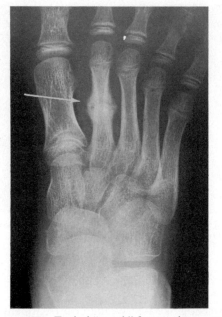

Figure 627. Typical "march" fracture in a young athlete. Note complete absence of any fracture line as such. Uneventful healing.

proximal interphalangeal joint. Painful corns may result. Hammer toes may come from unrecognized poliomyelitis, from a high arched, cavus type foot, as a result of short shoes or socks, or from previous injury. Proper care of the primary condition should minimize the deformity. Hammer toes can be successfully treated and athletics can be resumed. In the meantime, a properly fitted shoe with the leather split at the pressure point, or the application of suitable pads may add materially to the patient's comfort. A very frequent instance of disabling hammer toe involves the fifth toe. In fact, this toe is very frequently in the hammer toe position which presents the knuckle of the proximal interphalangeal joint dorsally and the tip of the toe on the plantar surface, each of which may develop a very painful corn. A simple method for treatment

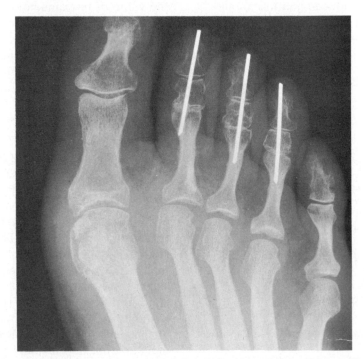

Figure 628. Hammer toes, corrected by fusion of the proximal interphalangeal joints. The severe hallux valgus has been corrected. The wires may be removed once fusion is solid.

of this condition may save many months and even years of discomfort. The head of the proximal phalanx should be resected and tenotomy of the extensor tendon performed. This does not leave any residual deformity; in fact, the toe looks more normal than its previous hammer-toe condition. It almost always relieves the corn on the dorsum on the inner side of the head of this proximal phalanx and on the tip of the distal phalanx.

Subungual Exostosis

This is a painful condition of the distal phalanx, usually of the first toe, which is not uncommon in athletes (Fig. 629). The pathology is the development of an exostosis on top of the distal phalanx extending up under the nail bed. Trauma may be a definite etiological factor. The condition may develop in a basketball player as a result of having his toe repeatedly trampled. Once the exostosis develops it is extremely sensi-

tive to pressure or trauma. The patient will present himself with a very painful, swollen, edematous toe. In many instances the nail has been cut away to permit the tumor mass to push up without the pressure of the nail over it. While these lesions look vicious clinically, they are always benign and may be cured by removal of the exostosis. If it is extensive and the nail bed has been destroyed, removal of the distal one-half of the distal phalanx with plastic closure of the toe after removal of the entire nail and nail bed may be the best solution. This condition is often confused with ingrown toenail or simple contusion and hematoma. The frightening appearance may suggest a malignant type tumor.

Ingrown Toenail

Ingrown toenail may occur on any toe but is most severe on the first. Basically, the cause is a rolling of the toenail in a scroll-like fashion so that the two lateral margins tend to roll under the

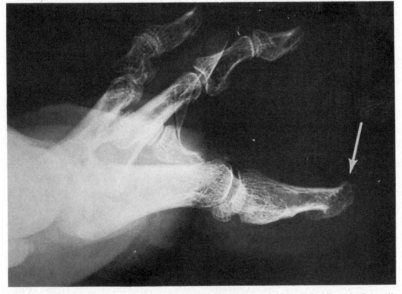

Figure 629. Subungual exostosis. Note the sharp spurring upward of the distal end of the distal phalanx. This was treated by resection of the tuft of the distal phalanx. It should be emphasized that the entire tip of the distal phalanx should be removed. To simply remove the spur invites recurrence.

central portion to make a tube rather than a flat plane. This is a natural tendency of the nail as evidenced in some species of mammals in which a conical claw is formed by a complete circling of the toenail. The resulting convexity causes the edge of the nail to dig into the side of the toe. The paronychial fold bulges to the outside and extends out over the dorsum of the nail.

Treatment. In the early stages ingrown toenail can usually be managed conservatively. Prophylaxis is of prime importance; well fitted shoes and socks, careful hygiene to avoid inflammation and proper trimming of the nail will many times prevent serious deformity. The nail should be trimmed straight across without the rounding off and pointing of the nail that is so popular in the hand. If the nail tends to be heavy, the center portion may be thinned by the emory board or suitable nail file so that, in the middle of the nail extending from the root to the tip, the substance is quite thin. This permits the lateral margins to roll upward by breaking the arc of the nail. A similar thing has been done by misguided individuals who split the nail down its center, but this often results in serious complications. The flattening may be aided by placing very small pledgets of cotton under the nail corners, once the tendency for ingrowing is noted. This must be carefully done, otherwise the pledgets may break off the corner of the nail and do more harm than good. They should not be made large enough to lift the nail away from the nail bed lest the problem be further complicated. If infection occurs, it should be adequately treated by drainage, application of hot packs and suitable antibiotics, both local and general. The patient should be barred from the general dressing room while his toe is acutely infected. Surgery of the toenail can usually be avoided by adequate attention in the early stages.

If the deformity persists and defies conservative treatment, surgery will usually give very satisfactory results. I cannot condemn too strongly the prevalent custom of simply removing the nail. In the first place this is not simple, and in the second place, when the nail regenerates it is even more curled than before so that the problem is only magnified. A suitable procedure is illustrated in Figure 630, great care being taken to eliminate all of the nail root and nail bed lest a recurrence or spur formation occurs that will require further treatment.

Active competition in the presence of a serious ingrown toenail is scarcely permissible since excruciating pain may result from the foot being trod upon. Active forcible flexion and extension may cause pain and increased inflammation.

Ingrown toenail involving the smaller toes is much less serious but should receive essentially the same treatment. This, however, is more difficult to carry out in the small toes. Surgical removal of all or part of the nail bed is not a mutilating operation and is far more acceptable in the small toes than a similar procedure on the first toe.

Corns

The best way to prevent disability in an athlete from a corn is to prevent the corn. The shoe must be carefully fitted and no pressure points permitted to develop. The most common locus is the toes where definite pressure occurs between the toe and shoe. The little toe particularly is an offender since it will frequently tend to curl up in the hammer toe position. Many athletes have a very high arch with some degree of hammer toe in all the small toes. These tend to get corns along the dorsum of the proximal interphalangeal joints. It does little

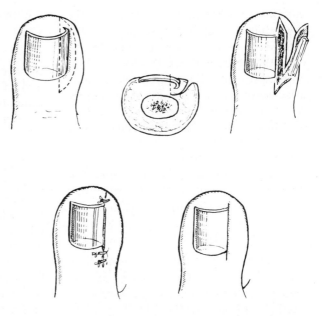

Figure 630. Surgical treatment of ingrown toenail. Care is taken to eliminate all the nail root and nail bed to prevent recurrence or spur formation. This may be done on each side of the nail if indicated. There should be no permanent disability if properly done.

good to remove a corn and not eliminate the situation that caused it. The area should be padded to protect it from pressure. The corn should be softened up by lanolin. If necessary, judicious trimming may be done. Careless application of medicated corn plasters has often resulted in painful ulcers. Careful fitting of the shoe and sock and avoidance of wrinkles are important.

Calluses

Calluses of the foot are the result of friction and pressure. They tend to be extremely disabling since the piling up of keratin, presumably as a protective measure, results in interposition of a very hard mass between the bone and the shoe. Painful bruising of the underlying tissues or periosteum may result. The obvious measure is to prevent the imbalance of the foot and get more even distribution of weight by building up or padding the shoe in such a manner as to relieve the weight on the involved area. The most frequent pressure on the foot is under the metatarsal heads. Painful callus under the first head may be re-

lieved by shifting the weight to the lateral side of the foot. An anterior heel or metatarsal bar may protect against direct weight bearing. In running on the toes, however, the metatarsal bar which ordinarily protects a person by taking the weight off the metatarsal head is, of course, not functioning. Careful attention to the callus by buffing it down with an emory board, softening it with lanolin, and so forth, will pay dividends.

Athlete's Foot

Fungus infections of the foot are endemic in almost the entire population. They are particularly prevalent in the locker room where too often little attention is paid to ordinary precautionary measures. For details of prevention and treatment, see page 61. Enteric medication seems to offer definite promise in resistant cases.

Verrucae

The verruca or wart must be distinguished from callus. The callus arises as a direct result of too much pressure on a certain area. Multiple verrucae, on the other hand, is a skin disease probably caused by a virus which may spread over the entire sole of the foot and be extremely disabling. Confusion may arise when a verruca is at a weight-bearing point and is surrounded by callus. Treatment should be carried out by one especially proficient in the treatment of conditions of the foot. Radiation should be used only under the careful guidance of an expert and probably not more than one series given to any one area.

Freiberg's Disease

Freiberg's disease is an osteochondritis of the metatarsal head, usually before the epiphysis closes, similar to Perthes' disease at the hip (Fig. 631). Early Freiberg's disease should be treated by prevention of weight bearing but this condition is frequently not recognized until it is well advanced. If the bone is seriously deformed, the painful metatarsal head should be removed. If the lesion heals without deformity, it is of no consequence.

Congenital Deformities of the Foot

There are may other deformities of the foot that are simply developmental and of little significance. They may at times be the precursors of later disability due to static imbalance but should not bar participation in athletics. The congenital hallux valgus (Fig. 632) or bunion is amenable to surgical treatment if necessary (Fig. 633). In the male it usually can be handled without surgery. Congenital short first metatarsal (Fig. 634) may be helped by suitable padding of the shoe. Pronation or supination similarly can be improved by improving the weight-bearing stance. The accessory navicular (Figs. 635, 636 and 637) or prehallux may become symptomatic by pronation of the foot and may be completely relieved by application of a suitable arch support. The athletic shoes with little or no arch, often with no heel, may often give inadequate support to the pronated or flat foot and need to be supplemented by a molded arch support.

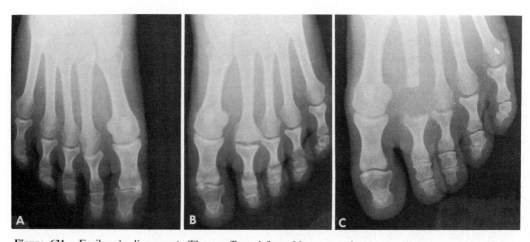

Figure 631. Freiberg's disease. *A,* The unaffected foot. Note extra long second metatarsal shaft with large head which bears undue proportion of the weight. This contributes to the osteochondritis. *B,* The healed osteochondritis of the metatarsal head (Freiberg's disease) with joint irregularity and pain. *C,* Removal of the second metatarsal head resulted in considerable improvement.

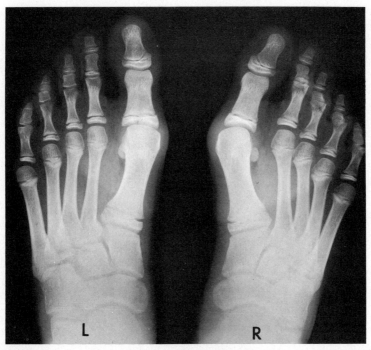

Figure 632. Congenital hallux valgus, right. Note bifid epiphysis on the proximal phalanx of first toe, left. This is not pathologic but may require treatment. The primary pathologic change here is the adduction of the first metatarsal, which is trying to act like a thumb. Correction of the "bunion joint" will fail unless the metatarsal adduction is corrected by osteotomy.

Fracture of a Sesamoid

Various sesamoid bones in the foot are subject to injury.

Accessory Navicular. The most common sesamoid injury occurs in the prehallux or accessory navicular. In an eversion injury with a tight posterior tibial tendon, an avulsion force is applied to the accessory bone and it is pulled away from its attachment to the navicular or, in the occasional case, pulled in two. This is similar to avulsion of the tendon attachment to the navicular. It may be misleading since the accessory navicular will be recognized as being an extra bone and the injury may be overlooked. A history of forceful eversion of the foot or of active contraction of the posterior tibial is characteristic. On examination, tenderness will be sharply localized to the accessory bone and to the navicular. Forced passive eversion or strong active inversion against resistance is painful. X-rays may be confirmatory.

Treatment for this condition may be nonsurgical. The patient is placed in a cast with the foot inverted for about three weeks, followed by inversion type strapping for another three weeks. However, if there is separation of the fragment or if the navicular is large, it will be advisable to remove the accessory navicular and complete the sling operation by positioning the posterior tibial tendon under the navicular. This type of operation is particularly gratifying since the arch is usually good and correction of the pronation will give markedly improved function of the foot.

While this condition may be overlooked, the contrary situation also must be guarded against. One must not interpret an accessory navicular as being a

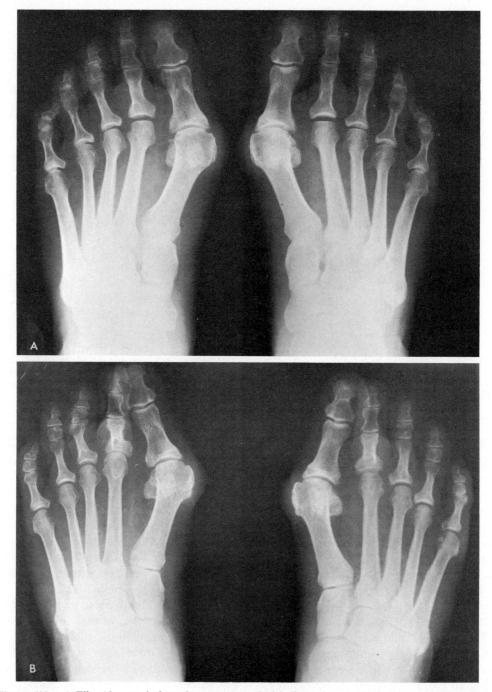

Figure 633. *A*, Film 13 years before shows very marked hallux valgus on both sides with formation of exostosis on the metatarsal head and widening of the space between the first and second metatarsals. Note the longer length of the second metatarsal. This should be classified as congenital adductus primus varus. *B*, Film 13 years later; note the marked advancement of the changes. No intervening treatment. Note the deformity of the proximal phalanx of the second toe on the left with considerable hammer toe and overlapping of the first and second toes. There is marked migration of the lateral sesamoid with extensive increase in the size of the exostosis and bursa. The prognosis would have been very much more favorable if surgery had been carried out when the patient was first seen.

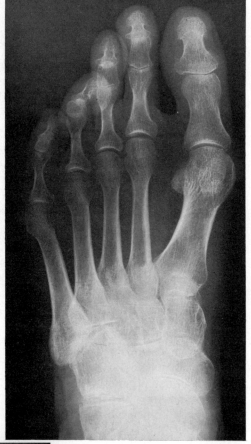

Figure 634. Congenital short first metatarsal with separation of the first and second heads. This throws unusual weight on the second head and is likely to cause a painful foot. The first metatarsal not only is short but is adducted. Correcting the deformity by open wedge osteotomy will give additional length to the first metatarsal.

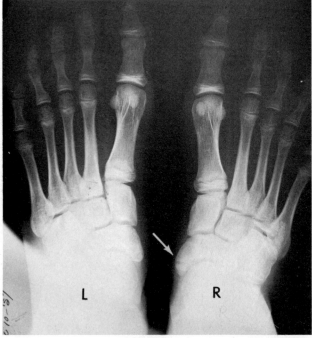

Figure 635. Note accessory navicular at the medial border of right foot. This should not be interpreted as an injury. Note the much smaller one on the left side. While the accessory navicular is not primarily traumatic, it is quite subject to injury either by a single episode with avulsion of the accessory bone or by repetitive strain. If symptomatic, the bone may be removed and the posterior tibial tendon placed under the navicular, the "sling operation."

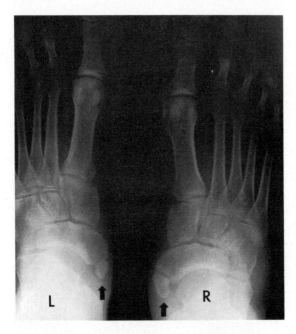

Figure 636. Patient has long-standing pronated feet with recent development of severe symptoms on the right over the medial portion of the navicular. No known history of injury although one might suspect there had been an avulsion of this bone with subsequent nonunion. Note the accessory bone is very much larger on the right. This should be treated by resection of the accessory bone and some of the protruding medial border of the navicular, transferring the posterior tibial tendon to a new course under the navicular.

fracture of the tubercle of the navicular. Careful comparison with the opposite foot and careful analysis of the clinical findings will usually distinguish between the two conditions. As indicated above, the two may coincide and require sharp diagnostic acumen. In case the accessory bone remains persistently painful, it should in any event be removed.

Sesamoid in the Flexor Tendon to the Big Toe. The medial sesamoid under the first metatarsophalangeal joint is subject to trauma when the toe is in forced dorsal flexion and a blow is ap-

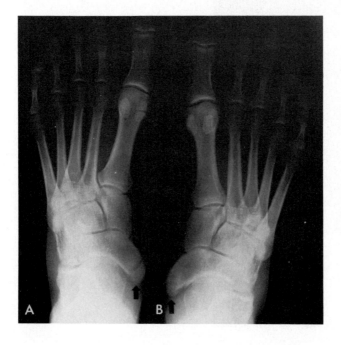

Figure 637. Acute injury simulating accessory navicular. *A,* This is actually a fracture of the medial tubercle of the navicular. *B,* Normal foot. This fracture may heal if properly protected. A painful fibrous union can be treated by resection of the fragment and repositioning the posterior tibial tendon.

plied to the ball of the foot. The mechanics of this injury resembles that of patellar fracture in which the combination of tension on the patella plus a localized blow fractures the bone. This injury can be extremely distressing, since it prevents the athlete from running on his toes. He may have very persistent pain and the true pathology is readily overlooked. This history of sudden, severe pain under the ball of the foot with tenderness and inability to "drive" are significant. Examination will reveal sharply localized tenderness with localized swelling, pain on dorsiflexion of the toe and pain on active plantar flexion of the toe. X-ray is confirmatory.

Treatment consists of immobilization of the foot for several weeks. Usually the acute condition is not recognized and it is seen as a chronic condition at which time the best treatment will be excision of the sesamoid (Fig. 638). In case nonsurgical treatment has been elected and has failed, or in certain instances when surgical treatment has

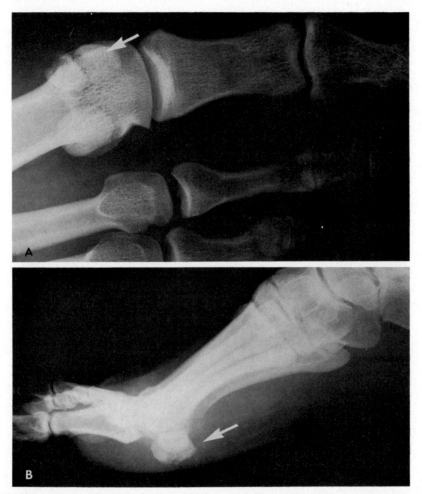

Figure 638. Unrecognized fracture of sesamoid. Note the difference from bipartite sesamoid. Here there is an irregular fracture line and calcification around the area. This sesamoid was removed. Note the high arched foot which probably contributed to the injury. A plantar fasciotomy was done at the time of the removal of the irregular sesamoid in order to reduce some of the stress caused by the high arch.

been elected as the primary treatment, it will be noted that the injury often occurs in a person with a high arch and a tight plantar ligament. In such a case, one should consider the advisability of carrying out a plantar fasciotomy at the time of the surgery for the sesamoid in order to relieve the tension of the plantar fascia. This would not unduly prolong the morbidity since the plantar fasciotomy could be done at the same time the sesamoid is removed and the recovery period would be parallel. There can be no question that the cavus type foot with a high arch and tight plantar fascia contributes to pressure on the metatarsal head. This should be considered in the management.

Bipartite Sesamoid

This is a congenital condition in which the medial and occasionally the lateral sesamoid will show transverse separation of the two segments at the midline (Fig. 613). This must not be confused with fracture, which is much less frequent. Since many fractures are not recognized until late, they may, indeed, under x-ray resemble the rounded-off margins of the partite bone. The history will be quite different as a rule, however, in that discomfort in the case of the bipartite sesamoid will be gradual in onset and mild in character. The symptoms are ordinarily those of accompanying metatarsal arch strain and the bipartite sesamoid is found coincidentally and usually is of no significance whatever. Careful analysis of the case and comparison with the opposite foot will give a lead as to the true nature of the condition. Chronic symptoms definitely localized in the sesamoid merit its surgical removal. Disappointment will follow removal without these clear indications.

CHAPTER 22

REHABILITATION FOLLOWING ATHLETIC INJURIES

FRED L. ALLMAN, JR., M.D.

INTRODUCTION

Rehabilitation of the athlete following injury and/or surgery is perhaps the most important aspect of treatment, for often the degree of rehabilitation determines the ability of the athlete to safely and effectively return to competition. Kraus (1959) has stated, "Injuries which are sustained during athletic participation are usually produced by circumstances inherent in respective athletic performance, and they are, therefore, characterized by exposure to recurrent identical trauma, making re-injury likely."

It is very unlikely that an athlete will be restored to a safe performance level unless specific measures are taken to regain normal function. Rarely is an injury so mild that some form of rehabilitation is not necessary, and as a rule the more serious the injury, the more prolonged and necessary is the rehabilitation.

Yet, in spite of the importance of adequate rehabilitation, many athletes either are never rehabilitated or are inadequately rehabilitated. Numerous studies have indicated that this inadequacy of rehabilitation is most certain to result in a very high incidence of re-injury and an unnecessary restriction of future participation by the athlete.

In order to overcome this inadequacy of proper rehabilitation, each individual who has the responsibility of determining whether a previously injured athlete should play must develop and fully understand certain basic guidelines to follow during the rehabilitative process.

It is hoped that this chapter on rehabilitation will help those involved with the treatment of athletes to be more specific and more knowledgeable in this regard.

Athletic injuries tend to occur in rather definite patterns and to certain parts of the body more than others. There are principles of rehabilitation that might be applied generally; however, there are certain parts of the body in which injury is particularly prevalent and in which rehabilitation is extremely important. These are grouped together as thigh and knee, calf and foot, shoulder and arm, forearm and wrist, and head and spine. Included in the text are further recommendations coordinated with the current discussion of the various areas of the body with suitable reference to this special chapter on rehabilitation.

GOAL OF REHABILITATION

The goal of rehabilitation is restoration of function to the greatest possible degree and in the shortest possible time. In order to reach this goal and achieve a safe performance level, the best protection is balanced bilateral muscular strength as well as antagonistic muscle balance.

Rehabilitation following injury is better when an exercise can be applied selectively and when resistance can be used where it is most needed and avoided where it is not needed or wanted.

Rehabilitation must be individualized, and the missing quality of muscle function must be identified and restored. Properly performed exercises to build strength not only will improve strength but also will improve speed, flexibility and functional ability. Neuromuscular reeducation is also an essential objective of training.

PROGRESSIVE RESISTIVE EXERCISE

In 1945, scientific experimentation and clinical application by DeLorme proved that the best way to build muscular strength and endurance was a program of progressive resistive exercise. This has been confirmed many times in the last 30 years.

More recently, Jones has proved that with properly performed progressive resistive exercise an increased range of motion and improved flexibility are not only possible but also highly desirable. This is because injury is far less likely when flexibility has improved as much as possible in association with good strength.

THE SAID PRINCIPLE

In reconditioning for vigorous sports activity following injury, it is necessary to understand the SAID principle (Wallis and Logan, 1964). The letters SAID stand for Specific Adaptation to Imposed Demands. Simply stated, this means that the training program must attempt to adapt the individual to the demands that may be made upon him during athletic performance. Adaptation is specific and refers to the alteration of the structure or function of an organ or part as a result of an altered environment. Function increases with use, and that which we do not use, we lose. The intensity, duration and frequency of activity are all related to the functional capacity that is developed.

Rehabilition of the athlete deals primarily with the restoration of muscle function; i.e., the missing quality of muscle function must be identified and restored (muscle strength, endurance and flexibility). Strength is general; however, the application of strength is selective. The proper use of strength in any activity comes only from the practice of the particular activity.

In formulating the exercise prescription, exercise should be applied selectively, depending upon the sport in which an athlete is involved.

Types of Rehabilitative Exercises

Rehabilitative exercises are prescribed body movements that help to restore or favorably alter specific functions in an individual following an injury. Active exercise is purposeful voluntary motion that is performed by the injured individual himself, with or without resistance and with or without the aid of gravity. Active exercise may be static, kinetic or isokinetic. Static exercise is that which is performed without producing joint motion. The muscle being utilized maintains a fixed length, which is an isometric contraction. Kinetic exercise is that which is performed to produce joint movement. The contracting muscle shortens, producing the movement which is an isotonic exercise. Isokinetic exercises are those in which joint motion occurs at a controlled rate. Concentric (positive) contraction occurs when a muscle is contracted from the extended to the shortened position. Eccentric (negative) contraction occurs when the tensed muscle lengthens.

In a positive contraction, tension develops in the muscle, a resistance is overcome, and the length of the muscle decreases. In isometric contraction, muscle length remains constant as muscle tension is developed. In negative contraction the muscle develops tension, and the muscle increases in length. Generally speaking, when a weight is lifted, "positive" work is performed. When a weight is lowered, "negative" work is involved.

It requires at least twice as much oxygen to do positive work as negative work (therefore, there is little or no training effect on the cardiovascular system).

Muscular soreness and discomfort usually accompany an intense bout of negative work. However, this soreness has proved to be more bearable if a break-in period of several days precedes the actual training, or if the actual training is continued for at least three consecutive days. Never should the trainee discontinue exercising and just rest. He will become even sorer in this case.

Strength increases are produced by exercises in proportion to the intensity of work, and "negative only" exercise provides an intensity of work that is impossible in any other manner.

The superiority of negative exercise for strength building can be seen in the studies of Doss and Karpovich, Olson's group, and Komi and Buskirk. Some attempts were made on the part of these researchers to equate the training routines of the positive and negative groups, and the quality of negative work is clearly seen.

High intensity of muscular contraction is undoubtedly the single most important factor in exercises performed for the purpose of increasing muscular strength.

Muscle Tension

Baer and associates concluded from a study they conducted that neither total work done nor power in the physical sense is a major factor in determining the improvement of muscular strength. They contended that the common denominator which explains strength improvement is the *tension developed* by the muscle during exercise. Earlier studies by others demonstrated that the tension which a muscle produces during contraction decreases as the speed of shortening increases. Thus, in isotonic exercise, greatest tension is developed at a slower rather than a faster rate of contraction, thereby establishing a condition which is conducive to greater improvement in muscular strength.

MAXIMUM INTENSITY OF CONTRACTION

Maximum intensity of contraction is produced when the highest possible percentage of the muscular mass is involved at a given moment, and certain factors are required to produce this situation.

Good form, or the style of performance, is very important if maximum benefit is to be obtained with progressive resistive exercise. Proper form includes the speed of movement, the range of movement and beginning the movement from a prestretched position. Also, the resistance should be moved in a smooth fashion and briefly stopped in the position of full muscular contraction. Jerking movements should be avoided.

1. The speed of movement must not be too fast or too slow. If it takes 2 to 3 seconds to raise a weight, then it should take 4 to 5 seconds to lower that same weight.

2. The range of movement must be as great as possible. Prevention of injury is most likely when the muscles have been strengthened in every position and over a full range of possible movement.

3. The movement must start from a prestretched position. Prestretching is involved when a relaxed muscle is pulled into a position of increased tension prior to the start of contraction. Prestretching properly applied enables one to handle heavier weights and thus bring into action a greater percentage of the muscle mass during each repetition. For example, the weight should be lowered from the contracted position in a controlled manner until the bar (or resistance arm) is about one inch from the position of full extension. At that point, there should be a very quick "twitch" or "thrust." Immediately following the quick "twitch," the movement should

be slowed down in a controlled manner. The only rapid movement of the bar or resistance arm should be during the first portion of the raising (positive) part of the repetition. The remaining portion of each repetition should always be smoothly performed.

4. The load must be heavy enough to require a maximum intensity of contraction. High-intensity exercise requires the repetitive performance of a resistance movement that is carried to the point of momentary muscular failure. When performing high-intensity exercise, at least 8 repetitions should be performed and usually not more than 12 to 15. If 8 repetitions cannot be completed then the resistance is too high, and if one can perform more than 12 to 15 it is too light. Consider a set completed when it is momentarily impossible to perform another full repetition in good form.

High-intensity contraction must be practiced on an infrequent basis, with adequate allowance for total recovery between training sessions (must not work too long or too often). Total recovery from a high-intensity training session requires at least 48 hours. *During the early stages of rehabilitation the intensity of the work is so low that training is possible on a daily basis.* Later, as the intensity increases, the workouts are reduced to three times per week, and during in-season training to only twice per week.

THE SEQUENCE OF EXERCISES

The sequence in which the various muscle groups are to be worked should be such that the largest muscle group is worked first, proceeding down to the smallest group last. Working the largest muscles first causes the greatest growth stimulus. Also, it is sometimes impossible to reach the required condition of momentary muscular exhaustion while working a large muscle group if the system has been previously exhausted by exercises for other smaller muscles.

NEUROMUSCULAR REEDUCATION

Neuromuscular reeducation primarily involves development of a proprioceptive awareness. Normal function will in most cases return more quickly to the athlete who is allowed to continue with activities that permit near normal function but do not interfere with the normal healing process.

EVALUATION FOR RETURN TO SPORTS ACTIVITY

Prior to being given permission to return to full activity, the athlete must be evaluated from the standpoint of strength, range of movement and girth, and finally there should be some form of functional evaluation of the involved body area (see Figures 639, 640 and 641).

It should be remembered that although normal strength may have been restored by a properly conducted therapeutic exercise program, skill is required for the proper use of strength, and skill is produced in only one way — by the practice of a particular activity. Therefore, the injured athlete must be evaluated on the athletic field while participating in order to fully evaluate his return to normal high-level performance.

Even after the athlete has achieved a safe performance level and is allowed to return to full participation, he should be recalled for periodic reevaluation at appropriate times. It is only through pe-

Date _____
Name _____
Record Number _____

	Right	Left
Girth		
Quadriceps		
at cc above patella......................		
midpatella................................		
Calf		
Strength		
Quadriceps...............................		
Hamstrings..............................		
Gastroc soleus..........................		
Hip flexor...............................		
Hip abductor............................		
Hip extensor............................		
Hip adductor............................		
Goniometric		
Extension................................		
Flexion....................................		

Comments

Figure 639. Knee evaluation form.

Date _____
Name _____
Record Number _____

	Right	Left
Girth		
Arm..		
Forearm		
Strength		
Hand		
Shoulder		
Internal Rotation.......................		
External Rotation......................		
Flexion....................................		
Extension		
Abduction...............................		
Goniometric		
Abduction...............................		
Flexion....................................		
Internal Rotation.......................		
External Rotation......................		
Extension		

Comments

Figure 640. Shoulder evaluation form.

riodic reevaluation that an athlete can maintain a safe performance level. While many will be able to maintain such a performance level with relative ease, others will have to continue with some form of rehabilitation even after their return to activity in order to maintain such a high level.

Further, it should be remembered that rehabilitation must deal with the total organism, not just with the involved injured part. Therefore, while most of the initial effort will be directed toward the injured area, attention must also be given to maintaining overall fitness as much as possible during the duration of rehabilitation. Measures that will enable uninvolved parts of the body

to remain active should be encouraged, and as soon as possible the overall program should include activities that will aid in cardiovascular-pulmonary reconditioning.

Stationary cycling and swimming are often possible long before the injured athlete is ready for return to full participation in his specific sports activity. Other similar activities can often be initiated at an early stage in the rehabilitation program.

The ability of the athlete to continue to use the uninvolved parts of his body to the fullest extent possible will surely shorten the recovery period and allow safe return to full sports participation at the earliest possible time.

REHABILITATION PROCEDURES FOR SPECIFIC AREAS

As indicated in the preceding discussion, it is of utmost importance that the entire musculoskeletal system be maintained at the optimal level. Interest in the injured area should not preclude general conditioning. However, it is obvious that the rehabilitation should be concentrated on the injured area. Specific measures are necessary for each different location.

We have grouped these areas in certain combinations which in general require similar measures. The following discussion takes up each of these areas in some detail and will be found to be quite valuable as rehabilitation proceeds.

HEAD AND SPINAL INJURIES

Head and spinal injuries are the number one cause of deaths directly related to athletic participation. While proper technique is very important, it is also mandatory that all athletes participating in contact sports provide themselves the greatest possible degree of protection by maintaining good strong musculature with a full range of painless unrestricted motion. Maximum strength and flexibility in the spinal muscles can be obtained with proper progressive resistive exercises.

Many less serious conditions involving the spine and low back respond very well to conservative measures when the appropriate exercise routine is utilized. Examples of the type used at

Date _____
Name _____
Record Number_____

Right   Left

Girth
  Foot ....
  Ankle...................................
Strength
  Plantar flexion ....
  Dorsiflexion ....
  Internal Rotation......................
  External Rotation......................
Goniometric
  Plantar flexion ....
  Dorsiflexion ....
  Inversion ....
  Eversion................................

Comments

Figure 641. Ankle evaluation form.

the Sports Medicine Clinic are shown below.

NECK EXERCISES

Phase 1. (Do these exercises as long as pain exists at the site of injury. Do not progress to more strenuous exercise.) These exercises consist of moving the neck and head through the entire range of motion and *then* continuing to contract the neck muscles at the completion of the movement for an additional 5 seconds. Repeat each movement 10 times. The movements are as follows.

1. Head rotation — to right; to left (Fig. 642, *A*).

2. Side tilt — ear toward right shoulder with head held erect; ear toward left shoulder with head held erect (Fig. 642, *B*).

3. Forward thrust — chin forward and down, touching low on chest (Fig. 642, *C*).

4. Head backwards — Note: *Do not* move head backwards past the neutral or "natural" position. That movement will aggravate most neck problems.

Phase 2. (Start these exercises only when pain and stiffness are no longer a problem.) This phase includes all the above exercises with the added resistance of an outside force such as:

1. Partner resisting movement in all directions with his hands.

2. Self-applied resistance with a towel or your hands.

3. Spring-loaded or weight-loaded head strap.

NECK BRIDGES

Perform this exercise only when injury is pain free (Fig. 643). Note the correct technique below!

1. Back of head or helmet contacts ground, *not* the top of head.

2. Push with neck muscles smoothly; do not jerk or arch into a balanced position.

3. Assist this effort by pushing with elbows if your neck is not strong enough to perform alone.

4. Hold 5 seconds; repeat 10 times.

Variation: turn over and use forehead or front of helmet as contact point.

WILLIAM'S FLEXION EXERCISES [LOW BACK]

Abdominal Curl. Regular sit-ups can aggravate back injuries. *Do not do them!* The following exercise should permanently replace regular sit-ups in your training. If need be, show these instructions to your coaches.

Assume the starting position shown in Figure 644, *A*: knees bent, arms folded on your chest, back flat on floor or mat. Now, roll your body up as one rolls a rug;

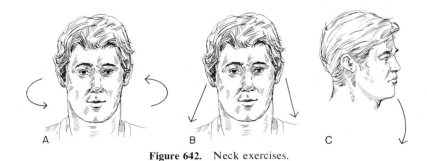

A   B   C

Figure 642.   Neck exercises.

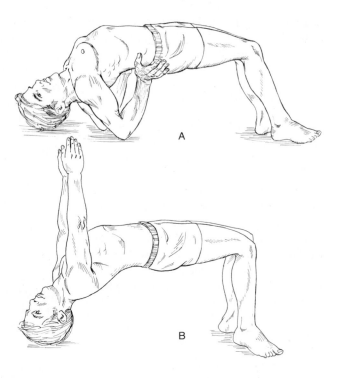

Figure 643. *A,* Back of head contacts ground; elbow assistance is used if necessary. *B,* Illustrates incorrect technique.

start by pulling the neck forward so your chin is on your chest. Now roll your shoulders forward (Fig. 644, *B*). Now attempt to push your head as far forward between your legs as possible. You will not go far, but if you try as hard as possible for 5 seconds, your abdominal muscles will get very good exercise. Relax; repeat as many times as desired. Athletes should do 25 to 40 repetitions. Others may perform at least 10 at a time and gradually build to 25.

Knees to Chest Stretching. Perhaps the worst exercise one can do, in terms of aggravating back problems, is the double leg raise, done lying on one's back. *Do not, under any circumstance, do this exercise.* Rather, perform the following:

Assume the same starting position as in Exericse A. Pull the knees as far into your chest as possible, while forcing your head toward your stomach (Fig. 644, *C* and *D*). Hold this position for 10

to 30 seconds. Repeat as many times as it takes to feel a relaxing stretch to the back.

Back Stretch on Chair. Sit on the edge of a chair that is supported against the wall. Drop your head and shoulders between your knees while attempting to touch your elbows to the floor (Fig. 644, *E* and *F*). Relax and stay in this position for 10 to 30 seconds. If your back is quite painful, do more of *C* and *D* and do not do this exercise until you have less pain.

Posture. Proper posture can be explained in terms of the relationship between the knees and the spine. When a person stands or walks continually with the knees held very straight (even locked-out), as in Figure 644, *G*, his spine will exhibit an excess curve. This will cause pain and weakness in the small of the back. If the individual maintains a slight bend at the knees (10–15 degrees) as in Figure 644, *H*, then back alignment is normal and stresses are reduced. Assume this posture and practice maintaining it.

SHOULDER AND ARM

The shoulder and arm play a critical role in all major sports, but most especially in the throwing sports. The action of throwing is an extremely complex activity, with a sequential pattern of movements in which each part of the body must perform a number of carefully timed and executed acts. Synergistic fluid agonist-antagonist function for each associated movement in the shoulder and arm is extremely important, but just as important is the coordinated footwork, leg action, hip motion and trunk rotation, plus some action of the other arm.

Fast body movements require the greatest muscle forces, and therefore throwing produces the highest forces at the most number of joints. It therefore becomes obvious that the entire body must be carefully and properly conditioned or reconditioned — not just the involved throwing arm.

REHABILITATION FOLLOWING SHOULDER INJURIES IN ATHLETES

The following program outlined is that used at the Sports Medicine Clinic in Atlanta, Georgia, by William Andrews, R.P.T.

Rotator Cuff Injuries

Early Rehabilitation. At this stage the rotator cuff is compromised by its subacute or postsurgical status. The shortness of the cuff muscles and the disproportionate strength of the other musculature of the pectoral girdle make conventional full range exercise inappropriate, even if active range of motion is possible. The following exercises are indicated.

GRIPPING EXERCISES. Gripping a hand dynamometer or tennis ball at several points along the arc from full (pain-free) abduction-flexion–external rotation to full adduction-extension–internal rotation. This brings the rotator cuff into synergistic (fixative) contraction, as well as conditions forearm muscles which have probably atrophied if inactivity has been of long duration.

CODMAN (PENDULUM) EXERCISES. This exercise increases the range of motion while stimulating contraction of the rotator cuff owing to the gentle traction applied to the muscle systems (see Fig. 161, *A*).

BENCH PRESS SUPPORTS. Lie supine on the bench, holding the barbell in a "locked-out" position. A freely held barbell or dumbbells are preferable to a statically held weight machine, since fourway control is stimulated by the free barbell and not by the weight machine. The weight should be only heavy enough to stimulate fixation of the cuff gently. Progression is accomplished by widening the grip gradually from about 20 to 30 inches (to pain tolerance). This increases the external rotation gradually. The weight is also increased gradually.

DEADLIFT SUPPORTS. Hold the barbell or corresponding lever of the multistation weight training apparatus with an overhand grip at the front of the thighs. The shoulders are held in a shrug position. Single efforts of 10 seconds are performed. Progression is obtained by widening the grip and increasing weight.

HANGING FROM CHINNING BAR. A bench or chair is used to elevate the body so that the bar can be grasped regardless of a deficient range of motion. The bar is gripped but no effort is made to support full or partial weight until the arms can be painlessly held over the head. The patient merely grips the bar and isometrically sets the latissimus muscle group in a comfortable range. Once full weight bearing is possible, progression is obtained by widening the grip.

Intermediate Rehabilitation. At this stage the rotator cuff should be able to contract fully without pain, but full range is not present and strength is not yet fully developed. The cuff is, however, adequate to take on conventional shoulder conditioning exercises that will develop strength and further increase range of motion. The following exercises are performed.

LIGHT DUMBBELL CIRCLES. This is a progression of the pendulum exercises. Done while standing upright, the dumbbell is directed upward and outward in a rotary manner, and then upward and inward in the opposite manner. These circles progress by widening the excursion of the circle and increasing the weight.

BENCH PRESSES. Progressing from supports, the patient gradually adds bending to the movement until a full range bench press is possible. More weight is added. Once again, because of the need to support the weight in all directions, freely held weights are preferable to weight machines. Dumbbell bench exercises, or "flyes," while they may present a safety problem, will offer a wider range of motion.

UPRIGHT ROWING. This is a progression of the deadlift supports, using the same grip, in which the weight is raised to a position high on the chest. Varying the width of the hand grips is desirable.

"LAT" MACHINE PULL-DOWNS TO THE REAR OF NECK. A shoulder-width grip is used at first with later progression to a wider grip. Weight is added until the patient is able to progress to behind the neck pull-ups (only if a minimum of six can be performed).

Advanced Rehabilitation. The progress of the intermediate stage has probably left the athlete at near normal development. To develop extra strength of the structures in question, along with increased flexibility, the following program might be utilized.

1. Alternate dumbbell presses or presses behind the neck.
2. Dumbbell benches, incline presses, "flyes," or parallel bar dips.
3. Bent-arm pull-overs.
4. High pulls with a snatch grip, or repetition "cleans."

All of the above are done for strength at a level of weight, repetitions, and number of sets to assure maximum development in accordance with the individual's potential. The exercises are done to the extremes of motion so that flexibility is improved. If properly done in this manner, no specific flexibility exercise is needed. To supplement any deficiency, however, the following exercises can be performed.

5. Straight arm pull-overs across the width of a bench, using a progressively wider grip. The weight is kept at a permanently light poundage (30 pounds).
6. Light dumbbell "flyes" with a medicine ball between the shoulder blades, or elastic cable stretching at pulley weights. In the latter, the cable is held in back of the shoulders with the palms facing forward at shoulder height; the cable is worked forward and backward, stretching the pectoral girdle and rib cage.

Glenohumeral Dislocations and Subluxations

All stages of rehabilitation are similar to the rotator cuff with the following exceptions.

1. If surgical intervention has not been instituted to correct the dislocation, no exercise should be done which

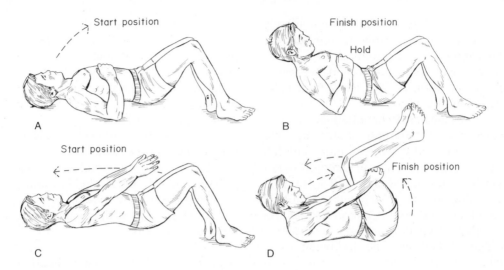

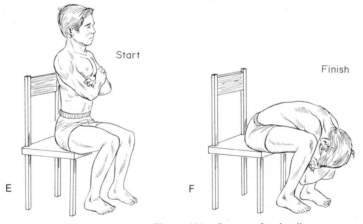

Figure 644.   See text for details.

places the shoulder in a compromised position (abducted and externally rotated). Thus, grips should never be wide, bench work should only be done in the top one-third of the movement, and presses are best performed in only the lower half of the range. To accomplish this, the use of a "power rack" is beneficial. If unavailable, the barbell with the assistance of two spotters is used.

2. The extent of damage to the cuff and surrounding structures may be such that progress is slower, and there is greater atrophy and limitation of range.

3. Special emphasis is given to strengthening the internal rotator muscles (subscapularis muscle).

Acromioclavicular Injuries

Early Rehabilitation. At the subacute or postoperative stage, pain is often a limiting factor, with associated tight-

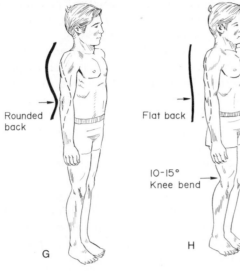

Rounded
back

Flat back

10-15°
Knee bend

G

H

Figure 644.   *Continued.*

ening of all the shoulder musculature (trapezius, pectoral, deltoid, latissimus, etc.) as well as the possibility of tightness and weakness in the adjacent arm muscles. For this reason, the following exercises are used.

1. Light, active range of motion for shoulder flexion, abduction and internal and external rotation for flexion and extension of the elbow, and for supination and pronation of the forearm.

2. Light resistive exercise for the trapezius (shrug).

3. Light resistive exercise for the anterior deltoid (upright row).

4. Resistive exercise, to tolerance, for the forearm, biceps and triceps muscles. All should be done in such a fashion that little or no downward pull is effected at the shoulder (lying or seated rather than standing).

5. Codman (pendulum) exercises are done to increase the tolerance of the shoulder to weight-support with a limited range of motion (see Fig. 161, *A*).

Intermediate Rehabilitation. Pain should be absent and the range of motion should be nearly full. The main goal is strengthening the muscular attachments of the trapezius and deltoids in

the area of the clavicle and acromion near the acromioclavicular joint. This is done by strengthening the entire deltoid-trapezius group. The following exercises should be done.

1. Dumbbell presses done alternately (emphasis on the anterior deltoid).

2. Wide grip press behind the neck (emphasis on the lateral deltoid and trapezius).

3. Shoulder shrug (emphasis on the trapezius).

4. Upright row (emphasis on the anterior deltoid and trapezius).

Advanced Rehabilitation. Increasing the general muscle bulk in the anterior shoulder area should have a strengthening effect on the acromioclavicular joint. All of the above exercises are appropriate when done intensively with a heavy progression of weight. Also beneficial are all incline presses, all "cleans," snatches and deadlifts, bench presses, and pull-overs.

Injuries Related to the Throwing Sports

The key is prevention. Assuring general fitness of the musculature through adequate strength training is important. More important, however, is the establishment of fluid agonist-antagonist function for each associated movement at the shoulder and elbow. Development of appropriate flexibility and coordination of movement, as well as of a proper kinesthetic sense by the athlete, is extremely important. The following general points are important.

1. Full range strength training, mostly with dumbbells. Done to extremes of stretch and with "ballistic" movement to assure the maintenance of quick, fluid reaction in the muscles.

2. Additional stretching movements for the entire shoulder-elbow area.

3. Maintenance of flexibility and fluid motion in the thoracic and lumbar spine. This can have a beneficial effect on the general state of flexibility in the extremities.

4. Thoughtful practice of the throwing skill to establish the most fluid and efficient pattern possible.

5. Always practicing proper warm-up, and not abusing the endurance and recovery capabilities of the structures involved (not throwing too often or too much at one time, or too soon after a lay-off).

STRETCHING FOR SHOULDERS AND UPPER BACK

Dead Hang. Grip overhead bar and hang (till grip fails) (Fig. 645, A).
Variations:
1. Pull knees to chest while hanging (Fig. 645, B).
2. Perform partial (not full) pull-ups while hanging (Fig. 645, C).
3. Swing side to side while hanging (Fig. 645, D).
4. Do "frog kick" while hanging (Fig. 645, E).
Bar Dips. Use 24-inch width parallel bars or chair backs (chairs sturdy!). Lower body into the stretched, fully

lowered position (Fig. 645, F). Remain in this position 15 seconds. Repeat 5 to 10 times.
Variations:
1. Use weight strapped about waist for added resistance.
2. Do "push-up" dips between chair seats (Fig. 645, F).
Upper Back Extension. Lie face down across an exercise bench or use the "hyperextension" unit on the Universal Gym. Bench supports you at level of rib-cage (Fig. 646). Do as follows:
1. Fold hands behind neck and point elbows outward (Fig. 646, A).
2. Lift body to fully extended (up) position.
3. Hold 2 seconds.
4. Lower and repeat 10 times.
Variations:
1. Maintain extended position while raising dumbbells to side; 10 repetitions (Fig. 646, B).
2. Maintain extended position while raising dumbbells forward (Fig. 646, C).
3. Maintain extended position while "rowing" barbell to chest (Fig. 646, D).

WRIST-ELBOW EXERCISES

Wrist Flexion. Place the wrist in a palms-up position, supported at the edge of a table or on your knee, so that only the hand will be allowed to move. Grasp the weighted dumbbell (_____ pounds)* or weighted bag. Perform the exercise as follows:
1. Flex (bend upward) the wrist as far as possible (Fig. 647, A).
2. Hold 2 to 3 seconds.
3. Lower fully; repeat up to 15 repetitions.
4. Increase weight if 15 proper rep-

---

*The initial starting weight must be determined. It will vary according to sex, size, disability and other factors. It is determined by trial and error.

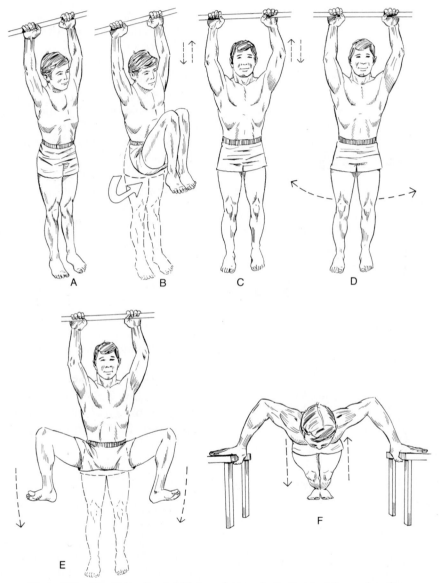

Figure 645.   Stretching for shoulders and upper back. See text for explanation.

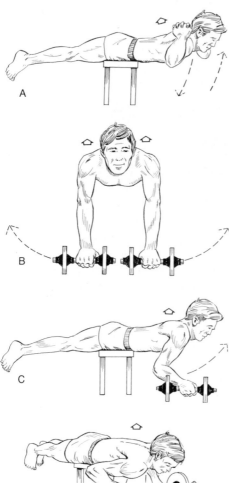

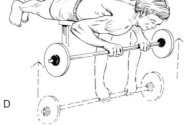

Figure 646. Upper back extension. See text for details.

etitions can be performed with no pain at the site of injury.

Wrist Extension. Performed in similar fashion to wrist flexion except that palm faces down. Start with _____ pounds.

Gripping Exercise. Use a tennis ball or other gripping-type device. Start with moderate intensity gripping, which is held 2 to 3 seconds and repeated 15 times. Increase intensity of grip corresponding to increased intensity in wrist flexion and wrist extension exercises.

Thumbs-Up Elbow Flexion. Hold a dumbbell or weighted bag (_____ pounds)* at your side so that your thumb points straight forward. Perform the exercise as follows:

1. Slowly bend elbow to 90 degrees only. Allow no upper arm movement (Fig. 647, _B_).

2. Hold in this position 2 to 3 seconds.

3. Lower slowly; repeat up to 12 repetitions.

4. Increase weight if 15 repetitions can be achieved without pain at your injury or a break in strictness of form.

Lever-Bar Rotation (In). Use a dumbbell bar arranged as shown in Figure 647, _C_).

Place wrist at edge of table as in wrist flexion exercise. Grip bar at nonweighted end with the weight (_____ pounds)* outboard. Perform as follows:

1. Rotate hand inward as far as possible (Fig. 647, _D_).

2. Hold momentarily.

3. Allow weight to return to starting position _slowly_ (2–3 seconds). Repeat up to 15 repetitions.

4. Effective weight can be increased by using a fixed weight and increasing distance A-B as your strength increases.

Lever-Bar Rotation (Out). Place wrist at edge of table as in wrist extension exercise. Use _____ pounds* to start, gripping the nonweighted end of the bar with the weights inboard. Perform as in previous exercise, except rotate wrist out rather than in during Step 1 (Fig. 647, _E_).

---

*The initial starting weight must be determined. It will vary according to sex, size, disability and other factors. It is determined by trial and error.

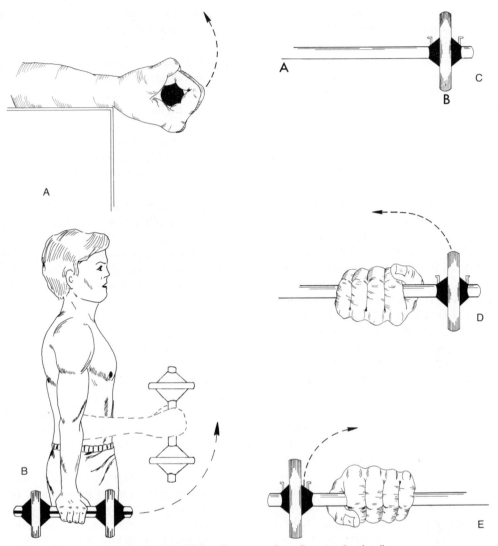

Figure 647. Wrist-elbow exercises. See text for details.

KNEE AND THIGH

Injury to the knee constitutes the most frequent disabling injury in sports. An increase in the number of participants, an increased tempo of most sports activities, and failure of adaptation to imposed demands all relate to the increase in the frequency of knee injuries in recent years. Although many factors are related to the incidence and severity of knee injuries, no other is more important than adequate musculature to provide maximum protection.

Also, no other area of the body is as prone to atrophy following injury as are the knee and thigh.

The muscular atrophy that usually follows injury or surgery is a neurological phenomenon. It causes a very rapid loss of strength and muscle bulk in the supporting musculature of the knee.

It is possible, however, to prevent a significant amount of this muscle atrophy through the use of preoperative and postoperative exercises. These exercises should be instituted as soon as possible, and in order to achieve the desired result in the shortest possible time, a definite plan with preestablished goals must be formulated.

Muscle action stabilizes the knee joint and helps to defend the ligaments against abnormal stress. The stretch effect of the normal ligament to which stress is applied is a proprioceptive stimulation to the surrounding musculature, causing these muscles to offer support to the stressed joint. The knee with ligamentous laxity and muscular weakness is much more injury prone than the knee without such laxity and weakness. It should also be remembered that although the response is much less visible or measurable, ligaments respond to a training program as do muscles, and over a period of time become stronger and thus more resistant to injury.

In rehabilitating knee and other lower extremity injuries, it is very important to seek equal bilateral strength as well as antagonistic muscle balance. Numerous studies have indicated that a disparity of 10 per cent or greater in the lower extremity makes injury or reinjury much more likely. Testing is therefore essential to determine the strength level of the various muscle groups about the knee, hip and leg.

REHABILITATION FOLLOWING KNEE INJURIES IN ATHLETES

The following program outlined is that used at the Sports Medicine Clinic in Atlanta, Georgia, by William Andrews, R.P.T.

Injury Classification

It is important to classify injuries by type and extent, since the course of rehabilitation will differ from one type to another. The injury classification and specified therapy routines should not be considered to be inflexible or to limit further detailing or specialization. Types of injury include:

1. Single ligament or uncomplicated meniscus injury.

2. Multiple ligament injury or complicated single ligament and/or meniscus injury.

3. Multiple ligament injury associated with other complicating factors, such as a fracture.

4. Chondromalacia of the patella and/or femoral condyle erosion, either alone or in combination with any of the above types.

Stages of Rehabilitation

Rehabilitation following knee injury and/or surgery can be divided into five stages: presurgical, immediate postoperative, early intermediate, late intermediate, and advanced.

Presurgical Stage. The presurgical stage is usually significant only when elective surgery is to be performed. If a specific diagnosis has not been made, therapeutic exercise may be instituted for purposes of aiding in diagnosis as well as for functional benefits. Therapeutic exercise at this stage is designed to build or maintain strength, while at the same time not to aggravate the existing injury. Thus, the exercise must be, for the most part, not through a full range of motion. Isokinetic exercise is especially desirable during this stage because of its readily controlled, noncompelling nature. The following exercises should be carried out.

1. Quadriceps setting: 10-second contractions for 5 minutes each hour while awake. See Figure 648, *D.*

2. Straight leg raising: 15 nonstop

repetitions with the maximum possible resistance each hour while awake. See Figure 648,*A*.

If due to pain and subsequent reflex inhibition of the quadriceps femoris muscle the athlete is unable to initiate quadriceps setting and/or straight leg raising, then the special "negative" resistance exercise as described in the following section should be utilized. In negative resistance exercises, the patient raises the leg with assistance, then actively lowers it without assistance.

3. Isometric knee extension (at or near full extension): 15 repetitions each hour while awake.

4. Isometric or isokinetic knee flexion: 15 repetitions (optional).

5. Hip extension (wall pulley): 20 to 25 repetitions (optional).

6. Hip flexion (wall pulley): 20 to 25 repetitions (optional).

7. Hip abduction (wall pulley): 20 to 25 repetitions (optional).

8. Hip adduction (wall pulley): 20 to 25 repetitions (optional).

The above routine should be performed daily for 10 to 14 days prior to surgery. In so doing, the preservation of muscle tone and the improved kinesthetic sense will help in preparation for the practice of similar exercises immediately postoperative. Instruction in three-point gait training should also be given during this stage. Touch weight bearing with the injured extremity is allowed; however, while the involved extremity is in the weight bearing phase of gait, the knee is fully extended and the quadriceps muscle is "set." Complicated or more serious injuries are usually treated by elective surgery and, therefore, are not included in this stage of therapy, since surgery is most often indicated immediately.

Immediate Postoperative or Postinjury Stage. The optimal time for commencement of therapeutic exercise is approximately 24 hours following surgery or injury. An earlier beginning is often met by an unreceptive and confused patient. Any beginning later than 24 hours must be considered a loss of valuable time. As soon as normal function ceases, atrophy and other debilitating mechanisms begin to occur and serve to delay further return of normal function. Exercises in this stage are similar to those in the presurgical stage, except for those movements that are precluded by the presence of a cast, dressing, or associated immobilization. The following exercises should be carried out.

1. Quadriceps setting: 10-second contractions for 5 minutes each hour while awake.

2. Straight leg raising: 10 repetitions each hour while awake with maximum possible resistance.

If due to pain and subsequent reflex inhibition of the quadriceps femoris muscle the athlete is unable to initiate quadriceps setting and/or straight leg raising, then the following routine should be used.

a. Manually, by using appropriate slings and pulleys or by using the opposite leg for assistance, passively elevate the involved extremity to a position of 90 degrees of hip flexion (or as much hip flexion as the patient will comfortably tolerate).

b. Have athlete "hold" the involved limb in this position by active contraction of the involved muscles. Slowly remove the passive support and have patient lower the limb to the starting position.

c. Repeat Step a, but this time elevate the limb only two-thirds the height obtained in Step a. Then slowly lower as described in Step b.

d. Repeat Step a, but this time elevate the involved limb only one-third the height obtained in Step a. Then slowly lower as described in Step b.

e. If the athlete is able to actively

hold the involved limb at 30 degrees, then he probably will thereafter be able to initiate elevation on his own without manual support or slings and pulley assistance.

f. If the athlete is unable to initiate elevation of the limb from the starting position, then have him "hold" at the lowest possible position that he can maintain actively and then raise the extremity as high as possible. Several such repetitions should enable the athlete to initiate quadriceps setting and straight leg raising with no assistance.

3. Isometric hip extension: 10-second "presses" onto the bed for 10 repetitions each hour while awake.

4. Abduction and adduction of the hip: 10-second presses against resistance for 10 repetitions each hour while awake.

5. Ankle plantar flexion: 10-second presses against resistance for 10 repetitions each hour while awake.

6. Ambulation. As soon as the patient is able voluntarily to elevate the involved extremity from the bed, he is allowed to ambulate on crutches, using a three-point gait, with touch weight bearing on the involved extremity. The touch weight bearing stimulates proprioceptive receptors that provide the central nervous system with an awareness of body segments (in the involved extremity). Proprioceptive awareness has been shown to be of primary importance in neuromuscular reeducation.

The goal during this stage of rehabilitation is maintenance of muscle mass, strength and function during the period of time that immobilization is indicated. These exercises should be progressive and continuous during the entire immobilization period. It is important that exercises be prescribed for the entire extremity as well as for other major body segments, since bed rest and immobilization deprive all of these segments of normal activity.

The above exercises are recommended for uncomplicated single ligament and meniscectomy cases. More complicated injuries introduce elements of increased instability, increased pain, increased potential for hemorrhage, and the need for more extensive tissue repair. These conditions are, therefore, indications for the most judicious choice of activity and dosage. In most cases, however, given time and proper supervision, the level of activity can approach that of less complicated cases. Careful control of the rate of exercise progression is the key to success, with the obvious testimony of pain and edema serving as primary guidelines. Thus, the following immediate postsurgery, or postinjury, routine is usually possible, even with very complicated cases:

7. Quadriceps setting: 10-second sets, for 5 minutes each hour while awake.

8. Straight leg raising: to tolerance for 30 seconds each hour while awake.

9. Hip extension (isometric): to tolerance for 30 seconds each hour while awake.

Early Intermediate Rehabilitation. At the end of the immobilization period, the patient proceeds immediately into the early intermediate stage of rehabilitation. This stage is a continuation of the postsurgical stage and the exercises are similar, but with added emphasis on progression. Exercises are also included to increase the active range of motion (ROM). Passive stretching is seldom used, as active ROM exercises usually provide full ROM within a reasonable period of time. In cases in which terminal extension is a problem, the patient is instructed in passive-active exercise to correct this deficit. The following exercises should be carried out:

1. Straight leg raising: using maximum possible resistance.

2. Pulley exercises:

Hip extension—progressive to 15 to 20 repetitions

Hip flexion—progressive to 15 to 20 repetitions

Hip abduction—progressive to 15 to 20 repetitions

Hip adduction—progressive to 15 to 20 repetitions

3. Knee extension-flexion utilizing isokinetic exercises, beginning with a relatively low speed and gradually increasing the speed.

Or, if using another type of weight loading apparatus, lift the weight or perform the exercise effort by using both legs in a steady lift fashion—taking two full seconds to lift the weight. In the "lifted" position, hold for 1 to 2 seconds. Then, lower with involved leg only, taking four full seconds: 2 Up—Hold 2—Lower 4.

4. Ankle plantar flexion: progressive to 15 to 20 repetitions.

5. Terminal extension exercise (hurdler's exercise): with the addition of a towel looped over the forefoot for additional stretching of the popliteal area (see Fig. 650, A, for details of exercise).

The above exercises are done once in a circuit during the first session, two sets at the next, three sets at the next, and never more than three sets subsequently. Progression is consistent and judicious. As soon as a pain-free ROM in excess of 90 degrees is present at the knee with no apparent swelling and no significant pain, the following changes are made:

6. Leg raises are eliminated.

7. Isotonic leg extension is added: one leg at a time, alternating legs. Resistance is added progressively, 15 to 20 repetitions.

8. Isotonic knee flexion: resistance is added progressively, 15 to 20 repetitions.

9. Terminal extension is continued if necessary.

10. Active stretching of the rectus femoris muscle, the hamstring muscles, and the Achilles tendon is initiated at the same time that isotonic exercises are introduced.

11. Stationary bicycling is added to tolerance, usually 2 to 4 miles at one sitting, with a resistance based upon the capability of the individual.

12. At this stage the leg press is added to tolerance. Resistance is progressive, 20 to 30 repetitions.

Each of these exercises is performed 2 to 3 times daily. The rationale at this stage is no longer one of maintenance of function but of building (rebuilding) muscle mass and function. Still, aggressiveness should not gain the upper hand over judicious choice of exercise dosage. Of primary importance at this stage is mobilization and achievement of pain-free flexion and full extension. Secondarily, proper form in the performance of exercise is indicated. Of third importance is the actual amount of resistance used in the exercise, although once motion and proper form have been achieved, the resistance load becomes all-important. More complicated or extensive injury may call for a slower beginning at this stage. By observing the signs of pain and swelling, however, as well as following basic precautions as far as the rate of progression is concerned, there is no reason to believe that most such cases cannot eventually progress to the same level of performance as less complicated ones. The difference is one of a slower rate of progress. *In many cases of extensive erosion of the joint surfaces on either the patella or the femoral condyle, resistive ROM exercise may be permanently contraindicated.* In these cases isokinetic types of exercise are usually helpful.

Late Intermediate Rehabilitation. The criteria for advancement to this stage are pain-free full range motion of the involved joint and a strength deficit in the quadriceps group of no more than 25 per cent. The following exercises should be carried out:

1. Leg extension: both legs simultaneously, 15 to 20 repetitions.

2. Leg flexion: both legs simultaneously, 15 to 20 repetitions.

3. Leg press: 15 to 20 repetitions. Accentuate the "negative." Take 2 full seconds to lift weight. In lifted position hold for 1 to 2 seconds. Then lower, taking 4 seconds.

4. Stationary bicycle: emphasize high speed and high resistance. Progress with distance up to 5 miles.

5. Running: preferably uphill, or if on the treadmill, with a grade of 5 to 10 per cent. Progress in distance and speed.

At this stage of rehabilitation the rationale becomes less one of therapy and more one of sports conditioning. Sports conditioning centers on a concern for "functional power." Considerations must include resistance, speed of movement, range of movement and repetitions. By this stage it has been determined whether or not intensive exercise is indicated. If not, then exercise is limited to nonresistive exercise of the isokinetic type, and to non-ROM exercises such as straight leg raises, isometrics at various angles, and full ROM hip and ankle movements.

Advanced Rehabilitation. The criteria for entry into this phase of rehabilitation are that the athlete be deemed able to participate in competitive sports and have no more than 5 to 10 per cent strength deficit in the quadriceps mechanism. The following exercises are to be carried out:

1. Warm-up using a stationary bicycle or jump rope. Maximum performance, 3 to 5 minutes' duration.

2. Leg press: to exhaustion, 15 to 20 repetitions. Accentuate the "negative" by tak-

ing twice as long to lower than was required to raise the weight.

3. Leg extension: to exhaustion, 15 to 20 repetitions.

4. Three-quarter knee bends: to exhaustion, 15 to 20 repetitions.

5. Leg curl: to exhaustion, 15 to 20 repetitions.

6. Toe raise: to exhaustion, 15 to 20 repetitions.

7. Stationary bicycle: taper off. Moderate resistance for 3 to 5 minutes' duration.

The above exercises should be performed with absolutely no rest between exercises and, with the exception of the stationary bicycle or jump rope, should be performed in approximately 5 minutes. The central focus of advanced rehabilitation is exactly the same as advanced sports conditioning. Done properly, sports conditioning should simultaneously provide maximum benefit in developing power, endurance and flexibility.

SPECIAL CIRCUMSTANCES THAT REQUIRE ALTERATION OF REHABILITATION PROCEDURES

Cruciate Ligament Instability

Following injuries to the anterior cruciate and/or capsular ligaments, varying degrees of anterior and rotary instability may be present. If so, maximum loading or fast, jerky extension of the knee may cause anterior subluxation of the tibia on the femur. It is therefore very important, following such injuries and following surgery for anterior cruciate ligament repair or reconstruction, that precautions be taken and the rehabilitation procedure be so modified that maximum loading and fast, jerky movement be avoided when performing knee extension exercises. This phenomenon is progressively less likely to occur as the range of motion approaches full extension.

TERMINAL EXTENSION EXERCISES

Occasionally following surgery or injury the patient has difficulty in obtaining full extension of his knee. This lack of complete extension is most often due to weakness in the extensor mechanism during the last 10 to 15 degrees of extension. If allowed to persist for a long period of time in addition to a subjective feeling of weakness or "instability," the loss of complete extension is prone to produce a "flexion contracture" due to shortening of the hamstring muscles. The injured knee with a weak quadriceps will require a special precaution. *In doing active extension exercises, one must be sure that the knee reaches complete extension at each level of weight.* If the exercises do not bring the knee to complete extension, a distressing extensor lag may develop with a devastating effect on the athlete. He must be able to lock his knee in complete extension to participate. Extensor lag means that the player can passively extend to zero degrees but can actively extend to only 15 or 20 degrees. The knee is completely unstable between zero and 15 or 20 degrees and so will tend to give way with every stride. This is a much more important handicap than a flexion contracture of the same degree. The latter case can be controlled by the quadriceps, whereas the extensor lag cannot. Also, if the athlete is allowed to participate in too much activity prior to regaining full extension, chronic synovitis is likely to occur. The existence of flexion contracture, quadriceps weakness and swelling usually results in pain, and in turn the pain is likely to cause continuation of the aforementioned conditions.

It is therefore very important to obtain full knee extension as soon as possible following surgery or injury.

The following exercises are recommended.

1. Sitting on floor with involved knee extended as much as possible, place bath towel around forefoot with foot dorsiflexed; while pulling the ends of the towel toward the body, set quadriceps muscle and simultaneously exert downward pressure on knee — stretching the posterior structures of the knee.

2. Place small rolled pad beneath involved knee. "Set" quadriceps muscle and elevate heel and leg while exerting downward pressure on the knee.

CHONDROMALACIA PATELLA

Rehabilitation of athletes with this condition necessitates alteration of the usual progressive resistive exercise program. If the condition is mild and there is no similar involvement of the underlying femur, then a continuation of straight leg raising exercises beyond the usual period of time is usually all that is necessary. However, in more severe cases or in those complicated by femoral involvement, the following exercises should be performed.

1. Straight leg raising as described earlier.

2. Isokinetic exercise using a "self-adjusting resistance" so that undue pressure will not be placed on the patella during maximum patella-femoral contact.

3. Isometric exercises performed at varying degrees of knee extension against a fixed object or the uninvolved limb.

4. Negative resistance exercise performed by lifting the weight with the

uninvolved extremity and lowering the weight with the involved extremity as described earlier under Intermediate Stage, Knee Rehabilitation.

5. Modified "Bench Technique" so that the starting position of the exercise permits only 10 to 15 degrees of knee flexion. As the legs are straightened, the major action of the patella is upward in line with the quadriceps mechanism and little pressure is placed on the patella against the femur in this terminal phase.

THE SINGLE BOOT PROGRESSIVE EXERCISE PROGRAM*

1. After a mild warm-up, determine the single maximum lift as follows. Determine the load which the muscle can lift to full extension and return to position, but which the muscle cannot lift a second time to full extension. If a second lift is accomplished with the initial load, allow a short rest and add weight to the boot; the amount of weight added depends on the ease of the second lift. Repeat the process again and readjust if necessary. The establishing of this single maximum lift is the most difficult part of the program. Accuracy here is necessary in the development of the total program. In the rebuilding of strength and bulk, it would be better to slightly underload rather than to overload.

2. Once this single lift factor has been determined, the exercise pattern may be developed as follows. Subtract five pounds from the single maximum lift (quadriceps) to establish the loading for ten repetitions of the exercise for the first set, for the quadriceps. This load should include the boot weight. If the muscle is only strong enough to lift the "boot" (5 pounds more or less), then it

is obvious that the muscle is very weak indeed. Removal of all the weight would leave only the weight of the leg, and possibly that would be enough weight during the initial workout period. In the first ten days to two weeks, moderate resistance exercise would be the best approach, that is, the lifting of the weight that is comfortable to the individual without undue stress.

3. The hamstring loading is determined by taking a percentage of the initial quadriceps loading (i.e., 50 to 55 per cent for upper high school and beginning college age level and 60 per cent for college varsity football age level). For example, quadriceps 10 repetition of motion load equals 30 pounds times 55 per cent or 16.50 pounds for the initial hamstring load. This would include the weight of the boot and clamp attachments. If the wall-pulley system is used, then the total 16.50 pounds would be placed on the pulley rack. If adjustments in the weight loading have to be made, an accurate initial loading program should be established during the first day or two. From this point the loading program follows an established weekly increase pattern. Occasionally, small adjustments will have to be made in the third to eighth week.

4. Each exercise week consists of three to four exercise periods, in which both muscle groups are exercised according to the individual's program.

5. At the beginning of each new week, a 10-pound increase in weight loading is added for both muscle groups. This addition is a constant factor and continues throughout the entire length of the program or as long as the person is able to do the work. In the latter few weeks it might be necessary to reduce each increment slightly, which would be indicative that the muscle groups are reaching their maximal strength. If the person is unable to complete the three sets of exercises at the beginning of the

---

*The Knee in Sports, Klein and Allman, Pemberton Press, 1969.

week, he should be able to do so by the latter part of the week. As strength and endurance are gradually raised, the program should be completed daily. This is a progressive challenge to the muscles and will be in effect throughout the program.

6. In quadriceps exercise, the most important point is full extension of the knee for maximal effect on the vastus medialis muscle. If the person is unable to fully extend the knee in all exercise sets, then the following adjustments should be made: (a) the total loading should be slightly reduced, or (b) specific terminal exercises should be added to the program.

HOME KNEE EXERCISES

1. Lie on back. Keep knee absolutely straight as you lift it to 45 degrees. Lower slowly. Do not relax the leg, but repeat 15 repetitions. As you get stronger, add weights by means of putting weight in a gym bag or "flight bag" and draping the handles over the ankles (Fig. 648, A).

2. Standing front leg raise is done exactly as above, only you stand to do the lift. Perform 15 repetitions. Add weight when you are able (Fig. 648, B).

Standing side raise is done exactly as above, only the weight is lifted to the side. Do 15 repetitions (Fig. 648, C).

3. This "Quad-Setting" exercise is performed seated on the floor. Place a couple of rolled-up towels under the knee. While pushing the back of the knee down into the towel as hard as possible, attempt to keep the entire surface of your leg in contact with the floor. Hold 5 seconds. Repeat 10 times (Fig. 648, D).

4. Sit on a high table, with the back of the knee just at the edge of the table. You may wish to use towels to pad the back of the knee. From the fully bent position, straighten the knee as much as possible. Hold for 3 seconds at the top. Repeat 15 times. As you get stronger, add weight by means of a weighted bag. Continue using this exercise only as long as no increased pain or swelling is caused as a result of the exercise (Fig. 648, E).

5. Stand erect and balance by holding onto a stable piece of furniture. Bend the exercising knee backwards. Use the weighted bag as in the above exercises. Do 15 repetitions (Fig. 648, F).

KNEE EXERCISES (Fig. 649)

Note: Because you will not be using your leg normally for some time, you will lose muscle size and strength. This loss must be regained by physical therapy after you are out of your cast or bandage. Much of the possible loss can be prevented by starting exercise *now*. You can speed your recovery and insure a more successful recovery by doing your best *now*.

Leg Push-Down. Push down as hard as you can with the entire leg; hold 5 seconds. Perform 10 times at once and repeat 10 times per day. Once home, this exercise should be done through the full range of motion (from overhead to floor) against a helper's resistance; i.e., you push down as helper pushes up (Fig. 649, A).

Straighten Knee. If in an elastic bandage, straighten your knee as hard *and as far* as you can; hold 5 seconds. Perform 10 times; repeat 10 times per day. If in cast, do same effort and imagine you are "breaking" the cast (Fig. 649, B).

Leg Lift. Lying *flat,* lift leg overhead as far as possible; hold 3 seconds; lower slowly. Perform 5 to 10 times and repeat up to 200 total lifts per day. Can be done against helper's resistance as in leg push-down exercise (Fig. 649, C).

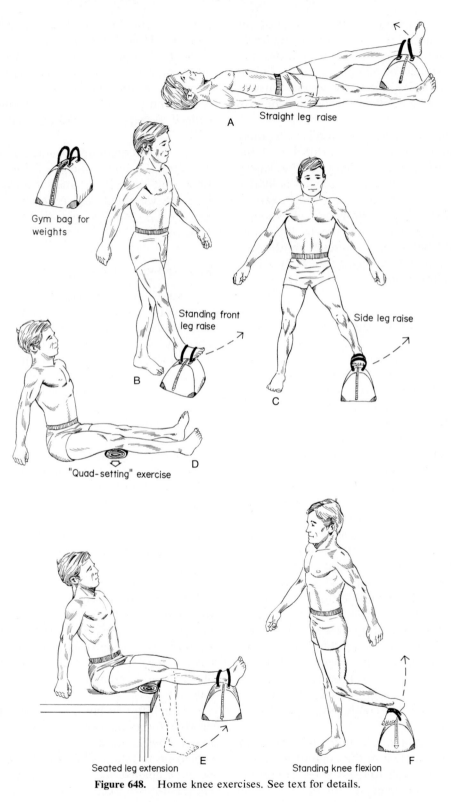

Straight leg raise

Gym bag for weights

Standing front leg raise

Side leg raise

B

C

"Quad-setting" exercise

D

Seated leg extension

E

Standing knee flexion

F

Figure 648. Home knee exercises. See text for details.

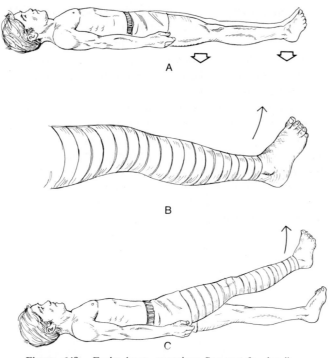

Figure 649. Early knee exercises. See text for details.

MYOSITIS OSSIFICANS TRAUMATICA REHABILITATION

During Stage I or the inflammatory phase of myositis ossificans traumatica, the involved extremity should be protected from further injury. Immobilization is usually helpful and limitation of motion at adjacent joints is usually beneficial. No active exercise should be given to the involved area during this stage. Ice and compression to aid in limiting the extent of the hematoma are indicated.

During Stage II or the proliferative stage, it is usually helpful to begin quadriceps setting exercises for the thigh; or, in case of myositis ossificans traumatica involving the arm, hand grip and upper extremity "setting" exercises are helpful. Active range of motion exercises are allowed as pain and soreness subside, but no attempt is made to forcibly increase motion.

During Stage III or the repair stage, it is usually possible to begin light resistive exercises through the available range of motion. Joint motion should be monitored daily, and if there is a decrease in motion or return of symptoms, then the exercises must be reduced or completely omitted. If the response to light resistive exercise is favorable, then gradually progress to normal progressive resistive exercise routine as outlined for rehabilitation elsewhere. In myositis ossificans these exercises must be carefully controlled. Pain in the involved muscle indicates overload. The exercises should be pain free.

STRETCHING EXERCISES FOR HIPS AND LEGS (Fig. 650)

Note: Before you do the following exercises, which are meant to be done intensely, you must warm up. This may include any light exercise and/or jogging, which does not cause pain. Allow ten minutes for warm-ups.

Ice Massage. You may wish to precede your stretching with ice massage if you are in real pain or if your muscles are in spasm. If you do the massage, omit the warm-ups mentioned above.

Use a large piece of ice frozen in a 10 or 12 ounce paper cup. Massage your injured muscle in firm, overlapping circles. Attempt to massage an area no greater than a softball, with the center being the point of most pain. Allow 15 minutes, then proceed directly to the stretching exercises below.

Hurdler's Stretch. Assume a seated position on the ground with one leg stretched straight in front of you and the other bent under itself in back of you (see Fig. 650, *A*).

Note: In any stretching exercise, it is more beneficial to assume a slow,

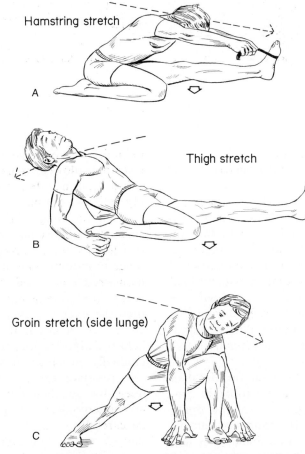

Figure 650.   Stretching exercises for hips and legs. See text for details.

steadily increasing stretch, which builds to a peak (will be quite painful) after 15 seconds; release slowly. Never jerk or fall into a stretched position.

This exercise is done in two parts. First is the hamstring stretch. While keeping the knee straight, attempt to bring the chin as close to the knee as possible. If need be, loop a belt over the foot and pull. Do one hamstring stretch and then one thigh stretch, as shown below.

Second is the thigh stretch. While keeping the point of the knee on the floor, and the ankle directly under your hips, bend your entire body backwards until you are as far as you can get (full range should be with your elbows resting on the floor in back of you (Fig. 650, *B*).

Now reverse your entire position and perform both exercises in the new position. Avoid overflexing the injured knee, i.e., deep knee bends.

Groin Stretch. Assume a stance with feet planted about double shoulder width and feet pointing forward and flat on the floor (keep them this way throughout). Now, lower your body to one side so that your fingertips support your balance by being placed on either side of your supporting leg. The opposite leg will experience a stretch from the inside of the knee clear into the groin area (Fig. 650, *C*). Release and do the other leg.

CALF AND FOOT

The susceptibility of the ankle to ligamentous injury in athletics necessitates complete rehabilitation following injury. Instability of the ankle joint cannot be tolerated in the athlete, and inadequately treated or poorly rehabilitated ankle injuries often result in instability. Also, regardless of the excellence of repair or the completeness of healing, any period of inactivity causes a progressive decline in the strength and flexibility of the involved part.

ANKLE AND LOWER LEG EXERCISES

Toe Raises. These can be done on the floor if your ankle is stiff or painful (Fig. 651, *A*). When it becomes more flexible, stand on the edge of a step or other elevated structure, so that your heel stretches below the level of your toes (Fig. 651, *B*).

Start doing this exercise using your body weight only and standing on both feet; do 20 to 25 repetitions. When able, switch to standing on one foot only, using the elevation as mentioned earlier. When able to perform 20 to 25 repetitions while standing on one foot only, you progress to holding a weighted object in one hand.

Heel Walking. Walk in such a manner as to keep your toes as far off the ground as possible. Take short "choppy" steps; use a shoe with good solid heels; walk on a firm surface (Fig. 651, *C*).

When able to walk in such a manner for two full minutes, or approximately 100 feet, progress to carrying weighted objects or walking in the same manner up a hill or incline (Fig. 651, *D*).

Isometric Ankle "Wrestling." Sit and place one ankle over the other (halfway through switch ankles). Exert an outward force with both ankles so that your feet are firmly pressing against each other. Hold for 10 seconds, release, and repeat 10 times (Fig. 651, *E*).

As your ankles become stronger and less painful or stiff, allow them to move in and out against each other as you exert. Make each full movement last 10 full seconds. Repeat 10 times.

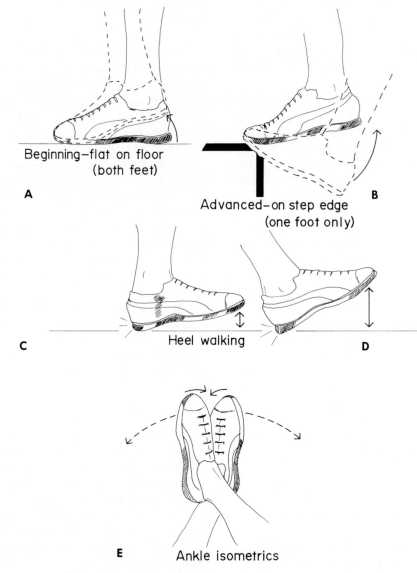

Beginning–flat on floor
(both feet)

A

Advanced–on step edge
(one foot only)

B

Heel walking

C

D

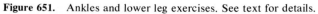

E Ankle isometrics

Figure 651. Ankles and lower leg exercises. See text for details.

REFERENCES

DeLorme, T. L.: Restoration of muscle power by heavy-resistance exercises. J. Bone Joint Surg. *27*:645–667, 1945.

Doss, W. S., and Karpovich, P. V.: A comparison of concentric, eccentric, and isometric strength of elbow flexors. J. Appl. Physiol. *20*:351–353, 1965.

Komi, P. V., and Buskirk, E. R.: Effect of eccentric and concentric muscle conditioning on tension and electrical activity of human muscle. Ergonomics. *15*:417–434, 1972.

Kraus, H.: Evaluation and treatment of muscle function in athletic injury. Am. J. Surg. *98*: 353–362, 1959.

Jones, A.: Metabolic cost of negative work. Ath. J. *56*:40–41; 80, 1976.

Olson, V. L., Smidt, G. L., and Johnston, R. C.: The maximum torque generated by the eccentric, isometric, and concentric contractions of the hip abductor muscles. J. Am. Phys. Ther. Assoc. *52*:149–157, 1972.

Wallis, E. L., and Logan, G. A.: Figure Improvement and Body Conditioning through Exercise. Englewood Cliffs, Prentice-Hall, 1964.

INDEX

Entries in **boldface** refer to figures; entries followed by (t) refer to tables.